Horse Diseases and Disorders: An Issue of Veterinary Clinics

Horse Diseases and Disorders: An Issue of Veterinary Clinics

Editor: Eliza Melton

STATES
ACADEMIC PRESS
www.statesacademicpress.com

States Academic Press,
109 South 5th Street,
Brooklyn, NY 11249, USA

Visit us on the World Wide Web at:
www.statesacademicpress.com

ISBN: 978-1-63989-272-3 (Hardback)

Cataloging-in-Publication Data

Horse diseases and disorders : an issue of veterinary clinics / edited by Eliza Melton.
p. cm.
Includes bibliographical references and index.
ISBN 978-1-63989-272-3
1. Horses--Diseases. 2. Veterinary hospitals. 3. Veterinary medicine. I. Melton, Eliza.
SF951 .H67 2022
636.108 9--dc23

Table of Contents

Preface

It is often said that books are a boon to mankind. They document every progress and pass on the knowledge from one generation to the other. They play a crucial role in our lives. Thus I was both excited and nervous while editing this book. I was pleased by the thought of being able to make a mark but I was also nervous to do it right because the future of students depends upon it. Hence, I took a few months to research further into the discipline, revise my knowledge and also explore some more aspects. Post this process, I begun with the editing of this book.

Horses are odd-toed ungulate mammals of commercial and domestic significance. The breed, environment and management of horses directly impact the lifespan of horses. They can be affected by several diseases and infections such as potomac horse fever, equine arthritis, botulism, laminitis, etc. The bacterial infection caused by an organism known as neorickettsia risticii is called potomac horse fever. Depression, fever and diarrhea are its most common symptoms. Equine arthritis is characterized by swelling, pain and redness of the joints. Osteoarthritis, septic arthritis and traumatic arthritis are some of its common forms. Botulism refers to a potentially fatal condition caused by a toxin producing bacteria. In horses, it may spread through wet or dry hay, a wound or hay which has been contaminated by an animas carcass. The inflammation of the laminae in a horse's hooves is called laminitis. It can be divided into developmental, acute, sub-acute and chronic stage. This book contains some path-breaking studies in the field of horse diseases and disorders. It consists of contributions made by international experts. Those in search of information to further their knowledge will be greatly assisted by this book.

I thank my publisher with all my heart for considering me worthy of this unparalleled opportunity and for showing unwavering faith in my skills. I would also like to thank the editorial team who worked closely with me at every step and contributed immensely towards the successful completion of this book. Last but not the least, I wish to thank my friends and colleagues for their support.

Editor

1

In vitro effects of platelet-rich gel supernatants on histology and chondrocyte apoptosis scores, hyaluronan release and gene expression of equine cartilage explants challenged with lipopolysaccharide

Jorge U. Carmona[1*], Diana L. Ríos[1], Catalina López[1], María E. Álvarez[1,2], Jorge E. Pérez[2] and Mabel E. Bohórquez[3]

Abstract

Background: Platelet-rich plasma (PRP) preparations are a common treatment in equine osteoarthritis (OA). However, there are controversies regarding the ideal concentration of platelets and leukocytes in these biological substances necessary to induce an adequate anti-inflammatory and anabolic response in articular cartilage. The aims were to study the influence of leukocyte- and platelet-rich gel (L-PRG) and pure platelet-rich gel (P-PRG) supernatants on the histological changes of cartilage, the degree of chondrocyte apoptosis, the production of hyaluronan (HA) and the gene expression of nuclear factor kappa beta (NFkβ), matrix metalloproteinase 13 (MMP-13), a disintegrin and metalloproteinase with thrombospondin motifs 4 (ADAMTS-4), collagen type I alpha 1 (COL1A1), collagen type II alpha 1 (COL2A1) and cartilage oligomeric matrix protein (COMP) in normal cartilage explants (CEs) challenged with lipopolysaccharide (LPS).

Results: Overall, 25 % L-PRG supernatant (followed in order of importance by, 50 % P-PRG, 25 % P-PRG and 50 % L-PRG) represented the substance with the most important anti-inflammatory and anabolic effect. 25 % P-PRG supernatant presented important anabolic effects, but it induced a more severe chondrocyte apoptosis than the other evaluated substances.

Conclusions: 25 % L-PRG supernatant presented the best therapeutic profile. Our results demonstrate that the biological variability of PRP preparations makes their application rather challenging. Additional in vivo research is necessary to know the effect of PRP preparations at different concentrations.

Keywords: Platelet-rich plasma, Cartilage explants, Chondrocyte apoptosis, Catabolic/anabolic gene expression, Growth factors

* Correspondence: carmona@ucaldas.edu.co
[1]Grupo de Investigación Terapia Regenerativa, Departamento de Salud Animal, Universidad de Caldas, Manizales, Colombia
Full list of author information is available at the end of the article

Background

Osteoarthritis (OA) is a chronic inflammatory disease that affects middle aged and older people worldwide [1]. This disease also affects horses and other animal species, which causes economic losses by diminishing the athletic potential of the affected animals and through the chronic use of anti-inflammatory drugs and nutraceuticals [2–4]. Thus, the horse is an important animal model to study both the pathophysiological mechanisms and the experimental treatments of OA [5, 6].

There are several extrinsic factors associated with OA development such as joint repetitive trauma, obesity, joint infection and osteochondrosis, amongst others [4]. During the OA developmental process, there are structural (histological) changes indicating the severity or degree of affectation of the articular cartilage [7]. This includes increased chondrocyte necrosis, cluster (complex chondrone) formation, fibrillation/fissuring, focal cell loss and diminished uptake of safranin-O fast green (SOFG) stain [8]. Furthermore, another important histological change associated with OA is chondrocyte apoptosis, which leads to loss of resident cells in the articular cartilage and results in severe alterations such as impaired extracellular matrix (ECM) remodelling [9]. This phenomenon has been described in both human and animal models of OA [10, 11]. Chondrocyte apoptosis could be detected by caspase-3 expression or terminal deoxynucleotidyl transferase dUTP nick end labelling (TUNEL) staining [12].

Together with the OA histological changes are several joint molecular alterations characterized by nuclear factor kappa beta (NFkβ) upregulation [13] that subsequently upregulates several catabolic and proinflammatory cytokines for cartilage such as interleukin-1 (IL-1) and tumour necrosis factor alpha (TNF-α), matrix metalloproteinases (MMPs - e.g. MMP-13), aggrecanases (i.e. a disintegrin and metalloproteinase with thrombospondin motifs 4 - ADAMTS-4), inducible synthases of nitric oxide and cyclooxygenase type 2 [14]. Consequently, a proinflammatory molecular milieu produces histological alterations in cartilage and induces molecular changes with clinical accompanying indicators such as pain and synovial effusion [4].

In the initial OA stages, joint tissues (e.g. cartilage) act by upregulating anabolic gene expression to induce cartilage ECM anabolism and to increase the synthesis of collagen type II alpha 1 (COL2A1), cartilage oligomeric matrix protein (COMP) and hyaluronan (HA) amongst other anabolic ECM components. However, as the OA progresses, the local expression and production of collagen type I alpha 1 (COL1A1) appears as a poor anabolic response by the osteoarthritic cartilage [15, 16].

Platelet-rich plasma (PRP) has been used as a therapy for OA in humans [17–19] and animals [20–23]. The rationale for the therapeutic use of PRP stems from the fact that platelets (PLTs) (but also white blood cells – WBC-) contained in PRP represent an important autologous source of some growth factors (GFs), which include transforming growth factor beta 1 (TGF-β_1), platelet derived growth factor isoform BB (PDGF-BB) [24, 25], and other anti-inflammatory cytokines such as interleukin 4 (IL-4) and the receptor antagonist of IL-1 (IL-1ra) [26, 27], which are implicated in the anabolic characteristics of OA [4, 28]. Furthermore, in vitro studies have revealed that PDGF-BB downregulates NFkβ [29, 30] and increases the proliferation of chondrocytes [29, 31], whereas TGF-β_1 increases the cartilage extracellular matrix (ECM) synthesis and promotes the differentiation of stem cells in chondrocytes [32].

Currently, there is controversy about which PRP preparation is ideal for the intra-articular treatment of patients with OA [33, 34]. Some in vitro [35–37] and clinical studies have suggested that leukoreduced PRP (also known as pure PRP [P-PRP]) preparations have better anabolic and anti-inflammatory effects for OA treatment than leukoconcentrate PRP (L-PRP) preparations, whereas other studies have described similar positive effects for both preparations [32, 38, 39].

Recently, we demonstrated in an in vitro system of cartilage inflammation that 50 % L-PRP releasate produced a more sustained temporal concentration of growth factors and anti-inflammatory cytokines than both 25 % L-PRP and P-PRP releasates and 50 % P-PRP releasate in relation to the concentration in culture media [40]. However, there is no information regarding the effects of these substances on the histology or ECM cartilage gene expression.

The study presented here shows complementary and novel information for the anabolic, anti-inflammatory effect of two supernatant concentrations (25 and 50 %) from both P-PRP and L-PRP preparations on equine cartilage explants (CEs) challenged with lipopolysaccharide (LPS). This research evaluates and compares the influence of both platelet-rich gel (PRG) supernatants on the histological changes of cartilage, the degree of chondrocyte apoptosis, the production of HA and the gene expression of NFkB, MMP-13, ADAMTS-4, COL1A1, COL2A1 and COMP in an in vitro system of cartilage inflammation and degeneration.

The hypothesis of this study is that L-PRG supernatants at a lower concentration (25 %) have better anti-inflammatory and anabolic effects than both PRG supernatants at the higher 50 % concentration and P-PRG supernatant at 25 % concentration in CEs challenged with LPS.

Methods

This study was approved by the committee on animal experimentation of the Universidad de Caldas, Manizales, Colombia.

Samples

Cartilage samples from the metacarpophalangeal joints from six horses, aged 4 to 9 years, were included in this study. The samples were taken from horses that were free from musculoskeletal disease and euthanised by a pentobarbital intravenous overdose for other medical reasons. All metacarpophalangeal joints were radiographed and macroscopically evaluated to exclude horses with OA-associated joint changes.

L-PRP and P-PRP preparation

Venous blood from one clinically healthy mare was used in order to avoid the great variability in the GF and cytokine concentrations in the PRG supernatants used in the experiments. Platelet concentrates were obtained through a manual double centrifugation tube method [41] that was previously validated and used clinically in horses with OA [21]. Blood was drawn from jugular venipuncture and immediately deposited in 4.5 mL tubes with sodium citrate solution (BD Vacutainer®, Becton Drive, Franklin Lakes, NJ, USA). After centrifugation at 120 × *g* for five minutes, the first 50 % of the top supernatant plasma fraction, adjacent to the buffy coat, was collected. This fraction was centrifuged at 240 × *g* for five minutes, and then the bottom quarter of the fraction was collected [41]. This fraction was considered as L-PRP. The upper plasma fraction was considered as P-PRP (Fig. 1). Whole blood and both PRP preparations were analysed for PLT and WBC counts using an impedance-based haematology device (Celltac-α MEK 6450, Nihon Kodhen, Japan).

Both PRP preparations were activated with calcium gluconate (Ropsohn Therapeutics Ltda®, Bogotá, Colombia) (ratio 1:10) and incubated at 37 °C for 1 h until clot retraction occurred. Fresh L-PRG and P-PRG supernatants were used to add to the culture media at two concentrations (25 % and 50 %). Aliquots of both PRG supernatants obtained were frozen at -86 °C for later quantification of PDGF-BB, TGF-β_1 and HA.

Cartilage explants culture and LPS challenge

Cartilage samples were obtained aseptically, and circular 4 mm diameter explants were obtained using a disposable biopsy punch (KAI Medical, Solingen, Germany). CEs were dissected from the articular surface without calcified cartilage layers and washed in phosphate-buffered saline.

CEs were stabilised in Dulbecco's Modified Eagle Medium (DMEM) (high glucose, 4500 mg/L) with L-glutamine and sodium bicarbonate and free of sodium pyruvate (DMEM, Lonza Group Ltd, Basel, Switzerland) and supplemented with streptomycin (100 μg/mL) and penicillin (100 μg/mL) without the addition of serum. Cultures were incubated in a 5 % CO_2 and water saturated atmosphere for 24 h and then replaced with fresh

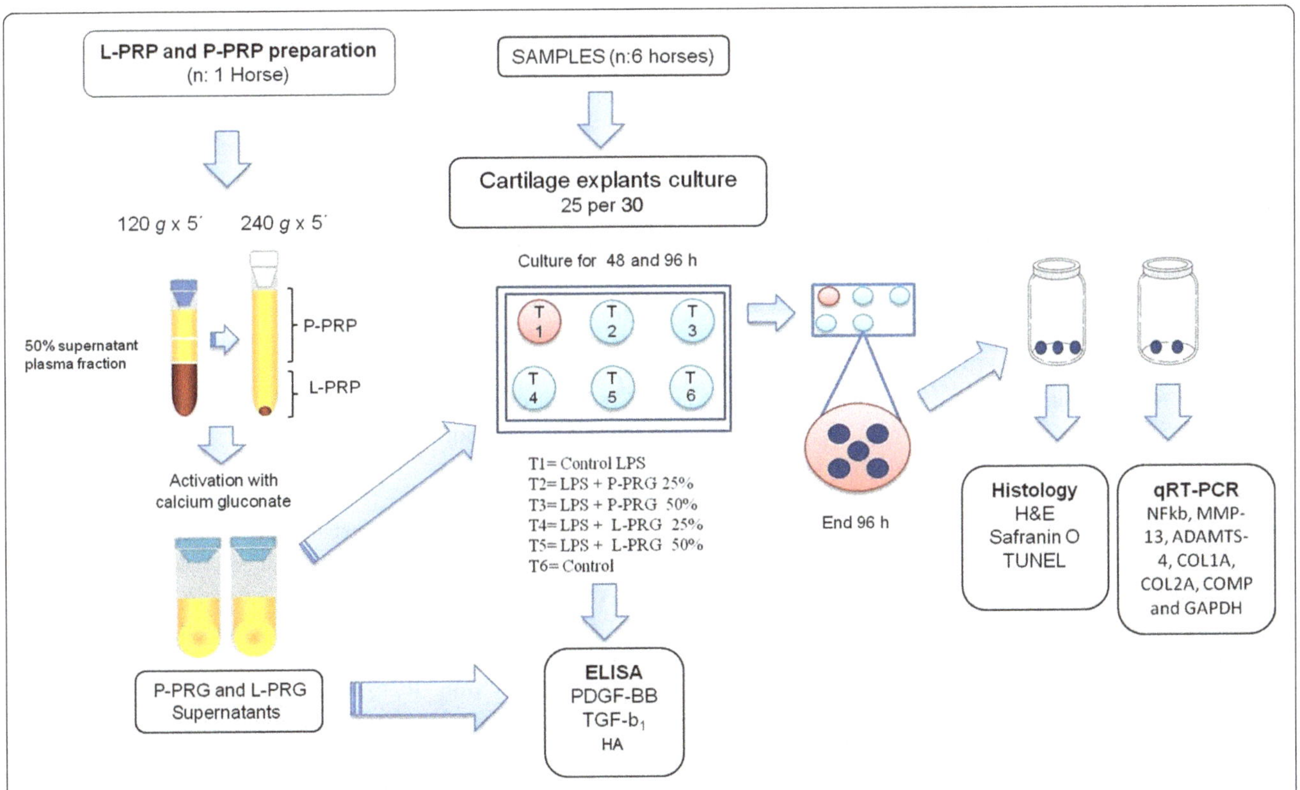

Fig. 1 Schematic workflow of the experiments of the study

culture media. At this time point (24 h), the CEs were challenged with 100 ng/mL of LPS (Sigma-Aldrich, St Louis, MO, USA) to induce inflammatory/catabolic damage of the cartilage [42, 43].

Study design

A total of 30 CEs were obtained from each horse. The study design included the evaluation of six experimental groups using five CEs per group from each horse as follows: one CE healthy control group without LPS and without addition of any PRG supernatant, one CE control group challenged with LPS and without addition of any PRG supernatant, and four CE groups cultured with L-PRG and P-PRG supernatants at two different concentrations (25 % and 50 %). After 1 h of incubation, L-PRG and P-PRG supernatants were added in order to obtain concentrations at 25 and 50 %. All CE groups were cultured at 96 h, after which the culture media were frozen in aliquots at -86 °C for later determination of HA concentration by ELISA. Furthermore, the CEs were deposited in buffered formaldehyde for histological analysis or in an RNA conserving solution (RNAlater, Life Technologies, Carlsbad, CA, USA) for quantitative gene expression of NFkB, MMP-13, ADAMTS-4, COL1A1, COL2A1 and COMP. The schematic diagram (Fig. 1) summarises the study design and methodology.

ELISA analysis

L-PRG and P-PRG supernatants and culture media at 96 h were used to determine the concentration of PDGF-BB, TGF-β_1 and HA via ELISA in duplicate. All proteins were assayed using commercial ELISA development kits from R&D Systems (Minneapolis, MN, USA). PDGF-BB (Human PDGF-BB DuoSet, DY220) and TGF-β_1 (Human TGF-β1 DuoSet, DY240E) were determined using human antibodies because there is a high sequence homology between these proteins in humans and horses [44, 45]. Furthermore, these kits have been used for the same purposes in other equine PRP studies [24, 25]. HA (Hyaluronan, DuoSet, DY3614) was determined using a multispecies detection ELISA kit. Standards provided for each ELISA kit were used to prepare each standard curve following the manufacturers' instructions. Absorbance readings were performed at 450 nm.

H&E histology evaluation

CEs were dehydrated in serial alcohol concentrations, fixed in wax blocks, cut into 3 μm slices and stained with either haematoxylin and eosin (H&E) or safranin O stains. The outcome parameters evaluated were: (1) chondrocyte necrosis, (2) cluster (complex chondrone) formation, (3) fibrillation/fissuring, (4) focal cell loss and (5) safranin-O stain uptake. All preparations were analysed using a light microscope in a 40× magnification following the OARSI histopathology initiative for histological assessments of osteoarthritis in the horse [8] (Table 1).

These variables were quantified using a 0–4 scale, with 0 being normal and 4 being abnormal (Table 1). Thus, a totally normal CE would score 0 and a maximally abnormal CE would score 15 [8]. Three sections randomly selected from each sample were evaluated blindly and the average score was used for comparison.

TUNEL assay for chondrocyte apoptosis

TUNEL staining was performed to detect DNA strand breakage using a commercial kit for cell and tissues (TACS TdT-Blue Label In situ Apoptosis Detection Kit, Trevigen, Inc., Gaitherburg, MD, USA). Briefly, the CEs were washed and dehydrated in serial alcohol concentrations, fixed in wax blocks and cut into 3 μm slices. The tissue sections were deparaffinised with xylene and ethanol and washed with PBS. The samples were covered with 50 μl of proteinase K solution and incubated for 15 min at 37 °C in a humidity chamber. The samples were washed with PBS and covered with 50 μl of labelling reaction mix. After this, the samples were immersed in a stop buffer solution for 5 min at room temperature to stop labelling reaction and once more washed twice with PBS for 2 min at room temperature. The samples were covered with 50 μl of antibody solution and incubated for 30 min at 37 °C then washed with PBS and covered with 50 μl of TACS Blue Label™ (Trevigen, Inc., Gaitherburg, MD, USA). These samples were washed with deionised water and counterstained with nuclear fast red. The controls were treated similarly except that terminal deoxynucleotidyl transferase was substituted by distilled water [46].

After the reaction, stained chondrocytes (grey-black) were analysed under a light microscope. Chondrocyte apoptosis was scored by a semiquantitative approach using a 0-4 scale, where 1 = 6–25 % of chondrocyte apoptosis; 2 = 26–50 % of chondrocyte apoptosis; 3 = 51–75 % of chondrocyte apoptosis and 4 = 76–100 % of chondrocyte apoptosis [47].

Molecular evaluation

CE samples were pulverised in liquid nitrogen and mixed with TRIzol reagent (Life Technologies, Carlsbad, CA, USA) for 5 min. The samples were centrifuged for 10 min at 10,000 × g, and the supernatant was mixed with 20 % chloroform (volume/volume) and then centrifuged for 15 min at 12,000 × g. The aqueous phase of the samples was removed and transferred to special columns (PureLink RNA Mini Kit, Life Technologies, Carlsbad, CA) for RNA extraction according to the manufacturer's instructions. RNA concentrations were

Table 1 Microscopic grading system for articular cartilage histology [8]

Articular cartilage		
Outcome parameter	Score	Description
Chondrocyte necrosis*	0	Normal section without necrosis
	1	No more than one necrotic cell located near the articular surface per 20x objective
	2	1e2 necrotic cells located near the articular surface per 20x objective
	3	2e3 necrotic cells located near the articular surface per 20x objective
	4	3e4 necrotic cells located near the articular surface per 20x objective
Cluster (complex chondrone) formation	0	No cluster formation throughout section
	1	Two chondrocytes (doublets) within same lacunae along superficial aspect of the articular cartilage section
	2	2e3 chondrocytes (doublets & triplets) within same lacunae along superficial aspect of the articular cartilage section
	3	3e4 chondrocytes within same lacunae along superficial aspect of the articular cartilage section
	4	Greater than four chondrocytes within same lacunae along superficial aspect of the articular cartilage section
Fibrillation/fissuring	0	No fibrillation/fissuring of the articular cartilage surface
	1	Fibrillation/fissuring of the articular cartilage restricted to surface and superficial zone
	2	Fissuring that extends into the middle zone
	3	Fissuring that extends to the level of the deep zone
	4	Fissuring that extends into the deep zone
Focal cell loss*	0	Normal cell population throughout the section
	1	A 10e20% area of acellularity per 20x field
	2	A 20e30% area of acellularity per 20x field
	3	A 40e50% area of acellularity per 20x field
	4	A greater than 50 % area of acellularity per 20x field
Safranin-O stain uptake	0	Normal staining
	1	Less than 25 % loss of staining characteristics
	2	25e50% loss of staining characteristics
	3	50e75% loss of staining characteristics
	4	Greater than 75 % loss of staining characteristics

*Chondrocyte necrosis is used to grade presence of lacunae with necrotic nuclei still present compared to focal cell loss which is most likely an extension of the pathologic change but lacunae or nuclei are no longer present

measured using a spectrophotometer (Nanodrop 2000, Thermo Scientific, Wilmington, DE, USA). Samples were diluted to a concentration of 5 ng/μL of RNA.

The samples were assayed for quantitative gene expression levels in a qRT-PCR device (StepOnePlus Real-Time PCR System, Life Technologies, Carlsbad, CA, USA) using a SuperScript III platinum SYBR Green One-Step qRT-PCR kit (Life Technologies, Carlsbad, CA, USA). Primers for NFkB, MMP-13, ADAMTS-4, COL1A1, COL2A1, COMP and GAPDH (glyceraldehyde 3-phosphate dehydrogenase) were designed and validated in the Colombian Centre for Bioinformatics and Computational Biology (BIOS) (Table 2).

The relative change in gene expression was determined via the comparative $2^{-\Delta\Delta CT}$ method [48]. GAPDH was used as the internal control (housekeeping gene), and cartilage samples from all horses that were not incubated with any treatment were used as reference samples.

Statistical and data analysis

The statistical analysis was performed with SPSS 19.0 software (IBM, Chicago, IL, USA). The Shapiro–Wilk test was used to assess the fit of the data set to a normal distribution (goodness of fit). All the parameters evaluated, except CE histology and apoptosis scores, demonstrated a normal distribution ($p > 0.05$). However, these data were normalised by using a transformation log (Y).

Platelet and WBC counts in whole blood and both PRP preparations were evaluated through a one-way analysis of variance (ANOVA), followed by a Tukey test. PDGF-BB, TGF-β_1 and HA concentrations from both PRG supernatants were compared using a t-non-paired test. A generalised lineal model (GLM), followed (when necessary) by a Tukey test, was used for comparing HA concentrations in culture media and gene expression at 96 h. The HA concentrations in fresh culture media with PRG supernatants at 1 h and 96 h were compared using a t-paired test. A $p < 0.05$ was accepted as statistically significant for all tests. Data are presented as mean ± mean standard error (m.s.e).

Results

Cell, growth factor and HA in L-PRP/L-PRG and P-PRP/P-PRG

PLT counts were significantly ($p < 0.05$) different between whole blood, L-PRP and P-PRP, with the lowest

Table 2 Genes and sequence of primers evaluated in the study

Targeted genes	Primer sequences (5'- > 3')	Product size (bps)
GAPDH, glyceraldehyde-3-phosphate dehydrogenase 6	Forward TCCCTGCTTCTACTGGTGCT Reverse TGACAAAGTGGTCGTTGAGG	306
NFkβ, nuclear factor of kappa light polypeptide gene enhancer in B-cells-like 1	Forward CGATTTCGATATGGCTGTGA Reverse CACCTTCTTCAGCTCCTTGG	399
MMP 13, matrix metallopeptidase 13 (collagenase 3) 7	Forward GCATTCAAAAAGGCCTTCAA Reverse GGAAGCACAAAGTGGCTTTT	356
ADAMTS 4, metallopeptidase with thrombospondin type 1 motif 4	Forward TGTCAGCTTGGTGGTGACTC Reverse GTTGAAGACATGGCCCAGTT	322
COL1A1, collagen, type I, alpha 1 11	Forward AGCCAGCAGATCGAGAACAT Reverse CTGGCCACCATACTCGAACT	309
COL2A1, collagen, type II, alpha 1 6	Forward primer ACGTCCAGATGACCTTCCTG Reverse primer GTCCACACCAAATTCCTGCT	326
COMP, cartilage oligomeric matrix protein 21	Forward CCACGTGAATACGGTCACAG Reverse TAGGAACCAGCGGTAGGATG	301

concentration for P-PRP (98.7 00 ± 4.600 PLT/μL), followed by whole blood (125.900 ± 3.400 PLT/μL) and L-PRP (312.800 ± 19.600 PLT/μL). WBC counts were also significantly different between the evaluated groups, with a higher concentration for L-PRP (35.100 ± 3.500 WBC/μL), followed by whole blood (8.300 ± 3.700 WBC/μL) and P-PRP (110 ± 40 WBC/μL). TGF-β_1 concentration was similar between L-PRG (1676.3 ± 312.4 pg/mL) and P-PRG (1356.9 ± 20.8 pg/mL). PDGF-BB had a significantly ($p < 0.05$) higher concentration in L-PRG (3053. 8 ± 956.7 pg/mL) when compared to P-PRG (372.7 ± 79.6 pg/mL). HA concentration was significantly ($p < 0.05$) higher in L-PRG supernatant (4.3 ± 1.7 pg/mL) in comparison to P-PRG supernatant (1.1 ± 0.21 pg/mL).

H&E histology evaluation

Chondrocyte necrosis scores were significantly ($p < 0.05$) worse (higher) for CEs from the control group with LPS and those treated with 25 % L-PRG and 50 % P-PRG supernatants when compared to CEs of the control group and those treated with 50 % LPRG and 25 % P-PRG supernatants (Fig. 2a). Cluster formation was significantly higher for CEs from the control group plus LPS when compared to the rest of the CE groups evaluated. This histology parameter was similar among CEs from the healthy control group and those treated with both L-PRG supernatants and 25 % P-PRG supernatant, whereas CEs treated with 50 % P-PRG supernatant presented a significantly worse score than the aforementioned CE groups (Fig. 2b).

Fibrillation/fissuring scores were significantly ($p < 0.05$) higher in both control groups, although there was a statistical trend ($p = 0.10$) showing CEs of the healthy control group with lower score in comparison to CEs of the control group treated with LPS. In general, CEs treated with all PRG supernatants presented significantly ($p < 0.05$) lower scores. However, CEs treated with 50 % L-PRG and 25 % P-PRG supernatants were significantly lower than CEs of healthy control group (Fig. 2c).

Focal cell loss scores were significantly ($p < 0.05$) worse for the CEs of control group treated with LPS and those treated with 50 % P-PRG supernatant. CEs from the healthy control group and those treated with both 25 % PRG supernatants presented significantly ($p < 0.05$) lower scores than the rest of the CE groups (Fig. 2d). SOFG stain uptake score were significantly ($p < 0.05$) worse for CEs treated with 50 % L-PRG supernatant, followed by CEs of the control group challenged with LPS and both 25 % PRG supernatants. The best score for this histology parameter was found in CEs of the healthy control group and those treated with 50 % P-PRG supernatant (Fig. 2e).

The general histology total score was significantly ($p < 0.05$) higher in CEs of the control group challenged with LPS when compared to CEs of the healthy control group and those treated with both L-PRG and 25 % P-PRG supernatant. In general, CEs treated with both 25 % PRG supernatants showed significantly ($p < 0.05$) better general histology score than the rest of the groups evaluated (Fig. 2f).

TUNEL assay for chondrocyte apoptosis

No chondrocyte apoptosis was detected in CEs of the healthy control group and those treated with both 50 % PRG supernatants. However, this cellular phenomenon was detected (and it was significantly higher [$p < 0.05$]) in CEs of the control group challenged with LPS and those treated with both 25 % PRG supernatants; although, the score for this parameter was apparently lower for those CEs treated with 25 % L-PRG supernatant (Fig. 2g).

Concentration of HA in culture media at 1 h and 96 h

At 1 h, HA concentrations varied significantly ($p < 0.05$) between all PRG supernatant groups evaluated. At 96 h, HA was released by all CE groups. However,

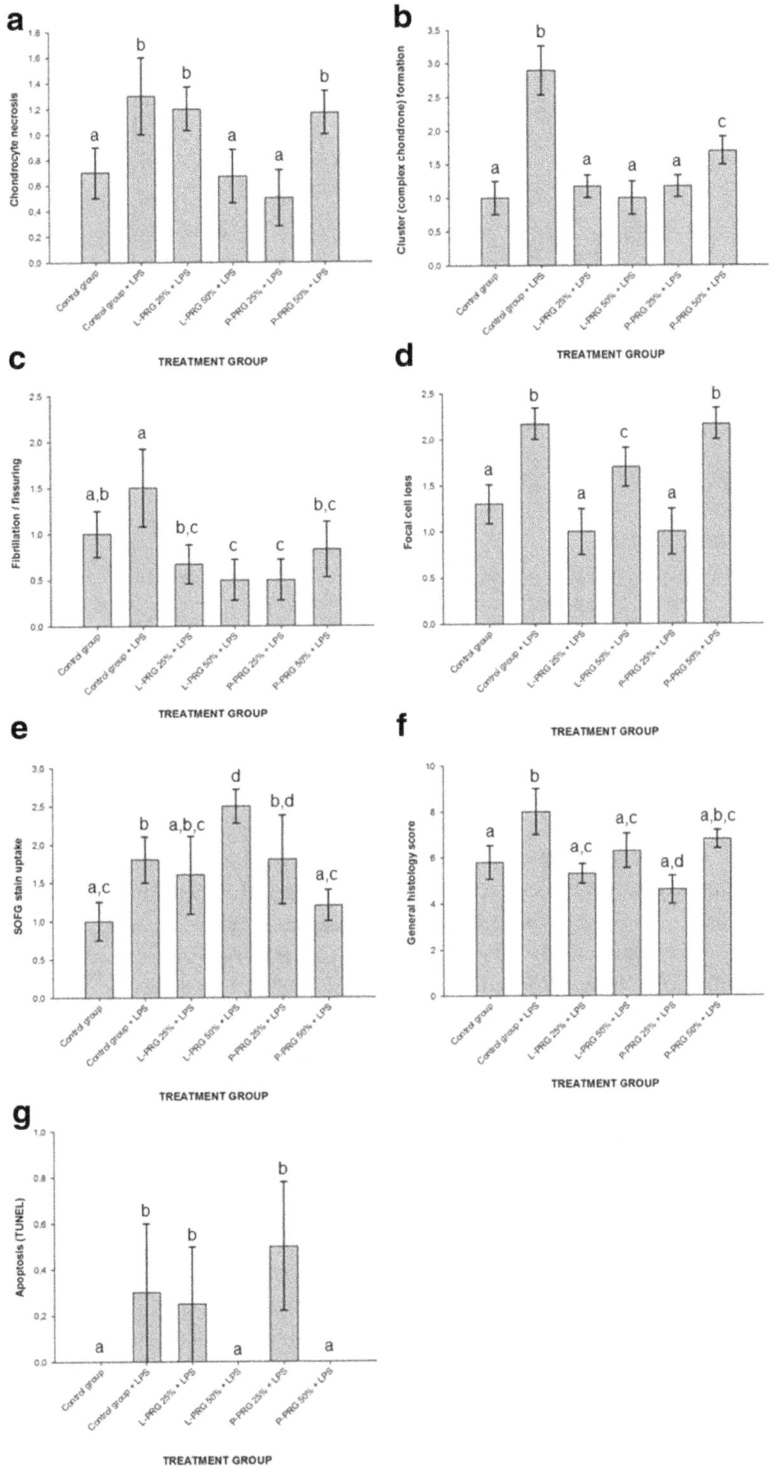

Fig. 2 Means (±standard error of the mean [s.e.m]) of the cartilage histology and chondrocyte apoptosis scores. **a** Chondrocyte necrosis. **b** Cluster formation. **c** Fibrillation/fissuring. **d** Focal cell loss. **e** SOFG stain uptake. **f** Total histology score. **g** Chondrocyte apoptosis. [a-b]Different lowercase letters denote significant ($p < 0.05$) differences between the groups evaluated by the Tukey test

the CE group cultured with 25 % P-PRG supernatant presented the highest significant ($p < 0.05$) HA release in comparison with the CE control group and the other CE PRG-treated groups. Notably, HA concentrations were different between CE PRG treated groups at 1 h and 96 h (Fig. 3).

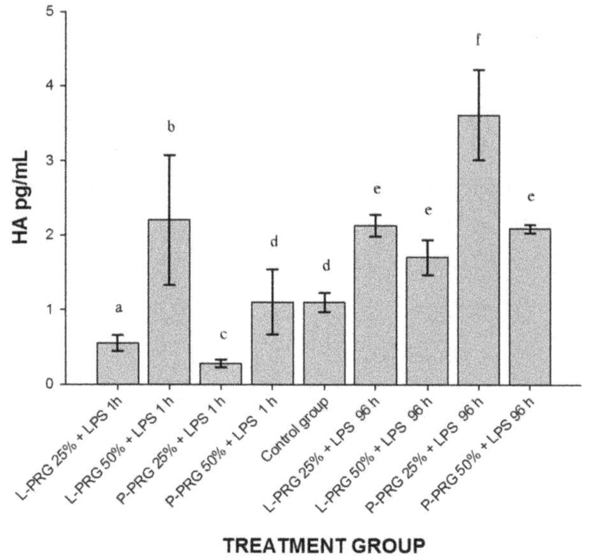

Fig. 3 Means (± s.e.m) of HA concentration in culture media from cartilage explant (CE) groups at 1 h and 96 h. [a-b] Different lowercase letters denote significant ($p < 0.05$) differences between the groups evaluated by the Tukey test over the same period of time. * Denotes significant differences between the same variable at different time periods by the t-paired test

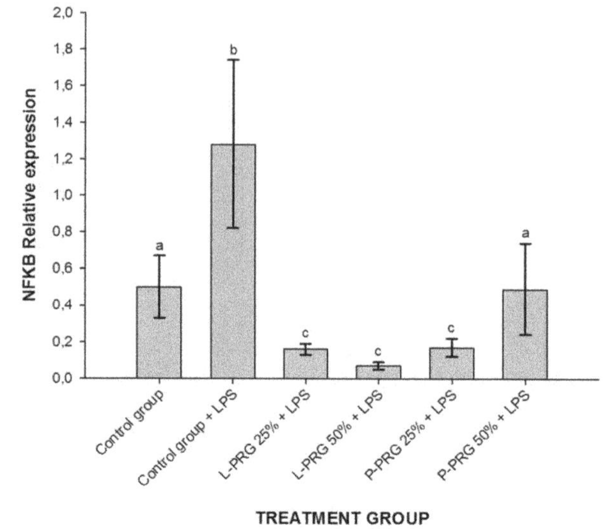

Fig. 4 Means (± s.e.m) of NFkB gene expression in CE groups at 96 h. [a-b] Different lowercase letters denote significant ($p < 0.05$) differences between the groups evaluated by the Tukey test

Gene expression

NFkB gene expression was significantly ($p < 0.05$) increased in CEs from the control group challenged with LPS in comparison to the rest of the CE groups evaluated. NFkB gene expression was significantly ($p < 0.05$) diminished in CEs treated with both 25 % PRG supernatants and 50 % P-PRG supernatant in comparison to the CEs from the healthy control group and those treated with 50 % P-PRG (Fig. 4).

CEs from the healthy control group and all PRG supernatant treatments presented a significant ($p < 0.05$) decrease of MMP-13 expression (Fig. 5). However, 25 % L-PRG supernatant induced a lesser expression of this gene in CEs when compared to CEs treated with 50 % P-PRG supernatant ($p < 0.05$). No significant differences were noticed for the expression of this catabolic gene in the CEs from the healthy control group and those treated with 50 % L-PRG, and 25 and 50 % P-PRG supernatants (Fig. 5).

All PRG supernatant treatments significantly ($p < 0.05$) decreased ADAMTS-4 gene expression in CEs when compared to CEs of both control groups (Fig. 6). Furthermore, CEs from the healthy control group and all PRG supernatant treatments showed significant ($p < 0.05$) COL1A1 gene downregulation when compared to CEs of the control group challenged with LPS (Fig. 7). L-PRG supernatants at different concentrations significantly ($p < 0.05$) diminished the COL2A1 gene expression in CEs in comparison to CEs treated with both P-PRG supernatant concentrations and the control group. Notably, there were not significant differences between these last three groups and CEs from the healthy control group for COL2A1 gene expression (Fig. 8). However, although this gene expression was statistically ($p = 0.09$) similar among CEs from both control groups, COL2A1gene expression was apparently higher in CEs from the healthy control group than in CEs challenged only with LPS (Fig. 8).

COMP gene expression was significantly ($p < 0.05$) diminished in CEs from the control group challenged with LPS and those treated with the 50 % L-PRG supernatant

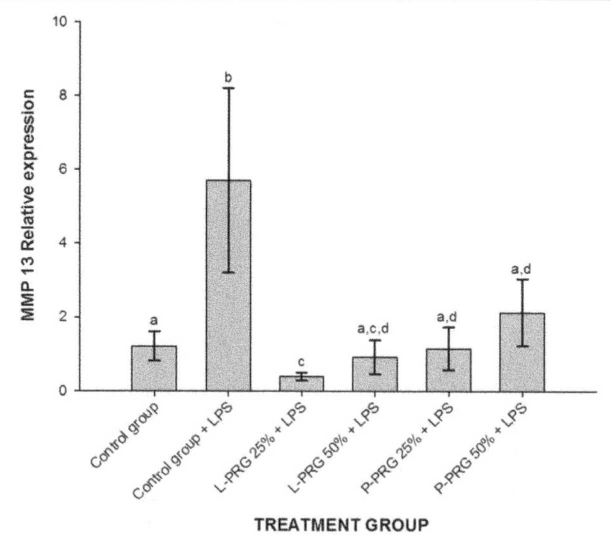

Fig. 5 Means (± s.e.m) of MMP-13 gene expression in CE groups at 96 h [a-b] Different lowercase letters denote significant ($p < 0.05$) differences between the groups evaluated by the Tukey test

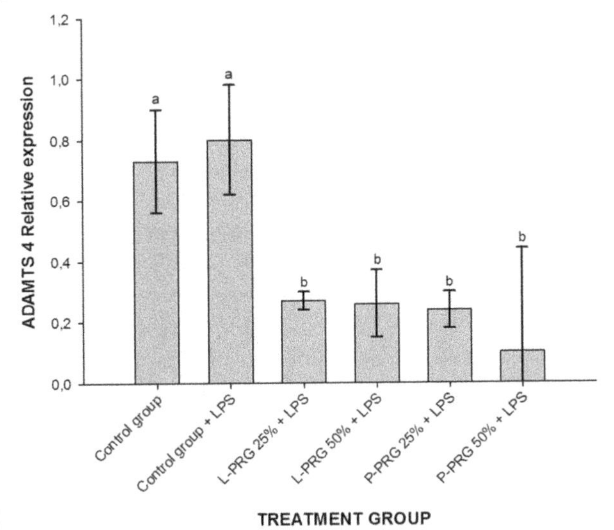

Fig. 6 Means (± s.e.m) of ADAMTS-4 gene expression in CE groups at 96 h. [a-b] Different lowercase letters denote significant ($p < 0.05$) differences between the groups evaluated by the Tukey test

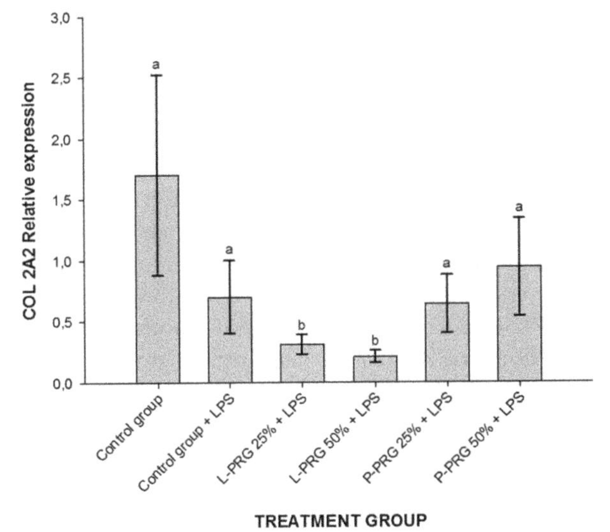

Fig. 8 Means (± s.e.m) of COL2A1 gene expression in CE groups at 96 h. [a-b] Different lowercase letters denote significant ($p < 0.05$) differences between the groups evaluated by the Tukey test

in comparison to CEs treated with both the 25 % PRG supernatants and the 50 % P-PRG supernatant. CEs from the healthy control group and those treated with both 25 % PRG supernatants presented similar increased COMP gene expression. However, CEs treated with both 25 % PRG supernatants demonstrated a significantly higher CE gene expression when compared to CEs treated with 50 % P-PRG supernatant (Fig. 9).

Discussion

Diverse PRP effects on cells and tissues are well recognised as depending on their varying preparations [38]. Thus, the molecular profile of a PRG supernatant is associated with the type and quantity of WBCs and PLTs initially present in PRP [25, 28]. However, after PRP is activated in a joint, it becomes a fibrin mesh or PRG that releases growth factors and cytokines and acts as an immune node inside the joint [49]. We currently believe that the cell ratio (PLT:WBC) in PRP is not as critical as the GF:GF or GF:cytokine ratios and concentrations

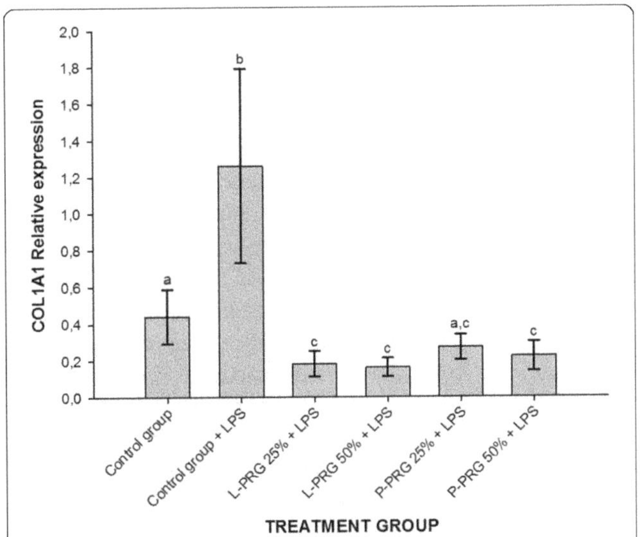

Fig. 7 Means (± s.e.m) of COL1A1 gene expression in CE groups at 96 h. [a-b] Different lowercase letters denote significant ($p < 0.05$) differences between the groups evaluated by the Tukey test

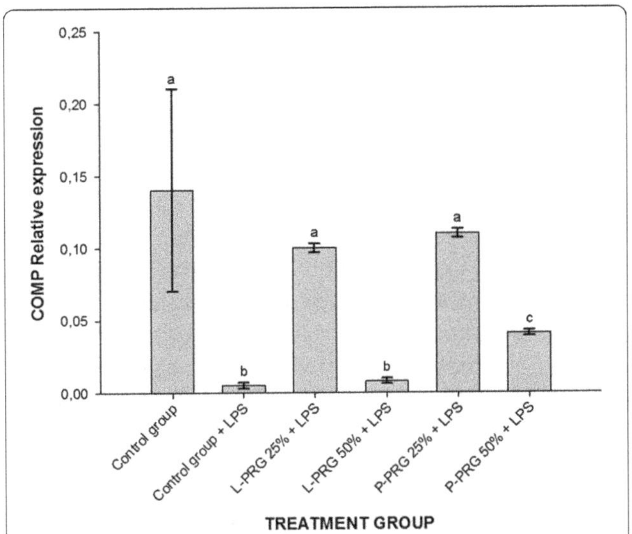

Fig. 9 Means (± s.e.m) of COMP gene expression in CE groups at 96 h. [a-b] Different lowercase letters denote significant ($p < 0.05$) differences between the blood component groups obtained with the same anticoagulant by the Tukey test

released into the joint fluid [50]. However, we also wish to clarify that this assumption could possibly be valid for the use of PRP in joints and not for the infiltrative use of this substance in tendons, ligaments or muscles, where not only is the growth factor concentration important, but also the fibrin mesh to allow growth factor storage, cell migration and cell proliferation [51].

Strong debates continue about the ideal PLT:WBC ratio and concentration in PRP [51]. Currently, there are several studies indicating that plasma with a poor quantity of PLTs and negligible WBs could be the best "PRP" preparations to treat OA and other musculoskeletal pathologies [35, 36, 52]. However, a recent in vitro study described molecular positive effects for several commercial kits which have concentrates at different PLT:WBC ratios and are used for OA treatment [39].

Thus, we decided to conduct an independent study to evaluate the effect of two different PRP preparations (obtained by a homemade lab method) at different concentrations on cartilage histology, chondrocyte apoptotic scores, HA release and catabolic and anabolic gene expression of CEs challenged with LPS. Exposure of CEs to LPS resulted in marked changes in the expression of genes involved in matrix formation and degradation as well as inflammation of which many were reduced by the addition of both PRG supernatants at different concentrations.

The use of LPS for inducing cartilage inflammation/degeneration is a classical methodological approach to perform diverse in vitro studies by simulating a system of inflammatory/degenerative arthropaty [42, 43, 53]; although, the use of recombinant IL-1β to induce in vitro articular cartilage degradation could be more suitable [54, 55]. However, it is important to clarify that the cellular receptors for LPS and IL-1β are closely interlinked and described as the TLR-IL-1 receptor (IL-1R) superfamily of receptors. When activated they induce a series of intercellular signalling pathways that converge on the activation of the transcription NFkB resulting in pro-inflammatory cytokine expression [55, 56].

It is important to mention that the evaluation of the anti-inflammatory effect of PRG supernatants by measuring the relative expression of the NFkB gene in the present study represents a very limited approach to understanding the activity signalling of this important inflammatory process [57]. However, an in vitro study in human chondrocytes revealed that activated PRP induced the expression and production of inhibitor-κBα (IκBα) (directly mediated by hepatocyte growth factor), which is responsible for the inhibition of the transcription of NFkB [58]. This finding has also been consistent for gingival fibroblasts and alveolar osteoblasts challenged with LPS and cultured with PRP preparations [59].

Notably, LPS challenge induced important structural (degenerative) changes accompanied with chondrocyte apoptosis in CEs, which were reverted or ameliorated in diverse degrees by PRG supernatants. However, the general histology score was significantly lower (better) for CEs treated with PRG supernatants, and some individual outcome parameters, such as chondrocyte necrosis, focal cell loss and SOFG uptake, were affected by some of these substances.

Chondrocyte necrosis was mostly observed in CEs treated with 25 % L-PRG and 50 % P-PRG supernatants. This finding could indicate that these substances at these specific concentrations were not able to reverse the catabolic effect mediated by endotoxin in CEs. Furthermore, it is also important to consider that both 25 % PRG supernatants presented chondrocyte apoptosis reaction similar to those observed in CEs from the control group challenged with LPS; although, CEs treated with 25 % P-PRG supernatant presented the highest score for this parameter. This last finding could possibly indicate that this substance at lower concentration is not able to reverse the cartilage catabolic effects of LPS and can induce additional chondrocyte apoptosis.

Focal cell loss was more evident for both 50 % PRG supernatants, possibly due to that chondrocytes being able to migrate inside the CEs towards the periphery through a chemotactic attractive stimulus in the culture media [60], such as the milieu of growth factors released from PRP [61–63]. In contrast, another explanation to demonstrate the cause of focal cell loss in the groups of CEs treated with higher concentrations of PRG supernatants could be attributed to chondrocyte necrosis or even chondrocyte apoptosis [64]. However, this lack of significant increase of these parameters occurred only for CEs treated with 50 % P-PRG supernatant, which could indicate that P-PRG preparations were not chondroprotective.

The SOFG uptake score was higher in CEs treated with 50 % L-PRG and 25 % P-PRG supernatants, and apparently this parameter was worst for CEs treated with 50 % L-PRG supernatant. This parameter is associated with the structural content of proteoglycans in the cartilage ECM [8], which indicate the quality and integrity of this structure. It is important to consider that 50 % L-PRG supernatant also induced downregulation of anabolic ECM genes, such as COL2A1 and COMP. Taken together, these histology and molecular findings indicate that higher concentrations of L-PRP preparations could be deleterious for osteoarthritic cartilage. One pitfall of the present research was that the release or accumulation of proteoglycans was not measured in the culture media of CEs. However, we consider that the combination of histology parameters and gene expression could be valid indicators for the degree of affection of ECM of the CEs of this study.

The combination of the general histology score, chondrocyte apoptosis findings, HA release to the culture media and the catabolic and anabolic cartilage ECM gene expression demonstrated that all PRG supernatants are "biosubstances" with mixed biological effects. In general, all PRG supernatants presented a potential anti-inflammatory effect and decreased the catabolic effects of LPS on CEs at the cellular and molecular level. However, the overall analysis of our results indicates that 25 % L-PRG supernatant (followed in order of importance by 50 % P-PRG, 25 % P-PRG and 50 % L-PRG) represented the substance with the most important anti-inflammatory and anabolic effect with lower affection of CEs at the histology level. Furthermore, 25 % P-PRG supernatant presented important anabolic effects, but it induced a more severe chondrocyte apoptosis than the other of the evaluated substances. This detrimental cell effect limits the potential clinical use of this substance at this concentration.

The present results can be complemented with the previous findings obtained by us in two in vitro studies, in which the production of anti-inflammatory and catabolic cytokines was measured in the culture media of synovial membrane explants (SME) [27] and CEs [40] challenged with LPS over 48 h and 96 h. In general, 25 % L-PRG and 50 % L-PRG supernatants presented the best anabolic and anti-inflammatory profile. However, in both studies, 25 % L-PRG supernatant produced a most significant reduction of TNF-α production and a total higher production of IL-1ra over time than 50 % L-PRG [27, 40].

Currently, we use 3-5 mL doses of PRP to treat fetlock osteoarthritis in horses with a body weight of 300-450 kg. This PRP volume has also been used for other researches with good results [22]. Notably, the complete volume capacity for an equine fetlock joint has been calculated at 12.5 ± 1.0 mL [65]. Thus, if the PRP volume used is adjusted in relation to the volume capacity of this specific joint [65], the effective concentration of PRP in clinical conditions could be near to 40 %, without considering the additional volume of synovial fluid (2-2.5 mL), which could represent a final PRP/synovial fluid concentration of 40-60 %. In line with this, the PRP dose for this joint could possibly be adjusted at 25 % using between 1.5-2.0 mL. However, this hypothesis should be probed in patients with osteoarthritis or experimentally induced synovitis.

Our findings are in line with the results of Cavallo et al. [39] and Kreuz et al.[38], who found diverse and positive effects for L- and P-PRP preparations in human osteoarthritic chondrocytes and subchondral mesenchymal progenitor cells. Conversely, our results are different from other in vitro studies [34–36], which have concluded that only P-PRP preparations induce an anabolic effect in cartilage and L-PRP preparations only induce an opposite (catabolic) joint state.

This study had several limitations. First, this is an in vitro study, which does not reflect the exact biological phenomena occurring in the osteoarthritic joint. However, this in vitro system of cartilage inflammation and degeneration could be useful to demonstrate that L- and P-PRG supernatants could act in function of their concentration and could have different mechanisms of action to induce cartilage joint anabolism and, potentially, diminish pain and inflammation. Another limitation of this study was that blood of only one animal was used to produce the PRG supernatants evaluated to avoid the great variability in the CE responses to several PRP preparations. This situation is not practical in clinical conditions because autologous PRP should be used. However, the response of each patient in particular will depend in some measure on the concentration of the cells' proteins in PRP.

Conclusions

This study demonstrates that both L- and P-PRP preparations at different concentrations can induce different anti-inflammatory, anti-catabolic, anabolic and even catabolic responses in an in vitro system of cartilage inflammation and degeneration.

Apparently, 25 % L-PRG supernatant presented the best therapeutic profile when compared to the other PRP preparations examined, because it presented anti-inflammatory and anabolic effects with minimal cellular and structural changes in CEs. Our results once more demonstrate that the biological variability of PRP preparations makes their application rather challenging. Additional studies in animal models and in patients with OA should be performed to know the in vivo effect of PRP preparations at different concentrations.

Abbreviations

ADMTS-4, A disintegrin and metalloproteinase with thrombospondin motifs 4; ANOVA, analysis of variance; CEs, cartilage explants; COL1A1, collagen type I alpha 1; COL2A1, collagen type II alpha 1; COMP, cartilage oligomeric matrix protein; DMEM, Dulbecco's modified Eagle medium; ECM, extracellular matrix; ELISA, enzyme-linked immunosorbent assay; GF, growth factor; HA, hyaluronan; IL-1, interleukin 1; L-PRG, leukoconcentrated platelet-rich gel; L-PRP, leukoconcentrated platelet-rich plasma; LPS, lipopolysaccharide; MMP-13, matrix metalloproteinase 13; NFkβ, nuclear factor kappa beta; OA, osteoarthritis; PDGF-BB, platelet derived growth factor isoform BB; PLT, platelet; P-PRG, pure platelet-rich gel; P-PRP, pure platelet-rich plasma; PRG, platelet-rich gel; PRP, platelet-rich plasma; RBC, red blood cell; TGF-β_1, transforming growth factor beta-1; TNF-α, tumor necrosis factor alpha; WBC, leukocyte.

Acknowledgments

The authors thank Wilson Gómez and Fabio Robayo for their assistance and thank Policía Nacional de Colombia.

Funding

This project was supported by grant No.397-2011 of the National Program of Biotechnology from COLCIENCIAS, Bogotá D.C and by grant No 0250911 of the Vicerrectoría de Investigaciones y Postgrados of the Universidad de Caldas, Manizales, Colombia. D.L.R's PhD scholarship was funded by COLCIENCIAS.

Authors' contributions

JUC had full access to all of the data in the study and takes responsibility for the decision to submit this work for publication. JUC designed the study and participated in data analysis and interpretation, manuscript drafting and critical revision. CL, DLR, MEA, JEP and MEB performed laboratory work and contributed to data collection, data analysis and interpretation and critical revision of the manuscript. All of the authors read and approved the final version of the manuscript to be published.

Competing interests

The authors declare that they have no competing interests.

Consent for publication

Not applicable.

Author details

[1]Grupo de Investigación Terapia Regenerativa, Departamento de Salud Animal, Universidad de Caldas, Manizales, Colombia. [2]Grupo de investigación Biosalud, Departamento de Ciencias Básicas para la Salud, Universidad de Caldas, Manizales, Colombia. [3]Grupo de Investigación en Citogenética, Filogenia y Evolución de Poblaciones, Universidad del Tolima, Ibagué, Colombia.

References

1. Marshall DA, Vanderby S, Barnabe C, MacDonald KV, Maxwell C, Mosher D, Wasylak T, Lix L, Stat P, Enns E, et al. Estimating the burden of osteoarthritis to plan for the future. Arthritis Care Res. 2015;4(10):22612.
2. Aragon CL, Hofmeister EH, Budsberg SC. Systematic review of clinical trials of treatments for osteoarthritis in dogs. J Am Vet Med Assoc. 2007;230(4):514–21.
3. Vandeweerd JM, Coisnon C, Clegg P, Cambier C, Pierson A, Hontoir F, Saegerman C, Gustin P, Buczinski S.Systematic review of efficacy of nutraceuticals to alleviate clinical signs of osteoarthritis. J Vet Intern Med. 2012;26(3):448–56.
4. Carmona JU, Prades M. Pathophisiology of osteoarthritis. Comp Equine. 2009;4(1):28–40.
5. McIlwraith CW, Fortier LA, Frisbie DD, Nixon AJ. Equine models of articular cartilage repair. Cartilage. 2011;2(4):317–26.
6. McCoy AM. Animal models of osteoarthritis: comparisons and key considerations. Vet Pathol. 2015;10:0300985815588611.
7. Neundorf RH, Lowerison MB, Cruz AM, Thomason JJ, McEwen BJ, Hurtig MB. Determination of the prevalence and severity of metacarpophalangeal joint osteoarthritis in Thoroughbred racehorses via quantitative macroscopic evaluation. Am J Vet Res. 2010;71(11):1284–93.
8. McIlwraith CW, Frisbie DD, Kawcak CE, Fuller CJ, Hurtig M, Cruz A. The OARSI histopathology initiative - recommendations for histological assessments of osteoarthritis in the horse. Osteoarthritis Cartilage. 2010;18 Suppl 3:S93–105.
9. Zamli Z, Sharif M. Chondrocyte apoptosis: a cause or consequence of osteoarthritis? Int J Rheum Dis. 2011;14(2):159–66.
10. Chang CH, Hsu YM, Chen YC, Lin FH, Sadhasivam S, Loo ST, Savitha S. Anti-inflammatory effects of hydrophilic and lipophilic statins with hyaluronic acid against LPS-induced inflammation in porcine articular chondrocytes. J Orthop Res. 2014;32(4):557–65.
11. Franciozi CE, Tarini VA, Reginato RD, Goncalves PR, Medeiros VP, Ferretti M, Dreyfuss JL, Nader HB, Faloppa F. Gradual strenuous running regimen predisposes to osteoarthritis due to cartilage cell death and altered levels of glycosaminoglycans. Osteoarthritis Cartilage. 2013;21(7):965–72.
12. Otsuki Y, Li Z, Shibata MA. Apoptotic detection methods–from morphology to gene. Prog Histochem Cytochem. 2003;38(3):275–339.
13. Marcu KB, Otero M, Olivotto E, Borzi RM, Goldring MB. NF-kappaB signaling: multiple angles to target OA. Curr Drug Targets. 2010;11(5):599–613.
14. Ownby SL, Fortuno LV, Au AY, Grzanna MW, Rashmir-Raven AM, Frondoza CG. Expression of pro-inflammatory mediators is inhibited by an avocado/soybean unsaponifiables and epigallocatechin gallate combination. J Inflamm (Lond). 2014;11(1):8. doi:10.1186/1476-9255-1111-1188.
15. Ishijima M, Kaneko H, Kaneko K. The evolving role of biomarkers for osteoarthritis. Ther Adv Musculoskelet Dis. 2014;6(4):144–53.
16. Aigner T, Bartnik E, Zien A, Zimmer R. Functional genomics of osteoarthritis. Pharmacogenomics. 2002;3(5):635–50.
17. Campbell KA, Saltzman BM, Mascarenhas R, Khair MM, Verma NN, Bach Jr BR, Cole BJ. Does intra-articular platelet-rich plasma injection provide clinically superior outcomes compared with other therapies in the treatment of knee osteoarthritis? A systematic review of overlapping meta-analyses. Arthroscopy. 2015;29(15):00353–9.
18. Say F, Gurler D, Yener K, Bulbul M, Malkoc M. Platelet-rich plasma injection is more effective than hyaluronic acid in the treatment of knee osteoarthritis. Acta Chir Orthop Traumatol Cech. 2013;80(4):278–83.
19. Jang SJ, Kim JD, Cha SS. Platelet-rich plasma (PRP) injections as an effective treatment for early osteoarthritis. Eur J Orthop Surg Traumatol. 2013;23(5):573–80.
20. Brossi PM, Moreira JJ, Machado TS, Baccarin RY. Platelet-rich plasma in orthopedic therapy: a comparative systematic review of clinical and experimental data in equine and human musculoskeletal lesions. BMC Vet Res. 2015;11:98.
21. Carmona JU, Argüelles D, Climent F, Prades M. Autologous platelet concentrates as a treatment of horses with osteoarthritis: a preliminary pilot clinical study. J Equine Vet Sci. 2007;27(4):167–70.
22. Pichereau F, Décory M, Cuevas Ramos G. Autologous platelet concentrate as a treatment for horses with refractory fetlock osteoarthritis. J Equine Vet Sci. 2014;34(4):489–93.
23. Silva RF, Carmona JU, Rezende CM. Intra-articular injections of autologous platelet concentrates in dogs with surgical reparation of cranial cruciate ligament rupture: a pilot study. Vet Comp Orthop Traumatol. 2013;26(4):285–90.
24. Giraldo CE, Alvarez ME, Carmona JU. Effects of sodium citrate and acid citrate dextrose solutions on cell counts and growth factor release from equine pure-platelet rich plasma and pure-platelet rich gel. BMC Vet Res. 2015;11:60.
25. Giraldo CE, Lopez C, Alvarez ME, Samudio IJ, Prades M, Carmona JU. Effects of the breed, sex and age on cellular content and growth factor release from equine pure-platelet rich plasma and pure-platelet rich gel. BMC Vet Res. 2013;9:29.
26. Rios DL, Lopez C, Carmona JU. Platelet-rich gel supernatants stimulate the release of anti-inflammatory proteins on culture media of normal equine synovial membrane explants. Vet Med Int. 2015;2015:547052.
27. Rios DL, López C, Álvarez ME, Samudio I, Carmona JU. Effects over time of two platelet gel supernatants on growth factor, cytokine and hyaluronan concentrations in normal synovial membrane explants challenged with lipopolysaccharide. BMC Musculoskelet Disord. 2015;16:153.
28. Andia I, Maffulli N. Platelet-rich plasma for managing pain and inflammation in osteoarthritis. Nat Rev Rheumatol. 2013;9(12):721–30. doi:10.1038/nrrheum.2013.1141. Epub 2013 Oct 1031.
29. Stewart K, Pabbruwe M, Dickinson S, Sims T, Hollander AP, Chaudhuri JB. The effect of growth factor treatment on meniscal chondrocyte proliferation and differentiation on polyglycolic acid scaffolds. Tissue Eng. 2007;13(2):271–80.
30. Montaseri A, Busch F, Mobasheri A, Buhrmann C, Aldinger C, Rad JS, Shakibaei M. IGF-1 and PDGF-bb suppress IL-1beta-induced cartilage degradation through down-regulation of NF-kappaB signaling: involvement of Src/PI-3 K/AKT pathway. PLoS One. 2011;6(12):e28663.
31. Brandl A, Angele P, Roll C, Prantl L, Kujat R, Kinner B. Influence of the growth factors PDGF-BB, TGF-beta1 and bFGF on the replicative aging of human articular chondrocytes during in vitro expansion. J Orthop Res. 2010;28(3):354–60.
32. Zhai G, Dore J, Rahman P. TGF-beta signal transduction pathways and osteoarthritis. Rheumatol Int. 2015;15:15.
33. Russell RP, Apostolakos J, Hirose T, Cote MP, Mazzocca AD. Variability of platelet-rich plasma preparations. Sports Med Arthrosc. 2013;21(4):186–90.
34. Sundman EA, Cole BJ, Fortier LA. Growth factor and catabolic cytokine concentrations are influenced by the cellular composition of platelet-rich plasma. Am J Sports Med. 2011;39(10):2135–40.
35. Kisiday JD, McIlwraith CW, Rodkey WG, Frisbie DD, Steadman JR. Effects of platelet-rich plasma composition on anabolic and catabolic activities in equine cartilage and meniscal explants. Cartilage. 2012;3(3):245–54.
36. Sundman EA, Cole BJ, Karas V, Della Valle C, Tetreault MW, Mohammed HO, Fortier LA. The anti-inflammatory and matrix restorative mechanisms of platelet-rich plasma in osteoarthritis. Am J Sports Med. 2014;42(1):35–41.

37. Braun HJ, Kim HJ, Chu CR, Dragoo JL. The effect of platelet-rich plasma formulations and blood products on human synoviocytes: implications for intra-articular injury and therapy. Am J Sports Med. 2014;42(5):1204–10.
38. Kreuz PC, Kruger JP, Metzlaff S, Freymann U, Endres M, Pruss A, Petersen W, Kaps C. Platelet-rich plasma preparation types show impact on chondrogenic differentiation, migration, and proliferation of human subchondral mesenchymal progenitor cells. Arthroscopy. 2015;13(15):00260-1.
39. Cavallo C, Filardo G, Mariani E, Kon E, Marcacci M, Pereira Ruiz MT, Facchini A, Grigolo B:. Comparison of platelet-rich plasma formulations for cartilage healing: an in vitro study. J Bone Joint Surg Am. 2014;96(5): 423–9.
40. Ríos DL, López C, Carmona JU. Evaluation of the anti-inflammatory effects of two platelet-rich gel supernatants in an in vitro system of cartilage inflammation. Cytokine. 2015;76(2):505–13.
41. Arguelles D, Carmona JU, Pastor J, Iborra A, Vinals L, Martinez P, Bach E, Prades M. Evaluation of single and double centrifugation tube methods for concentrating equine platelets. Res Vet Sci. 2006;81(2):237–45.
42. Bolt DM, Ishihara A, Weisbrode SE, Bertone AL. Effects of triamcinolone acetonide, sodium hyaluronate, amikacin sulfate, and mepivacaine hydrochloride, alone and in combination, on morphology and matrix composition of lipopolysaccharide-challenged and unchallenged equine articular cartilage explants. Am J Vet Res. 2008;69(7):861–7.
43. Byron CR, Orth MW, Venta PJ, Lloyd JW, Caron JP. Influence of glucosamine on matrix metalloproteinase expression and activity in lipopolysaccharide-stimulated equine chondrocytes. Am J Vet Res. 2003;64(6):666–71.
44. Penha-Goncalves MN, Onions DE, Nicolson L. Cloning and sequencing of equine transforming growth factor-beta 1 (TGF beta-1) cDNA. DNA Seq. 1997;7(6):375–8.
45. Donnelly BP, Nixon AJ, Haupt JL, Dahlgren LA. Nucleotide structure of equine platelet-derived growth factor-A and -B and expression in horses with induced acute tendinitis. Am J Vet Res. 2006;67(7):1218–25.
46. Furuta N, Yoshioka I, Fukuizumi T, Tominaga K, Nishihara T, Fukuda J. Morphological features of cartilage observed during mandibular distraction in rabbits. Int J Oral Maxillofac Surg. 2007;36(3):243–9.
47. Fraser A, Fearon U, Reece R, Emery P, Veale DJ. Matrix metalloproteinase 9, apoptosis, and vascular morphology in early arthritis. Arthritis Rheum. 2001; 44(9):2024–8.
48. Livak KJ, Schmittgen TD. Analysis of relative gene expression data using real-time quantitative PCR and the 2(-Delta Delta C(T)) Method. Methods. 2001;25(4):402–8.
49. Dohan DM, Choukroun J, Diss A, Dohan SL, Dohan AJ, Mouhyi J, Gogly B. Platelet-rich fibrin (PRF): a second-generation platelet concentrate. Part III: leucocyte activation: a new feature for platelet concentrates? Oral Surg Oral Med Oral Pathol Oral Radiol Endod. 2006;101(3):e51–55.
50. Giusti I, D'Ascenzo S, Manco A, Di Stefano G, Di Francesco M, Rughetti A, Dal Mas A, Properzi G, Calvisi V, Dolo V. Platelet concentration in platelet-rich plasma affects tenocyte behavior in vitro. Biomed Res Int. 2014;2014: 630870. doi:10.1155/2014/630870. Epub 632014 Jul 630823.
51. Dohan Ehrenfest DM, Bielecki T, Mishra A, Borzini P, Inchingolo F, Sammartino G, Rasmusson L, Evert PA. In search of a consensus terminology in the field of platelet concentrates for surgical use: platelet-rich plasma (PRP), platelet-rich fibrin (PRF), fibrin gel polymerization and leukocytes. Curr Pharm Biotechnol. 2012;13(7):1131–7.
52. McCarrel TM, Minas T, Fortier LA. Optimization of leukocyte concentration in platelet-rich plasma for the treatment of tendinopathy. J Bone Joint Surg Am. 2012, 94(19):e143(141-148).
53. Pearson W, Fletcher RS, Kott LS, Hurtig MB. Protection against LPS-induced cartilage inflammation and degradation provided by a biological extract of Mentha spicata. BMC Complement Altern Med. 2010;10(19):1472–6882.
54. Santoro A, Conde J, Scotece M, Abella V, Lopez V, Pino J, Gomez R, Gomez-Reino JJ, Gualillo O. Choosing the right chondrocyte cell line: Focus on nitric oxide. J Orthop Res. 2015;27(10):22954.
55. Bougault C, Gosset M, Houard X, Salvat C, Godmann L, Pap T, Jacques C, Berenbaum F. Stress-induced cartilage degradation does not depend on the NLRP3 inflammasome in human osteoarthritis and mouse models. Arthritis Rheum. 2012;64(12):3972–81.
56. Vezina Audette R, Lavoie-Lamoureux A, Lavoie JP, Laverty S. Inflammatory stimuli differentially modulate the transcription of paracrine signaling molecules of equine bone marrow multipotent mesenchymal stromal cells. Osteoarthritis Cartilage. 2013;21(8):1116–24.
57. Brenner D, Blaser H, Mak TW. Regulation of tumour necrosis factor signalling: live or let die. Nat Rev Immunol. 2015;15(6):362–74.
58. Bendinelli P, Matteucci E, Dogliotti G, Corsi MM, Banfi G, Maroni P, Desiderio MA. Molecular basis of anti-inflammatory action of platelet-rich plasma on human chondrocytes: mechanisms of NF-kappaB inhibition via HGF. J Cell Physiol. 2010;225(3):757–66.
59. Anitua E, Zalduendo M, Troya M, Padilla S, Orive G. Leukocyte inclusion within a platelet rich plasma-derived fibrin scaffold stimulates a more pro-inflammatory environment and alters fibrin properties. PLoS One. 2015;10(3):e0121713.
60. Morales TI. Chondrocyte moves: clever strategies? Osteoarthritis Cartilage. 2007;15(8):861–71.
61. O'Connell GD, Tan AR, Cui V, Bulinski JC, Cook JL, Attur M, Abramson SB, Ateshian GA, Hung CT. Human chondrocyte migration behaviour to guide the development of engineered cartilage. J Tissue Eng Regen Med. 2015, 28(10). doi:10.1002/term.1988.
62. Kruger JP, Hondke S, Endres M, Pruss A, Siclari A, Kaps C. Human platelet-rich plasma stimulates migration and chondrogenic differentiation of human subchondral progenitor cells. J Orthop Res. 2012;30(6):845–52.
63. Schar MO, Diaz-Romero J, Kohl S, Zumstein MA, Nesic D. Platelet-rich concentrates differentially release growth factors and induce cell migration in vitro. Clin Orthop Relat Res. 2015;473(5):1635–43.
64. Thomas CM, Fuller CJ, Whittles CE, Sharif M. Chondrocyte death by apoptosis is associated with the initiation and severity of articular cartilage degradation. Int J Rheum Dis. 2011;14(2):191–8.
65. Ekman L, Nilsson G, Persson L, Lumsden JH. Volume of the synovia in certain joint cavities in the horse. Acta Vet Scand. 1981;22(1):23–31.

2

Effects of controlled hypoxemia or hypovolemia on global and intestinal oxygenation and perfusion in isoflurane anesthetized horses receiving an alpha-2-agonist infusion

Klaus Hopster[1,2*], Liza Wittenberg-Voges[1], Florian Geburek[1], Charlotte Hopster-Iversen[1] and Sabine B. R. Kästner[1]

Abstract

Background: Aim of this prospective experimental study was to assess effects of systemic hypoxemia and hypovolemia on global and gastrointestinal oxygenation and perfusion in anesthetized horses. Therefore, we anesthetized twelve systemically healthy warmblood horses using either xylazine or dexmedetomidine for premedication and midazolam and ketamine for induction. Anesthesia was maintained using isoflurane in oxygen with either xylazine or dexmedetomidine and horses were ventilated to normocapnia. During part A arterial oxygen saturation (SaO_2) was reduced by reducing inspiratory oxygen fraction in steps of 5%. In part B hypovolemia was induced by controlled arterial exsanguination via roller pump (rate: 38 ml/kg/h). Mean arterial blood pressure (MAP), heart rate, pulmonary artery pressure, arterial and central venous blood gases and cardiac output were measured, cardiac index (CI) was calculated. Intestinal microperfusion and oxygenation were measured using laser Doppler flowmetry and white-light spectrophotometry. Surface probes were placed via median laparotomy on the stomach, jejunum and colon.

Results: Part A: Reduction in arterial oxygenation resulted in a sigmoid decrease in central venous oxygen partial pressure. At $SaO_2 < 80\%$ no further decrease in central venous oxygen partial pressure occurred. Intestinal oxygenation remained unchanged until SaO_2 of 80% and then decreased. Heart rate and pulmonary artery pressure increased significantly during hypoxemia. Part B: Progressive reduction in circulating blood volume resulted in a linear decrease in MAP and CI. Intestinal perfusion was preserved until blood loss resulted in MAP and CI lower 51 ± 5 mmHg and 40 ± 3 mL/kg/min, respectively, and then decreased rapidly.

Conclusions: Under isoflurane, intestinal tissue oxygenation remained at baseline when arterial oxygenation exceeded 80% and intestinal perfusion remained at baseline when MAP exceeded 51 mmHg and CI exceeded 40 mL/kg/min in this group of horses.

Trial registry number: 33.14-42,502-04-14/1547.

Keywords: Gastrointestinal tract, Hypoxemia, Hypovolemia, Laser Doppler flowmetry, Microperfusion

* Correspondence: Klaus.hopster@gmx.de
[1]Equine Clinic, University of Veterinary Medicine Hanover, Foundation, Bünteweg 9, D-30559 Hanover, Germany
[2]Department of Clinical Studies-NBC, School of Veterinary Medicine, University of Pennsylvania, 382 West Street Road, Kennett Square, PA 19348, USA

Background

Global oxygen delivery ($\dot{D}O_2$) is determined by total blood flow or cardiac output, and arterial oxygen content, which depends on hemoglobin concentration and its saturation with oxygen as well as the arterial oxygen partial pressure (PaO_2). Impaired $\dot{D}O_2$ to the periphery might contribute to the high prevalence of equine fatalities directly related to anesthesia and/or surgery [1, 2] by drug induced reduction of cardiovascular function, hemorrhage and arterial hypoxemia.

During general anesthesia, particularly if in dorsal recumbency, horses may develop a large alveolo- arterial oxygen partial pressure gradient and become hypoxaemic [3]. Hypoxemia (defined as an arterial partial pressure of oxygen <60 mmHg) leading to inadequate $\dot{D}O_2$ to peripheral tissues during anesthesia would seem a potential cause of increased mortality [4] and an impairment of splanchnic oxygenation can contribute to alterations in intestinal integrity and to postoperative colic. During severe hypoxemia $\dot{D}O_2$ may become diminished so that oxygen consumption (VO_2) becomes linearly dependent on $\dot{D}O_2$. As a linear relationship develops between both, $\dot{D}O_2$-becomes inadequate to maintain aerobic metabolism leading to tissue hypoxia and necrosis. To our knowledge there are no studies investigating effects of arterial hypoxemia on regional gastrointestinal oxygenation in horses.

Dose-dependent cardiovascular depression by isoflurane has been well described and decreased cardiac index (CI) is a direct effect of isoflurane on myocardial contractility, leading to a reduction in stroke volume and consequent, in combination with its vasodilatory effects, to a reduction in mean arterial blood pressures (MAP) [5]. In horses it has been shown, that states of low blood pressure and low cardiac output will lead to impaired intestinal perfusion [6]. However, information on the influence of acute blood loss on gastrointestinal microperfusion is limited in this species. In man, severe hemorrhage is associated with redistribution of cardiac output to vital organs (brain, heart) but reduced perfusion and oxygen delivery to others, such as the gut [7]. Impairment of splanchnic perfusion and/or oxygenation can contribute to alterations in intestinal motility [8] and breach of the intestinal mucosal barrier [9] leading to septicemia and ileus. In horses, studies investigating effects of acute blood loss on global and intestinal perfusion during anesthesia are missing.

Aim of this study was to evaluate effects of hypoxemia and hypovolemia on global perfusion and oxygenation and microperfusion and oxygenation of the gastrointestinal tract in anesthetized horses using surface lightguide tissue spectrophotometry combined with laser Doppler flowmetry.

Results

Part A: Hypoxemia

There were no differences between horses receiving either dexmedetomidine or xylazine. At the beginning of the experiment all horses were sufficient oxygenated with an arterial oxygen saturation values (SaO_2) > 95% and PaO_2 ranging between 82 mmHg and 389 mmHg. Due to the high variation in lung function at the beginning of the experiment, inspiratory oxygen concentrations resulted in different SaO_2 during the down titration of FiO_2.

Reducing the inspiratory oxygen concentration resulted in a decrease in $\dot{D}O_2$, PaO_2 and mixed venous oxygen partial pressure ($P\bar{V}O_2$) in all horses (Fig. 1). As expected by the shape of the oxygen dissociation curve

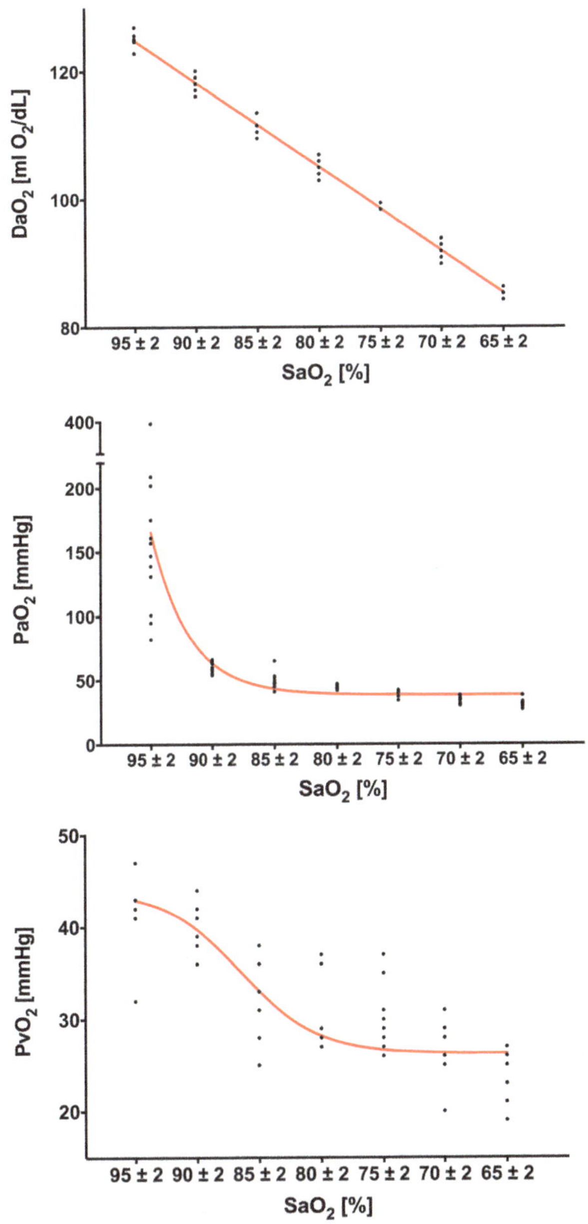

Fig. 1 Oxygen delivery ($\dot{D}O_2$), arterial oxygen partial pressure (PaO_2) and mixed venous oxygen partial pressure ($P\bar{V}O_2$) at different arterial oxygen saturation values (SaO_2) in anaesthetized horses during controlled hypoxemia

relation between decrease in SaO_2 and PaO_2 was not linear. The reduction in SaO_2 resulted in a non-linear decrease in intestinal tissue oxygenation (Fig. 2) and in $P\check{V}O_2$ (Fig. 1). MAP and CI remained stable but heart rate increased significantly when SaO_2 decreased below 72% (Table 1). There was a constant, but non-significant increase in pulmonary artery pressure (PAP) (Table 1). Gastrointestinal tissue oxygenation (sO_2) decreased rapidly and significantly when SaO_2 dropped below values 80 ± 2% (Fig. 2).

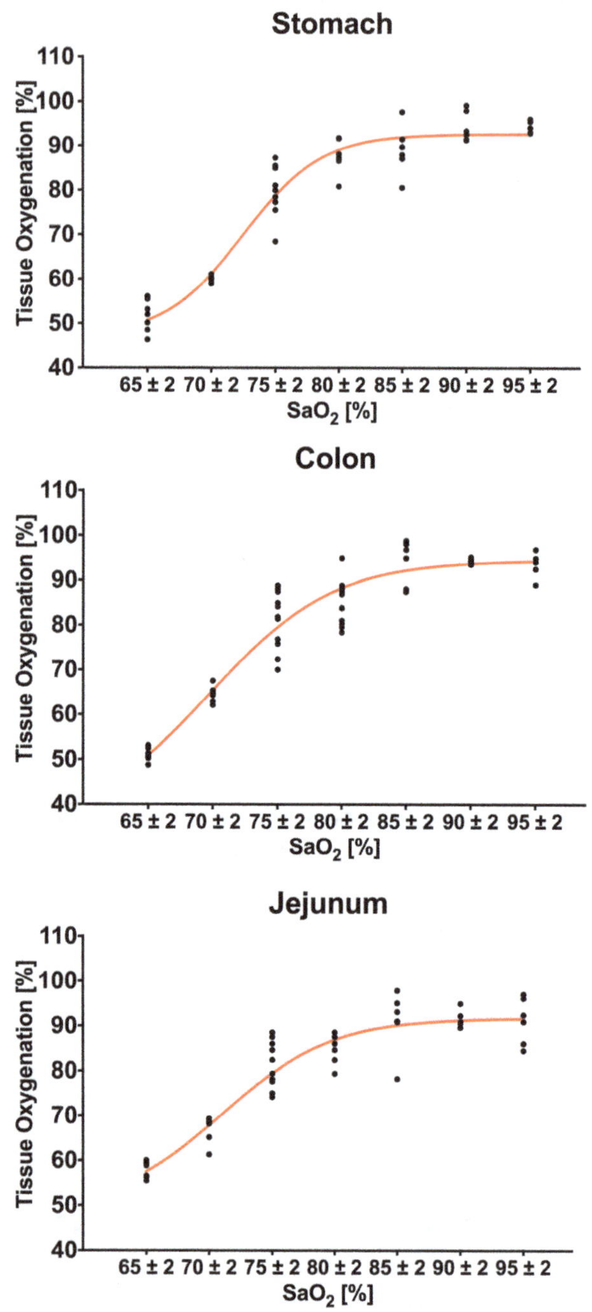

Fig. 2 Non-linear relation between tissue oxygenation of the stomach (gastric oxygenation), the jejunum (jejunal oxygenation) and the colon (colonic oxygenation) and the arterial oxygen saturation (SaO_2)

Part B: Hypovolemia

Measurements during exsanguination were performed at baseline blood volume and at 88%, 75%, 63%, 50% and less than 45% of that value. All horses died after a total blood loss of 55 to 62% (no pulse and no cardiac output detectable). Exsanguination resulted in a continues decrease in CI and MAP (Fig. 3). Intestinal perfusion remained stable for the first 3 measurements; at a total blood volume of less than 63% (CI and MAP lower 40 ± 3 mL/kg/min and 51 ± 5 mmHg, respectively) a significant decrease of tissue blood flow of stomach, jejunum and colon occurred (Figs. 4 and 5). No significant differences were found between horses receiving either dexmedetomidine or xylazine.

Discussion

In horses, especially in non-healthy colic patients, adequate oxygenation is regularly a problem [10]. One aim of this study was to evaluate effects of severe hypoxemia during anesthesia on gastrointestinal oxygenation in horses. Reducing inspiratory oxygen fraction resulted in a decrease in PaO_2 and SaO_2 and therefore in a decrease in arterial oxygen content (CaO_2) and $\dot{D}O_2$, as CI remained constant during FiO_2 reduction. Under physiologic steady-state conditions, intestinal VO_2 is independent of $\dot{D}O_2$ and determined by cellular metabolic needs [11–13]. A moderate decrease in $\dot{D}O_2$ is compensated by an increase in oxygen extraction by the tissue [14]. In our study, a decrease in $SaO_2 < 90\%$ resulted in a decrease in SvO_2 and PvO_2. At this point the oxygen extraction ratio increased as well and therefore maintained VO_2 and oxygenation of the tissue. When $\dot{D}O_2$ is severely compromised in situations of severe hypoxia or ischemia, VO_2 becomes limited by and therefore dependent on $\dot{D}O_2$ [15, 16]. Intestinal oxygenation was initially stable when starting the reduction of FiO_2 and SaO_2 and therefore reducing O_2, but decreased rapidly when SaO_2 dropped below values of less than 80%, and the compensatory increase in oxygen extraction reached the limit. During progressive hypoxia in resting dogs, $\dot{D}O_2$ needed to decrease below 50% of baseline before VO_2 and jejunal tissue oxygenation decreased [14, 17]. In other animals (rats, pigs, lambs) critical values also ranged between 50 and 60% [15, 18, 19] whereas in our study a $\dot{D}O_2$ reduction of more than 30% resulted in a decrease in tissue oxygenation. Intestinal tissue oxygenation is relatively resistant to hypoxemia as compared to ischemia and the capacity to tolerate pure hypoxemia is dependent on perfusion being preserved to intestinal tissue [17]. All previous measurements were either performed in isolated organs or in previous equipped and awake animals. Our horses were anesthetized and therefore, had per se a reduced cardiovascular function

Table 1 Mean and standard deviation of cardiac index (CI), mean arterial blood pressure (MAP), heart rate (HR) and pulmonary artery pressure (PAP), central venous oxygen saturation ($S\check{V}O_2$) and oxygen extraction ratio (O_2ER) at different arterial oxygen saturation values (SaO_2) in anesthetized horses during controlled hypoxemia

	SaO_2 (%)						
	95 ± 2	90 ± 2	85 ± 2	80 ± 2	75 ± 2	70 ± 2	65 ± 2
CI (ml/kg/min)	61 ± 16	62 ± 15	63 ± 16	61 ± 11	67 ± 14	73 ± 18	75 ± 13 [a]
MAP (mmHg)	72 ± 9	75 ± 8	76 ± 12	77 ± 11	76 ± 10	75 ± 11	78 ± 9
HR (beats/min)	30 ± 2	30 ± 3	31 ± 5	31 ± 4	33 ± 6	37 ± 6 [a]	42 ± 8 [a]
PAP (mmHg)	16 ± 4	18 ± 3	20 ± 3	21 ± 4	22 ± 4	23 ± 5	25 ± 6
$S\check{V}O_2$ (%)	74 ± 2	67 ± 4	61 ± 2 [a]	57 ± 3 [a]	55 ± 3 [a]	53 ± 2 [a]	49 ± 4 [a]
O_2ER (%)	21 ± 2	23 ± 2	26 ± 2 [a]	29 ± 3 [a]	25 ± 3	25 ± 2	22 ± 4

[a]Statistically significant different from baseline (SaO_2 95%)

(lower CI and MAP) but also reduced oxygen requirements compared to standing and resting animals.

Decreasing $\dot{D}O_2$ resulted in a significant increase in heart rate but blood pressure and CI did not change. The increase in heart rate can be explained by an increase in sympathetic tone by hypoxemia [20]. Despite an increase in sympathetic nerve activity, acute systemic hypoxemia leads to decreased blood pressure due to vasodilation [21]. In contrast to these findings blood pressure remained stable in our study which can be explained by the use of constant rate infusion of alpha-2-agonists during anesthesia masking/reducing vasodilative effects of hypoxia by their vasoconstrictive properties [22]. Under hypoxic conditions a depression of the myocardium is observed resulting in a reduction of myocardial performance and cardiac ejection fraction [23, 24]. The fact that there were no significant changes in cardiac index can be explained by a partial compensation of the reduced myocardial performance by the sympathetic-mediated increase of the heart rate. Further the time of hypoxemia was probably too short to cause severe myocardial changes. The fact that we had no changes in either CI or MAP further might explain the lack in changes in gastrointestinal perfusion during hypoxemia in this study [6]. We cannot exclude that longer or more severe periods of hypoxemia may affect the gastrointestinal perfusion in horses.

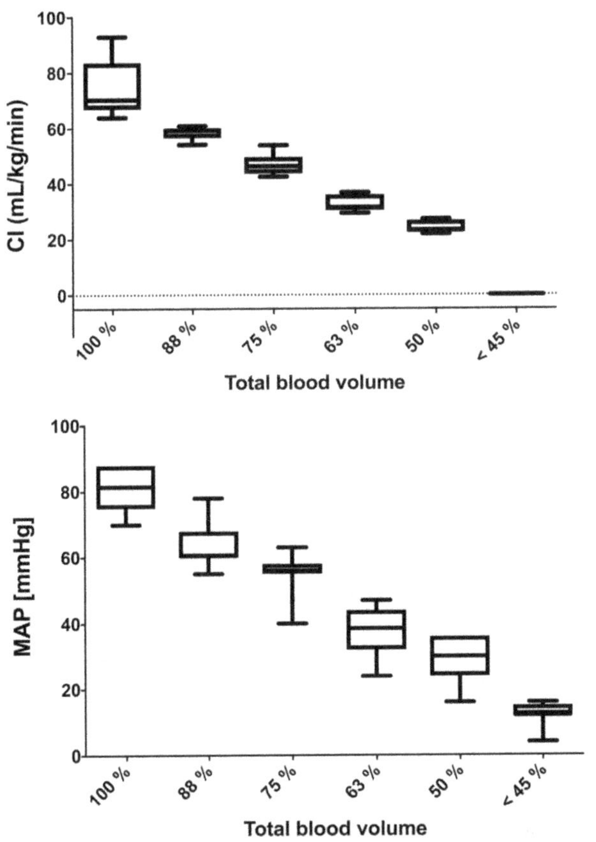

Fig. 3 Box and whiskers plots of cardiac index (CI) and mean arterial blood pressure (MAP) during controlled exsanguination at different states of total blood loss; the boxes are indicating the 75% quantile, the whiskers min to max and the bar the mean value

The second part of this study was performed to investigate effects of a hemorrhagic shock on central and intestinal perfusion in anesthetized horses. All animals responded very similar to the acute blood loss. There was a close inverse and linear correlation of arterial blood pressure and cardiac index with the amount of blood loss as indices of global perfusion. The pathophysiological response to hemorrhagic shock is characterized by vasoconstriction with an initial increase in MAP followed by a marked decrease in MAP and CI when acute loss of 20% of the total blood volume is exceeded [25–27]. In the presence of cardiovascular diseases, anemia or otherwise compromised cardiovascular function or by using different drugs as alpha-2-agonists these responses can vary.

In our horses a drop in MAP and CI was already apparent when total blood loss exceeded 10%. A study in horses anesthetized with halothane or isoflurane showed that severe hemorrhage leads to a significant drop in

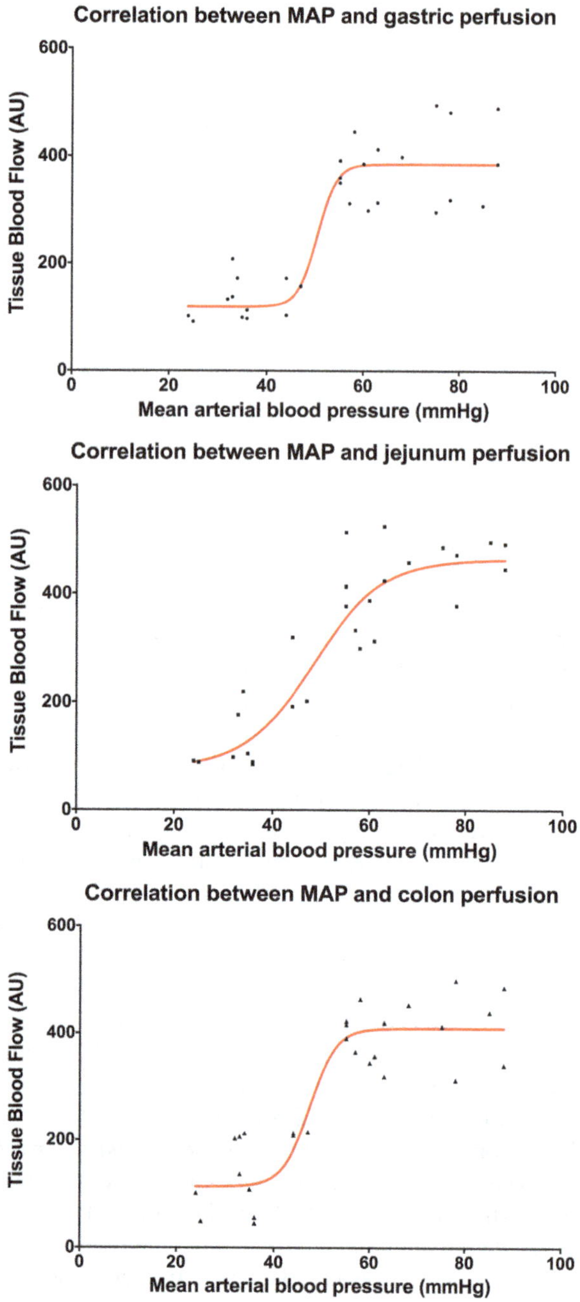

Fig. 4 Non-linear relation between mean perfusion of the stomach (total gastric blood flow), the jejunum (total jejunal blood flow) and the colon (total colonic blood flow) and mean values of mean arterial blood pressure (MAP) during controlled exsanguination in anaesthetized horses

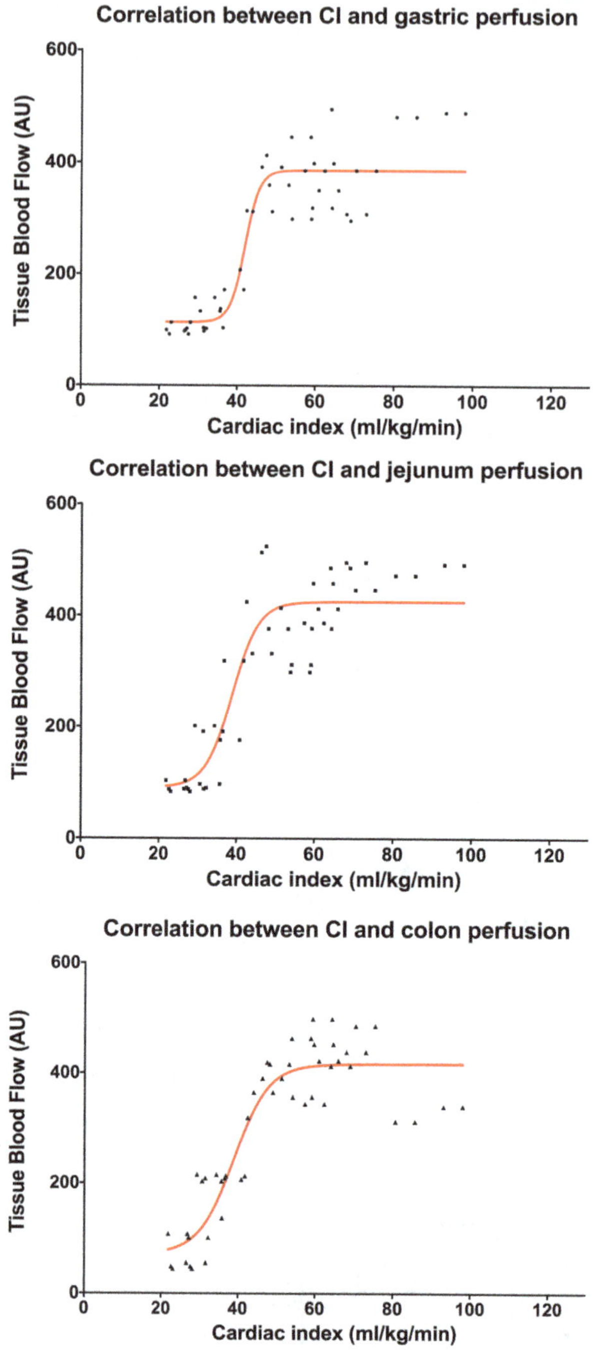

Fig. 5 Non-linear relation between mean perfusion of the stomach (total gastric blood flow), the jejunum (total jejunal blood flow) and the colon (total colonic blood flow) and mean values of the cardiac index (CI) during controlled exsanguination in anaesthetized horses

blood pressure that is most prominent in the initial phase [28] and less linear than observed in non-anesthetized horses. This can be explained by the influence of isoflurane leading to a reduction in stroke volume as well as causing vasodilation [5]. In our study heart rate remained stable until blood loss exceeded 25%. This is also consistent with results decribed by Wilson et al. [28]. Other studies describe an increase in heart rate with progressive hypovolemia. Often, tachycardia is one of the first clinical signs with blood loss [29–31], but in human medicine between 7% and 28% of patients in hypovolemic shock are presented with bradycardia [32, 33]. Common causes for bradycardia are drugs or an increase in the parasympathetic drive. An explanation for the delayed tachycardia might be the presence of high doses alpha-2-agonists in our horses leading to a high parasympathic tone or the isoflurane-induced depression of the sympathetic tone. Further this response could also vary between species.

The perfusion of the intestinal organs remained unchanged until a total blood loss of 37% of the calculated total blood volume resulted in cardiac index and blood pressure values of less than 40 ± 3 ml/kg/min and 51 ± 5 mmHg, respectively. In dogs, pigs and rats it has been shown that in a hypovolemic situation the perfusion of the skin, the skeletal muscles and the gastrointestinal tract is not a priority and is disproportionally reduced compared to the muscle tissue [34–36]. In contrast a study with nine healthy horses under isoflurane anesthesia showed that gastrointestinal perfusion was preserved until a threshold blood pressure of about 60 mmHg or cardiac output lower 50 mL/kg /min were reached [6]. These authors assumed that differences in the regulation of large and small vessel tone [37]. As well as differences between species could be the reason for this. Therefore, it is possible that in our horses despite this reduced blood flow in the larger vessels the local microperfusion of the gastrointestinal perfusion is maintained for a wider range. We further claim that in horses under general anesthesia the intestinal perfusion is sustained for a longer period of acute blood loss.

One limitation of the method we used for measuring the perfusion, the laser Doppler flowmetry, is that this method only allows measurements in arbitrary units and not in quantifiable units. This is because calibration of the output voltage of a laser Doppler flowmeter is difficult, due to the small sample volume size and variations in the optical properties of the tissues [38]. Therefore, interpreting the horses local blood flow technically is only possible in comparison to baseline values, which is one of the reasons for the numerous baseline measurements in between each drug in this experiment. Comparing the results directly to other studies is thereby limited to comparing a trend rather than actual numerical data. Further the used device is calibrated for human blood characteristics, and it is possible that absolute values measured by the O2C were different from real tissue oxygenation. Nonetheless, changes in oxygenation measured in our study were considered reliable because all measurements were performed over time with the same probe in the same animal. Another limitation is that we used a balanced anesthesia protocol with Isoflurane in combination with an alpha-2-agonist. The use of vasoactive drugs including during the anesthetic maintenance phase might have an influence on perfusion parameters and the response of the horses to hypoxemia and exsanguination. We decided to evaluate these effects on a clinical acceptable anesthesia protocol. Inhalational agents like isoflurane are accompanied by dose-related cardiovascular depression affecting cardiac output, blood pressures and muscle perfusion and therefore often combined with alpha-2-agonists like xylazine or dexmedetomidine due to their great potential to reduce the MAC of inhalation agents. However, the lack of a control group not receiving alpha-2-agonists makes interpretation of this difficult. All horses were part of another experiment making the use of two different alpha-2-agonists necessary. Both drugs were used in equipotent doses [39] and infusion time was long enough to assume a steady state.

Another point that needs to be addressed is anesthetic preconditioning, a mechanism referring to changes on a biomolecular level to improve tissue tolerance for hypoxemic conditions. It has been shown that isoflurane as well as different alpha-2-agonists can lead to drug induced preconditioning [40, 41]. Whether this had contributed to our results and to which amount cannot be clarified with our results.

Although there is clear evidence that hemodynamic parameters are stable and time-independent during isoflurane anesthesia in horses [5, 6], it is possible that the hypovolemia experiment was effect first by the long duration of anesthesia and second by the hypoxemia experiment. Due to ethical reasons, we decided to use these horses for multiple experiments as euthanasia was necessary in these animals for tissue sampling of an associated surgical study.

Conclusion

Under isoflurane anesthesia in combination with an alpha-2-agonist constant rate infusion the intestinal tissue compensates a decrease in $\dot{D}O_2$ initially by an increase in oxygen extraction but becomes dependent on $\dot{D}O_2$ during severe hypoxemia with $SaO_2 < 80\%$.

During acute blood loss in anesthesia intestinal perfusion seems to be preserved until a threshold blood pressure (< 50 mmHg) or CI (< 40 mL/kg/min) is reached. With high doses of alpha-2-agonists heart rate might not be a good predictor of hemorrhage in the early state of blood loss. Maintaining perfusion pressure is important for intestinal perfusion.

Methods

Animals

The study was approved by the Ethics Committee for Animal Experiments of Lower Saxony, Germany, number 33.14-42,502-04- 14/1547. Twelve experimental horses (six mares, three geldings and three stallions) with a body weight of 540 ± 41 kg (mean ± SD) and an age of 7 ± 6 years were used for this study. All horses were systemically healthy based on physical examination and routine haematological and biochemical blood work. They were part of an additional anesthesia study and a terminal, experimental surgery study and were euthanized for tissue sampling at the end of anesthesia using pentobarbital (60 mg/kg i.v.).

Anesthesia

Horses were sedated with xylazine (0.5 mg/kg, Xylavet, CP-Pharma, Burgdorf, Germany) or dexmedetomidine (3.5 µg/kg, Dexdomitor, Pfizer Tiergesundheit GmbH, Germany). Induction of anesthesia with midazolam (0.05 mg/kg, Midazolam-ratiopharm, ratiopharm, Ulm, Germany) and ketamine (2.2 mg/kg, Narketan, Vetoquinol, Ravensburg, Germany) was identical in all horses. Anesthesia was maintained with isoflurane (IsofluranCP, CP-Pharma, Burgdorf, Germany) in pure oxygen in combination with a constant rate infusion of 1 mg/kg/h xylazine or 7 µg/kg/h dexmedetomidine. The end tidal isoflurane concentration was maintained between 1.1 and 1.2 Vol.% and kept constant during the experimental procedure and horses received lactated Ringer's solution (B. Braun, Melsungen, Germany) at a rate of 10 ml/kg/h. After induction and intubation horses were positioned on a surgical table in dorsal recumbency. Controlled mechanical ventilation was performed with a pressure cycled large animal ventilator (Model JAVC 2000 J.D. Medical Distributing Company Phoenix, USA) using intermittent positive pressure ventilation with an inspiratory pressure of 25 cm H_2O. Respiratory rate was adjusted to maintain arterial partial carbon dioxide pressure ($PaCO_2$) between 40 and 45 mmHg.

Instrumentation

Before anesthesia the skin over the right and left jugular vein was clipped and subcutaneously infiltrated with mepivacaine (Scandicain 2%, AstraZeneca GmbH, Germany). One 12 G catheter (EquiCathTM Fastflow®, Brau, Melsungen, Germany) was placed into the left jugular veins and two 8F catheter (BD CritiCath; BD Critical Care Systems, USA) introducers in the right jugular vein to facilitate the placement of two balloon tipped catheters. A Swan-Ganz standard thermodilution pulmonary artery catheter (BD CritiCath; BD Critical Care Systems, USA) with a length a 110 cm was placed into the pulmonary artery and a second balloon tipped catheter (Arrow 5 Fr 110 cm Balloon Wedge Pressure Catheter, Teleflex, Germany) was placed into the right atrium. Correct placement was confirmed by visual inspection of the pressure waveforms and by transthoracic ultrasonography.

During anesthesia, the transverse facial artery was cannulated with a 20 G catheter (VenocanTM IV Catheter, Kruuse, Langeskov, Denmark) for invasive blood pressure monitoring and arterial blood sampling. The catheters were connected to calibrated pressure transducers (Gould Statham Transducer, PD 23 ID, USA) via fluid-filled extension lines. The pressure transducers were positioned at the level of the sternal manubrium. A combined spectrophotometry and laser-doppler flow probe of the micro-lightguide spectrophotometer O2C (Oxygen to See, LEA Medizintechnik) was placed via median laparotomy on the serosal surface of the stomach, the jejunum and the pelvic flexion of the colon.

Measured variables

Recording and evaluation of the data started 180 min after induction of anesthesia and after finishing another conducted study. MAP, PAP, heart rate (HR), respiratory rate, end tidal isoflurane concentration (E_TIso) and FiO_2 were measured continuously with a standard anesthesia monitor° and recorded.

For cardiac output measurements, the bolus thermodilution (BTD) technique was used. Therefore iced 5% dextrose solution (one mL per 15 kg bodyweight) was injected into the right atrium and the temperature change was measured via an inline temperature probe positioned in the pulmonary artery. Five injections were performed and the average of the closest three values was used. The CO was measured and the CI was calculated.

Arterial and mixed venous blood samples were taken and arterial pH, PaO_2, $P\grave{V}O_2$ and $PaCO_2$ as well as arterial and mixed venous hemoglobin concentrations and arterial and mixed venous oxygen saturation (SaO_2, $S\grave{V}O_2$) and measured immediately after sampling (AVL995, AVL Medizintechnik, Germany).

Oxygen delivery to the tissue was calculated using the standard formula:

$$\dot{D}O_2 = CO \times (1.34 \times [\text{hemoglobin concentration}] \times SaO_2) + (0.0031 \times PaO_2)$$

Oxygen extraction ratio was calculated using the standard formula:

$$O_2ER = \left[\left(CaO_2 - C\grave{V}O_2\right)/CaO_2\right] \times 100\%$$

With CaO_2 = 1.34 × [hemoglobin concentration] × SaO_2) + (0.0031 × PaO_2).

And with $C\grave{V}O_2$ = 1.34 × [hemoglobin concentration] × $S\grave{V}O_2$) + (0.0031 × $P\grave{V}O_2$)

Tissue oxygenation and blood flow

Gastrointestinal tissue oxygenation (sO_2 in %) and blood flow (flow) were measured by the micro-lightguide spectrophotometer O2C as described previously [42]. This device uses the laser Doppler shift to measure tissue blood flow and white light spectroscopy for measuring the tissue oxygenation (sO_2). A probe with a penetration depth of 2.5 mm was used for all measurements. The surface of this probe was placed on the mucosa of the stomach, the jejunem (about 3 m orally from the ileum) and the pelvic flexure of the large colon. Flow and saturation were recorded for at least 30 s at every measuring time point. Before each recording, quality of the laser Doppler signal was evaluated on a monitor so that identification of incorrect probe positioning or movement artefacts was possible.

Experimental protocol

Part A: Hypoxemia

After equilibration and instrumentation two baseline measurements were performed at a stable plane of anesthesia with an inspiratory oxygen concentration of >95%. Thereafter FiO_2 (constant fresh gas flow of 8 l per minute) was stepwise decreased to 75%, 55%, 40%, 30%, 20%, 15% and 10% by mixing inspiratory oxygen with nitrogen up stream of the vaporizer. Measurements were performed 10 min after reaching the new inspiratory oxygen concentration. Decreasing inspiratory oxygen concentration was terminated when a horse had SaO_2 of 65% or less. About 10 min after reaching the targeted FiO_2 the MAP and CI as well as the sO2 were measured and arterial and central venous blood samples were taken.

For comparison of global oxygenation (SaO_2) and peripheral oxygenation (tissue oxygenation) SaO_2 values were grouped as follows: 95 ± 2%, 90 ± 2%, 85 ± 2%, 80 ± 2%, 75 ± 2%, 70 ± 2% and 65 ± 2% independent from FiO_2.

After completion of hypoxic measurements, nitrogen flow was stopped and pure oxygen was used. After 30 min inspiratory oxygen concentration was 90% or higher and no horse showed signs of hypoxemia (SaO_2 > 95%). Gastrointestinal oxygenation recovered back to baseline values.

Part B: Hypovolemia

Surgical preparation of the carotid artery was performed and an 8G catheter was placed into the artery. The catheter was connected to a roller pump (IP 65, Ismatec, Germany) to ensure controlled and continuous exsanguination and Ringer-Lactate-Infusion was stopped.

Total blood volume of the horses was estimated being about 7.6% of the total body weight (bwt) or 76 mL/kg bwt [43]. After calculation total blood volume of each horse pumping rate was set to get an exsanguination rate of 50% total blood volume loss per hour (38 mL/kg bwt/h).

The HR, MAP, PAP and CI as well as the intestinal blood flow were measured every 15 min starting at baseline blood volume and at 88%, 75%, 63%, 50% and less than 45% of that value. Central and peripheral perfusion parameters measurements were continued until horses had no detectable pulse or cardiac output.

Statistical analysis

Statistical significance was attributed when $p < 0.05$. Analyses were carried out with the statistical software SAS, version 9.1.3 (SAS Institute, Cary, NY, USA) and GraphPad Prism 5 (GraphPad Software, Inc., USA). For the analysis of the linear model, the procedure MIXED was used. The parameters sO_2 and flow were sampled with 2 Hz. Measurements were performed over at least 25 to 30 s resulting in 50 to 60 values for each parameter and time point. The mean of these single measurements was calculated and used for this set time point. Normal distribution of model residuals of dependent variables was confirmed by Shapiro-Wilks-Test. Data is presented as mean ± standard deviation. A two way analysis of variance and Tukey's post hoc test were used for comparing the measured parameters by period of time (repeated measurements). The non-linear curve fitting was used to construct the curve that has the best fit to the data points in Figs. 1, 2, 4 and 5.

Abbreviations

BTD: Bolus thermodilution; CaO_2: Arterial oxygen content; CI: Cardiac index; CO: Cardiac output; $C\bar{v}O_2$: Mixed venous oxygen content; CVP: Central venous pressure; $\dot{D}O_2$: Oxygen delivery; E_TIso: End tidal isoflurane concentration; FiO_2: Inspiratory oxygen fraction; HR : Heart rate; IPPV: Intermittent positive pressure ventilation; MAP: Mean arterial blood pressure; O_2ER: Oxygen extraction ratio; $PaCO_2$: Arterial partial carbon dioxide pressure; PaO_2: Arterial partial oxygen pressure; PAP: Pulmonary artery pressure; $P\bar{v}O_2$: Mixed venous partial oxygen pressure; SaO_2: Arterial oxygen saturation; sO_2: Tissue oxygenation; $S\bar{v}O_2$: Mixed venous oxygen saturation; VO_2: Oxygen consumption

Acknowledgements

Not applicable.

Funding

No sources of funding for the research reported.

Authors' contributions

KH: Made substantial contributions to conception and design, and acquisition, analysis and interpretation of data and has been involved in drafting the manuscript; LWV: Made substantial contributions to acquisition of data and interpretation of data and has been involved in revising the manuscript critically for important intellectual content; FG: Made substantial contributions to acquisition of data and has been involved in revising the manuscript critically for important intellectual content; CHI: Made substantial contributions to acquisition of data and interpretation of data and has been involved in revising the manuscript critically for important intellectual content; SBRK: Made substantial contributions to design, interpretation of data and has been involved in drafting the manuscript. All authors read and approved the final manuscript.

Consent for publication

Not applicable as the manuscript does not contain data from any individual person.

Competing interests

The authors declare that they have no competing interests.

References

1. Johnston GM, Steffey E. Confidential enquiry into perioperative equine fatalities (CEPEF). Vet Surg. 1995;24(6):518–9.
2. Bidwell LA, Bramlage LR, Rood WA. Equine perioperative fatalities associated with general anesthesia at a private practice–a retrospective case series. Vet Anaesth Analg. 2007;34(1):23–30.
3. Hall LW, Gillespie JR, Tyler WS. Alveolar-arterial oxygen tension differences in anaesthetized horses. Br J Anaesth. 1968;40(8):560–8.
4. Hubbell JA, Muir WW. Oxygenation, oxygen delivery and anesthesia in the horse. Equine Vet J. 2015;47(1):25–35.
5. Steffey EP, Dunlop CI, Farver TB, Woliner MJ, Schultz LJ. Cardiovascular and respiratory measurements in awake and isoflurane-anesthetized horses. Am J Vet Res. 1987;48(1):7–12.
6. Hopster K, Hopster-Iversen C, Geburek F, Rohn K, Kästner SB. Temporal and concentration effects of isoflurane anesthesia on intestinal tissue oxygenation and perfusion in horses. Vet J. 2015;205(1):62–8.
7. Schlichtig R, Kramer DJ, Pinsky MR. Flow redistribution during progressive hemorrhage is a determinant of critical O2 delivery. J Appl Physiol 1985. 1991;70(1):169–78.
8. Buell MG, Harding RK. Effects of peptide YY on intestinal blood flow distribution and motility in the dog. Regul Pept. 1989;24(2):195–208.
9. Fink MP, Kaups KL, Wang HL, Rothschild HR. Maintenance of superior mesenteric arterial perfusion prevents increased intestinal mucosal permeability in endotoxic pigs. Surgery. 1991;110(2):154–61.
10. Hopster K, Kästner SB, Rohn K, Ohnesorge B. Intermittent positive pressure ventilation with constant positive end-expiratory pressure and alveolar recruitment manoeuvre during inhalation anesthesia in horses undergoing surgery for colic, and its influence on the early recovery period. Vet Anaesth Analg. 2011;38(3):169–77.
11. Cain SM. Peripheral oxygen uptake and delivery in health and disease. Clin Chest Med. 1983;4(2):139–48.
12. Gutierrez G. The relationship of tissue oxygenation to cellular bioenergetics. Adv Exp Med Biol. 1988;227:183–205.
13. Gutierrez G, Pohil RJ, Strong R. Effect of flow on O2 consumption during progressive hypoxemia. J Appl Physiol. 1988;65(2):601–7.
14. Grum CM, Fiddian-Green RG, Pittenger GL, Grant BJ, Rothman ED, Dantzker DR. Adequacy of tissue oxygenation in intact dog intestine. J Appl Physiol Respir Environ Exerc Physiol. 1984;56(4):1065–9.
15. Adams RP, Dieleman LA, Cain SM. A critical value for O2 transport in the rat. J Appl Physiol Respir Environ Exerc Physiol. 1982;53(3):660–4.
16. Stainsby WN, Otis AB. Blood flow, blood oxygen tension, oxygen uptake, and oxygen transport in skeletal muscle. Am J Phys. 1964;206:858–66.
17. Grum CM. Tissue oxygenation in low flow states and during hypoxemia. Crit Care Med. 1993;21(2):S44–9.
18. Edelstone DI, Holzman IR. Fetal intestinal oxygen consumption at various levels of oxygenation. Am J Phys. 1982;242(1):50–4.
19. Aliabadi-Wahle S, Choe EU, Flint LM, Ferrara JJ. Post-treatment dopexamine infusions partially reverse reductions in cranial mesenteric blood flow and mucosal oxygenation induced by hypoxia in newborn piglets. Am Surg. 1999;65(6):548–54.
20. Shirai M, Tsuchimochi H, Nagai H, Gray E, Pearson JT, Sonobe T, Yoshimoto M, Inagaki T, Fujii Y, Umetani K, Kuwahira I, Schwenke DO. Pulmonary vascular tone is dependent on the central modulation of sympathetic nerve activity following chronic intermittent hypoxia. Basic Res Cardiol. 2014; 109(5):432.
21. Leuenberger U, Gleeson K, Wroblewski K, Prophet S, Zelis R, Zwillich C, Sinoway L. Norepinephrine clearance is increased during acute hypoxemia in humans. Am J Phys. 1991;261(5):1659–64.
22. Louis WJ, Jarrott B, Conway EL. Sites of actions of alpha 2 agonists in the brain and periphery. Am J Cardiol. 1988;61(7):15–7.
23. Rosa AO, Movafagh S, Cleemann L, Morad M. Hypoxic regulation of cardiac Ca2+ channel: possible role of haem oxygenase. J Physiol. 2012;590(17): 4223–37.
24. Yumoto Y, Satoh S, Fujita Y, Koga T, Kinukawa N, Nakano H. Noninvasive measurement of isovolumetric contraction time during hypoxemia and acidemia: fetal lamb validation as an index of cardiac contractility. Early Hum Dev. 2005;81(7):635–42.
25. Abreu GF, Coelho AR, Aguiar JL, Moura Filho SA. Cardiocirculatory changes in hemorrhagic shock induced in pigs submitted to three distinct therapeutic methods. Acta Cir Bras. 2010;25(1):126–30.
26. Hardaway RM 3rd. Monitoring of the patient in a state of shock. Surg Gynecol Obstet. 1979;148(3):339–45.
27. Ledingham IM, Ramsay G. Hypovolaemic shock. Br J Anaesth. 1986;58(2): 169–89.
28. Wilson DV, Rondenay Y, Shance PU. The cardiopulmonary effects of severe blood loss in anesthetized horses. Vet Anaesth Analg. 2003;30:81–7.
29. Letson HL, Dobson GP. Unexpected 100% survival following 60% blood loss using small-volume 7.5% NaCl with adenocaine and mg(2+) in the rat model of extreme hemorrhagic shock. Shock. 2011;36(6):586–94.
30. Peterson KL, Hardy BT, Hall K. Assessment of shock index in healthy dogs and dogs in hemorrhagic shock. J Vet Emerg Crit Care (San Antonio). 2013; 23(5):545–50.
31. Pottecher J, Chemla D, Xavier L, Liu N, Chazot T, Marescaux J, Fischler M, Diemunsch P, Duranteau J. The pulse pressure/heart rate ratio as a marker of stroke volume changes during hemorrhagic shock and resuscitation in anesthetized swine. J Trauma Acute Care Surg. 2013;74(6):1438–45.
32. Barriot P, Riou B. Hemorrhagic shock with paradoxical bradycardia. Intensive Care Med. 1987;13(3):203–7.
33. Demetriades D, Chan LS, Bhasin P, Berne TV, Ramicone E, Huicochea F, Velmahos G, Cornwell EE, Belzberg H, Murray J, Asensio JA. Relative bradycardia in patients with traumatic hypotension. J Trauma. 1998;45(3): 534–9.
34. Nielsen PA, Secher NJ. Blood flow in adipose tissue and skeletal muscle during hemorrhagic shock in heparinized dogs. Life Sci I. 1970;9(2):75–82.
35. Lundeen G, Manohar M, Parks C. Systemic distribution of blood flow in swine while awake and during 1.0 and 1.5 MAC isoflurane anesthesia with or without 50% nitrous oxide. Anesth Analg. 1983;62(5):499–512.
36. Mellstrom A, Månsson P, Jonsson K, Hartmann M. Measurements of subcutaneous tissue PO2 reflect oxygen metabolism of the small intestinal mucosa during hemorrhage and resuscitation. An experimental study in pigs. Eur Surg Res. 2009;42(2):122–9.
37. Chou CC. Intestinal blood flow regulation. In: Dulbecco R, editor. Encyclopedia of human biology, vol. 4. San Diego: Academic Press; 1992. p. 547–56.
38. Borgos J. Principles of instrumentation: calibration and technical issues. In: Belcaro G, Hoffman U, Bollinger A, Nicolaides A, editors. Laser Doppler. London: Med-Orion; 1994. p. 3–16.
39. Hopster K, Müller C, Hopster-Iversen C, Stahl J, Rohn K, Kästner S. Effects of dexmedetomidine and xylazine on cardiovascular function during total intravenous anaesthesia with midazolam and ketamine and recovery quality and duration in horses. Vet Anaesth Analg. 2014;41:25–35.
40. Kersten JR, Schmeling TJ, Pagel PS, Gross GJ, Warltier DC. Isoflurane mimics ischemic preconditioning via activation of K(ATP) channels: reduction of myocardial infarct size with an acute memory phase. Anesthesiology. 1997;87:361–70.
41. London M. Beta blockers and alpha2 agonists for cardioprotection. Best Pract Res Clin Anaesthesiol. 2008;22:95–110.
42. Reichert C, Kästner SB, Hopster K, Rohn K, Rötting AK. Use of micro-lightguide spectrophotometry for evaluation of microcirculation in the small and large intestines of horses without gastrointestinal disease. Am J Vet Res. 2014;75:990–6.
43. Persson SGB. On blood volume and working capacities in horses. Acta Vet Scand. 1967;19:1–189.

Evaluation of six serological ELISA kits available in Italy as screening tests for equine infectious anaemia surveillance

Roberto Nardini[1], Gian Luca Autorino[1], Charles J. Issel[2], R. Frank Cook[2], Ida Ricci[1], Raffaele Frontoso[1], Francesca Rosone[1] and Maria Teresa Scicluna[1*]

Abstract

Background: ELISAs are known to have a higher diagnostic sensitivity than the agar gel immunodiffusion (AGID) when employed for serological diagnosis of equine infectious anaemia (EIA). For this purpose, an "in-house" and five commercial ELISAs available in Italy were assessed by the National Reference Centre for EIA for their analytic specificity (Sp); precocity, defined as capability of detecting first antibodies produced during a new infection; precision based on repeatability and reproducibility, estimated from the coefficient of variation (CV); accuracy, estimated from multiple K and relative Sp and sensitivity (Se). Two serum panels, positive for non-equine retroviruses and the most frequent equine viruses, were employed to measure analytic Sp. ELISA precocity was also compared to that of one "in-house" and three commercial AGID kits, employing a panel of sera, collected weekly from horses infected with modified EIA viruses. Precision and accuracy were defined using results of a panel containing positive and negative sera examined in an inter-laboratory trial with the participation of the ten Official Laboratories. Furthermore, a questionnaire was used to assess the appropriateness of each kit for routine use.

Results: Analytic Sp was 100%, while the 75th percentile of CVs for positive sera varied from 0.4% to 12.73% for repeatability and from 1.6% to 44.87% for reproducibility. Although CV of the negative serum was constantly high, its outcome was unaltered. Relative Se ranged from 98.2% to 100%, relative Sp was constantly 100% and multiple K ranged from 0.95 to 1. Precocity differed among the assays: three kits detected 4.8% and 42.9% positive samples on 21 days post infection (dpi), all assays detected positive samples on 28 dpi, between 47.6% and 95.2%. Precocity of ELISAs was superior to that of the AGIDs except for two assays. In view of the feedback obtained from the questionnaires, all kits were considered appropriate for routine use.

Conclusion: All ELISAs having high Se and precocity are preferable as a screening test in EIA surveillance programmes to the AGID tests examined. These two tests can be incorporated in a serial diagnostic pathway to improve the efficacy of a surveillance plan.

Keywords: Equine infectious anaemia, ELISA, AGID, Comparison, Commercial assays, In-house assays, Surveillance

Background

EIA is a blood-borne disease of equids caused by EIA virus (EIAV) of the Retroviridae family, subfamily Orthoretrovirinae, genus Lentivirus. EIA has a nearly worldwide distribution and causes sanitary and economic repercussions on the horse industry. In view of this, it is among the eleven equine diseases listed by the World Organisation for Animal Health (OIE). In addition, in several countries it is included in national and international Regulations defining the sanitary conditions for horse trade and movement and is also subjected to regional or national control programmes.

EIAV detection is generally problematical [1, 2], hence diagnosis of suspect cases and screening during surveillance programmes are based on antibody detection [3]. At present, for surveillance purposes, the OIE

* Correspondence: teresa.scicluna@izslt.it
[1]Istituto Zooprofilattico Sperimentale del Lazio e della Toscana "M. Aleandri", Via Appia Nuova 1411, 00178 Rome, Italy
Full list of author information is available at the end of the article

considers ELISA as a secondary method to the AGID, reporting that various factors limit its use. Nevertheless, it is also indicated as suitable for the declaration of population freedom from disease and for the evaluation of the efficiency of eradication programmes. The OIE also recommends that samples positive in ELISA are to be confirmed using either the AGID or the immunoblot (IB) [4]. These three methods have been proposed in a three-tier system that increases the diagnostic efficacy of EIA [5].

Since 2007, a surveillance programme for the identification and removal of EIA positive animals is on-going in Italy. In its initial phases, the AGID was employed both as screening and as confirmatory method respectively by the network of the ten Official Laboratories and the National Reference Centre (NRC) for EIA. In recent years, scientific reports [6–8], including those from Canada [9] and the USA [5], have demonstrated that ELISA-based tests are potentially more sensitive than AGID. The NRC adopted a similar approach to that described in these studies to evaluate, on the basis of their key diagnostic characteristics, the possibility of employing ELISA kits available in Italy for the serological screening of equid serum samples examined within the National surveillance programme. The results obtained, including a comparison with four different AGID kits, are presented and discussed especially in terms of the implications of the use of the ELISAs on the efficacy of the EIA surveillance.

Methods

A summary of the technical characteristics of the ELISAs employed in the present study are presented in Table 1. One ELISA is an "in-house" assay while the remaining are commercially produced. Following invitation to participate to the present evaluation, each producer kindly provided a kit of the batch that was at that time available on the market. ELISA #1 [10] and #2 [Scicluna, personal communication, 2016] were the kits that at the time of the study were already validated according to the OIE guidelines [11]. All the immunoassays were performed according to the manufacturer's instructions.

The AGID assays included in the comparison analysis were performed according to the OIE procedure [4] and consisted in one in-house and three commercially available AGIDs. Two AGIDs employed a recombinant EIAV p26 antigen, the third reported the use of a highly purified recombinant viral protein without providing further information and the remaining kit did not include details relative to the source of the antigen employed.

The composition and characteristics of the four panels of sera employed in the evaluation of the ELISAs are described in Table 2 and these will be referred throughout by an identification number accompanied by a brief description.

The parameters by which the ELISAs were assessed are: analytic Sp that was defined employing serum samples containing antibodies to non-equine retroviruses (Panel 1), along with a set of sera, positive for the most common equine viral diseases (Panel 2) [12]. Each serum sample included within these panels was examined in 30 replicates.

Precocity of both ELISA and AGID tests, defined as the capability to detect the first amounts of antibodies produced during the onset of an infection, was assessed using equine serum samples collected at weekly intervals (day 0 to 28 dpi), from 3 groups of eight horses infected with one of the following EIAV attenuated strains [10]: $EIAV_{D9}$, $EIAV_{Trivalent}$ and $EIAV_{Consensus}$. Three of the 24 horses, two infected with $EIAV_{Consensus}$ and one with $EIAV_{D9}$, seroconverted after 28 dpi (Issel CJ, personal

Table 1 Principal characteristics of the ELISAs employed in the study

	ELISA #1	ELISA #2	ELISA #3	ELISA #4	ELISA #5	ELISA #6
Type	Competitive	Indirect	Competitive	Competitive	Indirect	Indirect
Antigen	Recombinant p26	Recombinant *gag* and *env* antigens	Purified p26	Recombinant p26	Recombinant antigen-not specified	Recombinant p26
Run time (′)	160	135	45	90	20	35
Interpretation Criterion/Formula	$PI = 100 - (\overline{OD_S}/\overline{OD_{K-}} * 100)$	$S/P = \frac{(\overline{OD_S} - \overline{OD_{K-}})}{(\overline{OD_{K+}} - \overline{OD_{K-}})} * 100$	Compared to OD_{K+}	$S/P = \frac{(\overline{OD_S} - \overline{OD_{K-}})}{(\overline{OD_{K+}} - \overline{OD_{K-}})} * 100$	Compared to OD_{K+}	Compared to OD_{K+}
	PI <30: Neg	$S/P \leq 40$: Neg	$OD_S > OD_{K+}$: Neg	$S/P \leq 50$: Neg	$OD_S < OD_{K+}$: Neg	$OD_S < OD_{K+}$: Neg
Outcome definition	$30 \leq PI \leq 50$: Equivocal	$40 < S/P < 50$: Equivocal	$OD_S \leq OD_{K+}$: Pos	$50 < S/P < 60$: Equivocal	$OD_S \geq OD_{K+}$: Pos	$OD_S \geq OD_{K+}$: Pos
	PI >50: Pos	$S/P \geq 50$: Pos		$S/P \geq 60$: Pos		

Gag and *env:* genes of EIAV respectively coding for nucleocapsid and envelope antigens, PI: percentage inhibition, S/P: Corrected Sample /Positive Ratio; OD_S: Optical Density of Sample; OD_{K-}: Optical Density of Negative Control; OD_{K+}: Optical Density of Positive Control; Neg: Negative; Pos: Positive

Table 2 Characteristics of the panels of sera employed in the study

Panel #	Characteristics
1: Sera positive for non-equine retroviruses	20 sera for feline immunodeficiency virus
	20 for feline leukemia virus
	20 for enzootic bovine leukosis virus
	20 for maedi visna virus
2: Sera positive for other equine viruses	20 sera positive for equine influenza
	20 sera positive for equine viral arteritis
	20 positive for equine herpes virus −1
	20 sera positive for equine herpes virus −4
3: Sera of 21 horses experimentally infected[b,c]	84 sera sampled at 0, 14, 21, 28 days post infection (dpi)
4: Interlaboratory test panel[a]	30 sera: 22 positive and 8 negative

[a]Available at the EIA National Reference Centre and at the National Reference Centre for Equine Diseases as secondary reference sera
[b]Provided by Gluck Equine Research Center University of Kentucky Lexington, Kentucky
[c]Infected with EIA attenuated virus $EIAV^{D9}$ $EIAV^{Trivalent}$, $EIAV^{Consensus}$ (further information is provided in the text)

communication, 2014), therefore for this study only the samples of the 21 positive horses were included in Panel 3.

For the statistical analysis, the Chi Square test was used to compare the proportions of reactive samples (positive and equivocal) detected by each method and in case of a statistical significant difference, the Marascuilo procedure was employed to investigate for which pair of assays this occurred. Samples with an equivocal result to the screening test were reclassified as positive since these, as for the positively reacting samples, are also forwarded to the NRC for confirmation.

XLStat (Addinsoft®, 2011) was the software utilized for the statistical analysis and a test obtaining a p value ≤0.05 was considered significant.

The results obtained for panel 4, used in the interlaboratory trial (IT) to which the ten Official Laboratories participated [13], were analysed to assess precision and accuracy. The panel was examined blindly and consisted of one negative reference serum, included as eight replicates, and 11 positive samples each provided as two replicates. The positive samples were prepared from one positive reference serum diluted with a negative one to obtain three different reactivity levels that were arbitrarily defined as follows by the NRC, on the basis of the percentage inhibition (PI) obtained in ELISA #1: strong positive (SP) with a PI ≥95% (n = 2), medium positive (MP) with a PI between 75% and 94% (n = 3) and weak positive (WP) with a PI between 51% and 74% (n = 6). The positive sera were also confirmed, except for one WP, in the in-house AGID described above. Both in-house tests, in use at the NRC, are accredited according to ISO/IEC 17025 [14].

Precision was assessed using repeatability and reproducibility, which were calculated as follows. Repeatability was measured using the CV of the results of the two replicates of each positive serum and of the eight replicates of the negative obtained in each ELISA run by every IT participant. The CVs were calculated using the percentage inhibition (PI) or corrected sample/positive ratio (S/P) values (see formulae in Table 1). For those assays without an interpretation formula, the results were normalized according to their set-up, using either the PI (ELISA #3) or the S/P (ELISA #5 and ELISA #6).

Reproducibility of the assays was evaluated using the CVs estimated from the gathered results of the IT.

The accuracy of the ELISA kits was defined from the values obtained for multiple K and relative Sp and Se. The latter were calculated as the percentage of samples identified over the total number of expected results, respectively for the negative and positive sera, independently from the different reactivity level. For the reason mentioned previously, sera with equivocal results were also here reclassified as positive.

Concordance with the expected results was estimated, for each laboratory, using K coefficient [15] for those assays (ELISA #3, #5 and #6) with two possible outcomes (positive and negative) and with a modified K coefficient, i.e. weighted K [16] for those ELISAs (#1, #2 and #4) with three expected outcomes: positive, equivocal and negative, arbitrarily assigning a weight of 0.33 to a partial concordance. The results of all the laboratories were then aggregated to calculate the multiple K value [17] of each assay, which was interpreted as reported in literature [18].

Furthermore, the laboratory personnel participating in the IT also replied to a questionnaire to investigate the suitability of the ELISA kits for routine use. This survey contained 17 questions covering 15 criteria, with preset answers represented by a scale of 1 (lowest rating) to 5 (highest rating). The questions focused on ease of interpretation of procedures, reagents characteristics, ease and time of execution, straightforwardness of result formula and result interpretation. Overall rating for each question was assigned using the mode obtained from all the scores reported by the laboratories and summed for each kit. In addition, the questionnaire also included two open questions requesting advice and recommendations for improvements of each kit.

Results

Analytical Sp was 100% for all ELISAs as no cross-reactivity was detected for sera of Panel 1 (positive for non-equine retroviruses) and Panel 2 (positive for common equine diseases). Data on the analytical Se is presented in Fig. 1 and was assessed by the precocity of antibody detection in the horse sera (Panel 3) collected at weekly intervals following infection with modified live viruses. The results of this parameter are expressed as the percentage of the number of samples detected positive/equivocal out of the total samples expected as positive. Positive samples were detected from 21 dpi, in ELISA #1 and ELISA#4 identifying each a different positive sample (4.8%) and ELISA #2, identifying 9 positive samples (42.9%), including the two detected by ELISAs #1 and #4; on 28 dpi all assays detected a percentage of positive/equivocal samples, ranging from 47.6% (ELISA #6) to 100% (ELISA #2).

Positive samples were also detected at 28 dpi by the different AGID assays with percentages ranging between 28.6% (AGID #4) and 61.9% (AGID #1). In comparing the precocity of the two different methods, for ELISA #6 this was equal (47.6%) to those of AGIDs #2 and #3 and for ELISA #4 it was equal (61.9%) to that of AGID #1 (Fig.1).

No statistical differences were observed among the AGID kits in terms of percentage of positive/equivocal samples detected. For the ELISAs, differences were detected at 21 dpi with a p value of <0.0001 for the Chi Square test and with the Marascuilo procedure showing a statistical difference between the proportions of positives detected by ELISA #2 with those of ELISAs #3, #5 and #6. Even on 28 dpi, the p value was statistically significant with a value of 0.018 and differences were detected between the proportions of ELISA #2 and ELISAs #4 and #6.

The distribution of the CV values for repeatability and reproducibility for each of the assays and for all laboratories are shown in Fig. 2. The 75th percentile of the CVs of the positive sera did not exceed 12.73% for repeatability (Fig. 2a) and 44.87% for reproducibility (Fig. 2b). Conversely, for the negative serum, CVs at the 75th percentile were high with a maximum of 137.54% for repeatability (Fig. 2c) and 534.31% (Fig. 2d) for reproducibility, without ever modifying the expected outcome.

The results of the accuracy and total scores obtained from the questionnaires are reported in Table 3. Relative Sp was 100% for all the ELISAs while relative Se ranged from 96.8% (ELISA #5) to 100% (ELISA #6), with all the remaining kits having a relative Se of >98%. Three laboratories misclassified sixteen sera represented by 1 SP, 2 MP and 13 WP (7 of which corresponded to that negative in the AGID).

Values of Multiple K ranged from 0.95 (ELISA #3) to 1 (ELISA #6), resulting in an "almost perfect" concordance according to the adopted classification. Scores for kit quality perception were very high for all the ELISAs and varied from 56 (ELISA #1) to 63 (ELISA #4) on a maximum score of 65.

Comments provided by laboratory participants were reporting as critical the small sample volume used in ELISA #2, the absence of hazard and safety statements for kit reagents in ELISAs #3, #4 and #5, the quality of the reagent containers used in ELISAs #1 and #2, as they were prone to leaking, and the orientation of the well-

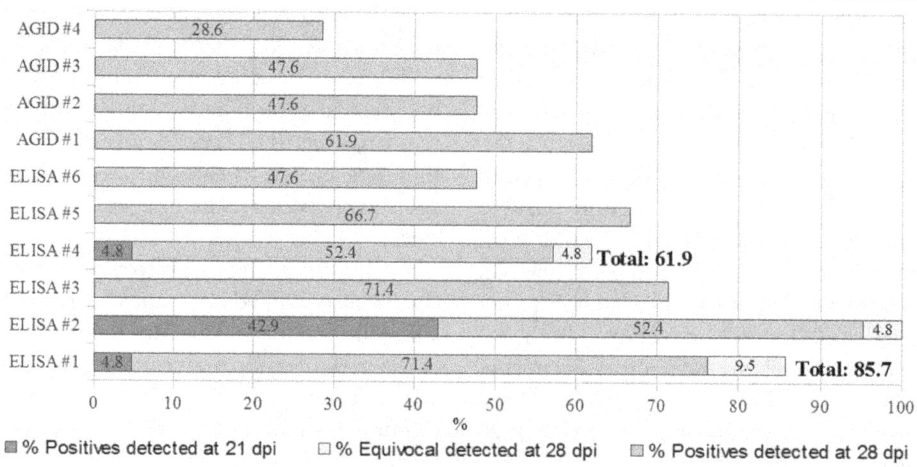

Fig. 1 Percentage of positive and equivocal samples detected by each ELISA and AGID assay for sera sampled at 21, 28 dpi with attenuated EIAV strains ($EIAV_{D9}$, $EIAV_{Trivalent}$ and $EIAV_{Consensus}$)

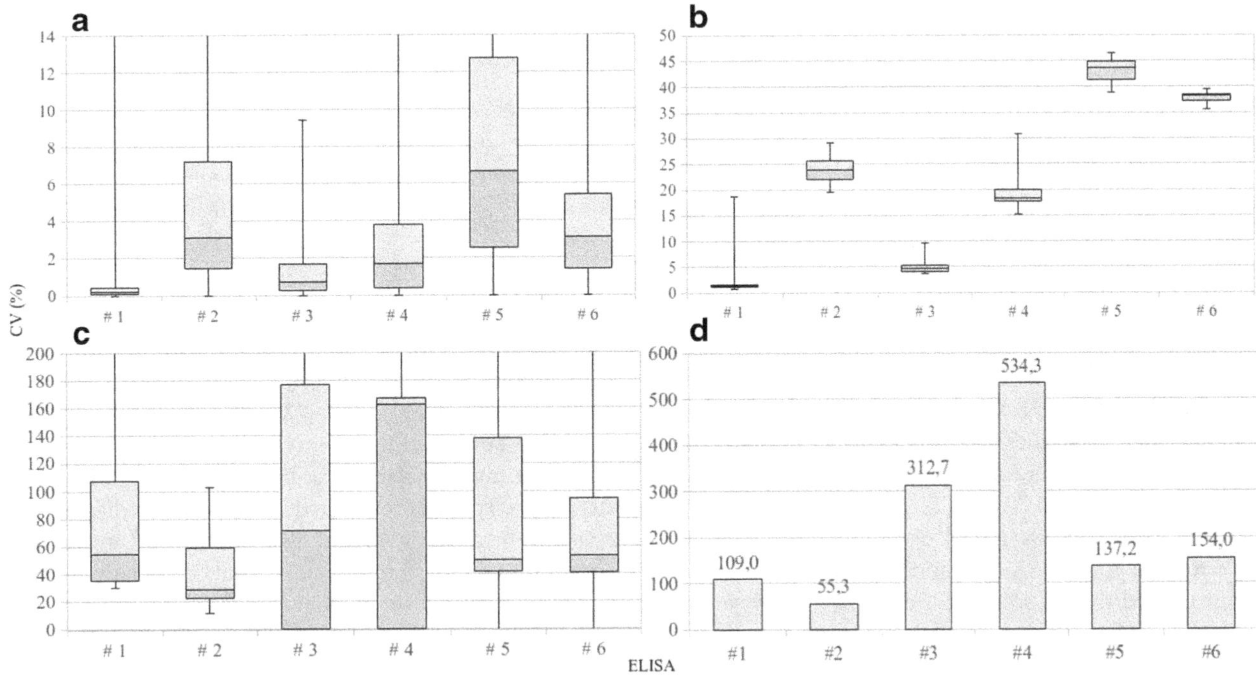

Fig. 2 Box plot graphs of CVs of repeatability and reproducibility, respectively for positive (**a**, **b**) and negative (**c**, **d**) sera for each assay. Lower box represents difference between first quartile and median and upper box difference, between third quartile and median. Y bars represent minimum and maximum values (due to the graphical representation some values are out of scale). Graph D represents the CVs of the negative serum considering all laboratories

strips of ELISA #3. In contrast to all other assay formats, the individual strips of this kit were made up of twelve wells instead of the more often available format of eight wells and therefore considered impractical when used in preset instruments such as automated washers.

Discussion

Results of the present study demonstrated that, except for precocity, the ELISA kits currently available in Italy for serological diagnosis of EIA offered similar performance levels. All exhibited high analytical Sp (100%) and accuracy, with a relative Se between 98.2% and 100%, a relative Sp of 100% and multiple K values ranging from 0.95 to 1 (see Table 3). Sera misclassification mostly occurred for the WP (81.3%), with 43.8% of these corresponding to the WP-AGID negative serum. A misclassified sample could be due either to the test sensitivity or to the laboratory's technical capability. In particular, the WP-AGID negative sample was detected as negative by 3 laboratories in one or more of the following ELISAs: #1, #2, #3, and #5. For the latter two ELISAs, misclassification could be related to their low precocity. Differently for the other two kits, which demonstrated a high precocity, the use of relatively small serum volumes could influence their sensitivity, especially when using uncalibrated instrumentation.

All assays were sufficiently repeatable and reproducible as CV values obtained for the positive sera are similar to those described in the literature [19–21]. The higher magnitude of the CVs observed for the negative serum is due to the low values that this assumes when using the PI and S/P formulae. In this case, small numerical differences have a greater weight when calculating the CV [9].

Screening tests in a surveillance programme should detect all levels of true positivity, especially those at borderline level, as a false negative serum would immediately be lost and consequently diminish the efficacy of the control programme.

Sensitivity, which in this study was also assessed through precocity, is essential for avoiding the persistence of EIA, not only through the early detection of new cases that are still mounting their antibody response but also by the identification of animals with a low serological response [8] that may occur during the chronic or inapparent phases of AIE and which was evaluated by the inclusion of WP sera in the IT panel. The best performing kit for precocity was ELISA #2, which could be ascribed to the use of *env* gene-derived recombinant antigen in combination with the p26, employed by all the other assays [22]. Previous studies report that antibodies against the glycoproteins (transmembrane -gp45 and surface unit -gp90) expressed by the *env*-gene are produced earlier than those against the p26 [23–26].

Table 3 Values of accuracy, multiple K, and total scores obtained from the questionnaire

ELISA	Re_{Se} (%)	Re_{Sp} (%)	Multiple K	Score (maximum score 65)
#1	99.5	100	0.99	56
#2	99.1	100	0.98	57
#3	98.2	100	0.95	59
#4	99.1	100	0.98	63
#5	96.8	100	0.96	58
#6	100	100	1	60

Re_{Se}: relative sensitivity; Re_{Sp}: relative specificity

Lacking complete information on the immunological reagents employed in the ELISAs, this hypothesis requires further investigation, considering also that a previous study describes that an assay containing just the gp45 had a lower performance than those using the p26 [9].

Further investigations are also required to verify the data obtained for ELISAs #4 and #6, as their precocity did not exceed that of some of the AGIDs. However, the performance of these assays relative to the other parameters was perceived as good with relative Sp and Se values equal to 100% for the first and respectively 99.1% and 100% for the second, while those of multiple K were 1 for ELISA #4 and 0.98 for ELISA #6. The evaluation of ELISA kits described here, together with results reported by other authors [5–9], confirm that most of these test-formats have higher or equal levels of overall sensitivity than the AGID assay, even if this method is still considered as the "Gold Standard" by many governmental regulatory authorities and is also indicated as an appropriate screening test by the OIE [4]. In addition to the present data, a limit of detection (LOD) for the AGID of at least 0.9 Log_{10} lower than that of the ELISA was already reported by the same authors [10]. Laboratories employing this method as screening test are strongly advised to replace it with a more sensitive ELISA to increase the benefits of their control programmes.

The approach presented here for the evaluation of the performance of the ELISA kits provides the technical basis for establishing the criteria of choice of a diagnostic assay within the context in which it is be employed. However, further to the evaluation of the diagnostic parameters that rely on laboratory data, the ease of use of a kit in the routine is also critical in determining its choice. For this, questionnaires are valid tools [27, 28] for considering aspects that are not directly dependant on the assay's diagnostic performance, such as the availability and completeness of the validation data, clarity of the manufacturer's instructions and practicability of execution.

The implications of the questionnaire go even beyond the purpose of this study, as the recommendations provided through these means are also useful to the manufactures. Worthy of note are the replies provided in the open questions section, relative to the 5 μl sample volume analysed by ELISA #2, which was judged as too small and perceived as a source of variability, even if this assay was highly performing in all aspects and especially for precocity. Further to what previously discussed, a cost benefit analysis should also be included in the decisional process for the choice of a kit, especially in terms of time of execution in view of the high turnover required in surveillance programmes where a large number of samples are generally examined.

The validation of diagnostic kits, based on the criteria included in international guidelines, such as those indicated by the OIE [29], provides essential information for their comparison. Such an approach is adopted in some countries, as prior to the first release of the diagnostic kits on the market official laboratories either directly validate the kit or verify the technical data provided by the manufactures. Further to this, every released batch has to be approved by the appointed laboratory through the verification of the performance of some of the key diagnostic parameters or from the data presented by the producer.

Validation, according to the international guidelines for those ELISAs (#3 to #6) which at the time of the present study was unavailable, would have required a consistent amount of resources, especially in terms of time and costs. For this reason, only parameters considered as critical were evaluated for the assessment of the diagnostic performance of the assays, especially those that define the kits' sensitivity, fundamental characteristic for a screening test. The advantage of the simultaneous comparison of the ELISAs kits was that the sera panels used were the same for all of them, differently from what would have been the case in an independent evaluation, therefore increasing the objectivity of the data produced. In addition, it also gave the opportunity of using an assessment questionnaire that represents an innovative method of evaluation. Also, on completion of this study, a final report was provided to each manufacturer participating to this study, offering them the opportunity of an independent performance appraisal in relation to the other kits available on the market.

As the results of the present study are exclusively related to the batches that were provided at that time by the manufactures, the NRC established a set of verification criteria for monitoring batch-to-batch variability based on the results obtained in this study. The verification parameters consist in the comparison of the LOD of the ELISA to that of AGID, estimation of specificity and CV respectively assessed from a statistically representative number of certified negative and positive samples. The batches of the kits that are approved are then published on the NRC website so that the Official Laboratories may procure any one of them.

In view of the parameters evaluated, all the ELISAs had an equal analytic Sp of 100%, while the best performing kits were ELISA#2 for precocity, ELISAs #1 and #2, respectively for repeatability and reproducibility, which were a measure of precision, and ELISA #1 and ELISA #4 for accuracy.

Conclusions

The present study demonstrates that in general, the six ELISAs available in Italy have similar performance characteristics except for precocity. In view of the points discussed, the EIA Italian surveillance programme adopted this method as screening test, instead of the former AGID based-system, to guarantee a major efficacy of the on-going surveillance programme. The results presented corroborate those obtained in similar studies and provide evidence to national and international regulatory bodies, including the OIE, to reconsider the use of high performing ELISAs for the estimation of prevalence infection and also as screening method for surveillance purposes. The other advantages of the use of this test to the AGID, are its standardization, automation, high turnover of samples, cost per determination, and objective reading of sample outcomes [10].

Also, according to the different Sp and Se characterizing the kits, the authors support the parallel use of different ELISAs, already proposed in the "multitier system" [5], which would enhance the sensitivity of the diagnostic system and, as reported in a previous study conducted by the authors, would require that only 1 ‰ of the examined samples be subsequently submitted to a higher level of diagnosis in IB [5].

Further to the diagnostic quality of the ELISAs, the technical capability of the laboratory network conducting the serological surveillance of EIA employing different tests should also undergo verification. This aspect, together with the certification of kits for their use within a diagnostic system, is among the institutional duties of a NRC. In view of this, the official laboratories are periodically evaluated through the organization of ITs where the sensitivity limits of the diagnostic system that is subject to verification are set through the inclusion of weak positive and/or equivocal sera.

This double aspect, made up of high performing laboratories and methods, guarantees the efficiency of a surveillance system.

Abbreviations

AGID: Agar gel immunodiffusion; CV: Coefficient of variation; Dpi: Days post infection; EIA: Equine infectious anaemia; EIAV: Equine infectious anaemia virus; IB: Immunoblot; IT: Inter-laboratory trial; LOD: Limit of detection; MP: Medium positive; NRC: National Reference Centre; OIE: World Organisation for Animal Health; PI: Percentage inhibition; Re_{Se}: Relative sensitivity; Re_{Sp}: Relative specificity; S/P: Corrected sample/positive ratio; Se: Sensitivity; Sp: Specificity; SP: Strong positive; WP: Weak positive

Acknowledgements

The authors would like to acknowledge the manufacturers for supplying the assays employed in the study and laboratories of Istituto Zooprofilattico Sperimentale delle Venezie, Padua; Istituto Zooprofilattico Sperimentale Piemonte Liguria e Valle d'Aosta, Turin; Istituto Zooprofilattico Sperimentale della Puglia e della Basilicata, Foggia; Istituto Zooprofilattico Sperimentale Lombardia ed Emilia Romagna "Bruno Ubertini", Brescia; Istituto Zooprofilattico Sperimentale del Mezzogiorno, Naples; Istituto Zooprofilattico Sperimentale della Sicilia "A. Mirri", Palermo; Istituto Zooprofilattico Sperimentale Abruzzo e Molise "G. Caporale", Teramo; Istituto Zooprofilattico Sperimentale Umbria e Marche, Perugia; Istituto Zooprofilattico Sperimentale della Sardegna "G. Pregreffi", Sassari; which participated in the inter-laboratory trial.

Funding

ELISAs and AGIDs were supplied by manufacturers free of charge. This study was conducted within the research project "Evaluation of concordance of results between ELISA assays for EIA"- LT 07/08" funded by the Italian Ministry of Health.

Authors' contributions

RN, GLA and MTS were involved in the conception and design of the experiment, in the drafting and supervision of the manuscript elaboration of the manuscript and its critical revision for its intellectual content. IR, RF and FR coordinated the acquisition of the data. RN and MTS were responsible for the analysis of the data. CJI and RFC were involved in the design of the experiment and in the drafting and critical revision of the manuscript. All authors read and approved the final manuscript.

Competing interests

The Istituto Zooprofilattico Sperimentale del Lazio e della Toscana "M. Aleandri", Via Appia Nuova 1411, 00178 Rome, Italy, having as authors R. N., G. L. A., I. R., R. F., F. R., and M. T. S., receives royalties from the manufactures of ELISA #2 for having collaborated in its development.

Consent for publication

Not applicable.

Author details

[1]Istituto Zooprofilattico Sperimentale del Lazio e della Toscana "M. Aleandri", Via Appia Nuova 1411, 00178 Rome, Italy. [2]Department of Veterinary Science, Gluck Equine Research Center, University of Kentucky, Lexington, KY, USA.

References

1. Hines R, Maury W. DH82 cells: a macrophage cell line for the replication and study of equine infectious anemia virus. J Virol Methods. 2001;95:47–56.
2. Leroux C, Cadoré J-L, Montelaro R. Equine Infectious Anemia Virus (EIAV): what has HIV's country cousin got to tell us? Caroline. Vet Res. 2004;35:485–512.
3. Issel CJ, Cook SJ, Cook RF, Cordes TR. Optimal paradigms to detect reservoirs of equine infectious anemia virus (EIAV). J Equine Vet Sci. 1999;19:728–32.
4. World Organization For Animal Health: Manual of Diagnostic Tests and Vaccines for Terrestrial Animals 2015. www.oie.int/fileadmin/Home/eng/Health_standards/tahm/2.05.06_EIA.pdf. Accessed 12 Feb 2016.
5. Issel CJ, Scicluna MT, Cook SJ, Cook RF, Caprioli A, Ricci I, Rosone F, Craigo JK, Montelaro RC, Autorino GL. Challenges and proposed solutions for more accurate serological diagnosis of equine infectious anaemia. Vet Rec. 2013; 172:210.
6. Lew AM, Thomas LM, Huntington PJ. A comparison of ELISA, FAST-ELISA and gel diffusion tests for detecting antibody to equine infectious anaemia virus. Vet Microbiol. 1993;34:1–5.
7. Matsushita T, Hesterberg LK, Porter JP, Smith BJ, Newman LE. Comparison of diagnostic tests for the detection of equine infectious anemia antibody. J Vet Diagn Investig. 1989;1:50–2.
8. Scicluna MT, Issel CJ, Cook FR, Manna G, Cersini A, Rosone F, Frontoso R, Caprioli A, Antognetti V, Autorino GL. Is a diagnostic system based exclusively on agar gel immunodiffusion adequate for controlling the spread of equine infectious anaemia? Vet Microbiol. 2013;165:123–34.
9. Paré J, Simard C. Comparison of commercial enzyme-linked immunosorbent assays and agar gel immunodiffusion tests for the serodiagnosis of equine infectious anemia. Can J Vet Res. 2004;68:254–8.
10. Nardini R, Autorino GL, Ricci I, Frontoso R, Rosone F, Simula M, Scicluna MT. Validation according to OIE criteria of a serologic competitive enzyme-linked immunosorbent assay as screening method in surveillance programs for the detection of Equine infectious anemia virus antibodies. J Vet Diagnostic Invest. 2016;28:88–97.
11. World Organization for Animal Health (OIE). Manual of Diagnostic Tests and Vaccines for Terrestrial Animals, Chapter 1.1.5. Paris: OIE; 2010.
12. Slater J. Findings from the National Equine Health Survey, 2013. Vet Rec. 2014;175:271–2.
13. Langton SD, Chevennement R, Nagelkerke N, Lombard B. Analysing collaborative trials for qualitative microbiological methods: Accordance and concordance. Int J Food Microbiol. 2002;79:175–81.
14. ISO/IEC 17025 General requirements for the competence of testing and calibration laboratories. International Organization for Standardization, 2005.
15. Cohen J. A Coefficient of Agreement for Nominal Scales. Educ Psychol Meas. 1960;20:37–46.
16. Cohen J. Weighted kappa: nominal scale agreement with provision for scaled disagreement or partial credit. Psychol Bull. 1968;70:213–20.
17. Fleiss JL. Measuring nominal scale agreement among many raters. Psycological Bull. 1971;76:378–82.
18. Landis JR, Koch GG. The measurement of observer agreement for categorical data. Biometrics. 1977;33:159–74.
19. Chung C, Wilson C, Timoney P, Adams E, Adams DS, Chung JS, Evermann JF, Shuck K, Lee SS, McGuire TC. Validation of an improved competitive enzyme-linked immunosorbent assay to detect Equine arteritis virus antibody. J Vet Diagn Investig. 2013;25:727–35.
20. Colling A, Morrissy C, Barr J, Meehan G, Wright L, Goff W, Gleeson LJ, van der Heide B, Riddell S, Yu M, Eagles D, Lunt R, Khounsy S, Than Long N, Phong Vu P, Than Phuong N, Tung N, Linchongsubongkoch W, Hammond J, Johnson M, Johnson W, Unger H, Daniels P, Crowther JR. Development and validation of a 3ABC antibody ELISA in Australia for foot and mouth disease. Aust Vet J. 2014;92:192–9.
21. Paweska JT. Jansen van Vuren P, Swanepoel R: Validation of an indirect ELISA based on a recombinant nucleocapsid protein of Rift Valley fever virus for the detection of IgG antibody in humans. J Virol Methods. 2007;146:119–24.
22. Issel CJ, Cook RF, Mealey RH, Horohov DW: Equine infectious anemia in 2014: live with it or eradicate it? Vet Clin North Am Equine Pract 2014, 30: 561–577.
23. Ball JM, Henry NL, Montelaro RC, Newman MJ. A versatile synthetic peptide-based ELISA for identifying antibody epitopes. J Immunol Methods. 1994; 171:37–44.
24. Carpenter S, Alexandersen S, Long MJ, Perryman S, Chesebro B. Identification of a Hypervariable Region in the Long Terminal Repeat of Equine Infectious Anemia Virus. J Virol. 1991;65:1605–10.
25. Chong YH, Ball JM, Issel CJ, Montelaro RC, Rushlow KE. Analysis of equine humoral immune responses to the transmembrane envelope glycoprotein (gp45) of equine infectious anemia virus. J Virol. 1991;65:1013–8.
26. Hussain KA, Issel CJ, Schnorr KL, Rwambo PM, West M, Montelaro RC. Antigenic mapping of the envelope proteins of equine infectious anemia virus: identification of a neutralization domain and a conserved region on glycoprotein 90. Arch Virol. 1988;98(3-4):213–24.
27. Crowther JR, Unger H, Viljoen GJ. Aspects of kit validation for tests used for the diagnosis and surveillance of livestock diseases: producer and end-user responsibilities. Rev Sci Tech. 2006;25:913–35.
28. Johnson AM, Roberts H, Tenter AM. Evaluation of a recombinant antigen ELISA for the diagnosis of acute toxoplasmosis and comparison with traditional antigen ELISAs. J Med Microbiol. 1992;37:404–9.
29. World Organization For Animal Health: Manual of Diagnostic Tests and Vaccines for Terrestrial Animals 2015. www.oie.int/fileadmin/Home/eng/Health_standards/tahm/1.01.06_VALIDATION.pdf. Accessed 12 Feb 2016.

Lawsonia intracellularis in the feces of wild rodents and stray cats captured around equine farms

Jeong-Min Hwang[1], Myung-Ji Seo[2,3] and Jung-Yong Yeh[4,5*]

Abstract

Background: Proliferative enteropathy is a global enteric disease of particular importance in pigs. The causative bacterium, *Lawsonia intracellularis*, has a wide range of susceptible host species. Recently, *L. intracellularis* has been recognized as an etiologic agent of an emerging enteric disease in foals called equine proliferative enteropathy (EPE). The presence of *L. intracellularis* in nonruminant wildlife has raised questions regarding the role of these species in EPE transmission.

Results: This study investigated exposure to *L. intracellularis* in wild rodents and feral cats from eight farms with confirmed EPE. Serum (42) and fecal (40) samples from resident foals and fecal samples (131), intestinal mucosa tissues (14), and mesenteric lymph nodes (14) from wild and feral animals were collected for the evaluation of the farm status and the molecular detection of *L. intracellularis* following the diagnosis of EPE in index cases. Fresh feces from wild rodents and feral cats were collected from the ground while walking the premises or after trapping the animals using live traps. A total of 3 brown rats, 7 house mice, 1 striped field mouse, 2 grey red-backed voles, and 3 feral cats showed evidence of prior exposure to *L. intracellularis*.

Conclusions: Our data add to increasing evidence demonstrating the potential for *L. intracellularis* transmission and infection in wild rodents and feral cats and provide possible evidence of interspecies transmission. The exposure of wild rodents and feral cats provides potential evidence for the spillover of *L. intracellularis* to wildlife species and raises the question of spillback to horses. Additionally, these animals may represent an indicator of environmental exposure or may be actively involved in the transmission of *L. intracellularis* to foals by acting as potential reservoir/amplifier hosts. This study is the first to demonstrate the magnitude of *L. intracellularis* shedding in the feces of wild rodents and feral cats and to indicate the significant infection risk that wild rodents and feral cats pose to naïve horses in South Korea.

Keywords: *Lawsonia Intracellularis*, Infection, Prevalence, Wildlife, Exposure, Equine proliferative enteropathy

Background

Lawsonia intracellularis is the etiologic agent of porcine proliferative enteropathy (PPE). PPE is considered a disease of particular importance in the pig because it usually affects growing pigs and has a large impact on performance [1]. Proliferative enteropathy, which is also known to be due to enteric disease induced by *L. intracellularis* infection, was first described in 1931 in pigs [2]. Since that time, the microbe itself or its DNA has been identified in numerous warm-blooded species [3–7] and in chickens [8] but never in humans [9, 10]. *L. intracellularis* has also been recognized as an etiologic agent in an enteric disease in foals called equine proliferative enteropathy (EPE) [11, 12], and an increasing number of clinical cases have been reported in horses [11, 13].

At present, the transmission of *L. intracellularis* is generally thought to occur through the ingestion of feed or water contaminated with *L. intracellularis*-infected feces from free-living or domestic animals [4]. Regarding transmission within a herd or between herds, wild

* Correspondence: yehjy@inu.ac.kr
[4]Department of Life Sciences, College of Life Sciences and Bioengineering, Incheon National University, Academy-ro 119, Yeonsu-gu, Incheon 22012, Republic of Korea
[5]Previous address: Emerging & Exotic Diseases Research Laboratory, Foreign Animal Diseases Division, Animal, Plant, and Fisheries Quarantine and Inspection Agency, Anyang-ro 175, Manan-gu, Anyang-si, Gyeonggi-do 14089, Republic of Korea
Full list of author information is available at the end of the article

animals can contribute to endemic infections in livestock and to the introduction, reintroduction and maintenance of pathogens [14]. For endemic diseases such as EPE, the source of introduction to foals may not be known, and the extent of wildlife contribution to local spread is largely unexplored.

Previous studies have shown that a variety of wild and domestic animals, including house mice, brown rats, striped field mice, yellow-necked mice, and common voles in pig farms in the Czech Republic [6], wild rats in Australian pig farms [15], and dogs, jackrabbits, opossums, skunks and coyotes in horse farms located in California and Kentucky [16], can shed *L. intracellularis* on farms with diagnosed PPE and EPE cases. However, no previous assessment of evidence or magnitude demonstrate of *L. intracellularis* shedding in the feces of wild rodents and feral cats has been conducted in South Korea. Thus, from the perspective of a vector/reservoir for *L. intracellularis*, the goal of the present study was to expand recent epidemiological findings to wild and feral animals from farms with EPE in an attempt to determine their role in the spread of *L. intracellularis* in South Korea.

Methods

Farm selection

Criteria for farm selection in this study were followed according to the previous study performed in Unites States of America [17]. Farms were chosen based on voluntary involvement following the diagnosis of EPE in foals on the basis of age, clinical signs, hypoalbuminemia, a thickened small intestinal wall, and the detection of *L. intracellularis* by PCR or serology [11, 12]. Farmers were explained the study purposes and procedures and upon agreeing to participate, they provided a written consent prior to study procedures and sample collection from their animals or captured animals. Within 7–10 days of diagnosing EPE in index cases, each farm was visited to begin the collection of study samples. A total of 8 breeding farms in South Korea were enrolled over a 26-month period (Table 1). Blood was collected from 3 to 8 resident foals from each horse farm by direct venipuncture, and fecal samples were collected from every five foals and tested for *L. intracellularis* DNA by real-time PCR. Blood for the serological analysis was collected from 42 resident foals. Fecal samples were collected from 40 resident foals. After collection, the samples were kept on ice and processed within 24 h.

Animals

Fresh feces from free-living animals were collected after trapping the animals using live traps. The traps were laid in trap-lines within the farm's boundaries, inside and outside of the horse stable, and in the farm's surroundings in a 0.5-km radius. The surrounding habitats

Table 1 Serology and fecal shedding of resident foals in the farms investigated in this study tested for *Lawsonia intracellularis* (LI)

Farm ID	Location	Date diagnosing EPE	Foal serum samples (seropositive/total)	Fecal samples from foals (PCR positive/total)	Mean number of LI shed per gram of fecal samples	Main clinical findings in weanling foals at the occurrence of EPE
A	Gyeonggi	January 2011	2/5 (40%)	1/5 (20%)	1.2×10^5	Anorexia, fever (rectal temperature > 38.5 °C), weight loss, watery diarrhea
B	Gangwon	December 2012	1/3 (33%)	1/5 (20%)	1.0×10^3	Lethargy, anorexia, weight loss, and watery diarrhea (fecal staining of distal limb)
C	Chungnam	September 2011	3/4 (43%)	2/5 (40%)	1.4×10^4	Lethargy and diarrhea varying from cow pie to watery (fecal staining of distal limb)
D	Chungnam	February 2013	1/6 (17%)	1/5 (20%)	1.2×10^4	Mild lethargy, anorexia, fever, severe weight loss, and watery diarrhea
E	Jeonbuk	November 2012	1/4 (25%)	1/5 (20%)	1.3×10^5	Peripheral edema (ventrum, sheath, and distal limbs), weight loss, and diarrhea
F	Jeonnam	December 2012	6/7 (86%)	3/5 (60%)	1.7×10^6	Lethargy, fever (rectal temperature > 38.5 °C), severe weight loss, and diarrhea varying from cow pie to watery
G	Gyeongnam	January 2011	4/5 (80%)	2/5 (40%)	1.2×10^5	Fever (rectal temperature > 38.5 °C), peripheral edema (ventrum and distal limbs), severe weight loss, watery diarrhea
H	Jeju	February 2013	6/8 (75%)	4/5 (80%)	1.7×10^7	Lethargy, anorexia, fever (rectal temperature > 38.5 °C), severe weight loss, and watery diarrhea

All farms involved in this study had known occurrences of equine proliferative enteropathy (EPE)

included agricultural fields (seasonal vegetation, rice paddies, and vegetable patches), groves, roadside ditches, forests, riversides, and low mountains. The interval between two traps was more than at least approximately 1 m. The live traps were baited with pieces of bacon, carrot, apple, and acorn. The traps were set for durations of one to three nights and checked every day. The bait was refreshed every second day.

After determining the species, the trapped animals, including grey red-backed voles (*Myodes rufocanus*), Eurasian flying squirrels (*Pteromys volans*), and Eurasian red squirrels (*Sciurus vulgaris coreae*), were released unharmed, and the feces dropped in the cage during the confinement period were collected. Trapped animals determined to be pests regulated under the authority of the Korea Ministry of Health and Welfare (Infectious Disease Prevention and Management Act) were euthanized. A small number of animals (4 brown rats (*Rattus norvegicus caraco Pallas*), 7 house mice (*Mus musculus*), 3 grey red-backed voles, and 1 striped field mouse (*Apodemus agrarius*) were killed by professional trappers to control pests on certain farms independent of the traps set for this study. When the animals were killed as part of routine rodent control, the animals were stored at −20 °C on the farm. Frozen rodents were thawed, and their intestines were removed from the body cavity. The intestinal mucosa was scraped with the blade of a sterile scalpel to obtain approximately 0.2–0.3 g of both tissue and feces. When animals were euthanized because they were classified as pests, the intestinal mucosa (ileum, cecum, and, colon) was scraped as mentioned above. The mesenteric lymph nodes were taken for DNA isolation and real-time PCR assays if the intestinal tissues or mesenteric lymph nodes were sufficient for sampling. Samples were collected under sterile conditions from each animal and from each part of the intestine (or mesenteric lymph node). The scraped mucosa or mesenteric lymph node was combined with 2 mL of sucrose-phosphate-glutamate solution with 5% fetal bovine serum and homogenized in a blender for 2 min. All cats trapped during the study period were anesthetized and neutered or spayed in accordance with local regulations (Trap-Neuter-Return policy), and released unharmed. Fecal samples were collected at the same time. To prevent potential cross-contamination between fecal and intestinal tissue samples, separate disposable gloves were worn for each collected sample. When possible, the samples were immediately sent to the laboratory and examined. Otherwise, the samples were kept at −20 °C at the farm until proper testing could be undertaken in the laboratory.

All animal handling, trapping, euthanasia and blood collection procedures were conducted in compliance with the regulations of the "Animal Care and Use Manual" of the Animal, Plant, and Fisheries Quarantine and Inspection Agency (No. 75/2011) and the "Animal Protection Law" of the Ministry of Agriculture, Food and Rural Affairs (No. 10310/2010).

Serology

Sera from the resident foals were used to measure *L. intracellularis*-specific antibodies in the immunoperoxidase monolayer assay (IPMA) [18] in order to obtain information on EPE status of the farms involved in this study. The cultivation of *L. intracellularis* and serology using the IPMA technique were performed as described previously [18–20]. The pathogenic isolate PHE/KK421 (Korean Collection for Type Cultures 10686BP, Daejeon, South Korea) was used to infect murine fibroblast-like McCoy cells (American Type Culture Collection CRL 1696, VA, USA). Briefly, a *L. intracellularis* culture plate was incubated with sera diluted 1:60 in phosphate-buffered saline (PBS) for 30 min at 37 °C and washed 5 times with PBS (pH 7.2). Peroxidase-labeled goat anti-horse IgG was diluted 1:500 (KPL, MD, USA) in 2% bovine serum albumin and 0.08% Tween 80 in PBS and then added at a concentration of 50 μL/well. The plate was incubated for 45 min at 37 °C. The plate was washed again, and chromogen (3-amino-9-ethyl-carbazole, Dako Corporation, CA, USA) solution was added to each well. Then, the plate was incubated at room temperature for 20 min. The plate was washed with distilled water 3 times, allowed to dry, and examined using a BX50 microscope (Olympus, Tokyo, Japan). Positive samples had red-labeled bacteria in both the cytoplasm of the infected McCoy cells and the extracellular space [21–24].

DNA extraction

Feces or intestinal tissues collected in the field that arrived at the laboratory were kept refrigerated at 4 °C prior to processing for nucleic acid purification within 48 h of collection. First, 2 mL of PBS was added to 0.2 g of feces or intestinal tissue homogenate in a conical tube. In case of fecal samples, the samples were vortexed for 10 s and centrifuged at 16,000×*g* for 1 min to remove fecal debris. To minimize contamination, all pipetting steps were performed in a laminar flow cabinet. Next, 200 μL of PBS and feces (or tissue homogenate) was processed for DNA purification using a BioRobot M48 workstation apparatus (Qiagen, GmBH, Hilden, Germany) with a MagAttract DNA Mini M48 Kit (Qiagen) according to the manufacturer's recommendations. One negative extraction sample of other bacterial cells (*E. coli*) and 1 positive extraction sample of *L. intracellularis* were included in each experiment to check for any contamination in the DNA extraction process. The DNA concentrations were measured on the NanoDrop ND-1000 v.3.1 Spectrophotometer (NanoDrop Technologies, Inc., USA) according to the manufacturer's instructions. The concentrations of pure chromosomal DNA were used to calculate the genome equivalents (GEs) used in the standard curves. Nucleic acids were eluted in 50 μL of buffer and stored at −70 °C.

DNA amplification

All purified DNA samples were assayed for the presence of the aspartate ammonia lyase (aspA) gene of *L. intracellularis* by real-time PCR. All purified DNA samples from the feces or tissue homogenates were assayed in triplicate for the presence of the *L. intracellularis* aspA gene by real-time PCR as described previously (Additional file 1: Appendix 1) [16]. This real-time TaqMan PCR assay used is based on the detection of a specific 104-base pair product of the aspA gene of *L. intracellularis* (GenBank accession no. AM180252).

Precautions were taken to minimize contamination during the precipitation, preamplification, and amplification steps, including performing all pipetting steps in a laminar flow cabinet and including positive (DNA from cell-grown *L. intracellularis*) and negative (*L. intracellularis*-free DNA from fecal samples) DNA controls. Furthermore, swabs were taken from centrifuges, laminar flow cabinets, and countertops and assayed for the *L. intracellularis* aspA gene by real-time PCR to assess potential contamination. A real-time PCR assay that targeted a universal sequence of the bacterial 16S rRNA gene was used as a quality control (i.e., efficiency of DNA purification and amplification) and as an indicator of fecal inhibition as described previously [25, 26].

Bacterial quantification

The amount of *L. intracellularis* in the feces was determined. For the absolute quantification of *L. intracellularis*, a standard curve was generated from 10% horse feces that was negative by real-time PCR and spiked with a 10-fold dilution of the reference strain *L. intracellularis* (strain PHE/KK421) as described previously [27]. Standard curves were made by spiking 0.9 mL of 10% *L. intracellularis*–free equine feces with a 0.1 mL suspension of the reference *L. intracellularis* PHE/KK421 strain (derived from cell culture in McCoy cells (mouse fibroblast cells)) in 10-fold dilutions prior to DNA extraction. The bacterial numbers were assessed by direct counting under a microscope after indirect immunoperoxidase staining using the *L. intracellularis*-specific antibody O6 [28]. Three μL of extracted DNA was used as a template in the real-time PCR assays. Each subsequent real-time PCR experiment included the same reference concentrations of pure DNA in triplicate, which facilitated the adjustment of the standard curves to each new real-time PCR run [27]. The final quantitation for each sample was expressed as the average of the triplicate results.

Repeatability

The biological repeatability was determined by taking double samples of feces from 16 *L. intracellularis*-positive samples as described previously [27]. The fecal or intestinal tissue samples were diluted to 10% in PBS. DNA was also extracted using a BioRobot M48 workstation apparatus (Qiagen) with a MagAttract DNA Mini M48 Kit and subsequently analyzed by real-time PCR as parallel samples. The technical repeatability was determined by measuring the concentration of *L. intracellularis* in one DNA extract from spiked feces in parallel real-time PCR samples.

Statistical analysis

Statistical significance was set at the 5% level, and two-sided p-values were calculated for the analysis of the correlation between the data from the farms and the detection rates of *L. intracellularis* DNA in fecal samples from the captured wild rodents and feral cats. The statistical analysis was performed via the paired t-test, and a p-value <0.05 was accepted as significant. All data were analyzed using the GraphPad PRISM software (version 6.07 for Windows; GraphPad Software Inc.).

Results

All farms enrolled in this study experienced EPE between September and February from 2011 to 2013. The proportion of tested foals with antibodies against *L. intracellularis* in each farm ranged from 17 to 86%, and the proportion of foals with fecal shedding in each farm ranged from 20 to 80% (Table 1). For this study, sampling was conducted for 2–3 months on each farm. Feces were collected for the bacterial shedding analysis from a total of 131 free-living animals from 8 farms with diagnosed EPE cases. The total number of captured animals in each farm ranged from 9 to 26. The highest proportion of positive wild animals was identified on farm F (25%), whereas relatively low proportions of positive animals were found on farms C, E, and H (less than 12%) (Table 2). No positive wild animals were identified on farms B or D. All animals with evidence of exposure to *L. intracellularis* in this study were clinically normal when the feces were sampled. In most cases, the feces were formed, firm, and typical of the particular species. The feces were soft (diarrheic) in one case from a feral cat captured on farm A.

Significant associations ($p < 0.05$) were found between the proportions of positive wild animals among the total animals captured from each horse farm enrolled in this study and the serological results for each farm. The proportion of positive wild animals was somewhat correlated with the positive rate in fecal samples from foals from each farm ($p = 0.051$). However, the correlation between the mean number of *L. intracellularis* shed per

Table 2 Wild rodents and feral cats tested for *Lawsonia intracellularis* (LI) from eight horse farms with known occurrences of equine proliferative enteropathy

Farm ID	Total no. of samples (positive/total)	Sampling period (start-end)	Family	Species	Common name	No. of samples (positive/total)
A	2/15 (13.3%)	January 2011	Muridae	*Rattus norvegicus caraco Pallas*	Brown Rat	2/5
		-		*Apodemus agrarius*	Striped Field Mouse	0/5
		February 2011	Cricetidae	*Myodes rufocanus*	Grey Red-backed Vole	0/3
			Sciuridae	*Pteromys volans*	Eurasian Flying Squirrel	0/1
			Felidae	*Felis catus*	Feral Cat	0/1
B	0/8 (0%)	December 2012	Muridae	*Rattus norvegicus caraco Pallas*	Brown Rat	0/3
		-		*Mus musculus*	House Mouse	0/2
		February 2013		*Pteromys volans*	Eurasian Flying Squirrel	0/1
			Felidae	*Felis catus*	Feral Cat	0/2
C	2/17 (11.8%)	September 2011	Muridae	*Rattus norvegicus caraco Pallas*	Brown Rat	0/1
		-		*Mus musculus*	House Mouse	1/6
		October 2011		*Apodemus agrarius*	Striped Field Mouse	0/4
			Cricetidae	*Myodes rufocanus*	Grey Red-backed Vole	0/4
			Sciuridae	*Sciurus vulgaris coreae*	Eurasian Red Squirrel	0/1
			Felidae	*Felis catus*	Feral Cat	1/1
D	0/10 (0%)	February 2013	Muridae	*Mus musculus*	House Mouse	0/7
		-	Cricetidae	*Myodes rufocanus*	Grey Red-backed Vole	0/2
		April 2013	Felidae	*Felis catus*	Feral Cat	0/1
E	1/13 (7.7%)	November 2012	Muridae	*Mus musculus*	House Mouse	1/2
		-		*Apodemus agrarius*	Striped Field Mouse	0/6
		January 2013	Cricetidae	*Myodes rufocanus*	Grey Red-backed Vole	0/4
			Sciuridae	*Sciurus vulgaris coreae*	Eurasian Red Squirrel	0/1
F	4/16 (25.0%)	December 2012	Muridae	*Rattus norvegicus caraco Pallas*	Brown Rat	1/2
		-		*Mus musculus*	House Mouse	2/7
		January 2013		*Apodemus agrarius*	Striped Field Mouse	0/4
			Cricetidae	*Myodes rufocanus*	Grey Red-backed Vole	0/1
			Felidae	*Felis catus*	Feral Cat	1/2
G	4/26 (15.4%)	January 2011	Muridae	*Rattus norvegicus caraco Pallas*	Brown Rat	0/4
		-		*Mus musculus*	House Mouse	1/7
		February 2011		*Apodemus agrarius*	Striped Field Mouse	1/6
			Cricetidae	*Myodes rufocanus*	Grey Red-backed Vole	1/5
			Sciuridae	*Sciurus vulgaris coreae*	Eurasian Red Squirrel	0/1
			Felidae	*Felis catus*	Feral Cat	1/3
H	3/26 (11.5%)	February 2013	Muridae	*Rattus norvegicus caraco Pallas*	Brown Rat	0/6
		-		*Mus musculus*	House Mouse	2/8
		April 2013		*Apodemus agrarius*	Striped Field Mouse	0/6
			Cricetidae	*Myodes rufocanus*	Grey Red-backed Vole	1/3
			Felidae	*Felis catus*	Feral Cat	0/3

gram of fecal sample and the detection rate of *L. intracellularis* DNA in the fecal samples from the captured wild animals in each horse farm was not significant.

The prevalence of PCR-positive animals varied substantially between farms. *L. intracellularis* DNA was detected by PCR in the feces of 3 out of the 21 examined brown rats, 7 out of the 39 examined house mice, 1 of the 31 examined striped field mice, 2 of the 22 examined grey red-backed voles, and 3 of the 13 examined feral cats from a total of 6 horse farms (Table 3). The *L.*

Table 3 Total numbers of wild rodents and feral cats caught at eight horse farms and the positive rates of *Lawsonia intracellularis* assessed using real-time PCR

Family	Species	Common name	No. of samples (positive/total)	Correlation (*p* value)		
				Positive percentage in captured animals vs. serology of resident foals	Positive percentage in captured animals vs. fecal shedding rate of resident foals	Positive percentage in captured animals vs. mean number of LI shed per gram of fecal samples
Muridae	*Rattus norvegicus caraco Pallas*	Brown Rat	3/21 (14%)	0.0052	0.0364	*ns*[a]
	Mus musculus	House Mouse	7/39 (18%)	0.0134	0.0423	*ns*
	Apodemus agrarius	Striped Field Mouse	1/31 (3%)	0.0009	0.0034	*ns*
Cricetidae	*Myodes rufocanus*	Grey Red-backed Vole	2/22 (9%)	0.0008	0.0009	*ns*
Sciuridae	*Pteromys volans*	Eurasian Flying Squirrel	0/2 (0%)	-	-	-
	Sciurus vulgaris coreae	Eurasian Red Squirrel	0/3 (0%)	-	-	-
Felidae	*Felis catus*	Feral Cat	3/13 (23%)	*ns*	*ns*	*ns*
Total			16/131 (12%)			

[a]*ns*, no statistically significant association between two evidences
Statistical significance was set at the 5% level, and two-sided *p*-values were calculated for the analysis of the correlation between data from the farms and the detection rates of *L. intracellularis* DNA in fecal samples from captured wild rodents and feral cats

intracellularis DNA-positive proportion of each animal species except for the feral cats was significantly associated with the serological results and the fecal shedding rates of the resident foals ($p < 0.005$).

A large number of *L. intracellularis* was shed (more than 1×10^7/g of feces) by a rat from farm F and a mouse from farm G. A small proportion of wild rodents from farms F and H shed 10^5–10^7 *L. intracellularis* per gram of feces (Additional file 1: Appendix 2). However, the majority of the wild rodents trapped on the 6 horse farms shed less than 10^5 *L. intracellularis*/g of feces, and *L. intracellularis* could not be detected in more than 90.0% of the wild rodents trapped on farms B, C, D, and E. All feral cats that tested positive for *L. intracellularis* shedding shed 10^5–10^7 *L. intracellularis* per gram of feces.

Gastrointestinal tissue samples from 11 animals that tested PCR-positive for *L. intracellularis* in the feces were investigated (Table 4). The adenomatous lesions typical of *L. intracellularis* infection were not observed in any of the necropsied animals investigated in this study. Intestinal mucosal tissues and mesenteric lymph nodes were not available for testing in another five animals that tested PCR-positive for *L. intracellularis* because the animals were released unharmed after the fecal samples were collected.

Two of the 6 horse farms in which brown rats were captured and tested had brown rats with evidence of exposure to *L. intracellularis*. Four of the 7 horse farms in which house mice were captured and tested had house mice with evidence of exposure to *L. intracellularis*. In contrast, only 2 of the 6 horse farms in which grey red-backed voles were captured and tested had grey red-backed voles with evidence of exposure to *L. intracellularis*. Although striped field mice were captured on 6 horse farms, only 1 farm had striped field mice with evidence of exposure to *L. intracellularis*. Likewise, 3 farms had feral cats with evidence of exposure to *L. intracellularis*, although only 7 feral cats were captured.

Based on fecal shedding and the detection of *L. intracellularis* DNA by real-time PCR in the intestinal mucosal tissue and mesenteric lymph node samples, a total of

Table 4 The detection of *Lawsonia intracellularis* DNA by real-time PCR in the intestinal mucosal tissues and mesenteric lymph nodes of 10 wild mammals with confirmed *L. intracellularis*-positive test results in fecal samples that were available for additional tests

	Ileum			Cecum			Colon			MLN[b]			No. of examined animals		
Animal species	*n.*	Pos[a]	%	*n.*	Pos	%	*n.*	Pos	%	*n.*	Pos	%	*n.*	Pos	%
Brown Rat (*Rattus norvegicus caraco Pallas*)	3	0	0.0	3	1	33.3	3	0	0.0	3	1	33.3	3	2	66.7
House Mouse (*Mus musculus*)	7	2	28.6	7	1	14.3	7	2	28.6	7	2	28.6	7	3	42.9
Striped Field Mouse (*Apodemus agrarius*)	1	1	100	1	0	0.0	1	0	0.0	1	0	0.0	1	1	100
Total	11	3	27.3	11	2	18.2	11	2	18.2	11	3	27.3	11	6	54.5

[a]Positive; [b]In some animals, corresponding mesenteric lymphatic nodes (MLN) were examined

3 brown rats from 2 farms, 7 house mice from 5 farms, 1 striped field mouse from 1 farm, 2 grey red-backed voles from 2 farms, and 3 feral cats from 3 farms had evidence of prior exposure to *L. intracellularis*. On farms F, G, and H, 25%, 15%, and 12% of the captured wild mammals had evidence of exposure to *L. intracellularis*, respectively. The largest number of PCR-positive *L. intracellularis* fecal samples was observed in the house mice (7), followed by brown rats (3), feral cats (3), grey red-backed voles (2) and striped field mice (1).

Discussion

Our results correlate with previous findings demonstrating similar exposure rates to *L. intracellularis* in weanling foals from farms with EPE in a study on horse farms located in California and Kentucky, with a serological prevalence for each farm that ranged from 11 to 100% [16]. Our finding also indicates that the exposure rates to *L. intracellularis* in foals from farms with EPE were moderate to high at the time point when the first clinical EPE case were diagnosed on each farm.

Based on individual identification or the detection of only 1 positive animal for a specific species, an exact prevalence of 23% was determined for feral cats and 3% for striped field mice. Among the wild animals captured in this study, the highest detection rate of *L. intracellularis* DNA was found in feral cats. The relatively high prevalence determined for feral cats may be influenced by the small sample size; thus, additional samples are needed to assign a more accurate prevalence. However, this study showed a low detection rate of *L. intracellularis* DNA in the total number of striped field mice (3%) compared with a previous report on the prevalence in wild rodents from pig farms with PPE (16%) [6]. None of the fecal samples from Eurasian flying squirrels or Eurasian red squirrels had detectable *L. intracellularis*. The lack of molecular pathogen detection in these species may be related to the small sample size, a potential intermittent mode of pathogen shedding, or the inability of *L. intracellularis* to infect these species as previously described [16].

Collectively, three rodent species and 1 feral cat species were positive for *L. intracellularis* at farms A, C, E, F, G, and H, suggesting that the bacterium had been introduced into the surrounding environments of these particular farms. The presence of *L. intracellularis* in wild rodents and feral cats living in close proximity to the farm led us to assume that this pathogen might be shed into the natural environment and spread as previously described [6]. The transmission of the bacterium may occur not only between wild rodents or feral cats themselves but also to other free-living animals, such as wild boars, deer and carnivores.

From the perspective of herd prevalence in wild animals, the proportion of positive feces from the wild animals captured in this study ranged from 0 to 25% for each farm. Differences in habitat, the number of trapping events between farms, and the total numbers of each captured animal species between the farms might be at the source of this discrepancy. Additionally, the results of this study highlight the variety of animal species that are potentially involved in the shedding of *L. intracellularis* on farms with documented EPE cases in South Korea. Based on our results, a number of free-living rodents and feral cats can be considered host or reservoir species of *L. intracellularis*. Furthermore, we identified a new *L. intracellularis*-infected host: the grey red-backed vole. This species may be an important vector/reservoir of *L. intracellularis* in the Far East region, including South Korea, because this species ranges across northern Eurasia, including the Korean Peninsula, and is frequently found in South Korea.

The parallel finding of the causative agent in the intestinal mucosal membrane and the corresponding mesenteric lymph nodes in one of the brown rats and two of the house mice was suggestive of the earlier findings in domestic pigs [29]. Our observations seem to suggest that *L. intracellularis* infection among wild rodents and feral cats around horse farms can spread through the oro-fecal route similar to domestic pigs on farms with intensive breeding [30].

The importance of EPE transmission by vectors is unknown. Following experimental inoculation, histological lesions develop in laboratory mice, rats and hamsters but not in sparrows or chickens [6, 7, 15, 31–34]. Natural infection has been described in rats and mice, but the importance of these vectors for transmission within a herd or transmission between herds under natural conditions is uncertain. However, rats, mice, and cats have been considered important reservoirs of *L. intracellularis* on pig or horse farms, with the prevalence of PCR-positive animals varying substantially between farms from 4 to 83% [6, 7, 15, 17, 31].

Evidence of exposure to *L. intracellularis* in wild rodents and feral cats captured on farms with EPE was higher than previously reported, possibly due to differences in regions or sampling methods; for instance, surveys reporting prevalence rates of 1.0 and 0%, respectively, have used PCR analysis of tissue or fecal samples, respectively [17, 35].

A random sampling-based study previously performed in South Korea reported that 15.7 and 12.5% of tissue samples from wild rodents and stray cats, respectively, tested PCR-positive for *L. intracellularis* [31]. Because the detailed species investigated in this previous study were not determined, information on the prevalence of each rodent species was limited. Interestingly, the overall rates of *L. intracellularis* DNA detection in wild rodents and feral cats were not significantly different, although the research design in terms of farm selection was different between our study and the study by Truong et al. This difference might explain why the previous study by Troung et al. investigated animals captured on pig farms regardless of consideration of farm selection based on PPE outbreak by *L. intracellularis* infection, which was in contrast to our method. Additionally, Lee et al. reported an extraordinarily high nationwide prevalence of PPE-positive pig farms (100%) in South Korea [36].

Regardless of the affected species, the antemortem diagnosis of proliferative enteropathy is based on the detection of *L. intracellularis*–specific IgG by serology and the molecular identification of *L. intracellularis* DNA in feces by PCR [22, 37]. Positive serology characterizes exposure to infection rather than disease, whereas positive PCR results indicate shedding of the bacteria and active infection. However, to date, epidemiologic studies that have determined the exposure rate of free-living animals to *L. intracellularis* have been hampered by the lack of established and validated serological assays [16]. Difficulties associated with in vitro cultivation of this organism related to its ubiquitous presence and ability to cause disease in a variety of animal species also highlight the need for higher resolution diagnostics to provide a better understanding of the interspecies transmission dynamics and the realistic importance of the disease in different species [38]. Among a variety of diagnostic methods, the molecular detection of *L. intracellularis* in the feces of animals generally does not provide any conclusive evidence regarding the biological state of the organism or its origin. The direct link between wild animals and EPE still needs to be proven by either characterization of the detected bacterial isolates or experimental challenges using isolates from free-living hosts. To overcome these difficulties, good diagnostic methods and increased knowledge of epidemiology and immunity are required for the *L. intracellularis* bacterium.

A major limitation of this study was the lack of widely-accepted serological assay to evaluate *L. intracellularis*-specific antibodies in cat or rodent species. Although IPMA could be available in our laboratory in this study and actually performed for sera from some animals, the serological data for cats and rodents is not shown in this paper because the assay was not fully evaluated and still not widely accepted for sera from cats and rodents. Another limitation was the study design, which was based on voluntary enrollment instead of randomized selection. Similar limitations were reported by Pusterla et al., [16] in the United States. Likewise, no farms with EPE over the study period refused participation in this study. In addition, one of the limitations of this study was that the study lacked control farms. However, we did not try to determine the risk factors associated with the occurrence of EPE but instead focused solely on the exposure rates of *L. intracellularis* in wild and feral animals.

The mode of transmission of *L. intracellularis* to susceptible weanlings remains speculative. However, foals most likely become exposed to *L. intracellularis* after the ingestion of feed or water contaminated by *L. intracellularis*-containing feces from domestic or free-living animals. Potential reservoir hosts must be abundant on the premises, have unlimited access to feeding and drinking areas of the susceptible weanlings, and be able to maintain the agent indefinitely within their populations. From the study results, brown rats, house mice, striped field mice, grey red-backed voles, and feral cats would be considered prime reservoir host candidates in South Korea. At the very least, these wild animal species may play a role in the circulation of *L. intracellularis* in the natural habitats around EPE-affected horse farms in the Far East, including South Korea. Additional domestic or free-living animals might have played a role in the transmission of *L. intracellularis* on the horse farms enrolled in this study. Therefore, the role of clinically and subclinically infected foals in the feco-oral transmission of *L. intracellularis* requires further investigation.

Conclusions

In summary, the infection source of *L. intracellularis* in foals remains speculative worldwide, and only limited information on epidemiological findings in wild and feral animals from farms with EPE has been reported in the United States in an attempt to determine their role in the spread of *L. intracellularis*. This study is the first report to describe the identification of five wild mammalian hosts that are potentially associated with the shedding of *L. intracellularis* on farms with a known EPE status in South Korea. Additionally, this study is the first to demonstrate the magnitude of *L. intracellularis* shedding in the feces of wild rodents and feral cats and to indicate the significant infection risk that wild rodents and feral cats pose to naïve horses in South Korea. These results also demonstrate the importance of understanding the role of wildlife species in the development of management strategies for EPE in weanling foals in South Korea. The findings emphasize the need to enforce biosecurity measures to prevent wild animals, including wild rodents and feral cats, from entering horse stables.

Additional file

Additional file 1: Appendix 1. Oligonucleotide primers and probe used for the real-time PCR detection of Lawsonia intracellularis in the fecal samples used in this study. **Appendix 2.**The total percentages of wild and feral animals shedding Lawsonia intracellularis and the percent shedding at high (more than 1×10^7), medium (10^5–10^7) or low (10^3–10^5) numbers of L. intracellularis/g of feces or with undetectable numbers in each horse farm. (DOC 100 kb)

Abbreviations

EPE: Equine proliferative enteropathy; IPMA: Immunoperoxidase monolayer assay; PBS: Phosphate-buffered saline; aspA: aspartate ammonia lyase; PCR: Polymerase chain reaction; PPE: Porcine proliferative enteropathy

Acknowledgements

The author is very grateful to the local government veterinary officers and equine veterinary clinicians for their expertise and help in the review of the cooperative research design. The authors also thank the farm staff for coordinating the wild animal capture and collecting samples on selected horse farms. We are grateful to the two anonymous reviewers that reviewed the first draft of the manuscript for their critical comments and suggestions.

Funding

This work was supported by the Incheon National University Research Grant to Jung-Yong Yeh and Myung-Ji Seo in 2014.

Authors' contributions

Conceived and designed the study: JYY and MJS. Laboratory testing: JYY and JMH. Drafted the manuscript: JYY and JMH. The authors read and approved the manuscript.

Consent for publication

Not applicable.

Competing interests

None of the authors of this paper had a financial or personal relationship with other people or organizations that could inappropriately influence or bias the content of the paper.

Author details

[1]Veterinary Research Center, Green Cross Veterinary Products Co., Ltd., Kugal-dong 227-5, Giheung-gu, Yongin-si, Gyeonggi-do 17066, Republic of Korea. [2]Division of Bioengineering, Incheon National University, Academy-ro 119, Incheon 22012, Republic of Korea. [3]Department of Bioengineering and Nano-Bioengineering, Graduate School of Incheon National University, Academy-ro 119, Incheon 22012, Republic of Korea. [4]Department of Life Sciences, College of Life Sciences and Bioengineering, Incheon National University, Academy-ro 119, Yeonsu-gu, Incheon 22012, Republic of Korea. [5]Previous address: Emerging & Exotic Diseases Research Laboratory, Foreign Animal Diseases Division, Animal, Plant, and Fisheries Quarantine and Inspection Agency, Anyang-ro 175, Manan-gu, Anyang-si, Gyeonggi-do 14089, Republic of Korea.

References

1. Kroll JJ, Roof MB, Hoffman LJ, Dickson JS, Harris DL. Proliferative enteropathy: a global enteric disease of pigs caused by Lawsonia Intracellularis. Anim Health Res Rev. 2005;6(2):173–97.
2. Biester HE, Schwarte LH. Intestinal adenoma in swine. Am J Pathol. 1931; 7(2):175–85. 176
3. Klein EC, Gebhart CJ, Duhamel GE. Fatal outbreaks of proliferative enteritis caused by Lawsonia Intracellularis in young colony-raised rhesus macaques. J Med Primatol. 1999;28(1):11–8.
4. Lawson GH, Gebhart CJ. Proliferative enteropathy. J Comp Pathol. 2000; 122(2–3):77–100.
5. Herbst W, Hertrampf B, Schmitt T, Weiss R, Baljer G. Diagnosis of Lawsonia Intracellularis using the polymerase chain reaction (PCR) in pigs with and without diarrhea and other animal species. Dtsch Tierarztl Wochenschr. 2003;110(9):361–4.
6. Friedman M, Bednar V, Klimes J, Smola J, Mrlik V, Literak I. Lawsonia Intracellularis in rodents from pig farms with the occurrence of porcine proliferative enteropathy. Lett Appl Microbiol. 2008;47(2):117–21.
7. Murakata K, Sato A, Yoshiya M, Kim S, Watarai M, Omata Y, et al. Infection of different strains of mice with Lawsonia Intracellularis derived from rabbit or porcine proliferative enteropathy. J Comp Pathol. 2008;139(1):8–15.
8. Ohta T, Kimura K, Katsuda K, Kobayashi H, Mikami O, Haritani M, et al. Proliferative Enteropathy caused by Lawsonia Intracellularis in chickens. J Comp Pathol. 2016;
9. Michalski CW, Di Mola FF, Kummel K, Wendt M, Koninger JS, Giese T, et al. Human inflammatory bowel disease does not associate with Lawsonia Intracellularis infection. BMC Microbiol. 2006;6:81.
10. Jacobson M, Rasback T, Floistrup H, Benz M, Braun-Fahrlander C, Riedler J, et al. Survey on the occurrence of Brachyspira species and Lawsonia Intracellularis in children living on pig farms. Epidemiol Infect. 2007; 135(6):1043–5.
11. Pusterla N, Gebhart CJ. Equine proliferative enteropathy–a review of recent developments. Equine Vet J. 2013;45(4):403–9.
12. Pusterla N, Gebhart C. Lawsonia Intracellularis infection and proliferative enteropathy in foals. Vet Microbiol. 2013;167(1–2):34–41.
13. McGurrin MK, Vengust M, Arroyo LG, Baird JD. An outbreak of Lawsonia Intracellularis infection in a standardbred herd in Ontario. Can Vet J. 2007; 48(9):927–30.
14. Pearson HE, Toribio JA, Lapidge SJ, Hernandez-Jover M. Evaluating the risk of pathogen transmission from wild animals to domestic pigs in Australia. Prev Vet Med. 2016;123:39–51.
15. Collins AM, Fell S, Pearson H, Toribio JA. Colonisation and shedding of Lawsonia Intracellularis in experimentally inoculated rodents and in wild rodents on pig farms. Vet Microbiol. 2011;150(3–4):384–8.
16. Pusterla N, Mapes S, Rejmanek D, Gebhart C. Detection of Lawsonia Intracellularis by real-time PCR in the feces of free-living animals from equine farms with documented occurrence of equine proliferative enteropathy. J Wildl Dis. 2008;44(4):992–8.
17. Pusterla N, Mapes S, Gebhart C. Further investigation of exposure to Lawsonia Intracellularis in wild and feral animals captured on horse properties with equine proliferative enteropathy. Vet J. 2012;194(2):253–5.
18. Guedes RM, Gebhart CJ, Deen J, Winkelman NL. Validation of an immunoperoxidase monolayer assay as a serologic test for porcine proliferative enteropathy. J Vet Diagn Investig. 2002;14(6):528–30.
19. Yeh JY, Kim TJ, Park SY, Song CS, Yoon YD, Kim SK, et al. Isolation of Lawsonia Intracellularis in Korea and reproduction of proliferative enteropathy in pigs and hamsters. J Vet Med Sci. 2006;68(5):499–501.
20. Guedes RM, Gebhart CJ. Comparison of intestinal mucosa homogenate and pure culture of the homologous Lawsonia Intracellularis isolate in reproducing proliferative enteropathy in swine. Vet Microbiol. 2003;93(2):159–66.
21. Page AE, Slovis NM, Gebhart CJ, Wolfsdorf K, Mapes SM, Pusterla N. Serial use of serologic assays and fecal PCR assays to aid in identification of subclinical Lawsonia Intracellularis infection for targeted treatment of thoroughbred foals and weanlings. J Am Vet Med Assoc. 2011;238(11):1482–9.
22. Pusterla N, Jackson R, Wilson R, Collier J, Mapes S, Gebhart C. Temporal detection of Lawsonia Intracellularis using serology and real-time PCR in thoroughbred horses residing on a farm endemic for equine proliferative enteropathy. Vet Microbiol. 2009;136(1–2):173–6.
23. Frazer ML. Lawsonia Intracellularis infection in horses: 2005-2007. J Vet Intern Med. 2008;22(5):1243–8.
24. Guimaraes-Ladeira CV, Palhares MS, Oliveira JS, Ramirez MA, Guedes RM. Faecal shedding and serological cross-sectional study of Lawsonia Intracellularis in horses in the state of Minas Gerais, Brazil. Equine Vet J. 2009;41(6):593–6.
25. Mapes S, Rhodes DM, Wilson WD, Leutenegger CM, Pusterla N. Comparison of five real-time PCR assays for detecting virulence genes in isolates of Escherichia Coli from septicaemic neonatal foals. Vet Rec. 2007;161(21):716–8.
26. Windsor RC, Johnson LR, Sykes JE, Drazenovich TL, Leutenegger CM, De Cock HE. Molecular detection of microbes in nasal tissue of dogs with idiopathic lymphoplasmacytic rhinitis. J Vet Intern Med. 2006;20(2):250–6.
27. Stahl M, Kokotovic B, Hjulsager CK, Breum SO, Angen O. The use of quantitative PCR for identification and quantification of Brachyspira pilosicoli, Lawsonia Intracellularis and Escherichia Coli fimbrial types F4 and F18 in pig feces. Vet Microbiol. 2011;151(3–4):307–14.
28. Hwang JM, Lee JH, Yeh JY. Generation of a monoclonal antibody against Mycoplasma spp. following accidental contamination during production of a monoclonal antibody against Lawsonia Intracellularis. Appl Environ Microbiol. 2012;78(6):2046–8.
29. Jordan DM, Knittel JP, Roof MB, Schwartz K, Larson D, Hoffman LJ. Detection of Lawsonia Intracellularis in swine using polymerase chain reaction methodology. J Vet Diagn Investig. 1999;11(1):45–9.

30. Knittel JP, Jordan DM, Schwartz KJ, Janke BH, Roof MB, McOrist S, et al. Evaluation of antemortem polymerase chain reaction and serologic methods for detection of Lawsonia Intracellularis-exposed pigs. Am J Vet Res. 1998;59(6):722–6.
31. Truong QL, Seo TW, Yoon BI, Kim HC, Han JH, Hahn TW. Prevalence of swine viral and bacterial pathogens in rodents and stray cats captured around pig farms in Korea. J Vet Med Sci. 2013;75(12):1647–50.
32. Collins AM, Love RJ, Jasni S, McOrist S. Attempted infection of mice, rats and chickens by porcine strains of Lawsonia Intracellularis. Aust Vet J. 1999; 77(2):120–2.
33. Gabardo MP, Sato JPH, Daniel AGS, Andrade MR, Pereira CER, Rezende TP, et al. Evaluation of the involvement of mice (Mus Musculus) in the epidemiology of porcine proliferative enteropathy. Vet Microbiol. 2017;205:75–9.
34. Viott AM, França SA, Vannucci FA, Cruz ECC Jr, Costa MC, Gebhart CJ, et al. Infection of sparrows (Passer Domesticus) and different mice strains with *Lawsonia intracellularis*. Pesq Vet Bras. 2013;33(3):372–8.
35. Pusterla N, Higgins JC, Smith P, Mapes S, Gebhart C. Epidemiological survey on farms with documented occurrence of equine proliferative enteropathy due to Lawsonia Intracellularis. Vet Rec. 2008;163(5):156–8.
36. Lee SW, Kim TJ, Park SY, Song CS, Chang HK, Yeh JK, et al. Prevalence of porcine proliferative enteropathy and its control with tylosin in Korea. J Vet Sci. 2001;2(3):209–12.
37. Guedes RM, Gebhart CJ, Winkelman NL, Mackie-Nuss RA. A comparative study of an indirect fluorescent antibody test and an immunoperoxidase monolayer assay for the diagnosis of porcine proliferative enteropathy. J Vet Diagn Investig. 2002;14(5):420–3.
38. Vannucci FA, Gebhart CJ. Recent advances in understanding the pathogenesis of Lawsonia Intracellularis infections. Vet Pathol. 2014;51(2):465–77.

5

Comparison of computed tomography and high-field (3.0 T) magnetic resonance imaging of age-related variances in selected equine maxillary cheek teeth and adjacent tissues

Christin Schoppe[1*], Maren Hellige[1†], Karl Rohn[2], Bernhard Ohnesorge[1†] and Astrid Bienert-Zeit[1†]

Abstract

Background: Modern imaging techniques such as computed tomography (CT) and magnetic resonance imaging (MRI) have the advantage of producing images without superimposition. Whilst CT is a well-established technique for dental diagnostics, MRI examinations are rarely used for the evaluation of dental diseases in horses. Regarding equine endodontic therapies which are increasingly implemented, MRI could help to portray changes of the periodontal ligament and display gross pulpar anatomy. Knowledge of age-related changes is essential for diagnosis, as cheek teeth and surrounding structures alter with increasing age. The aim of the present study was to highlight the advantages of CT and MRI regarding age-related changes in selected equine cheek teeth and their adjacent structures.

Results: The CT and MRI appearances of the maxillary 08 s and 09 s and adjacent structures were described by evaluation of post-mortem examinations of nine horses of different ages (Group A: <6 years, B: 6–15 years, C: ≥16 years). Most of the tissues selected were imaged accurately with MRI and CT. Magnetic resonance imaging gives an excellent depiction of soft endo- and periodontal units, and CT of hard dental and bony tissues. Negative correlation between dental age and pulpar sizes was found: 71.3% of the changes in pulp dimensions can be explained by teeth aging. Pulpar sizes ranged from 14.3 to 1.3 mm and were significantly smaller in older horses ($p < 0.05$). A common pulp chamber was present in 33% of the teeth with a mean dental age of 2.25 years. Ninety-four percent of the 08 and 09 alveoli of all groups were in direct contact with the maxillary sinus. An age-related regression was found ($R^2 = 0.88$) for the distance between alveoli and the infraorbital canal.

Conclusions: The present study provides information about the dental and periodontal age-related morphology and its visibility using different imaging techniques. These results aid in evaluating diagnostic images and in deciding which is the superior imaging modality for clinical cases.

Keywords: Horse, Ct, 3 tesla, High-field MRI, Equine maxillary cheek teeth, Age-related variances, Endodontic disease, Periodontal

* Correspondence: Christin.Schoppe@tiho-hannover.de
[†]Equal contributors
[1]Clinic for Horses, University of Veterinary Medicine Hannover, Foundation, Buenteweg 9, 30559 Hannover, Germany
Full list of author information is available at the end of the article

Background

Radiography has been the primary imaging modality historically for evaluating the heads, paranasal sinuses, and dental and periodontal structures [1]. Modern imaging techniques, such as computed tomography (CT) and magnetic resonance imaging (MRI), offer the benefit of producing three-dimensional (3D) images without superimposition and the possibility of multiplanar reconstructions (MPRs). Both CT and MRI are viable imaging modalities for evaluating the head in human [2–4] and veterinary medicine [5–10]. The well-established CT provides a good spatial resolution and excellent delineation of bony tissue [11], but is limited due to its inability to visualise pulpar and periodontal tissue with detailed resolution [12]. Whilst MRI, with its detailed depiction of soft tissues, has already become a valuable tool for diagnosing oro-dental diseases in humans [13–16], it is rarely used in equine dentistry [17]. Applications reported in the human medical sector include the evaluation of the temporomandibular joint [18, 19] and the nerve channels [20–22], as well as orthodontic utilisation for the assessment of impacted teeth [23], dental pulps or caries diagnosis [13] and apical periodontitis [24]. In accordance with these findings, a 1.5 Tesla MRI was used to portray physiological and pathological cheek teeth [17, 25] and their surrounding structures in equine dentistry [26]. Good MR image acquisition holds enormous potential for radiation-free diagnostic orthodontic workups [27], especially in times when endodontic procedures in conjunction with pulp infection become more common in equine clinical practice [28, 29].

Knowledge of age-related changes and their presentation in 3D imaging modalities is essential for diagnosis and surgical planning since the anatomy of equine hypsodont cheek teeth and neighbouring structures alters with increasing age. While CT, cone-beam CT and 3 Tesla-MRI dental imaging have been directly compared in humans [14], little is known about the dental head-to-head comparison of CT and high-field MRI in different age stages of equine patients.

The purpose of this study was to analyse the visualisation of anatomical landmarks (endo-, periodontal and adjacent structures) and their changes with increasing age in CT and MR images, aiming to highlight the best imaging technique for each structure at different ages. The maxillary 08 s and 09 s were chosen for the examinations because they belong to the cheek teeth with the most frequent pathologies [30].

Methods

Specimens

Nine horses of different breeds (eight warmbloods, one standardbred) were examined to acquire CT and high-field MRI scans of selected equine cheek teeth, their periodontal tissues and adjacent structures. The horses were clinic-owned (TiHo Hannover, Clinic for horses, Germany). The study population was divided into three groups according to age classes: Group A "young" (2–5 years), B "middle-aged" (6–15 years) and C "old to senile" (≥ 16 years), each with n = 3 horses. The age of the selected horses ranged from 2.4 to 21.7 years (median 8.5 years). All horses were subjected to euthanasia on human grounds for non-dental reasons and for health purposes not related to this study. When evaluating the CT and MR images, the Triadan system was used for numbering the cheek teeth [31]. A total of 36 maxillary cheek teeth were examined. The sample pool included eighteen Triadan 08 s and eighteen Triadan 09 s. Owing to eruption time, dental age was determined by subtracting the earliest possible eruption age of the tooth from the age of the horse [32]. An eruption time of 3.5 years for the 08 s and six months for the 09 s was assumed [33]. The population included selected teeth between 0.9 and 20.95 years (median age 7.95 years).

Diagnostic imaging techniques and image evaluation

The imaging processes were carried out at the University of Veterinary Medicine Hannover, Foundation. Images were taken within six hours after euthanasia. The horses were first placed on a stationary CT table in right lateral recumbency and afterwards in dorsal recumbency on a non-stationary MRI table. Dorsal and transversal scan series of the head were acquired (Table 1). The

Table 1 Imaging techniques and settings

Imaging technique	Sequence	Orientation	Matrix	TR (ms)	TE (ms)	ST (mm)
MRI	T1w	3D	1024	8.5	3.9	0.9
	T2w	transverse	1024	4500	80	3.1
	T2w	dorsal	1024	3000	80	4
	PDw	dorsal	1024	6400	30	4
	STIR	transverse	960	8872	30	3
CT	Helical Scan	transverse	1024			1.5

TE echo time, *TR* time to repetition, *ST* slice thickness

orientation for transverse planes was perpendicular and dorsal planes were orientated parallel to the hard palate.

The CT image acquisition was performed with a Brilliance™ CT – Big Bore Oncology Scanner (Philips Medical System, Best, The Netherlands). Images of the head were acquired using a modified dental scanning protocol with 140 kV and 300 mAs. A Philips Achieva™ 3.0TX-Series® was used for MRI acquisition. Surface coils (Philips SENSETM FlexM® and Philips SENSETM FlexL®) were positioned around the region of interest (ROI), between the rostral margin of the facial crest and the orbital cavity. The MRI sequences obtained were: T1 weighted (T1w), T2 weighted (T2w), proton density weighted (PDw) and PD fat-suppressed short-tau-inversion-recovery (STIR) images.

Visualisation and measurements

The CT and MR images were examined and visualisation of the dental and adjacent structures depicted was performed. All examinations were observed by M.H., an experienced radiologist, A.B.-Z., Diplomate EVDC (Equine), and C.S., a trained veterinarian.

Anatomical landmarks (endo-, periodontal and adjacent structures) and their visualisation in CT and MRI were described (Tables 2 and 3).

Special attention was paid to age-related changes. The positional relations between the dental roots and the floor of the paranasal sinuses were described. Pulpar sizes and the positional relation between the dental alveoli and the infraorbital canal (IOC) were portrayed. Each pulp was measured in the mid-tooth section of the cheek tooth selected (Fig. 1a) after each tooth's half-length was determined in the transverse MRI scans. The distance between the dental alveoli and the IOC was portrayed in transverse sections of the CT images. Therefore, the line between the dental alveolus above the pulp position five and the inner border of the IOC was measured (Fig. 1b). Pulpar sizes and the distance between the IOC and the dental alveoli were measured by one of the examiners (C.S.) using easyVET image editor (easy Vet, IFS Informationssysteme GmbH, Hannover, Germany). All measurements were repeated three times under the same conditions and the median value for each pulp or each distance (between the dental alveoli and IOC) was obtained. Moreover, the IOC's shape was assessed.

Statistical analysis

Data were collected on spreadsheets (Excel® 2010, Microsoft® Corporation Redmond, Washington, USA). SAS® software (SAS Institute, Cary North Carolina, USA) was used for statistical analysis and GraphPad Software, Inc.® (La Jolla, California, USA) was used for graphical and statistical representations. Data were tested for normal distribution with the Kolmogorov-Smirnov test. Correlation between dental ages and pulp sizes or alveolar-infraorbital distance was tested by Spearman's rho. A Wilcoxon matched pairs signed rank test was chosen to calculate whether there were significant differences in the pulp sizes or alveolar-infraorbital distances between both sides of the maxilla. The Kruskal-Wallis test and Dunn's multiple comparison test were performed to validate significant differences of pulp dimensions between different age groups. A p value <0.05 was considered statistically significant.

Results

Nine horses were examined immediately after euthanasia. Images of the entire head were acquired by CT

Table 2 Anatomical landmarks of dental structures depicted in MRI and CT referring to imaging advantages

Anatomical region		CT	MRI
Endodontic system	Dental sac	Low attenuated tissue surrounding the reserve crown of growing cheek teeth (transverse)	High signal intensity, marked off by the alveolar bone with low signal intensity (T2w and STIR, both transverse)*
	Common pulp cavity	Low attenuated pulp tissue in young maxillary teeth (transverse)	Hyperintense soft tissue, present in young cheek teeth (T2w transverse, PDw dorsal)*
	Pulps	Generally five pulp horns with very low density visible, moderate to well distinguishable from the hyperdense hard dental tissue; Pulp: −350 to 500 HU (transverse)	Generally five hyperintense pulp horns visible Very good distinction from the hard dental tissue (T2w, STIR transverse; PDw dorsal)*, especially in young cheek teeth
Anatomical crown	Tooth root	Isodense root (transverse)*	Isointense: with good alignment of the MRI scan, well demarcated structure (T2w transverse)
Clinical crown	Hard dental tissue, distinction to the oral cavity	Dentine, cement and enamel: distinction possible through the different grade of attenuation; Hyperdense enamel and dentine; slightly less opaque cement (transverse, dorsal)*	Dentine, cement and enamel: signal free, not distinguishable (T2w and STIR transverse) Distinction to the oral cavity not displayable, only visible where tongue with moderate signal intensity is in contact with the dental crown or saliva surrounds the tooth (T2w and STIR, transverse)

*superior imaging modality by comparison of the respective structure in CT and MR images (in brackets: the best imaging modalities and section planes)

Table 3 Anatomical landmarks of periodontal and adjacent structures depicted in MRI and CT referring to imaging advantages

Anatomical region		CT	MRI
Periodontal apparatus	Periodontal space: Periodontal ligament (PDL)	Slightly blurry, isodense gap between hard dental tissue and alveolar bone, moderate distinction from hard dental and bony tissue (transverse, dorsal)	Hyperintense gap, good distinction of hard dental tissue and alveolar bone* (T2w and PDw dorsal)
	Alveolar bone	Hyperdense bone* (transverse, dorsal)	Hypointense cortical bone, marked off by the PDL (T2w and STIR transverse)
Maxillary sinus	Mucosa and cortical bone	Respiratory epithelium: not visible; sinus: air-filled and hypodense; hyperdense thin-walled cortical bone* (transverse)	Signal free cortical bone, delineated by a hyperintense line of mucosa* (T2w and STIR transverse)
IOC	Soft tissue inside and bony structures	Soft tissue inside the canal: low attenuated IOC*: high attenuated, very well distinguishable (transverse)	IOC: signal free, becomes evident through the bright mucosa covering the bony surface of the maxillary sinus (T2w and STIR transverse) Soft tissue*: inhomogeneous, high to moderate signal, intense structures inside: nerve with moderate signal intensity, blood vessels with high or low signal intensity (T2w and STIR transverse)

*superior imaging modality by comparison of the respective structure in CT and MR images (in brackets: the best imaging modalities and section planes)

and MRI settings were adapted to accomplish maximum image quality within a reasonable examination time. The field of view (FOV) in the MRI scans was limited from a transverse line caudal to the 09 maxillary teeth to the rostral end of the 08 upper cheek teeth. It ranged from 180 to 250 mm in dorsally orientated sequences and from 180 to 220 mm in transversely orientated MR images. The duration of the CT scans was short (mean ± SD, 2 ± 5 min); the MRI examination took between 80 and 98 min (mean ± SD, 89 ± 9 min). While dorsally orientated MR image acquisition took between 10 (T2w) and 16 min (PDw), transversal scan duration took between 18 (T2w) and 24 min (STIR). The T1w 3D image scan for MPR lasted approximately 14 min.

Imaging modalities

Anatomical landmarks and imaging advantages comparing CT and MR images regarding the maxillary 08 s and 09 s and their adjacent structures were evaluated and summarised in Tables 2 and 3. Acquisition by CT proved to be the best imaging technique for the representation of the bony non-dental structures (alveolar bone, cortical and cancellous maxillary bone and the IOC). These bony structures were well delineated against the low attenuated soft tissues. Dental enamel, dentine and cementum were also detected as structures of specific density, marked with different greyscales by CT imaging, but the differentiation between them was not as clear as the line between the alveolar bone and the periodontal space due to their different opacity. Regarding

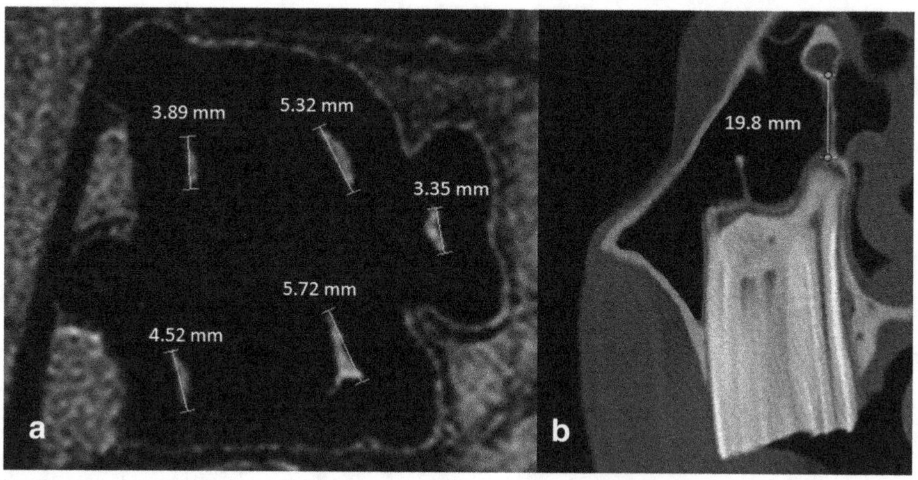

Fig. 1 Measurements of pulpar sizes and distance between alveolus and infraorbital canal (IOC). Pulp dimensions of an 8.5-year-old tooth (108, dorsal plane) in PDw magnetic resonance images (**a**); distance between the alveolar socket and the IOC in a 6-year-old tooth (209, transversal plane) using CT imaging (**b**)

the endodontic system, CT images revealed not only hypodense pulp horns and chambers, but also hypodense funnel-like infundibula. The infundibula could not be detected on the MR images. Marked hypoattenuating stripes were visible adjacent to the infundibula in some of the CT slices, that could be determined as gas. Compared with slightly blurred pulpar CT imaging, the pulp tissue appeared as bright, sharp, hyperintense pulp on the MR images. Other soft tissues, such as the periodontal ligament, respiratory mucosa and the infraorbital nerve, were also better visualised with MRI compared to CT images.

Age-related pulpar sizes

A total of 177 dental pulp measurements were acquired in the upper 08 s and 09 s on dorsally oriented PDw sequences of the MR images. Calculated dental ages for the equine age groups are documented in Table 4. One of the pulp horns was not visible (always pulp 5) in each of three older cheek teeth of the age group B and C (a 10-year-old 209 and a 15.75-year-old 109 and 209). A differentiation between the hypointense hard dental and the normally hyperintense soft pulp tissue could not be performed in any of these MRI sequences because both tissues appeared hypointense in these teeth. Thus, three pulps were excluded from the pulp measurements. The cheek teeth in all other maxillary 08 s and 09 s contained five pulp horns, named pulp 1 to pulp 5 (P1-P5) [34].

Negative correlation between dental age and pulpar dimensions was found ($r = -0.9$). Pulpar size decrease can be explained by dental aging in 71% of the teeth examined: the older the selected cheek teeth of clinically healthy horses became, the smaller the measurements of the pulps (Fig. 2). The sizes of all five pulps varied with age between 14.31 and 1.7 mm for the 08 s and between 14.05 and 1.3 mm for the 09 s. Other pulpar sizes are documented in Table 5. Comparing the pulp horns, pulp 4 was the largest and pulp 5 was the smallest, except for two teeth (Triadan 109) of age group C, where pulp 3 showed the smallest size. Whilst young teeth showed wide pulpar size variations, the range of size differences regarding all pulps became smaller with increasing age; this is visualised by the boxes in Fig. 4. There was no significant difference in the pulpar dimensions between both sides of the maxilla. Significant differences were measurable for the same pulp horn position in all teeth by comparing of the pulp sizes between age group A and C. Pulp 4 also showed a significantly smaller pulpar size between group A and B (Fig. 3). The percentage reduction of mean pulpar size comparing both age classes was between 40 (for all P5) and 56% (for all P4). Pulpar size decrease was smaller considering the same comparisons between the pulps of group B and C, with values ranging from 42 (P3, P2) to 53% (Fig. 4).

Common pulp chambers

The common pulp chambers (CPCs) were evaluated in dorsally orientated PDW sequences of MR images. A CPC was encountered in all cheek teeth of age group A (n = 12). The median dental age for these cheek teeth was 2.025 years and the maximum age was 3.75 years. Cheek teeth of the other age groups showed no CPC.

Positional relations between the maxillary sinus and the dental alveoli

Only two dental alveoli (upper 08 s of age group A) out of all 36 cheek teeth were not located below the maxillary sinus. Positional relations of the structures could be seen in both imaging modalities. Whilst CT images highlighted the bony alveoli, the MRI scans delineated the differentiation of sinus and alveolus through the hyperintense periodontal ligament (PDL) and the sinus mucosa. Eight of the 34 teeth roots located within the boundaries of the sinus cavity were only located below the maxillary sinus with their caudal aspect (08 s), including pulp horn 2 and 4. Fifty percent of these teeth (n = 4) partly contacting the sinus floor contained a CPC. The percentage of teeth that were positioned below the maxillary sinus with all five pulps (n = 26) consists of 08 s (n = 8) and 09 s (n = 18).

Age-related changes of the infraorbital canal and its distance to the dental alveoli

Age-related changes of the IOC were analysed in transverse CT scans showing the positional relation between tooth and bony canal, on the one hand, and the canals' shape, on the other (Fig. 1b). Where the bony IOC was not in contact with the alveolar bone, it was oval-shaped and held in position by a free bone bridge. If the cheek tooth alveolus and the IOC were in close contact, the bony canal was irregularly shaped. Age-related positional changes of the IOC could be measured (Fig. 5). Two teeth roots (both 08 s) of the youngest horse in group A showed direct contact with the IOC, but the distance

Table 4 Calculated dental age of the upper 08 s and 09 s related to the horses' age

Age group	Horses' age in years	Dental age in years: 08 s (n)	Dental age in years: 09 s (n)
A	< 6	< 2.5 (6)	< 5.5 (6)
B	6–15	2.5–12.5 (6)	5.5–15.5 (6)
C	≥ 16	≥ 12.5 (6)	≥ 15.5 (6)

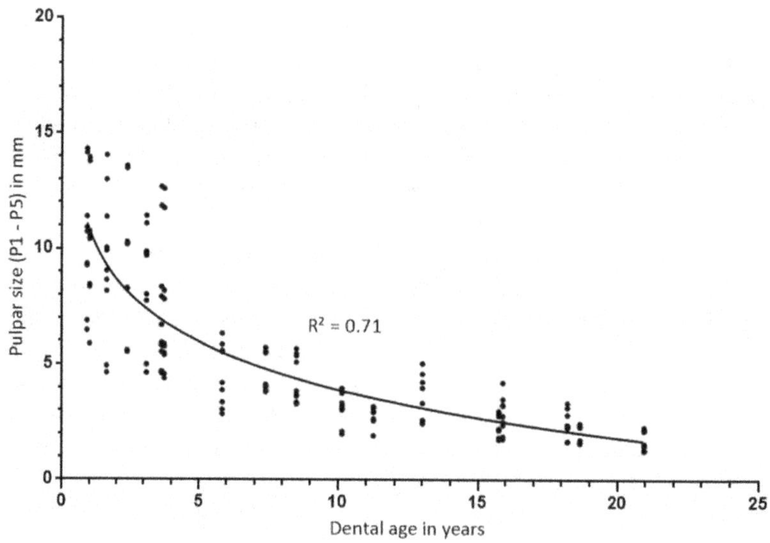

Fig. 2 Semi-logarithmic scale of age-related pulp horn sizes (pulp 1 - pulp 5). Pulps were measured in the mid-tooth section of the maxillary 08 s and 09 s in MR image scans (PDw, dorsal orientation); P1-P5: Pulp horn 1–5

between dental alveolus and IOC increased with dental age. The increase in distance in 88% could be explained by dental aging (R^2 = 0.88). There was no significant difference between both sides of the maxilla.

Discussion

Imaging modalities

As detailed evaluation of the internal and periodontal structures of the cheek teeth is important in deciding on treatment when pulpar or apical infection occurs [35], CT and MR images have been acquired in the present study, aiming to highlight the best imaging modality for each structure. The overview of the two techniques on the same head allows a direct comparison of the potential of both. There are several studies published in equine medicine describing the qualities of CT or MRI for the diagnosis of head pathologies without comparison of both techniques [1–6] and with lower MRI field strength of 0.5 to 1.5 T [17, 25, 36].

The image quality of MRI in the present study was comparable to that of CT, but was better for bony tissues in CT and for soft tissues in MRI. The present results correspond with the findings of Gerlach et al. [36] and Kaminsky et al. [10], who proved the excellent quality of MRI in portraying the dental pulp, PDL, bone-marrow, gingiva, facial soft tissue, sinus mucosa, infraorbital nerve and vessels, owing to a high water content and hydrogen atoms. There was no detectable MRI signal from hard dental tissues, cortical bone, lamina dura and the IOC, whereas these structures could be visualised with good detail resolution by CT acquisition. The best MR image quality in the present study could be achieved with T2w scans for an anatomical overview and with PDw or STIR scans for more detailed images; this is in line with the findings of Kraft and Gavin [37], where T2w, STIR and PDw scans appeared superior to T1w scans in all images evaluated. This is related to the thinner slice thickness of the 3D T1w sequences, which are more often affected by artefacts compared to the transversal and dorsal orientated sequences of the STIR, PD and T2 weighted images with thicker slices.

Compared to low-field tomography, 3.0 T MRI has a higher signal-to-noise ratio, leading to better resolution. Consequently, sequences can be taken with a lower

Table 5 Pulp parameters. MRI measurements were conducted in the mid-tooth section of the upper maxillary 08 s and 09 s. Results show pulp parameters independent of age; n = number of pulp horns; P1-P5: Pulp 1–5

	P1	P2	P3	P4	P5
n	35	36	34	36	36
Mean (mm)	4.89	5.81	5.57	7.32	3.45
s.d. (mm)	2.59	3.26	3.42	4.78	1.65
Median (mm)	3.89	3.75	5.24	5.67	3.17
Range (mm)	7.15	8.76	10.09	13.02	5.30
$x_{min} - x_{max}$ (mm)	2.19–9.34	2.16–0.91	1.3–11.39	1.28–14.31	1.57–6.87

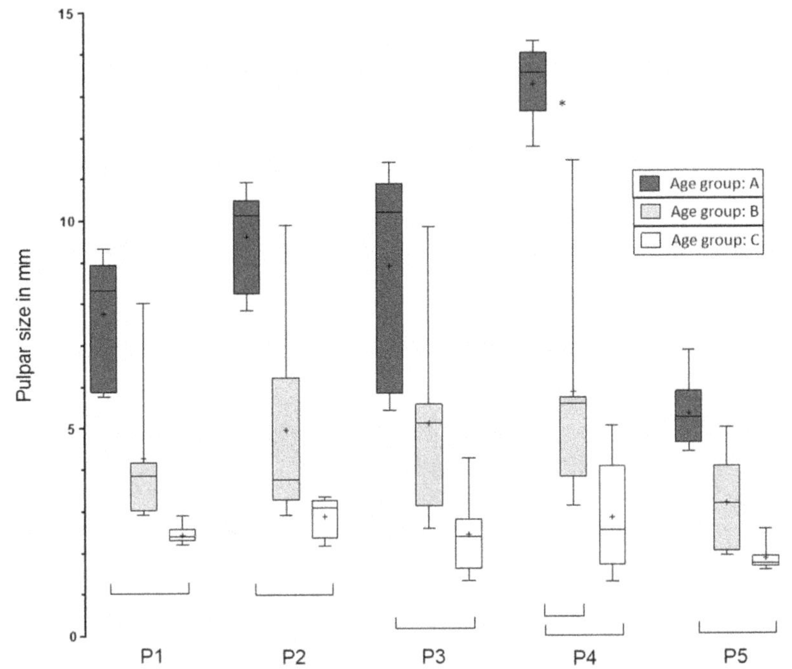

Fig. 3 Pulp measurements of MR images in different age groups. Examination was performed with PDw scans. Horizontal whiskers represent statistically significant differences in size between pulp horns. Boxes represent the interquartile range, vertical whiskers the range and "+" show mean in all boxplots; P1-P5: pulp horn 1–5

recording time and equal image quality compared to low-field MRI. The time for general anaesthesia for patients can be shortened and anaesthesia risk is reduced [38, 39]. The time required for imaging examination in the present study differed greatly between MRI and CT and between the different MRI scans. The CT was around 18 times faster than the entire MRI examination, due to the different imaging techniques and various MRI scans. The long MRI examination times were chosen to acquire images of excellent quality in the current study.

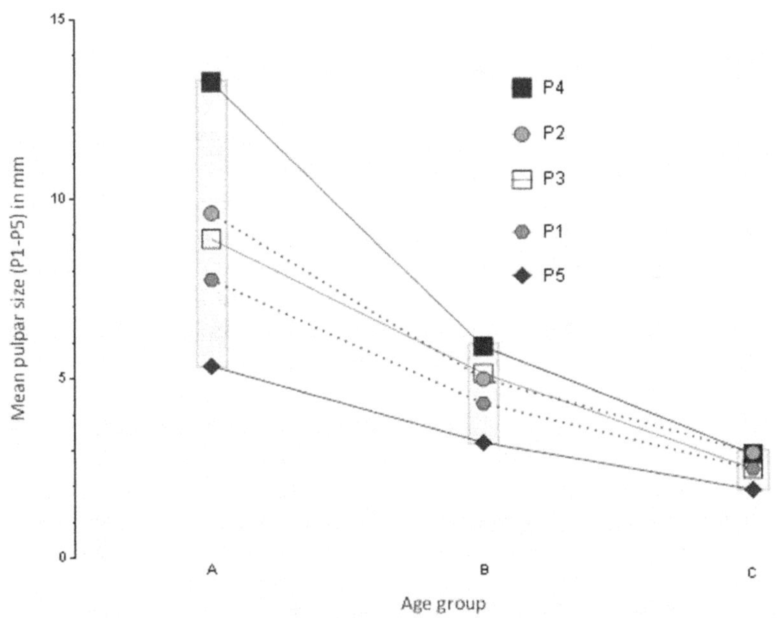

Fig. 4 Different mean reduction of each pulp between different age groups. Mean pulpar sizes presented in different age groups, measured in dorsally orientated MRI scans. Boxes show the range between the mean largest and smallest pulp in each age group. P1 – P5 present pulp horn 1 to pulp horn 5

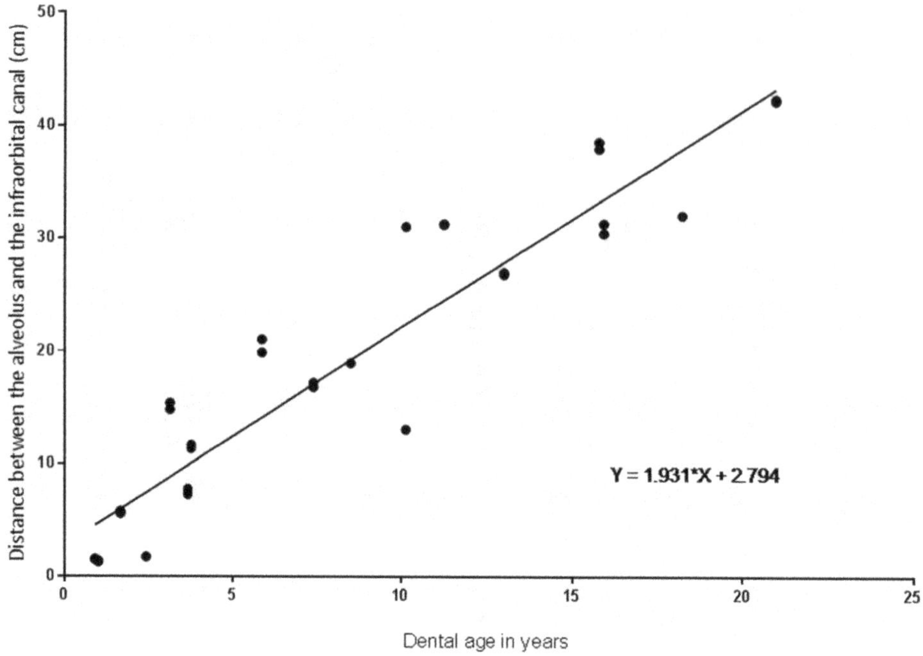

Fig. 5 Age-related distance between selected cheek teeth (n = 36) and the IOC. Scatterplot of the distance between dental alveoli of 08 s and 09 s and the bony IOC measured in transverse CT images

The number of image alignments (transverse, dorsally orientated), resolution, or FOV might be decreased for clinical use to reduce scan time.

Due to the differences in the alignment of teeth [40], the MR images obtained could include artefacts, because image alignment was chosen for the entire skull and not for each tooth. Finally, some pulps and PDLs appeared blurry only due to image angulation (T2w, PDw, STIR) in the current study, that might be mistaken for pathology [17]. The alignment for each tooth would take more time and anaesthetic risk in clinical patients would increase due to longer examination times [41]. T1w images with 3D datasets offer an exception: through MPR, this technique provides the possibility of producing image planes in alignment with the teeth depicted. The time for image acquisition in T1w sequences is prolonged in high-field MRI, as T1 relaxation time is longer [38]. Therefore, a short acquisition time for T1w images, as was applied in the current study, is always accompanied by worse image quality compared to the T2w scans.

In contrast to MRI, CT provides the possibility of different angulations through subsequent MPR and, thus, the potential to evaluate the dental and periodontal changes in alignment of every single tooth. Nevertheless, CT also shows limitations, as it is less useful in identifying early changes in the pulp [42] due to its inability to visualise soft tissues as excellently as T2w or PDw images.

Selected cheek teeth

As described in the literature, dental pathologies such as apical infections, dental fractures and infundibular caries occur predominantly in certain maxillary cheek teeth [43]. The upper 08 s and 09 s show clinical signs most frequently [44–46] and, therefore, they were chosen for examination in the current study.

Selected age groups

The planning of surgical procedures in cases of dental and associated pathologies requires accurate anatomical knowledge and imaging of the cheek teeth and adjacent structures, which are illustrated in this study. Selected equine groups of different ages were chosen in our study as dental changes can be influenced by morphological, functional and mechanical changes, which occur with increasing age [47]: Equine cheek teeth show second dentition and real longitudinal growth up to the horse's age of five years (Group A in the current study); afterwards, the tooth length decreases as teeth are pulled out of the alveoli in the oral direction and the cheek teeth abrasion continues (Group B in our study: 6–15 years) [48, 49]. In older horses (Group C from an age of 15 years onwards), cheek teeth have an exposition to higher dental forces [50]. All these aspects might influence changes of dental structures (e.g. pulpar size) or positional relations between dental and periodontal structures, which were examined in the current study.

Regarding the preselected horse groups (resulting in preselected dental age groups), the present evaluations should be treated with considerable caution: due to the small size of the study population, age distribution and image interpretation might not comply with the entire equine population.

Age-related variances

Common pulp chamber

It can be assumed that CPCs are more common in younger teeth [51], which is in line with the current results, as CPCs were displayed in all teeth evaluated of age group A with a mean dental age of 2.25 years. Dacre et al. [32] located a CPC in teeth with a mean dental age of 2 years (via microscopic examination), whereas Kopke et al. [52] stated the maxillary CPC to be evident in teeth with a mean dental age of 4 years (in high resolution micro-CT scans). While CT [28] and MRI studies [25] observed a CPC in cheek teeth up to 6 years and with micro-CT even up the dental age of 9 years [52] in the present study, the oldest teeth showing a CPC had a dental age of 3.75 years. The difference in results could be caused by the different imaging techniques, imaging settings or measuring techniques. More precise results could probably be achieved by micro-CT scans and histological investigations.

Pulps

Anatomical examinations of the endodontic system by Baker [53] and Dacre et al. [32], as well as MRI [25] and CT [28] imaging studies revealed a general pattern of five pulp horns in the maxillary 08 s and 09 s. These findings comply with the results of the current study, where five main pulp horns (P1-P5) were visible in 33 cheek teeth in the CT and MR images. Three out of all 36 cheek teeth evaluated showed only four pulps.

Contrary to the histological findings of Shaw et al. [54], which displayed an increase in pulpar sizes between 3.5- and 7-year-old teeth, the MRI measurements in the current study showed a continual reduction in size with age. This is consistent with MRI [25] and CT [28] studies demonstrating pulpar reduction with age. The reasons for the pulpar size decrease can be found in age-related physiological pulp modifications. Young equine pulp tissue consists of odontoblasts, connective tissue, nerves, vessels and different cell types. Attachment of secondary dentine is detected and the vital cell number decreases with age [51]. As secondary dentine contains fewer protons, the pulp appears smaller in older equine cheek teeth in the MR images. In the CT images, pulpar tissue does not appears as well delineated as in the MRI scans. Therefore, pulpar existence, dimension and pathologies might not be detected as well with CT imaging as in the MRI scans. Finally, both imaging modalities, CT and MRI, seem to be inferior to histological examinations, which could be the reason for different pulpar dimensions found by Shaw et al. [54] and in imaging studies such as the current one.

In the present study, three pulps could not be measured in the MR images: one pulp was missing completely in each of the 09 s affected (Age group B: n = 1; Age group C: n = 2). All three teeth with one missing pulp in the MRI scans showed a higher attenuated or a gas spot-filled pulp in the CT scans. Missing pulps have been described by Gasse et al. [55], who carried out research on pulpar changes of the 07 s and 09 s in horses of different ages. Due to the expansion and proliferation of secondary dentine, the number of vital pulps is reduced in horses aged between 15 and 23 years. Fewer hydrogen atoms might result in less pulp detection in MRI scans and secondary dentine might be the explanation for higher attenuated pulps in the CT images of the current study.

Reasons for the absence of pulp in the MRI scans can also be found in pathogenic mechanisms that become visible comparing both imaging techniques. Whilst the MRI showed no causes for the absence of the pulp, CT revealed indications for infundibular and pulpar gas spots that can be interpreted as infundibular caries in the 09 s affecting the pulp horn. While Veraa et al. [56] and Bühler et al. [43] argued that infundibular changes often appear as a singular dental change in CT without significant relationship with pulpitis, Dacre et al. [57] describe infundibular changes which can cause and result in pulpitis, collapsing into the adjacent pulp. Inflammatory cells proliferate as a consequence of the pulpitis, which leads to varied pulp capillary blood flow, arteriovenous anastomoses and ischemic necrosis of the pulp [58]. Finally, this initiates the reduction of pulp size through the production of tertiary dentine [59], decreasing the pulpar visibility in MRI.

Other processes, such as dental trauma [43] or haematogenous pulp infection [47], can result in secondary pulpitis. In addition to pulp stones, histologically referred to as intra-pulpar calcified structures without tubular configuration [32], all these mechanisms can cause decreased vascularity of the pulp itself [60], pulpar infection and destruction, and its inability to be visualised in MR images.

It is described in other studies that the pulps sometimes underwent an occlusal insult, resulting in occlusal necrosis and the production of repairing tertiary dentine, but more apically the horns were vital [57]. This is the reason that all dorsally orientated MRI section planes should be assessed and reviewed for vital pulp tissue.

As a pathologically decreased or missing pulp in MRI does not always allow any conclusions regarding the aetiopathogenesis [17], evaluation of the adjacent structures complemented by CT imaging of bony and hard dental structures and occlusal surfaces is important.

Although all the horses examined appeared to be clinically healthy in terms of their teeth, the missing pulps (MRI) or infundibular gas spots (CT) might be an indicator for the start of dental pathology.

Distance between dental alveoli and the maxillary sinus and the infraorbital canal

Precise anatomical knowledge is essential for the evaluation of dental ascending infections and planning of surgical procedures. If a tooth with apical infection is located within the boundaries of the sinus cavity and induces a sinusitis, treatment of the sinus affected may be indicated [61].

Various declarations referring to the contact between teeth and paranasal sinuses due to inter-individual skull anatomy and age-related variances exist in the literature. While Hillmann [62] revealed that only the last three cheek teeth are in contact with the sinus floor, Dyce et al. [63] mentioned that the last premolar tooth's alveolus is also in contact in young horses. In the current study, 94% of Triadan 08 and 09 showed contact with the maxillary sinus floor. The results obtained correspond to the increased risk of inducing secondary sinusitis in apically infected 08 s and 09 s that is described in literature [64].

Both the one-year-old teeth of Triadan 08 which did not show any contact with the sinus floor had direct contact to the IOC. If the IOC is in close contact with an infected tooth, local bony necrosis could occur due to facilitated expansion of proteolytic enzymes [65]. The distance between the alveoli of 08 s and 09 s and the IOC increased by an average of 1.9 mm per year with age. While a five-year-old tooth shows about 12 mm to the IOC, the distance is measured at 41 mm for a 20-year-old 08 or 09. Infraorbital nerve trauma, associated with neuritis and headshaking, is described as a complication of surgical tooth extraction and sinustomy [66]. Knowledge of the IOC's position, as outlined above, can be essential for the prevention of these complications.

Conclusions

The present study provides information about the dental and periodontal age-related morphology and its visibility via different imaging techniques in clinically healthy horses. Both 3 T MRI and CT provide a valuable tool for the visualisation and detection of dental and adjacent tissues. Both modalities complement each other, because MRI highlights soft dental and adjacent soft tissues and CT depicts hard dental and bony surrounding structures. The results aid in evaluating CT and MR images and in choosing the superior imaging modality. Although MRI is not applied as a routine diagnostic measure in dental pathologies, it provides some advantages that could be used for the detection of pulpar changes or before endodontic procedures. Future investigation is warranted to prove the opportunities of detecting and distinguishing pathological processes comparing MR and CT imaging. Knowledge about the age-related positional relations of the maxillary 08 s and 09 s and their adjacent structures expanded with imaging modalities (MRI, CT) might help to evaluate further clinical cases. False positive or negative results of dental pathologies can be avoided through optimal 3D imaging. Additionally, intra- or postoperative complications, such as IOC damage, can be prevented, as surgical planning is optimised.

Abbreviations

3D: three dimensional; CPC: Common pulp chamber; CT: Computed tomography; e.g.: exempli gratia = for example; FOV: Field of view; IOC: Infraorbital canal; ISS: Inter-slice spacing; min: minutes; MPR: Multiplanar reconstruction; MR: Magnetic resonance; MRI: Magnetic resonance imaging; PDL: Periodontal ligament; PDw: Proton density weighted; pulp 1–5: pulp horn 1–5: P1-P5; ROI: Region of interest; ST: Slice thickness; STIR: Short-time-inversion-recovery; T1w: T1 weighted; T2w: T2 weighted; TE: Echo time; TR: Repetition time; WL: Window level; WW: Window width

Consent to publish

Not applicable.

Authors' contributions

CS designed the study, optimised CT settings, acquired CT and MR data, analysed data, performed measurements and wrote the manuscript. MH supported and supervised the CT and MR data acquisition. AB and MH contributed to the study design, data and image analysis and interpretation of both. AB advised CS in dental nomenclature and preparing the manuscript. BO contributed to the study design. KR proofed the statistical analysis which CS performed. All authors read and approved the final manuscript.

Competing interests

None of the authors have any personal or financial relationships which could inappropriately influence or bias the content of this paper.

Author details

[1]Clinic for Horses, University of Veterinary Medicine Hannover, Foundation, Buenteweg 9, 30559 Hannover, Germany. [2]Institute for Veterinary Biometry and Epidemiology, University of Veterinary Medicine Hannover, Foundation, Buenteweg 2, 30559 Hannover, Germany.

References

1. Tremaine WH, Dixon PM. A long-term study of 277 cases of equine sinonasal disease. Part 1: details of horses, historical, clinical and ancillary diagnostic findings. Equine Vet J. 2001;33:274–82.
2. Hirschfelder U, Hirschfelder H. Imaging of the form and structure of the mandible by computed tomography. Fortschr Kieferorthop. 1985;46:138–48.
3. Fuhrmann R, Wehrbein H, Diedrich P: Dreidimensionale computertomographische Darstellung des bezahnten Alveolarkamms Fortschr Kieferorthop 1993;54:91–100.
4. Ordinola-Zapata R, Bramante CM, Duarte MH, Fernandes LMR, Camargo EJ, de Moraes IG, Bernardineli N, Vivan RR, Capelozza ALA, Garcia RB. The influence of cone-beam computed tomography and periapical radiographic evaluation on the assessment of periapical bone destruction in dog's teeth. Oral Surg Oral Med Oral Pathol Oral Radiol Endod. 2011;112:272–9.

5. Moore MP, Gavin PR, Kraft SL, DeHaan CE, Leathers CW, Dorn RV. MR, CT and clinical features from four dogs with nasal tumors involving the rostral cerebrum. Vet Radiol. 1991;32:19–25.
6. Arencibia A, Vazquez JM, Jaber R, Gil F, Ramirez JA, Rivero M. Magnetic resonance imaging and cross sectional anatomy of the normal equine sinuses and nasal passages. Vet Radiol Ultrasound. 2000;41:313–9.
7. Tucker RL, Sampson SN. Magnetic resonance imaging protocols for the horse. Clin Tech Equine Pract. 2007;6:2–15.
8. Bienert A. Digitalradiographische, computertomographische und mikrobiologische Untersuchungen bei Backenzahnerkrankungen des Pferdes. Dissertation. Hannover: Tierärztliche Hochschule Hannover; 2002.
9. Gerlach K, Gerhards H. Magnetresonanztomographische Merkmale von Zubildungen im Bereich der Nase, Nasennebenhöhlen und der angrenzenden Knochen: retrospektive Analyse von 33 Pferden. Pferdeheilkunde. 2008;24:565–76.
10. Kaminsky J, Bienert-Zeit A, Hellige M, Ohnesorge B. 3 tesla magnetic resonance imaging of the equine nasal cavities, paranasal sinuses and adjacent anatomical structures in 13 healthy horses. Pferdeheilkunde. 2014; 29:183–8.
11. Barbee DD, Allen JR, Gavin PR. Computed tomography in horses. Vet Radiol. 1987;28:144–51.
12. Newton CW, Hoen MM, Goodis HE, Johnson BR, McClanahan SB. Identify and determine the metrics, hierarchy, and predictive value of all the parameters and/or methods used during endodontic diagnosis. J Endod. 2009;35:1635–44.
13. Tymofiyeva O, Boldt J, Rottner K, Schmid F, Richter EJ, Jakob PM. High-resolution 3D magnetic resonance imaging and quantification of carious lesions and dental pulp in vivo. MAGMA. 2009;22:365–74.
14. Gaudino C, Cosgarea R, Heiland S, Csernus R, Beomonte Zobel B, Pham M, Kim TS, Bendszus M, Rohde S. MR-imaging of teeth and periodontal apparatus: an experimental study comparing high-resolution MRI with MDCT and CBCT. Eur Radiol. 2011;21:2575–83.
15. Idiyatullin D, Corum C, Moeller S, Prasad HS, Garwood M, Nixdorf DR. Dental MRI: making the invisible visible. J Endod. 2011;37:745–52.
16. Assaf AT, Zrnc TA, Remus CC, Schönfeld M, Habermann CR, Riecke B, Friedrich RE, Fiehler J, Heiland M, Sedlacik J. Evaluation of four different optimized magnetic-resonance-imaging sequences for visualization of dental and maxillo-mandibular structures at 3 T. J Craniomaxillofac Surg. 2014;42:1356–63.
17. Gerlach K, Ludewig E, Brehm W, Gerhards H, Delling U. Magnetic resonance imaging of pulp in normal and diseased equine cheek teeth. Vet Radiol Ultrasound. 2013;54:48–53.
18. Şener S, Akgünlü F. MRI characteristics of anterior disc displacement with and without reduction. Dentomaxillofac Radiol. 2014;33:245–52.
19. Orhan K, Nishiyama H, Tadashi S, Shumei M, Furukawa S. MR of 2270 TMJs: prevalence of radiographic presence of otomastoiditis in temporomandibular joint disorders. Eur J Radiol. 2005;55:102–7.
20. Nasel C, Gahleitner A, Breitenseher M, Czerny C, Glaser C, Solar P, Imho H. Localization of the mandibular neurovascular bundle using dental magnetic resonance imaging. Dentomaxillofac Radiol. 1998;27:305–7.
21. Kress B, Gottschalk A, Anders L, Stippich C, Palm F, Bähren W, Sartor K. High-resolution dental magnetic resonance imaging of inferior alveolar nerve responses to the extraction of third molars. Eur Radiol. 2004;14:1416–20.
22. Krasny A, Krasny N, Prescher A. Anatomic variations of neural canal structures of the mandible observed by 3-tesla magnetic resonance imaging. J Comput Assist Tomogr. 2012;36:150–3.
23. Tymofiyeva O, Proff PC, Rottner K, Düring M, Jakob PM, Richter EJ. Diagnosis of dental abnormalities in children using 3-dimensional magnetic resonance imaging. J Oral Maxillofac Surg 2013;71:1159–1169.
24. Geibel M, Schreiber E, Bracher A, Hell E, Ulrici J, Sailer L, Ozpeynirci Y, Rasche V. Assessment of apical periodontitis by MRI: a feasibility study. RöFo. 2015; 187:269–75.
25. Illenberger N, Brehm W, Ludewig E, Gerlach K. Darstellung altersabhängiger Veränderungen der Zahnpulpen ausgewählter Oberkieferbackenzähne des Pferdes mittels Magnetresonanztomographie. Pferdeheilkunde. 2013;29:183–8.
26. Gerlach K, Flatz K, Brehm W, Seeger J. Klinische Anatomie des Gesichtsbereiches des Pferdes in der Magnetresonanztomographie. Pferdeheilkunde. 2009;25:45–52.
27. Katti G, Ara SA, Shireen A. Magnetic resonance imaging (MRI)–a review. Internat J Dent Clin. 2011;3:65–70.
28. Windley Z, Weller R, Tremaine WH, Perkins JD. Two- and three-dimensional computed tomographic anatomy of the enamel, infundibulae and pulp of 126 equine cheek teeth. Part 2: findings in teeth with macroscopic occlusal or computed tomographic lesions. Equine Vet J. 2009;41:441–7.
29. Lundström T, Wattle O. Description of a technique for orthograde endodontic treatment of equine cheek teeth with apical infections. Equine Vet Educ. 2016;28:1–12.
30. Baker GJ. Dental decay and endodontic disease. In: Baker GJ, Easley J, editors. Equine dentistry. 1st ed. London: WB Saunders; 1999. p. 79–84.
31. Floyd M. The modified Triadan system: nomenclature for veterinary dentistry. J Vet Dent. 1991;8:18–9.
32. Dacre IT, Kempson S, Dixon PM. Pathological studies of cheek teeth apical infections in the horse. 1. Normal endodontic anatomy and dentinal structure of equine cheek teeth. Vet J. 2008;178:311–20.
33. Nickel R, Schummer A, Seiferle E. Eingeweide. Lehrbuch der Anatomie der Haustiere. 2nd ed. Stuttgart: Georg Thieme Verlag; 2004.
34. Du Toit N, Kempson SA, Dixon PM: Donkey dental anatomy. Part 1: gross and computed axial tomography examinations. Vet J 2008, 176:338–344.
35. Manso-Díaz G, García-López JM, Maranda L, Taeymans O. The role of head computed tomography in equine practice. Equine Vet Educ. 2015;27:136–45.
36. Gerlach K, Brehm W, Gerhards W, Ludewig E. Diagnostik von Erkrankungen der Backenzähne des Pferdes mittels Magnetresonanztomographie. Pferdeheilkunde. 2011;27:711–8.
37. Kraft SL, Gavin P. Physical principles and technical considerations for equine computed tomography and magnetic resonance imaging. Vet Clin North Am Equine Pract. 2001;17:115–30.
38. Merkle EM, Dale BM. Abdominal MRI at 3.0 T: the basics revisited. AJR Am J Roentgenol. 2006;186:1524–32.
39. Weishaupt D, Köchli VD, Marincek B. And Borut Marincek. Wie funktioniert MRI. 6th ed. Heidelberg: Springer Medizin Verlag; 2009.
40. Dixon PM. Du ToitN: dental anatomy. In: Easley J, Dixon PM, Schumacher J, editors. Equine dentistry. 3rd ed. Philadelphia: WB Saunders; 2011. p. 25–48.
41. Johnston GM, Eastment JK, Wood JLN, Taylor PM. The confidential enquiry into perioperative equine fatalities (CEPEF): mortality results of phases 1 and 2. Vet Anaesth Analg. 2002;29:159–70.
42. Casey MB, Pearson GR, Perkins JD, Tremaine WH. Gross, computed tomographic and histological findings in mandibular cheek teeth extracted from horses with clinical signs of pulpitis due to apical infection. Equine Vet J. 2015;47:557–67.
43. Bühler M, Fürst A, Lewis FI, Kummer M, Ohlerth S. Computed tomographic features of apical infection of equine maxillary cheek teeth: a retrospective study of 49 horses. Equine Vet J. 2014;46:468–73.
44. Staszyk C, Lehmann F, Bienert A, Ludwig K, Gasse H. Measurement of masticatory forces in the horse. Pferdeheilkunde. 2006;22:12–6.
45. Dacre I, Kempson S, Dixon PM. Equine idiopathic cheek teeth fractures. Part 1: pathological studies on 35 fractured cheek teeth. Equine Vet J. 2007;39:310–8.
46. Staszyk C. Anatomie. In: Vogt C, editor. Lehrbuch der Zahnheilkunde beim Pferd. 1st ed. Stuttgart: Schattauer; 2011. p. 1–29.
47. Dixon PM, Dacre I. A review of equine dental disorders. Vet J. 2005;169:165–87.
48. Becker E: Zähne. In: Joest E, editors. Handbuch der speziellen pathologischen Anatomie der Haustiere. Berlin-Hamburg: Paul Parey Verlag; 1970. p. 83–278.
49. Budras KD, Röck S. Atlas der Anatomie des Pferdes. 3rd ed. Schlütersche: Hannover; 1997.
50. Cordes V, Gardemin M, Lüpke M, Seifert H, Borchers L, Staszyk C. Finite element analysis in 3-D models of equine cheek teeth. Vet J. 2012;193:391–6.
51. Kirkland KD, Baker GJ, Manfra Marretta S, Eurell JAC, Losonsky JM. Effects of aging on the endodontic system, reserve crown, and the roots of equine mandibular cheek teeth. Am J Vet Res. 1997;57:8–31.
52. Kopke S, Angrisani N, Staszyk C. The dental cavities of equine cheek teeth: three-dimensional reconstructions based on high resolution micro-computed tomography. BMC Vet Res. 2012;8:1–16.
53. Baker GJ. Some aspects of equine dental disease. Equine Vet J. 1970;2:105–10.
54. Shaw DJ, Dacre IT, Dixon PM. Pathological studies of cheek teeth apical infections in the horse: 2. Quantitative measurements in normal equine dentine. Vet J. 2008;178:321–32.
55. Gasse H, Westenberger W, Staszyk C. The endodontic system of equine cheek teeth: a reexamination of pulp horns and root canals in view of age-related physiological differences. Pferdeheilkunde. 2004;20:13–8.

56. Veraa S, Voorhout G, Klein WR. Computed tomography of the upper cheek teeth in horses with infundibular changes and apical infection. Equine Vet J. 2009;41:872–6.
57. Dacre I, Kempson S, Dixon PM. Pathological studies of cheek teeth apical infections in the horse: 5. Aetiopathological findings in 57 apically infected maxillary cheek teeth and histological and ultrastructural findings. Vet J. 2008;178:352–63.
58. Syngcuk K, Trowbridge H. Pulpal reaction to caries and dental procedures. In: Cohen S, Burns RC, editors. Pathways of the pulp. 7th ed. St. Louis: Mosby; 1998. p. 414–33.
59. Dacre IT, Shaw DJ, Dixon PM. Pathological studies of cheek teeth apical infections in the horse: 3. Quantitative measurements of dentine in apically infected cheek teeth. Vet J. 2008;178:333–40.
60. Torneck CD. Dentin-pulp complex. In: Ten Cate AR, editor. Oral histology: development, structure and function. 5th ed. St. Louis: Mosby; 1985. p. 146–82.
61. Brinkschulte M. Morphologische Untersuchung der Apertura nasomaxillaris des Pferdes sowie deren Verzweigung in die Nasennebenhöhlen unter Anwendung dreidimensionaler Rekonstruktion computertomographischer Schnittbildserien. Doctoral dissertation. Hannover: Tierärztliche Hochschule Hannover; 2012.
62. Hillmann DJ. Skull. In: Getty R, editor. Sissons and Grossman's the anatomy of the domestic animals. 5th ed. Philadelphia: WB Saunders; 1975. p. 335–6.
63. Dyce KM, Sack WO, Wensing CJG. Anatomie der Haustiere – Lehrbuch für Studium und Praxis. Stuttgart: Enke; 1997.
64. Henninger W, Frame EM, Willmann M, Simhofer H, Malleczek D, Kneissl SM. CT features of alveolitis and sinusitis in horses. Vet Radiol Ultrasound. 2003; 44:269–76.
65. Waguespack RW, Burba DJ, Moore RM. Surgical site infection and the use of antimicrobials. In: Auer JA, Stick JA, editors. Equine surgery. 3rd ed. Philadelphia: Saunders; 2006. p. 70–87.
66. Gilsenan WF, Getman LM, Parente EJ, Johnson AL. Headshaking in 5 horses after paranasal sinus surgery. Vet Surg. 2014;43:678–84.

6

Appropriate threshold levels of cardiac beat-to-beat variation in semi-automatic analysis of equine ECG recordings

Mette Flethøj[1*], Jørgen K. Kanters[2,3], Philip J. Pedersen[4], Maria M. Haugaard[1], Helena Carstensen[1], Lisbeth H. Olsen[5] and Rikke Buhl[1]

Abstract

Background: Although premature beats are a matter of concern in horses, the interpretation of equine ECG recordings is complicated by a lack of standardized analysis criteria and a limited knowledge of the normal beat-to-beat variation of equine cardiac rhythm. The purpose of this study was to determine the appropriate threshold levels of maximum acceptable deviation of RR intervals in equine ECG analysis, and to evaluate a novel two-step timing algorithm by quantifying the frequency of arrhythmias in a cohort of healthy adult endurance horses.

Results: Beat-to-beat variation differed considerably with heart rate (HR), and an adaptable model consisting of three different HR ranges with separate threshold levels of maximum acceptable RR deviation was consequently defined. For resting HRs <60 beats/min (bpm) the threshold level of RR deviation was set at 20%, for HRs in the intermediate range between 60 and 100 bpm the threshold was 10%, and for exercising HRs >100 bpm, the threshold level was 4%. Supraventricular premature beats represented the most prevalent arrhythmia category with varying frequencies in seven horses at rest (median 7, range 2–86) and six horses during exercise (median 2, range 1–24).

Conclusions: Beat-to-beat variation of equine cardiac rhythm varies according to HR, and threshold levels in equine ECG analysis should be adjusted accordingly. Standardization of the analysis criteria will enable comparisons of studies and follow-up examinations of patients. A small number of supraventricular premature beats appears to be a normal finding in endurance horses. Further studies are required to validate the findings and determine the clinical significance of premature beats in horses.

Keywords: ECG analysis, Heart rate variability, Arrhythmias, Endurance horses

Background

Electrocardiography (ECG) is a valuable tool for the evaluation of cardiac arrhythmias in horses, yet analysis of the equine ECG is complicated by a lack of standardized criteria. Furthermore, the clinical interpretation of analysis results is challenged by limited knowledge of the clinical significance of various arrhythmias [1]. Both supraventricular and ventricular premature beats have raised concerns in equine cardiology as potential initiators of atrial fibrillation [2] and fatal ventricular arrhythmias [3]. In recent years, studies have therefore investigated the occurrence of premature beats in healthy horses [4–8], horses with poor performance [9, 10], and in both clinical [11, 12] and experimental settings [13]. These studies provide valuable information on the *prevalence* of premature beats, although a comparison of the results is problematic due to different study designs. The use of varying analysis criteria and ECG recordings of different duration impedes general conclusions about the *frequency* of premature beats in individual horses from the published studies. At what number, and under which circumstances premature beats become a clinical concern for the horse are questions which therefore remain. Consequently, large-scale frequency studies of equine arrhythmias – standardized in terms of recording duration, exercise intensity, and definitions of arrhythmia – are required.

* Correspondence: flethoj@sund.ku.dk
[1]Department of Large Animal Sciences, Faculty of Health and Medical Sciences, University of Copenhagen, Hoejbakkegaard Allé 5, 2630 Taastrup, Denmark
Full list of author information is available at the end of the article

Many arrhythmias are paroxysmal, and comprehensive evaluation of their frequency therefore requires long-term ECG recording for 24 h or more [14]. This makes ECG analysis very time-consuming and would constitute a substantial obstacle in conducting large-scale studies of equine arrhythmias. In human ECG studies, analysis of long-term recordings is commonly facilitated by automatic detection and classification of arrhythmias based on timing and morphology of ECG complexes [15]. However, no morphology algorithms are available for equine ECG analysis, as these would be impeded by the highly variable equine T-wave morphology. Computerized methods for the analysis of equine ECGs are therefore limited to timing algorithms, identifying beats with abnormal timing by assessing the variation in beat-to-beat intervals against an observer-specified threshold. These timing algorithms are, however, only an aid to the observer, who must still manually classify the arrhythmia category of every rhythm event detected by the algorithm, as well as manually assess the morphology of ECG complexes to identify any possible ectopic beats with normal timing. Nevertheless, with approximately 50,000–60,000 heartbeats in a 24-h ECG recording, timing algorithms represent an invaluable time-saving tool.

The aim of this study was to provide suggestions for a standardized approach to semi-automatic assessment of large equine ECG datasets. In order to achieve this, the following objectives were set: 1) to investigate the beat-to-beat variation of equine cardiac rhythm in order to determine appropriate threshold levels of maximum acceptable RR deviation, and 2) to evaluate a novel two-step timing algorithm for equine ECG analysis by quantifying the frequency of arrhythmias in a cohort of clinically healthy endurance horses both at rest for 24 h, as well as during moderate exercise training.

Methods

Horses

Eleven Arabian breed endurance horses were included in the study: 1 mare, 2 stallions and 8 geldings, with a median age of 11 years (range 8–15 years), and a median body weight of 415 kg (range 359–503 kg). A twelfth horse was excluded (see Results). All horses were in full training at the time of examination and successfully completed an endurance ride ≥80 km within 38 days of the examination (median, range 5–105 days). All horses were considered healthy, based on the performance history obtained from the owner and a clinical examination. A cardiac murmur exceeding grade 2/6 was considered an exclusion criterion [16]. Additionally, standardized echocardiography was used to rule out cardiac pathology [5]. The study conformed to the guidelines for non-invasive ethical animal research as dictated by Danish law (The Animal Experimentation Act 1306 of 23rd Nov 2007). Due to the non-invasive characteristics of the protocol, no blood samples were collected. Written informed consent was obtained from the horse owners.

ECG recordings

All ECG recordings were obtained with a Holter recording system at a sampling frequency of 500Hz.[1] Electrodes were placed in a modified base-apex lead and secured by adhesive foam pads.[2] Two bipolar leads (lead I and II) were recorded by two separate channels and a third lead (lead III) was computed by the Holter system. The ground electrode and the combined negative electrode of leads I and II were placed dorsally over the region of the left scapula. The positive electrode of lead I was placed in the left flank in the middle of the most caudal rib, and the positive electrode of lead II was placed caudomedial to the pectoral muscles and to the left of the ventral midline. Resting ECGs were obtained over a period of 24 h when the horses were confined to their stall or a small paddock. Exercise ECGs were obtained during a regular training session. The exercise protocol included six intervals of increasing velocities: one at walk, two in trot, two in canter and one in gallop. Each interval lasted for 3–10 min, or the equivalent of approximately 3,000 m. This ensured that a wide range of heart rates (HR) were included in the ECG recordings during exercise. The recordings were stored digitally and transferred to a computer using the software provided with the recorder.[1] All ECG recordings were manually reviewed in the first instance to assess the recording quality and the morphology of QRS complexes, so as to detect possible ventricular ectopic beats with normal timing that could potentially be "overlooked" by the timing algorithm later in the process. The RR intervals and associated time points were subsequently exported for further analyses in SAS.[3,4] Sequences with excessive noise and ECG artifact, caused for example by electrode detachment, were excluded separately in SAS, and exclusion of >10% of the recording duration resulted in exclusion of the entire recording. The heart rate was calculated as a moving average of 10 beats (arrhythmic beats excluded), and the mean, minimum and maximum heart rate of every hour of the 24-h ECG recording at rest was assessed. In addition, the following HRV time domain measures were calculated from the 24-h ECG recordings at rest: SDNN = standard deviation of NN (normal RR intervals) calculated over the entire 24-h period, SDANN = standard deviation of the means of NN intervals calculated over all 5-min sequences during the 24-h period, SDNN index = the mean of all 5-min standard deviations of NN, and pNN50 = proportion of successive NN intervals that differed more than 50 ms.

Cardiac beat-to-beat variation

For each individual horse, the percentage RR deviation ($RR_{dev(i)} = (RR_i - RR_{i-1})/RR_{i-1} * 100\%$) was plotted against the RR interval (RR_i) to display the beat-to-beat variation. This RR deviation plot is a modification of a Poincaré plot (RR_{i+1} against RR_i) and therefore results in a main cluster of sinus beats with normal timing around the line of identity [17], which in the case of the RR deviation plot is represented by the horizontal axis ($RR_{dev} = 0$). The margins of this main cluster were then visually assessed for each individual horse and plotted together in one superimposed plot to allow for comparison of the beat-to-beat variation among horses. Based on this superimposed plot, a general threshold model with three different HR ranges was defined: "*Rest*" HR <60 bpm; "*Transition*" HR = 60–100 bpm, and "*Exercise*" >100 bpm. According to the definition of RR deviation, intervals longer than the preceding interval ($RR_i > RR_{i-1}$) resulted in positive values of RR_{dev}, while shorter intervals ($RR_i < RR_{i-1}$) produced negative values of RR_{dev}. Premature beats would therefore obtain negative values of RR_{dev}, and the threshold level of maximum acceptable RR deviation ($RR_{max,dev}$) in each HR range was consequently determined by the largest negative RR deviation observed among the horses.

Two-step timing algorithm

A two-step timing algorithm incorporating the defined threshold model was then elaborated to identify beats with aberrant timing that were suspected of being arrhythmic (Fig. 1):

Step 1

This step served as a preliminary sorting where the beats with the most clearly aberrant timing (characterized by a $|RR_{dev}|$ >40%) were marked as "aberrant". These aberrant RR intervals were temporarily excluded and the remaining RR intervals linked together to create a temporary data series. This prevented excessively long intervals (i.e. blocks and pauses) from interfering with the calculation of a local mean in the next step.

Step 2

A modified Ho-Goldberger algorithm [18] was then run on the temporary data series to point out *additional* aberrant intervals. This algorithm compared each individual interval (RR_i) to a local mean of the four most proximal intervals ($RR_{mean(i)} = (RR_{i-2} + RR_{i-1} + RR_{i+1}RR_{i+2})/4$) against the threshold level of $RR_{max,dev}$. The relevant HR range in the threshold model was determined by $RR_{mean(i)}$ as an indicator of the underlying HR in the sequence.

Classification of arrhythmias

In order to evaluate the performance of the two-step timing algorithm, all RR intervals marked as "aberrant" were traced back to the ECG recordings for manual classification according to the following definitions:

- *Sinoatrial block:* a pause in the cardiac rhythm where the PP interval is equal to a multiple of the baseline PP interval [19].
- *Sinus arrest:* a pause in the cardiac rhythm where the PP interval is *not* a multiple of the baseline PP interval and is more than twice the baseline PP interval (i.e. longer than a sinoatrial block) [19].

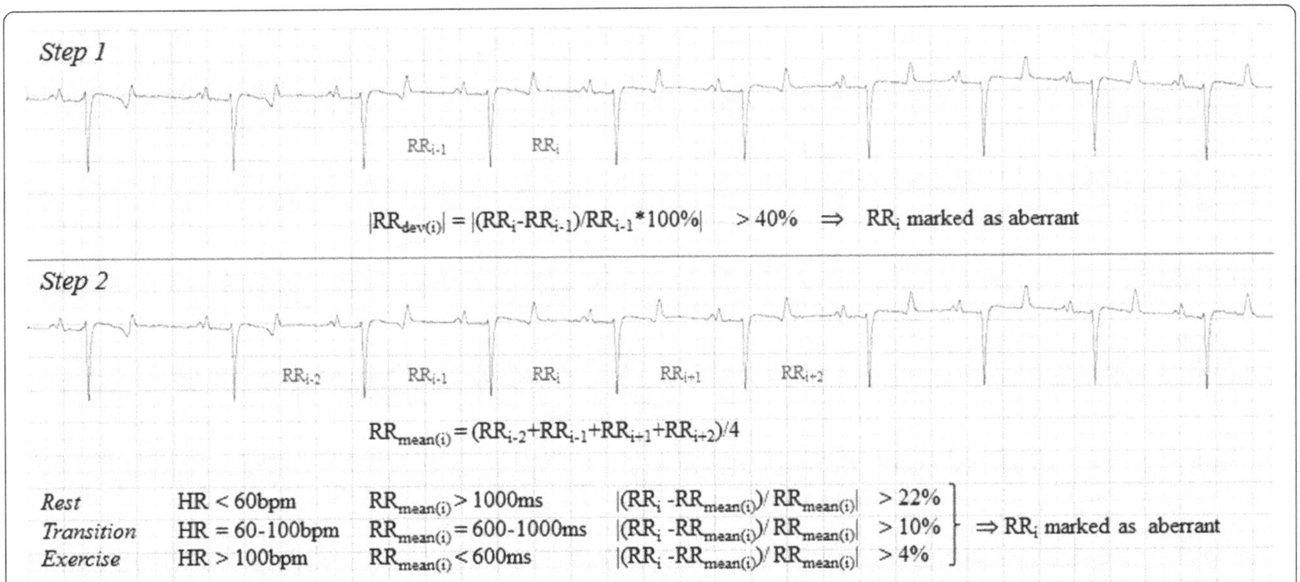

Fig. 1 Schematic presentation of the two-step algorithm

- *Delayed sinus beat:* a pause in the cardiac rhythm that is less than double the baseline PP interval (i.e. shorter than a sinoatrial block).
- *Sinus arrhythmia:* an irregularity of the cardiac rhythm (beyond what can be expected as normal beat-to-beat variation) with variable PP intervals that might show a cyclic pattern [19].
- *Wandering pacemaker:* an alternating P-wave morphology as the pacemaker function shifts between the sinus node and various ectopic foci in the atria [20].
- *2nd degree AV block:* the P wave is not succeeded by a QRS complex, as the electrical impulse is blocked in the AV node [19].
- *Supraventricular premature complex (SVPC):* an ectopic beat of atrial origin occurring too early (premature) according to the threshold of beat-to-beat variation [21]. The P-wave morphology may be changed depending on the location of the ectopic pacemaker. The SVPC might be followed by a *compensatory pause* if the ectopic impulse fails to enter and reset the sinus node [19].
- *Ventricular premature complex (VPC):* an ectopic beat from the ventricular myocardium occurring too early according to the threshold of beat-to-beat variation. The QRS complex is not related to a preceding P-wave and its morphology is often wide and bizarre, depending on the location of the ectopic pacemaker [22]. The VPC is often followed by a *compensatory pause*, but depending on the timing of the ectopic impulse, the VPC may also become *interpolated* between two sinus beats [19]. A special VPC variant is a *fusion beat* which occurs simultaneously with a sinus beat (not premature) [19].
- *False aberrant:* a normal RR interval in sinus rhythm incorrectly marked as aberrant by the two-step algorithm (e.g. due to neighboring arrhythmias).
- *Technical errors:* collective classification of aberrant RR intervals caused by QRS undersensing or ECG artifact.

Statistical analysis

The arrhythmia frequencies of the individual horses were calculated separately for rest and exercise ECG recordings. Values are given as median and range.

Results

One exercise ECG and one resting ECG (from different horses) were excluded from the arrhythmia classification as they were not considered to be of diagnostic quality. A twelfth horse was initially included in the study population, but showed excessive numbers of sinoatrial blocks and sinus arrests of up to 9 s long throughout the 24-h recording at rest. Although the condition resolved during exercise, this horse was suspected of sinus node dysfunction and excluded from the study. The hourly mean, minimum and maximum HR in the ECG recordings at rest is presented in Fig. 2. The HRV time domain measures were as follows (mean ± SD): SDNN was 233 ± 40 ms, SDANN was 160 ± 37 ms, SDNN index was 144 ± 30 ms, and pNN50 was 33 ± 12%. The maximum HR averaged over 10 beats during exercise was 188 bpm (156–209 bpm). Echocardiography revealed trivial aortic regurgitation in three horses, but no other valvular insufficiencies or abnormal cardiac dimensions were observed.

Threshold levels of beat-to-beat variation

The RR deviation plots showed a distinct pattern with a "club-shaped" main cluster surrounded by smaller clusters. Retracing the beats in different clusters to the ECG confirmed that the main cluster represented normal beats in sinus rhythm, while surrounding clusters revealed a consistent beat pattern associated with the different arrhythmia categories (Fig. 3). The club-shaped main cluster had its narrowest part ("the handle") at shorter RR intervals and was gradually enlarged with increasing RR intervals. Additionally, it was slightly asymmetric around the horizontal axis ($RR_{dev} = 0$) with wider dispersion of data points above the axis (Fig. 4). At RR intervals <600 ms (HR >100 bpm), the margins of the main cluster representing the normal RR_{dev} ranged from 3% to 4% in all horses. With intervals of 600-1000 ms (HR = 60–100 bpm), RR_{dev} gradually increased and ranged between 4% and 10% with the largest RR_{dev} at lower HRs. At RR intervals >1000 ms (HR <60 bpm), RR_{dev} showed considerable inter-horse variation and slight asymmetry with peak positive values ranging from 12% to 22% and peak negative values from 10% to 20%. Due to the apparent association between the beat-to-

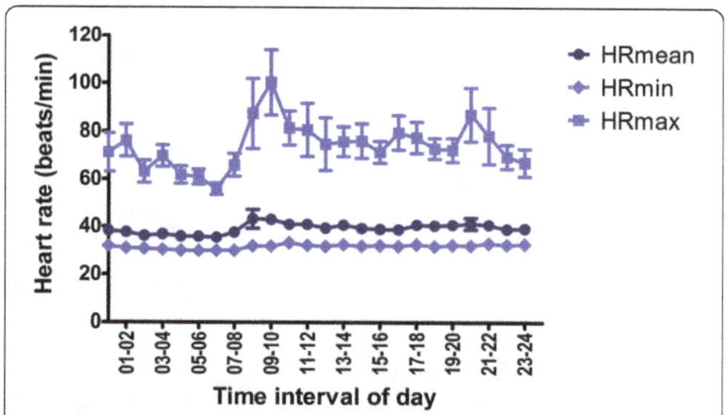

Fig. 2 The hourly heart rate during the 24-h EKG at rest. HRmean; average heart rate. HRmin; minimum heart rate. HRmax; maximum heart rate. Values presented as mean ± SEM

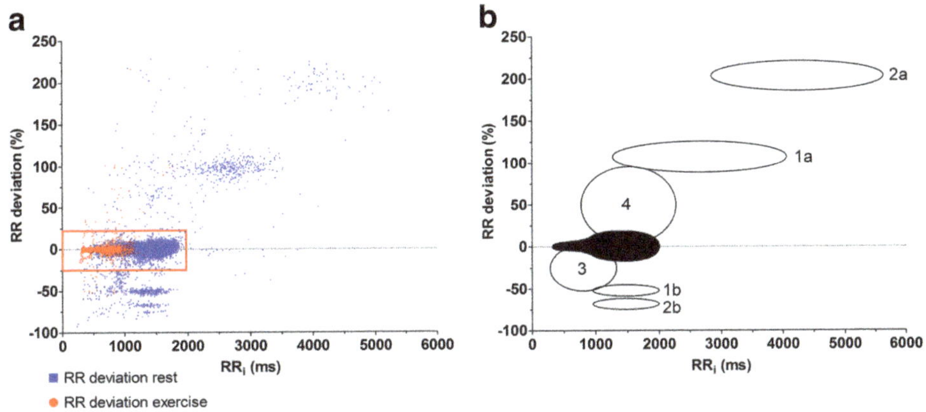

Fig. 3 RR deviation plot (**a**) and schematic presentation of beat patterning (**b**). Notice the main cluster (*red square*) surrounded by smaller clusters. The black area represents the main cluster of normal sinus beats. Area 1a represents sinoatrial blocks, second-degree AV blocks and QRS undersensing with double the length of normal RR intervals and $RR_{dev} \approx 100\%$. Similarly, area 2a describes QRS undersensing of two consecutive complexes. Areas 1b and 2b represent normal RR intervals succeeding the aberrant intervals of areas 1a and 2a and are therefore located below the main cluster with an RR_{dev} of approximately -50% and -66%, respectively. Area 3 refers to premature beats (both supraventricular and ventricular) while area 4 refers to *"Delayed sinus beats"*. Aberrant intervals caused by artifact were scattered throughout the plot

beat variation and HR, three different HR ranges ("Rest" <60 bpm; "Transition" = 60–100 bpm, and "Exercise" >100 bpm) were included in the threshold model. The threshold levels ($RR_{max,dev}$) of each HR range were defined based on the cluster margins described above and were evaluated by a trial-and-error approach, where the threshold value was adjusted multiple times and beats with an RR deviation just below and above the threshold were assessed. The final threshold values were then defined based on these observations and set at 20%, 10%, and 4%, respectively (Fig. 4b).

Arrhythmias

Aberrant intervals marked by the two-step algorithm constituted up to 1.7% of the total number of beats at rest and 3.8% during exercise. Manual classification of these intervals revealed that actual arrhythmias constituted up to 0.4% of the total beats in both the rest and exercise recordings (Table 1). The remaining aberrant intervals were: *delayed sinus beats*; *false aberrants* and *technical errors*. The hourly frequencies of arrhythmias during the 24-h ECG recordings at rest are displayed in Fig. 5. Seven horses had SVPCs in varying numbers (median 7, range 2–86) at rest, and six horses had

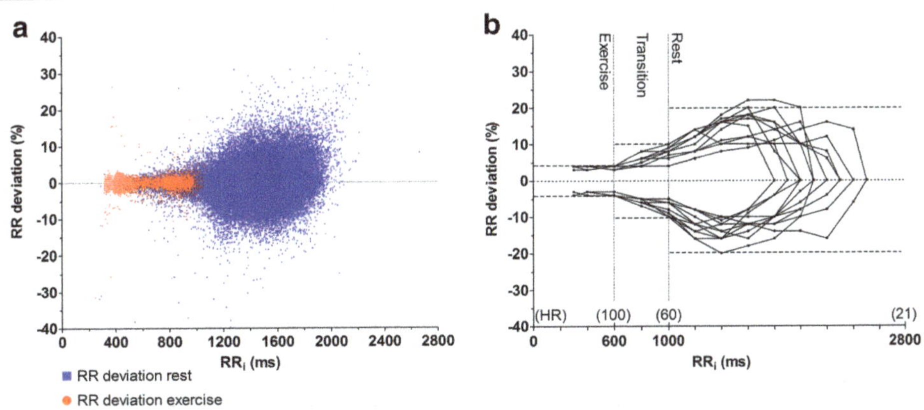

Fig. 4 Zoom in on the main cluster in the RR deviation plot of a representative horse (**a**). The club-shape clearly illustrates that RR intervals at rest (*blue*) show larger RR deviation (RR_{dev}) than RR intervals during exercise (*red*). Notice the slight asymmetry with a larger dispersion of positive values of RR_{dev} at rest. The visually extrapolated margins of the main cluster of individual horses were superimposed for direct comparison (**b**). The dashed lines indicate heart rate ranges and threshold levels of maximum acceptable RR deviation. Note the consistent pattern of small RR_{dev} with little inter-horse variation during exercise, gradual increase of RR_{dev} in the transition from exercise to rest, and large inter-horse variation at rest

Table 1 Frequency distribution of arrhythmias during rest and exercise

			Rest						Exercise	
Horse	Age (years)	Sex	Recording duration (hours)	Sinoatrial block	Sinus arrest	2nd degree AV block	SVPC	VPC	Recording duration (hours)	SVPC
1	11	G	24.0	1	0	0	0	0	1.6	0
2	14	G	23.3	0	0	0	6	0	1.6	1
3	9	G	22.9	0	0	211	7	0	N/A	N/A
4	15	S	N/A	N/A	N/A	N/A	N/A	N/A	1.3	5
5	8	G	24.0	0	0	1	0	0	1.4	1
6	8	G	24.0	7	0	3	4	0	1.8	2
7	15	G	24.0	0	0	0	86[a]	2	1.6	24
8	8	S	22.1	0	0	0	2	0	1.6	0
9	13	G	24.0	13	1	42	69	0	1.4	1
10	9	M	24.0	1	0	3	7	0	1.5	0
11	11	G	24.0	0	0	0	0	0	1.7	0

G gelding, *M* mare, *S* stallion. *SVPC* supraventricular premature complex, *VPC* ventricular premature complex. *N/A* not available. [a]Including three episodes of double SVPCs and one triple SVPC

SVPCs (median 2, range 1–24) during exercise (Fig. 6a–d). The two-step algorithm detected two VPCs (Fig. 6e), and no additional VPCs were detected during the initial manual review. A changed P-wave morphology indicating ectopy could be confirmed in 52% of the SVPCs at rest, and in 6% of the SVPCs during exercise. For the remaining SVPCs, the timing of the beat was the sole indicator of the arrhythmia. Varying P-wave morphology (Fig. 6e) suggesting a wandering pacemaker was observed in five horses, and pacemaker "shifts" occasionally

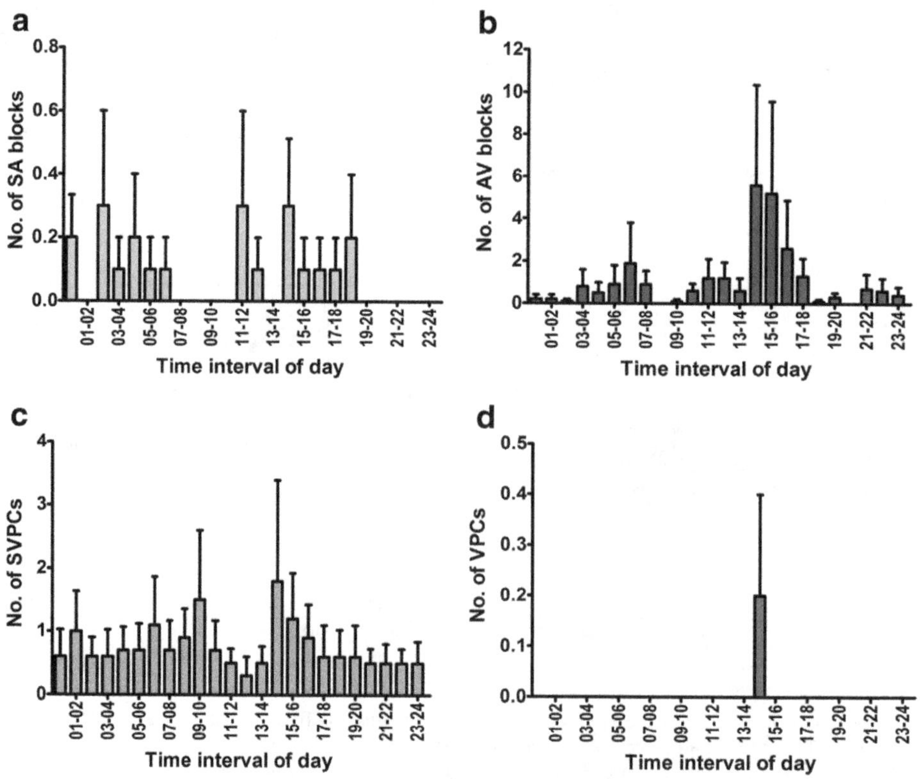

Fig. 5 The hourly frequency of arrhythmias during the 24-h ECG recordings at rest. **a** Sinoatrial (SA) blocks. **b** Second degree atrioventricular (AV) blocks. **c** Supraventricular premature complexes (SVPC). **d** Ventricular premature complexes (VPC). Bars indicate mean ± SEM. Note the different scales

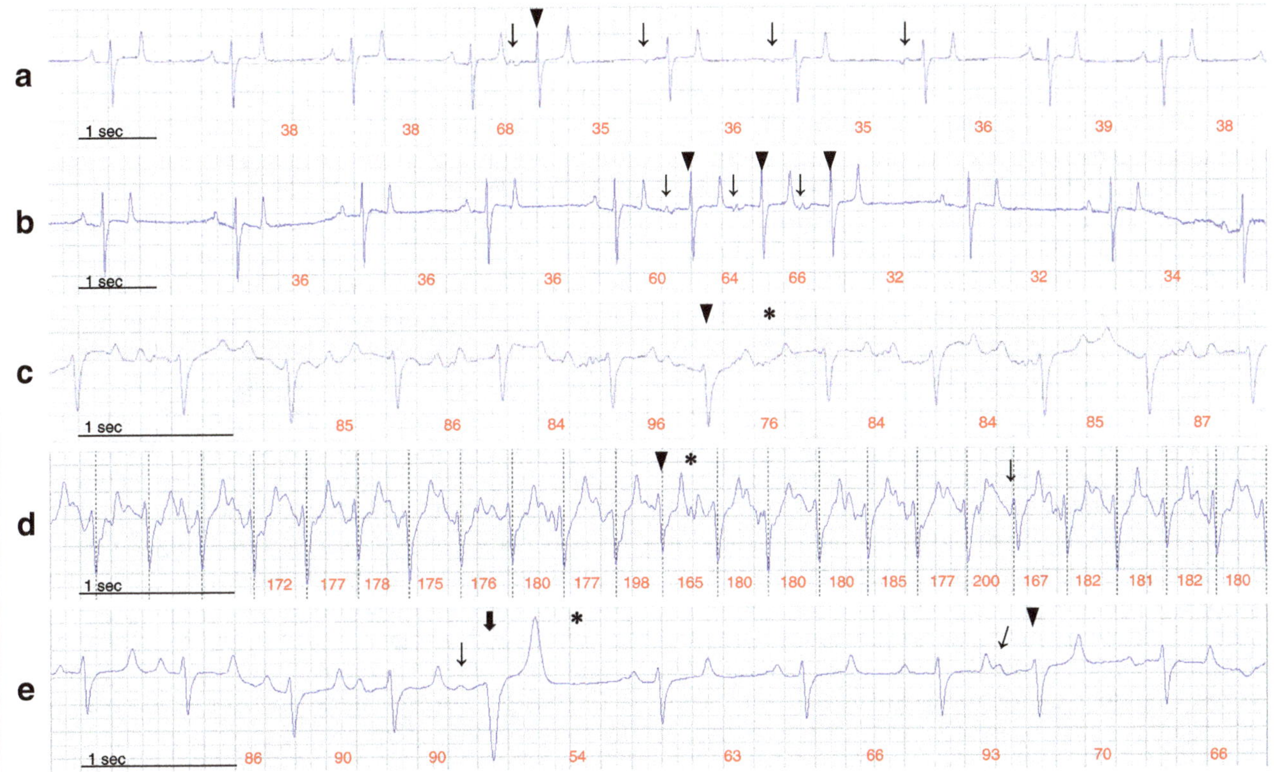

Fig. 6 Premature beats. **a** SVPC (arrowhead) without compensatory pause occurring at rest. Note the transient change in P-wave morphology (arrows). **b** Triple SVPC occurring at rest. Note the abnormal P-wave morphology (arrows). **c** and **d** SVPC (arrowhead) followed by a fully compensatory pause (*) occurring during walk and gallop, respectively. Note the presence of movement artifact on the baseline obscuring the P-wave, and the technical error in triggering the peak R-wave (arrow). **e**) VPC possibly a fusion beat (thick arrow) followed by a compensatory pause (*) and an SVPC (arrowhead) at rest. An abnormal and possibly unconducted P-wave (arrow) precedes the VPC. Note the varying P-wave morphology. The instantaneous heart rate is shown in red

coincided with SVPCs (Fig. 6a) or *"Delayed sinus beats"* (Fig. 7).

Discussion

This study is the first to provide recommendations on threshold levels of beat-to-beat variation for equine ECG analysis, and presents an adaptive model where threshold levels ($RR_{max,dev}$) are adjusted according to HR range. RR deviation is essentially a measure of heart rate variability (HRV), and in contrast to conventional measures of HRV such as SDNN (standard deviation of normal RR intervals), knowledge of the beat-to-beat RR_{dev} can be applied directly to the ECG analysis. The observation that beat-to-beat variation is larger at rest than during exercise agrees with existing knowledge that parasympathetic activity is responsible for equine HRs below 110–130 bpm, and that HRV is positively correlated with parasympathetic activity [23–26].

An interesting observation in the RR_{dev} plot was the asymmetric appearance of the main cluster with wider dispersion of positive values of RR_{dev} at rest (Fig. 4). This asymmetric distribution of RR_{dev} indicates a non-linear component in the beat-to-beat variation of equine cardiac rhythm, where the impulse formation in the

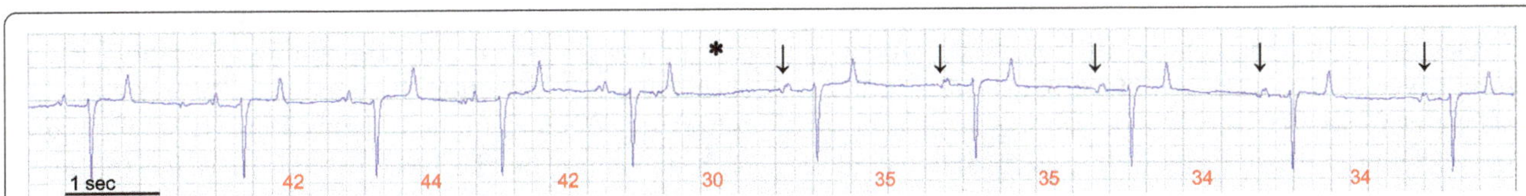

Fig. 7 Delayed sinus beat (*). This beat coincided with a change of pacemaker, indicated by altered P-wave morphology (arrows) in one horse with wandering pacemaker. Note the decrease in instantaneous heart rate (*red* numbers)

sinus node is more tightly regulated with regards to beats that appear "early" than beats that occur "delayed" (cf. the definition of RR_{dev}). Nonlinearity is a well-known trait of human HRV [27], and is rooted in the sympathetic/parasympathetic regulation of cardiac rhythm. In humans, short-term heart rate asymmetry has been shown to be dominated by heart rate decelerations (i.e. prolongations of the RR interval), whereas long-term and total heart rate asymmetry are primarily contributed by accelerations (i.e. RR interval shortenings) [28]. The exact causal mechanisms of heart rate asymmetry are unknown, but it is assumed be regulated by similar factor as HRV. These factors include the baroreceptor reflex and respiratory sinus rhythm modulations, but heart rate asymmetry has furthermore been linked to asymmetry in the myocardial conduction time between the atria and ventricles [29]. It remains unclear how heart rate asymmetry is modulated in horses. However, taking the dominant vagal tone of this species into consideration and the fact that the asymmetry in the RR_{dev} plot was only observed at resting hearts, it could be expected that heart rate deceleration (RR interval prolongations) might be the dominant contributor of both short-term and long-term heart rate asymmetry in horses – although this remains speculations. We chose to define the threshold levels based on the maximum negative peak beat-to-beat variation observed among the horses, in order to optimize the detection of premature beats. However, since the negative peak values of beat-to-beat variation were lower than positive peak values, a number of normal sinus beats with elongated RR intervals (delayed sinus beats) were consequently marked as aberrant. For this reason, traditional timing algorithms were rejected in favor of the Ho-Goldberger algorithm [18], which allows more physiological variation between two consecutive intervals than specified by $RR_{max,dev}$, providing the deviation from the local mean does not exceed the threshold. It is therefore less sensitive to minor physiologic rhythm variations such as sinus arrhythmia and delayed sinus beats, than traditional algorithms, where each RR interval (RR_i) is compared with only the preceding interval (RR_{i-1}). Nevertheless, timing algorithms merely identify beats with aberrant timing that are suspected of being arrhythmic, and the observer must still assess whether the "aberrant" beat is truly arrhythmic or simply caused by physiologic beat-to-beat variation. A higher level of accuracy in the threshold levels used will result in a more reliable timing algorithm. The algorithm presented in this study was very sensitive, and a number of the RR intervals marked as aberrant were not caused by actual arrhythmias, but instead by ECG artifacts, QRS undersensing or physiologic sinus arrhythmia (these beats were classified as technical errors, false aberrant or delayed sinus beat). However, ectopic beats could potentially go unnoticed should they occur within the "normal timing" defined by the $RR_{max,dev}$ (as is the case for *fusion beats*). Ideally, the observer should therefore evaluate the morphology of every single complex to check for undetected ectopic beats. This is relatively straightforward with beats of ventricular origin since they commonly have an unusual appearance (with the exception of those originating from the AV nodal area – i.e. *junctional beats* [22]). However, validation of the number of detected SVPCs is more complicated since the ectopic nature of these beats often cannot be confirmed by altered P-wave morphology. Without verifiable changes of the P-wave, it can be difficult to distinguish SVPCs from physiologic rhythm variations. Conversely, in horses with wandering pacemaker, a change of pacemaker can be associated with a shift in impulse rate and thereby mimic an SVPC (Fig. 6a). A number of beats classified as SVPCs in this study with obscured P waves were followed by a compensatory pause, and it is possible that some of these beats might actually be of ventricular origin, despite the normal appearance of the QRS complex. Other authors have refrained from classifying such "*isolated premature cycles*" as either supraventricular or ventricular which might be a more appropriate approach [7]. This again illustrates the need for more standardized analysis criteria in the assessment of equine ECGs.

Although a predisposition to arrhythmias has been demonstrated in human endurance athletes [30, 31], no studies have evaluated the occurrence of arrhythmias in endurance horses. The limited number of horses examined in this study is not sufficient to provide prevalence or frequency estimates for the general population. However, in agreement with previous studies in other types of horses [4–6, 8], the results suggest that SVPCs are relatively common in endurance horses. As stated in the Introduction, the appropriate clinical question is therefore related more to the *frequency* of premature beats in a given time period or under specific circumstances (e.g. exercise) than to their *prevalence*. However, the existing diverse study designs with inconsistent or inadequate definitions of premature timing prevent general conclusions on this matter. One human study has suggested a "normal range" for both SVPCs and VPCs of up to 200 per 24 h [32], though considering the low frequency of premature beats observed in this study, extrapolating this suggestion to horses is questionable. Large-scale frequency studies of arrhythmias in horses are therefore required.

The study presented here should be considered as a first practical step in defining suitable threshold values of normal RR deviation in equine ECG analysis. The cohort of horses examined in this study is small, and as such, it cannot be the basis of standards for the horse population in general. A number of limitations should therefore be addressed in future studies, and further investigations will require a larger number of animals in order to determine if the results can be extrapolated to larger populations and other breeds of horses. Ideally, future studies should also include a separate population for validation of the results. The ECG recording system used in this study is limited to three ECG leads. The P-wave morphology of an ectopic beat will therefore not necessarily appear abnormal on the surface ECG. Using more ECG leads from different angles could improve depiction of the P wave and thereby facilitate the classification of arrhythmias. Finally, it would be beneficial to include information on electrolyte levels and cardiac markers in the clinical evaluation of the horses.

Conclusions

This study presents a novel approach to semi-automatic ECG analysis in horses, with recommendations on threshold levels of beat-to-beat variation and a novel two-step timing algorithm which takes the physiological rhythm variation into account. Furthermore, the study provides preliminary results on arrhythmia frequencies in endurance horses during both rest and moderate exercise. The presented approach should be validated in a larger population of horses, but could be beneficial in future large-scale frequency studies which aim to determine the clinical significance of various arrhythmias in horses.

Endnotes

[1]Televet 100, Engel Engineering Services GmbH, Heusenstamm, Germany

[2]Animal Polster, Snøgg AS, Kristiansand, Norway

[3]Microsoft Excel 2010, Microsoft Corp, Redmond, WA, USA

[4]SAS Enterprise Guide 6.1, SAS Institute, Cary, NC, USA

Abbreviations

Bpm: Beats per minute; HR: Heart rate; HRV: Heart rate variability; RR_{dev}: Deviation of RR intervals; $RR_{max,dev}$: Maximum acceptable deviation of RR intervals

Acknowledgements

The horse owners are thanked for their participation in the study.

Funding

The study was funded by University of Copenhagen, Denmark.

Authors' contributions

MF planned the study, collected/analyzed the data and wrote the paper. JKK contributed to the data analyses and supervised the manuscript. PJP contributed to the data analyses. MMH participated in the planning and design of the study. HC contributed to the manuscript preparation. LHO supervised and edited the manuscript. RB supervised the entire project and contributed to the planning of the study and manuscript preparation. All authors read and approved the final manuscript.

Competing interests

R. Buhl is Associate editor of BMC Veterinary Research. None of the authors of this paper otherwise has a financial or personal relationship with other individuals or organizations that could inappropriately influence or bias the content of the paper.

Consent for publication

Not applicable.

Author details

[1]Department of Large Animal Sciences, Faculty of Health and Medical Sciences, University of Copenhagen, Hoejbakkegaard Allé 5, 2630 Taastrup, Denmark. [2]Laboratory of Experimental Cardiology, Department of Biomedical Sciences, Faculty of Health and Medical Sciences, University of Copenhagen, Blegdamsvej 3B, 2200 Copenhagen N, Denmark. [3]Department of Cardiology, Herlev & Gentofte University Hospitals, Copenhagen, Denmark. [4]Department of Veterinary Clinical and Animal Sciences, Faculty of Health and Medical Sciences, University of Copenhagen, Dyrlaegevej 100, 1870 Frederiksberg C, Denmark. [5]Department of Veterinary Disease Biology, Faculty of Health and Medical Sciences, University of Copenhagen, Groennegaardsvej 15, 1870 Frederiksberg C, Denmark.

References

1. Reef VB, Bonagura J, Buhl R, McGurrin MKJ, Schwarzwald CC, van Loon G, Young LE. Recommendations for Management of Equine Athletes with Cardiovascular Abnormalities. J Vet Intern Med. 2014;28(3):749–61.
2. Hiraga A, Kubo K. Two cases of paroxysmal atrial fibrillation during exercise in horses. Equine Vet Educ. 1999;11(1):6–10.
3. Lyle CH, Uzal FA, McGorum BC, Aida H, Blissitt KJ, Case JT, Charles JT, Gardner I, Horadagoda N, Kusano K, et al. Sudden death in racing Thoroughbred horses: An international multicentre study of post mortem findings. Equine Vet J. 2011;43(3):324–31.
4. Ryan N, Marr CM, McGladdery AJ. Survey of cardiac arrhythmias during submaximal and maximal exercise in Thoroughbred racehorses. Equine Vet J. 2005;37(3):265–8.
5. Barbesgaard L, Buhl R, Meldgaard C. Prevalence of exercise-associated arrhythmias in normal performing dressage horses. Equine Vet J. 2010;42:202–7.
6. Buhl R, Meldgaard C, Barbesgaard L. Cardiac arrhythmias in clinically healthy showjumping horses. Equine Vet J. 2010;42:196–201.
7. Physick-Sheard PW, McGurrin MKJ. Ventricular Arrhythmias during Race Recovery in Standardbred Racehorses and Associations with Autonomic Activity. J Vet Intern Med. 2010;24(5):1158–66.
8. Buhl R, Petersen EE, Lindholm M, Bak L, Nostell K. Cardiac Arrhythmias in Standardbreds During and After Racing—Possible Association Between Heart Size, Valvular Regurgitations, and Arrhythmias. J Equine Vet Sci. 2013;33(8):590–6.
9. Martin Jr BB, Reef VB, Parente EJ, Sage AD. Causes of poor performance of horses during training, racing, or showing: 348 cases (1992-1996). J Am Vet Med Assoc. 2000;216(4):554–8.
10. Jose-Cunilleras E, Young LE, Newton JR, Marlin DJ. Cardiac arrhythmias during and after treadmill exercise in poorly performing Thoroughbred racehorses. Equine Vet J. 2006;38(S36):163–70.
11. Morgan RA, Raftery AG, Cripps P, Senior JM, McGowan CM. The prevalence and nature of cardiac arrhythmias in horses following general anaesthesia and surgery. Acta Vet Scand. 2011;53:62.
12. Verheyen T, Decloedt A, De Clercq D, van Loon G. Cardiac changes in horses with atypical myopathy. J Vet Intern Med. 2012;26(4):1019–26.
13. Nostell K, Brojer J, Hoglund K, Edner A, Haggstrom J. Cardiac troponin I and the occurrence of cardiac arrhythmias in horses with experimentally induced endotoxaemia. Vet J. 2012;192:171–5.
14. Bass EB, Curtiss EI, Arena VC, Hanusa BH, Cecchetti A, Karpf M, Kapoor WN. The duration of Holter monitoring in patients with syncope. Is 24 h enough? Arch Intern Med. 1990;150(5):1073–8.
15. de Chazal P, O'Dwyer M, Reilly RB. Automatic classification of heartbeats using ECG morphology and heartbeat interval features. IEEE Trans Biomed Eng. 2004;51(7):1196–206.
16. Young LE, Wood JLN. Effect of age and training on murmurs of atrioventricular valvular regurgitation in young Thoroughbreds. Equine Vet J. 2000;32(3):195–9.

17. Esperer HD, Esperer C, Cohen RJ. Cardiac arrhythmias imprint specific signatures on Lorenz plots. Ann Noninvasive Electrocardiol. 2008;13(1):44–60.
18. Ho KK, Moody GB, Peng CK, Mietus JE, Larson MG, Levy D, Goldberger AL. Predicting survival in heart failure case and control subjects by use of fully automated methods for deriving nonlinear and conventional indices of heart rate dynamics. Circulation. 1997;96(3):842–8.
19. Verheyen T, Decloedt A, De Clercq D, Deprez P, Sys SU, van Loon G. Eletrocardiography in horses - part 2: how to read the equine ECG. Vlaams Diergeneeskundig Tijdschrift. 2010;79:337–44.
20. Kiryu K, Kaneko M, Satoh H. Cardiopathological observations on histopathogenesis of wandering pacemaker in horses. Nihon Juigaku Zasshi. 1978;40(2):131–40.
21. Miller MS, Bonagura JD. Atrial arrhythmias. J Equine Vet Sci. 1985;5(5):300–4.
22. Bonagura JD, Miller MS. Junctional and ventricular arrhythmias. J Equine Vet Sci. 1985;5(6):347–50.
23. Hamlin RL, Klepinger WL, Gilpin KW, Smith CR. Autonomic control of heart rate in the horse. Am J Physiol. 1972;222:976–8.
24. Kuwahara M, Hashimoto S-i, Ishii K, Yagi Y, Hada T, Hiraga A, Kai M, Kubo K, Oki H, Tsubone H, et al. Assessment of autonomic nervous function by power spectral analysis of heart rate variability in the horse. J Auton Nerv Syst. 1996;60(1-2):43–8.
25. Ohmura H, Hiraga A, Aida H, Kuwahara M, Tsubone H. Effects of repeated atropine injection on heart rate variability in Thoroughbred horses. J Vet Med Sci. 2001;63(12):1359–60.
26. Physick-Sheard PW, Marlin DJ, Thornhill R, Schroter RC. Frequency domain analysis of heart rate variability in horses at rest and during exercise. Equine Vet J. 2000;32(3):253–62.
27. Kanters JK, Højgaard MV, Agner E, Holstein-Rathlou NH. Short- and long-term variations in non-linear dynamics of heart rate variability. Cardiovasc Res. 1996;31(3):400–9.
28. Piskorski J, Guzik P. Asymmetric properties of long-term and total heart rate variability. Med Biol Eng Comput. 2011;49(11):1289–97.
29. Guzik P, Zuchowski B, Blaszyk K, Seniuk W, Wasniewski M, Gwizdala A, Wykretowicz A, Piskorski J. Asymmetry of the variability of heart rate and conduction time between atria and ventricles. Circ J. 2013;77(12):2904–11.
30. Andersen K, Farahmand B, Ahlbom A, Held C, Ljunghall S, Michaelsson K, Sundstrom J. Risk of arrhythmias in 52 755 long-distance cross-country skiers: a cohort study. Eur Heart J. 2013;34(47):3624–31.
31. Molina L, Mont L, Marrugat J, Berruezo A, Brugada J, Bruguera J, Rebato C, Elosua R. Long-term endurance sport practice increases the incidence of lone atrial fibrillation in men: a follow-up study. Europace. 2008;10(5):618–23.
32. Bjerregaard P. Premature beats in healthy subjects 40-79 years of age. Eur Heart J. 1982;3(6):493–503.

7

Evaluation of microRNA expression in plasma and skeletal muscle of thoroughbred racehorses in training

B. A. McGivney[1], M. E. Griffin[2], K. F. Gough[1], C. L. McGivney[1], J. A. Browne[1], E. W. Hill[1] and L. M. Katz[2*]

Abstract

Background: Circulating miRNAs (ci-miRNAs) are endogenous, non-coding RNAs emerging as potential diagnostic biomarkers. Equine miRNAs have been previously identified including subsets of tissue-specific miRNAs. In order to investigate ci-miRNAs as diagnostic tools, normal patterns of expression for different scenarios including responses to exercise need to be identified. Human studies have demonstrated that many ci-miRNAs are up-regulated following exercise with changes in expression patterns in skeletal muscle. However, technical challenges such as haemolysis impact on accurate plasma ci-miRNA quantification, with haemolysis often occurring naturally in horses following moderate-to-intense exercise. The objectives of this study were to identify plasma ci-miRNA profiles and skeletal muscle miRNAs before and after exercise in Thoroughbreds (Tb), and to evaluate for the presence and effect of haemolysis on plasma ci-miRNA determination. Resting and post-exercise plasma ci-miRNA profiles and haemolysis were evaluated in twenty 3 year-old Tbs in sprint training. Resting and post-exercise skeletal muscle miRNA abundance was evaluated in a second cohort of eleven 2 year-old Tbs just entering sprint training. Haemolysis was further quantified in resting blood samples from twelve Tbs in sprint training. A human plasma panel containing 179 miRNAs was used for profiling, with haemolysis assessed spectrophotometrically. Data was analysed using a paired Student's *t*-test and Pearson's rank correlation.

Results: Plasma ci-miRNA data for 13/20 horses and all skeletal muscle miRNA data passed quality control. From plasma, 52/179 miRNAs were detected at both time-points. Haemolysis levels were greater than the threshold for accurate quantification of ci-miRNAs in 18/25 resting and all post-exercise plasma samples. Positive correlations ($P < 0.05$) between haemolysis and miRNA abundance were detected for all but 4 miRNAs, so exercise-induced changes in plasma ci-miRNA expression could not be quantified. In skeletal muscle samples, 97/179 miRNAs were detected with 5 miRNAs (miR-21-5p, let-7d-3p, let-7d-5p, miR-30b-5p, miR-30e-5p) differentially expressed (DE, $P < 0.05$) between time-points.

Conclusions: The degree of haemolysis needs to be determined prior to quantifying plasma ci-miRNA expression from horses in high-intensity exercise training. Identification of DE miRNAs in skeletal muscle indicates modification of miRNA expression may contribute to adaptive training responses in Tbs. Using a human plasma panel likely limited detection of equine-specific miRNAs.

Keywords: Horse, miRNA, Exercise, Plasma, Haemolysis, Skeletal muscle

* Correspondence: lisa.katz@ucd.ie
[2]UCD School of Veterinary Medicine, Section of Veterinary Biomedical Sciences, University College Dublin, Belfield, Dublin 4, Ireland
Full list of author information is available at the end of the article

Background

MicroRNAs (miRNAs) are endogenous, non-coding RNAs with complex roles causing translational repression/degradation of bound mRNA [1], regulating many cellular processes [2]. They have intracellular effects, are extremely stable when secreted into the bloodstream [3] and have been identified in multiple body fluids [4]. MiRNAs are often tissue-specific and can be secreted from their tissue of origin into the bloodstream bound to lipoproteins [5] or packaged into extracellular microparticles [6]. When in blood they are termed circulating miRNAs (ci-miRNAs) [7] and are emerging as potential diagnostic biomarkers due to their stability [8] and ease of access for sample collection.

Human studies have identified a multitude of ci-miRNAs up-regulated following intense exercise training [9–12]. Furthermore, exercise training has been found to alter the expression pattern of miRNAs in skeletal muscle [11, 13, 14]. It has been hypothesised that skeletal muscle may contribute to changes in differentially expressed (DE) ci-miRNAs in response to exercise training by releasing exosomes into plasma [15, 16], supporting the possibility that DE plasma ci-miRNAs could be used to assess adaptive training responses of skeletal muscle.

MiRNA analysis in horses is an emerging area of research. To-date, >700 equine miRNAs have been identified with subsets of tissue-specific DE miRNAs isolated [17] including skeletal muscle and blood [18, 19]. Recently, 197 miRNAs were identified in equine skeletal muscle, with 76 found to be muscle-specific [20]. However, to-date there has only been one study evaluating ci-MRNA in exercising horses [21]. In this report, 167 DE miRNAs were identified from pre- and post-endurance exercise blood samples; however, whole-blood rather than plasma/serum was evaluated making it difficult to determine if ci-miRNAs were expressed from red blood cells (RBC) or other tissue sites such as skeletal muscle.

There are technical challenges involved in plasma/serum ci-miRNA measurement such as inaccurately quantifying plasma RNA due to low yields, haemolysis impacting on ci-miRNA quantification and a lack of validated stable reference miRNAs [22–25]. Since haemolysis may occur naturally in horses following moderate-to-intense exercise [26, 27], this needs to be considered when attempting to evaluate equine plasma/serum ci-miRNA expression.

The aim was to identify DE plasma ci-miRNAs and skeletal muscle miRNAs before and after exercise in Thoroughbreds (Tb), and to evaluate for the presence and effect of haemolysis on plasma ci-miRNA determination.

Methods

A Department of Health License (B100/3525), ethical approval from the University College Dublin Animal Research Ethics Committee and owner consent were obtained for all horses and procedures in this study.

Sample population

All horses in the study were from the same stable and were managed and trained in a similar way [28]. Horses trained 6 days per week with gradual introduction of 800–1000 m sprint training (work day [WD]) alternating with submaximal training, following which horses entered competitive racing.

Experimental protocol

Cohort A: Plasma ci-miRNA

Plasma lactate concentrations ([LA]) and ci-miRNA were evaluated in $n = 20$ sex- and fitness-matched 3 year-old Tbs ($n = 10$ males, $n = 10$ females) in active training and racing before (T_0) and 5 mins after (T_{5min}) a WD training session. The degree of haemolysis was evaluated in all samples.

Cohort B: Skeletal muscle miRNA

Resting (T_0) and T_{5min} plasma [LA] along with T_0 and 4 h (T_{4hr}) post-exercise skeletal muscle miRNAs were evaluated in $n = 11$ 2 year-old Tbs ($n = 7$ males, $n = 4$ females) before and after their first WD training session.

Cohort C: Degree of plasma haemolysis

The degree of haemolysis was further evaluated in T_0 plasma samples from an additional $n = 12$ Tbs in active training and racing ($n = 5$ males, $n = 7$ females, 2–4 years old).

Data collection

Prior to an exercise test horses were fitted with a heart rate (HR) telemetry system[1] and GPS unit[2] which recorded speed, HR and distance.

Resting jugular venous blood samples were collected before feeding and exercise. Samples for plasma [LA] and ci-miRNA measurement were placed into fluoride oxalate and ethylenediamine tetraacetic acid (EDTA) tubes, respectively. Once collected all blood tubes were immediately centrifuged with plasma separated. [LA] was measured on-site with an autoanalyser.[3] Plasma for haemoglobin concentrations [Hb] and ci-miRNA analysis was stored at 4 °C until transported to be stored at -80 °C (within 6 h of collection) and analysed as a batch at a later date.

Blood samples for miRNA

MiRNAs were extracted from plasma samples[4] with 4 μL amounts then reversely transcribed in 20 μL reactions.[5] Exogenous RNA spike-ins (UniSp2, UniSp4, UniSp5, cel-miR-39-3p) provided by the manufacturer of the human serum/plasma focus miRNA PCR panel kit were added during RNA extraction and analysed according to the manufacturer's instructions[5].

Haemolysis analysis

The degree of haemolysis was assessed by quantifying plasma [Hb] using a UV/VIS spectrophotometer,[6] measuring oxyhaemoglobin absorbance at k = 414 nm [22]. A value of ≤0.2 absorption units (AU) was used as the threshold for acceptable haemolysis and accurate quantification of ci-miRNA detection [22].

Skeletal muscle biopsy samples for miRNA

Skeletal muscle biopsies were obtained from the *gluteus medius* using a 6 mm-diameter, modified Bergstrom biopsy needle[7] according to previously described methods [29]. Samples were preserved in RNAlater[8] until further processing.

Total RNA was extracted from 50 to 100 mg of tissue using a protocol combining TRIzol reagent,[9] DNase treatment[10] and RNeasy.[11] RNA was quantified using a Qubit fluorimeter with the Qubit RNA HS assay. RNA quality was assessed using the 18S/28S ratio and RNA integrity number on an Agilent Bioanalyzer with the RNA 6000 Nano Lab-Chip kit.[12] RNA (2 µL@5 ng/ul) was reversely transcribed in 10 µL reactions[5]. UniSp6 (exogenous RNA spike-in) was added during cDNA conversion.

Real-time quantitative polymerase chain reaction measurements

cDNA was assayed in 10 µL PCR reactions[5]. All miRNAs were assayed once by RT-qPCR on the Exiqon Human Serum/Plasma Focus miRNA PCR panel I and II. Each panel consisted of a 96 well plate with 179 miRNAs of interest and 15 controls (inter-plate calibrators, negative and spike-in controls). Amplification was performed in an Applied Biosystems StepOnePlus™ Real-Time PCR System. Amplification curves were analysed using Applied Biosystems software to obtain raw PCR cycle threshold (C_t) values.

miRNA quantification

Quality control measures (inter-plate calibration, ommission of outliers, miRNAs with C_t values >34 from analysis) were carried out using GeneEx software. MiRNAs with >80% missing data were removed from the analysis, with missing values replaced with the mean value for that miRNA. Results from muscle biopsies were normalised to the global mean.

Statistical analysis

A paired Student's *t*-test was used to compare T_0 and T_{5min} plasma haemolysis and ci-miRNAs and T_0 and T_{4h} muscle miRNA abundance. A Shapiro-Wilk test was performed to confirm that the C_t data was normally distributed and the Benjamini and Hochberg method used to correct for multiple testing. Pearson's rank correlation was used to evaluate correlation between T_0 and T_{5min} ci-miRNA expression level and absorbance at 414 nm, and a paired Student's *t*-test used to assess the significance of that correlation. Significance was set at $P \le 0.05$.

Prediction and annotation of miRNA targets

Prediction of potential target genes and pathway analysis was completed using the DIANA-mirPath software [30] in the Diana Tools suite. The DIANA-microT-CDS algorithm was used to predict potential target genes for DE miRNAs; these were then utilised by miRPath for KEGG pathway analysis, enriched through analysis of all predicted targets. A 0.8 default setting was used as the MicroT prediction score threshold with species set to human since there was no equine option. Since there is a high conservation of miRNAs accross species suggesting the sharing of biological functions, it was believed that inferences could be made on the function of equine miRNAs based on their human homologues. Significance for over-represented KEGG pathways was set as $P \le 0.05$ following Benjamini and Hochberg correction for multiple testing.

Results

Quality control for miRNA quantification

The miRNA data for 7/20 horses from cohort A failed quality control and were omitted from analysis. All samples from cohort B passed quality control.

Physiological exercise parameters

For all horses undertaking an exercise test in the study, the average V_{peak} was 16.9 ± 0.98 m/s (range 15.2–18.5), the average HR_{peak} 221.4 ± 7.1 bpm (range 209–232) and the average total exercise distance 1130.19 ± 145.1 m/s (range 876–1471). The average pre- and 5 mins post-exercise plasma [LA] were 0.46 ± 0.09 mmol/l (range 0.33–0.63) and 26.3 ± 3.68 mmol/l (range 19.2–32.1), respectively. There were no significant differences between males and females regarding any of the exercise and physiological measurements.

Cohort A: Plasma ci-miRNA

In the equine plasma samples, 29% (52/179) of the miRNAs on the human plasma panel were detected at both timepoints, all of which had increased expression (3.23 ± 1.5 fold mean increase, 1.1–10.3 range increase) at T_{5min} when compared to T_0. However, absorbance >0.2 AU at 414 nm were detected in 11/13 T_0 and all T_{5min} plasma samples for horses in cohort A, with absorbance peaks significantly higher in the T_{5min} samples ($P = 1.2^{-05}$; Fig. 1). The T_0 absorbance ranged from

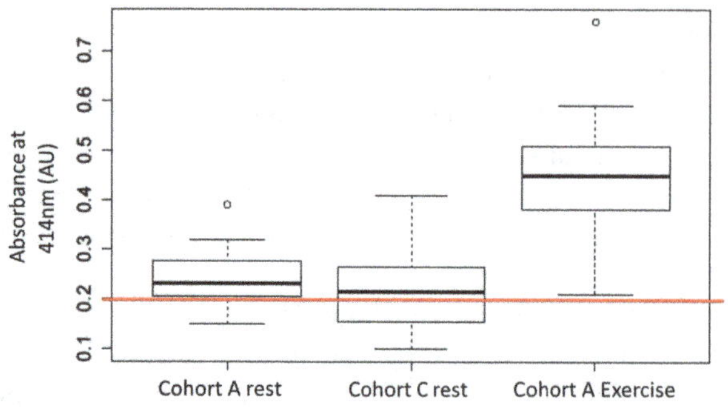

Fig. 1 Box and whiskers plot depicting the degree of haemolysis based on absorbance at 414 nm for $n = 13$ equine plasma samples before and after exercise (cohort A) and from $n = 12$ equine plasma sampes from horses at rest (cohort C). A value of ≤0.2 absorption units was used as the threshold for acceptable haemolysis and accurate quantification of ci-miRNA detection. The red line indicates the threshold above which accurate quantification of ci-miRNA is not possible

0.15–0.39 AU with an average of 0.25 ± 0.06 AU while the T_{5min} values ranged from 0.26–0.76 AU with an average of 0.46 ± 0.13 AU. The expression levels of 35 miRNAs were significantly correlated ($r > 0.55$, $P < 0.05$) with absorbance and thus haemolysis levels in both T_0 and T_{5min} samples while 13 miRNA expression levels were only significantly correlated with haemolysis in T_0 samples; 4 miRNAs were not correlated with haemolysis at either time point. Due to the high levels of haemolysis in the plasma samples and the strong positive correlation between haemolysis and miRNA abundance (Fig. 2), it was not possible to accurately quantify exercise-induced changes in plasma ci-miRNA expression in the present study. There were no significant differences between males and females regarding any of the haemolysis and ci-miRNA measurements.

Cohort B: Skeletal muscle miRNA

In the equine skeletal muscle biopsy samples, 55% (98/179) of the miRNAs on the human plasma panel were detected at both T_0 and T_{4h}. Following the Benjamini and Hochberg correction for multiple testing, 5 of these miRNAs were significantly DE at T_{4h} ($P < 0.05$; Fig. 3). The greatest expression difference was detected in miRNA miR-21-5p which increased 0.92 ± 0.2 fold. The expression of the miR-30b-5p and miR-30e-5p family members increased 0.52 ± 0.1 and 0.64 ± 0.2 fold, respectively. Expression of let-7d-3p and let-7d-5p decreased 0.68 ± 0.1 and 0.44 ± 0.1 fold, respectively. Using the DIANA-microT-CDS algorithm a total of 1687 gene targets for these 5 miRNAs were identified. The largest number of gene targets were identified for the miR-30 family members. In total 1077 of the predicted targets were unique to these 2 miRNAs while only 3 gene targets were predicted for let-7d-3p. The most over-represented KEGG pathways for each miRNA based on a predicted target gene list are summarised in Table 1 [31, 32]. Pathways previously implicated in the equine exercise response were significantly enriched among predicted targets of the DE miRNAs (Table 2). These included the Jak-STAT signaling, MAPK signaling, insulin signaling and mTOR signaling pathways and long-term potentiation.

Cohort C: Degree of plasma haemolysis

The average absorbance at 414 nm for this cohort was 0.21 ± 0.09 AU, ranging from 0.10–0.41 AU (Fig. 1); 7/12 samples had absorbtion peaks >0.2 AU. There was no significant difference in resting haemolysis levels between cohorts A and C, confirming that

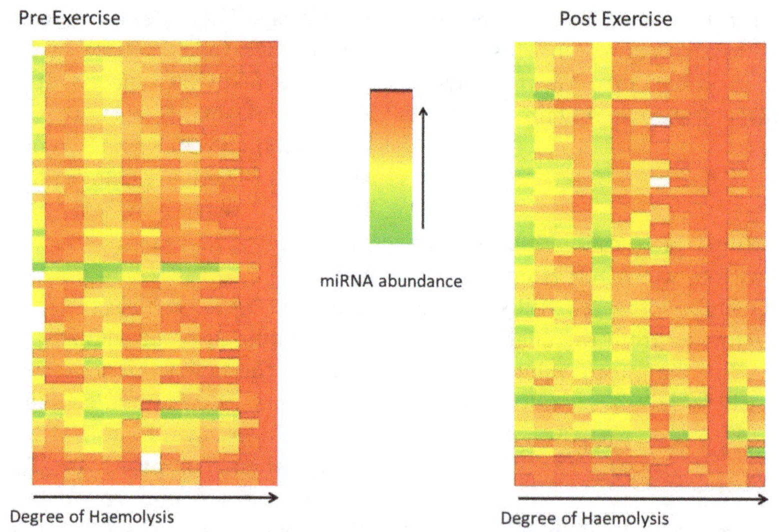

Fig. 2 Heatmap showing the levels of 52 miRNAs relative to the degree of haemolysis from $n = 13$ equine plasma samples before and after exercise. MiRNA abundance is presented as C_t values and degree of haemolysis is the absorbance at 414 nm for each plasma sample

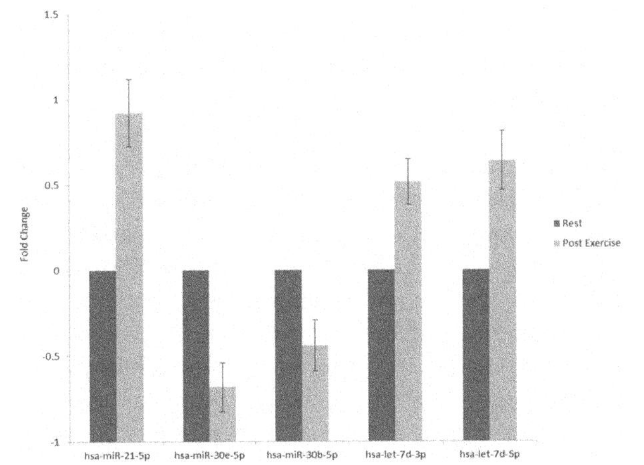

Fig. 3 Real time qRT-PCR results for miRNAs differentially expressed in skeletal muscle before and following exercise from $n = 11$ Thoroughbred horses. The standard 2-ΔΔCT method was used to determine mean fold changes in gene expression. All Ct values were normalised using the global normalisation function in the GeneEx software package. A Student's *t*-test was used to identify significant differences in mRNA abundance between time-points

haemolysis at rest is prevelant in Tb racehorses in high-intensity exercise training.

Discussion

The stability and ease of access for collecting samples for ci-miRNA measurement make them attractive as potential diagnostic biomarkers. However, in order to investigate ci-miRNAs as diagnostic tools it is vital to identify normal patterns of expression for different scenarios including responses to exercise. Furthermore, rigourous quality control measures must be in place to ensure reliable results. One adverse situation identified to cause variation in plasma ci-miRNA measurement is RBC haemolysis resulting in leakage of miRNAs into the plasma [22, 23, 33]. This is important to consider since there appears to be distinct miRNA profiles for the various cell types in blood [22]. Keeping this in mind, the use of stringent quality controls and careful sample handling has resulted in the accurate quantification of resting and post-exercise plasma ci-miRNAs from human subjects [12].

In the present study, haemolysis above the threshold for accurate quantification of ci-miRNAs was identified in the majority of the resting plasma samples as well as in all of the T_{5min} plasma samples. Intravascular haemolysis has been identified to occur in horses following racing [26], exercise on the treadmill [34–36] and after work on the gallops [27]. Exercise-induced haemolysis in horses primarily results from increased fragility of erythrocytes [37, 38], hypothesized to be due to the frequent accumulation of RBCs in the spleen [35, 37]. Changes in pH due to anaerobic exercise has also been associated with increased erythrocyte fragility [38], which also occurs in human althletes following maximal exercise [39]. It was interesting to note that in the present study even resting plasma samples had a degree of haemolysis above the threshold for accurate quantification of ci-miRNA detection [22]. We hypothesised that since the horses were in active training for 6 days of the week, which is typical for a flat racehorse training establishment, this resulted in almost daily and consistent exercise-induced insult to the RBCs resulting in persistent levels of haemolysis. Thus, the degree of plasma haemolysis and subsequent effect on miRNA abundance is important to consider when investigating plasma ci-miRNA levels in horses that are in active exercise programmes, even when evaluating pre-exercise samples.

In the present study plasma samples were analysed spectrophotometrically to determine levels of free Hb, as this is an extremely simple and accurate method to determine the extent of plasma haemolysis [22]. For the 48/52 miRNAs detected in plasma in the current study, miRNA abundance was significantly correlated with absorbance at one or both sampling time points supporting correlation between haemolysis and plasma ci-miRNA detection. Since measurement of ≥90% of the detected plasma ci-miRNAs in the current study was correlated with haemolysis, an accurate assessment of the changes in ci-miRNA abundance in response to exercise could not be made. It is believed, however, that this problem could be overcome through the quantification of exosomal ci-miRNAs (plasma miRNAs packaged in vesicles) rather than measurement of all plasma ci-miRNAs. This technique would exclude all unpackaged miRNAs which may have been leaked into the plasma from haemolysed erythrocytes.

Our research group previously demonstrated that mRNA in equine skeletal muscle responds to a single

Table 1 The most over-represented KEGG pathways for each miRNA based on a predicted target gene list

miRNA	Fold change	adjusted *P* value	*n* genes	Top KEGG pathway	*P* value
hsa-let-7d-3p	−0.68	0.002	3	NA	NA
hsa-miR-21-5p	0.92	0.002	243	Cytokine-cytokine receptor interaction	2.48E-06
hsa-let-7d-5p	−0.44	0.022	370	ECM-receptor interaction	9.22E-06
hsa-miR-30b-5p	0.52	0.023	1113	Ubiquitin mediated proteolysis	4.76E-10
hsa-miR-30e-5p	0.64	0.042	1153	Ubiquitin mediated proteolysis	2.92E-08

Table 2 Pathways previously implicated in the equine exercise response that were significantly enriched among predicted targets of the differntially expressed miRNAs

KEGG pathway	*P* value	*n* genes	*n* miRNAs
B cell receptor signalling pathway	1.4637E-06	16	4
Ubiquitin mediated proteolysis	1.4637E-06	25	4
Neurotrophin signalling pathway	3.75787E-06	22	4
T cell receptor signalling pathway	3.75787E-06	20	4
TGF-beta signalling pathway	9.00943E-06	15	4
PI3K-Akt signalling pathway	4.61509E-05	43	4
Long-term potentiation	0.000171436	13	4
Regulation of actin cytoskeleton	0.000171436	28	4
MAPK signalling pathway	0.000293552	34	4
Jak-STAT signalling pathway	0.000485158	22	4
Axon guidance	0.000671812	22	3
Arrhythmogenic right ventricular cardiomyopathy	0.000834821	13	3
Hepatitis B	0.000838527	21	4
Transcriptional misregulation in cancer	0.002038503	26	4
Hypertrophic cardiomyopathy	0.002113538	13	3
Insulin signalling pathway	0.002113538	19	4
Mucin type O-Glycan biosynthesis	0.002113538	6	3
Prostate cancer	0.0021797	13	4
mTOR signalling pathway	0.002349162	11	4
Acute myeloid leukaemia	0.003086604	9	4
Adherens junction	0.004193219	14	4

bout of exercise as well as exercise training [31, 32]. These results underpinned our interest in evaluating the effect that exercise may have on equine skeletal muscle miRNA expression. The initial profiling for equine skeletal muscle miRNA expression in the present study was carried out on horses just entering sprint training. This was based on results from previous studies in our laboratory in which Tb skeletal muscle was found to have the greatest transcriptional response to intense exercise at this training stage [31]. The 4 h post-exercise sampling time was also chosen based on previous work performed by our research group where it was identified to be the time-point exhibiting the most transcriptional activity [31]. These observations are in agreement with several human exercise studies [40–42].

In this study we observed changes in equine skeletal muscle miRNA abundance following exercise. All five of the DE miRNAs from skeletal muscle expressed at T_4 in the present study had been identified amongst the 48 miRNAs detected from haemolysed plasma samples from horses in cohort A. Furthermore, all five are known equine miRNAs with miR-30e-5p previously reported to be expresesed in muscle in a tissue-specific manner [20].

Of great interest is that these five DE miRNAs are amongst 167 DE miRNAs reported from pre- and 30 min post-endurance exercise whole-blood samples in a group of $n = 14$ pure-breed/half-breed Arabian horses [21].

In the present study, two members of the let-7 family of miRNAs, let-7d-3p and let-7d-5p, and miR-21-5p had increased expression following exercise. The Let-7 family of miRNAs are involved in the regulation of glucose homeostasis and insulin sensitivity [43], both key processes in energy metabolism during exercise. Mir-21 has been shown to be involved in the fibrogenic pathway and the progression of Duchenne muscular dystrophy [44], so may play a role in muscle remodelling during exercise training.

Two members of the miR-30 family, miR-30b-5p and miR-30e-5p, had decreased expression post-exercise. The miR-30 family has been shown to be down-regulated in *mdx4cv* mice (models for Duchenne muscular dystrophy), with in vitro analysis indicating that miR-30 miRNAs are decreased following injury and are increased during myoblast differentiation [45]. These findings suggest that these miRNAs may play an important role in skeletal muscle growth and repair [45]. The decreased expression in response to exercise may be related to repair of exercise-induced muscle damage. The over-representation of miRNA gene targets in exercise-related KEGG pathways certainly suggests that miRNAs play a key role in the modulation of gene expression in response to exercise.

Conclusions

In conclusion, our results indicate even resting plasma from horses in high-intensity training may not be suitable for ci-miRNA quantification due to haemolysis, although it is possible this problem could be overcome through the quantification of exosomal ci-miRNAs. However, identification of DE miRNAs in skeletal muscle indicates that modification of miRNA expression may contribute to adaptive training responses in Tbs. It is likely that additional miRNAs are differentially regulated in response to exercise but were undetectable due to the use of a human plasma panel. Future studies using a global platform such as miRNA sequencing will be required to generate a comprehensive profile of miRNAs in equine skeletal muscle at rest and following exercise. The most powerful approach to such an investigation would be an analysis of the miRNA-Seq transcriptome.

Endnotes

[1]Polar Equine S810i, Polar Electro Ltd., Warwick, UK
[2]GPSports Systems SPI10, Canberra, Australia
[3]YSI 2300 stat plus, YSI UK Ltd., Hampshire, UK

[4]biofluids miRCURYTM RNA Isolation Kit, Exiqon, Denmark
[5]miRCURY LNA™ Universal RT microRNA PCR, poly-adenylation and cDNA synthesis kit, Exiqon, Denmark
[6]NanoDrop™ Bioanalyzer ND2000, Labtech, Uckfield, UK
[7]Jørgen KRUUSE A/S, Langeskov, Denmark
[8]Ambion, ThermoFisher Scientific Inc., Darmstadt, Germany
[9]Invitrogen, ThermoFisher Scientific Inc., Darmstadt, Germany
[10]RNase-free DNase, Qiagen Ltd., Manchester, UK
[11]Mini-kit, Qiagen Ltd., Manchester, UK.
[12]Agilent Technologies Ireland, Ltd.

Abbreviations

[Hb]: Haemoglobin concentration; [LA]: Lactate concentrations; AU: Absorption units; ci-miRNAs: Circulating miRNAs; C_t: Cycle threshold; DE: Differentially expressed; EDTA: Ethylenediamine tetraacetic acid; HR: Heart rate; miRNAs: MicroRNAs; mRNA: Messenger ribonucleic acid; RBC: Red blood cells; RT-qPCR: Reverse transcription quantitative real-time polymerase chain reaction; T_0: before exercise (rest); T_{4hr}: 4 h after exercise; T_{5min}: 5 mins after exercise; Tb: Thoroughbreds; WD: Work day

Acknowledgements

The authors wish to express their appreciation to the trainer Mr. Jim Bolger and his staff.

Funding

This study has emanated from research conducted with the financial support of Science Foundation Ireland under Grant Number 11/PI/1166.

Authors' contributions

(i) BAMcG, EWH and LMK designed the experimental protocol; (ii) BAMcG, MEG, KFG, CLMcG and LMK collected all data; (iii) BAMcG, MEG, JAB, EWH and LMK performed all data analysis and interpretation; (iv, v) all authors contributed to the writing, revision and final approval of the manuscript.

Consent for publication

Not applicable.

Competing interests

None of the authors has any financial or personal relationships that could inappropriately influence or bias the content of the paper. E.W.H. is a shareholder in Plusvital Ltd., an equine nutrition and genetic testing company. Plusvital Ltd. has been granted a license for commercial use of data contained within patent applications: United States Provisional Serial Number 61/136553 and Irish patent application number 2008/0735, Patent Cooperation Treaty filing: A method for predicting athletic performance potential, September 7, 2009. E.W.H. and L.M.K. are named on the applications. The patent contents are not related to this manuscript. Plusvital Ltd. had no part in the research in the manuscript.

Author details

[1]UCD School of Agriculture and Food Science, Section of Animal & Crop Sciences, University College Dublin, Belfield, Dublin 4, Ireland. [2]UCD School of Veterinary Medicine, Section of Veterinary Biomedical Sciences, University College Dublin, Belfield, Dublin 4, Ireland.

References

1. Bartel DP. MicroRNAs: genomics, biogenesis, mechanism, and function. Cell. 2004;116:281–97.
2. Cai Y, Xiaomin Y, Songnian H, Yu JA. Brief review on the mechanisms of miRNA regulation. Genomics Proteomics Bioinformatics. 2009;7:147–54.
3. Cortez MA, Calin GA. MicroRNA identification in plasma and serum: a new tool to diagnose and monitor diseases. Expert Opin Biol Ther. 2009;9:703–11.
4. Chen X, Ba Y, Ma L, Cai X, Yin Y, Wang K, Guo J, Zhang Y, Chen J, Guo X, Li Q, Li X, Wang W, Zhang Y, Wang J, Jiang X, Xiang Y, Xu C, Zheng P, Zhang J, Li R, Zhang H, Shang X, Gong T, Ning G, Wang J, Zen K, Zhang J, Zhang C-Y. Characterization of microRNAs in serum: a novel class of biomarkers for diagnosis of cancer and other diseases. Cell Res. 2008;18:997–1006.
5. Vickers KC, Palmisano BT, Shoucri BM, Shamburek RD, Remaley AT. MicroRNAs are transported in plasma and delivered to recipient cells by high-density lipoproteins. Nat Cell Biol. 2011;13:423–33.
6. Turchinovich A, Weiz L, Langheinz A, Burwinkel B. Characterization of extracellular circulating microRNA. Nucleic Acids Res. 2011;39:7223–33.
7. Mitchell PS, Parkin RK, Kroh EM, Fritz BR, Wyman SK, Pogosova-Agadjanyan EL, Peterson A, Noteboom J, O'Briant KC, Allen A, Lin DW. Circulating microRNAs as stable blood-based markers for cancer detection. Proc Natl Acad Sci. 2008; 105:10513–8.
8. Reid G, Kirschner MB, van Zandwijk N. Circulating microRNAs: association with disease and potential use as biomarkers. Crit Rev Oncol Hematol. 2011; 80:193–208.
9. Baggish AL, Hale A, Weiner RB, Lewis GD, Systrom D, Wang F, Wang TJ, Chan SY. Dynamic regulation of circulating microRNAs during acute exhaustive exercise and sustained aerobic exercise training. J Physiol. 2011;589:3983–94.
10. Bye A, Rosjo H, Aspenes ST, Condorelli G, Omland T, Wisloff U. Circulating microRNAs and aerobic fitness–the HUNT-study. PLoS One. 2013;8:e57496.
11. Russell AP, Lamon S, Boon H, Wada S, Guller I, Brown EL, Chibalin AV, Zierath JR, Snow RJ, Stepto N, Wadley GD, Akimoto T. Regulation of miRNAs in human skeletal muscle following acute endurance exercise and short-term endurance training. J Physiol. 2013;591:4637–53.
12. Nielsen S, Akerstrom T, Rinnov A, Yfanti C, Scheele C, Pedersen BK, Laye MJ. The miRNA plasma signature in response to acute aerobic exercise and endurance training. PLoS One. 2014;9:e87308. doi:10.1371/journal.pone. 0087308.
13. Davidsen PK, Gallagher IJ, Hartman JW, Tarnopolsky MA, Dela F, Helge JW, Timmons JA, Phillips SM. High responders to resistance exercise training demonstrate differential regulation of skeletal muscle microRNA expression. J Appl Physiol. 2011;110:309–17.
14. Keller P, Vollaard NB, Gustafsson T, Gallagher IJ, Sundberg CJ, Rankinen T, Britton SL, Bouchard C, Koch LG, Timmons JA. A transcriptional map of the impact of endurance exercise training on skeletal muscle phenotype. J Appl Physiol. 2011;110:46–59.
15. Guescini M, Guidolin D, Vallorani L, Casadei L, Gioacchini AM, Tibollo P, Battistelli M, Falcieri E, Battistin L, Agnati LF, Stocchi V. C2C12 myoblasts release micro-vesicles containing mtDNA and proteins involved in signal transduction. Exp Cell Res. 2010;316:1977–2984.
16. Pedersen BK, Febbraio MA. Muscles, exercise and obesity: skeletal muscle as a secretory organ. Nat Rev Endocrinol. 2012;8:457–65.
17. Van der Kolk JH, Pacholewska A, Gerber V. The role of microRNAs in equine medicine: a review. Vet Q. 2015;35:88–96.
18. Barrey E, Bonnamy B, Barrey EJ, Mata X, Chaffaux S, Guerin G. Muscular microRNA expressions in healthy and myopathic horses suffering from polysaccharide storage myopathy or recurrent exertional rhabdomyolysis. Equine Vet J. 2010;42:303–10.
19. Gim JA, Ayarpadikannan S, Eo J, Kwon YJ, Choi Y, Lee HK, Park KD, Yang YM, Cho BW, Kim HS. Transcriptional expression changes of glucose metabolism genes after exercise in thoroughbred horses. Gene. 2014;547:152–8.
20. Kim MC, Lee SW, Ryu DY, Cui FJ, Bhak J, Kim Y. Identification and characterization of microRNAs in normal equine tissues by next generation sequencing. PLoS One. 2014;9:e93662.
21. Mach N, Plancade S, Pacholewska A, Lecardonnel J, Riviere J, Moroldo M, Vaiman A, Morgenthaler C, Beinat M, Nevot A, Robert C, Barrey E. Integrated mRNA and miRNA expression profiling in blood reveals candiate biomarkers associated with endurance exercise in the horse. Sci Rep. 2016;6:22932.
22. Kirschner MB, Kao SC, Edelman JJ, Armstrong NJ, Vallely MP, van Zandwijk N, Reid G. Haemolysis during sample preparation alters microRNA content of plasma. PLoS One. 2011;6:e24145.
23. McDonald JS, Milosevic D, Reddi HV, Grebe SK, Algeciras-Schimnich A. Analysis of circulating microRNA: preanalytical and analytical challenges. Clin Chem. 2011;57:833–40.

24. Blondal T, Jensby Nielsen S, Baker A, Andreasen D, Mouritzen P, Wrang Teilum M, Dahlsveen IK. Assessing sample and miRNA profile quality in serum and plasma or other biofluids. Methods. 2013;59:S1–6.
25. Kirschner MB, Edelman JJ, Kao SC, Vallely MP, van Zandwijk N, Reid G. The impact of hemolysis on cell-free microRNA biomarkers. Front Genet. 2013;4:94.
26. Masini AP, Tedeschi D, Badagli P, Sighieri C, Lubas C. Exercise-induced intravascular haemolysis in standardbred horses. Comp Clin Path. 2003;12: 45–8.
27. Cywinska A, Szarska E, Kowalska A, Ostaszewski P, Schollenberger A. Gender differences in exercise-induced intravascular haemolysis during race training in thoroughbred horses. Res Vet Sci. 2011;90:133–7.
28. Fonseca RG, Kenny DA, Hill EW, Katz LM. The association of various speed indices to training responses in thoroughbred flat racehorses measured with a global positioning and heart rate monitoring system. Equine Vet J. 2010;42:51–7.
29. Dingboom EG, Dijkstra G, Enzerink E, van Oudheusden HC, Weijs WA. Postnatal muscle fibre composition of the gluteus medius muscle of Dutch Warmblood foals; maturation and the influence of exercise. Equine Vet J. 1999;31:95–100.
30. Vlachos IS, Kostoulas N, Vergoulis T, Georgakilas G, Reczko M, Maragkakis M, Paraskevopoulou MD, Prionidis K, Dalamagas T, Hatzigeorgiou AGDIANA. miRPath v.2.0: investigating the combinatorial effect of microRNAs in pathways. Nucleic Acids Res. 2012;40:W498–504.
31. McGivney BA, Eivers SS, MacHugh DE, MacLeod JN, O'Gorman GM, Park SD, Katz LM, Hill EW. Transcriptional adaptations following exercise in thoroughbred horse skeletal muscle highlights molecular mechanisms that lead to muscle hypertrophy. BMC Genomics. 2009;10:638.
32. McGivney BA, McGettigan PA, Browne JA, Evans AC, Fonseca RG, Loftus BJ, Lohan A, MacHugh DE, Murphy BA, Katz LM, Hill EW. Characterization of the equine skeletal muscle transcriptome identifies novel functional responses to exercise training. BMC Genomics. 2010;11:398.
33. Pritchard CC, Kroh E, Wood B, Arroyo JD, Dougherty KJ, Miyaji MM, Tait JF, Tewari M. Blood cell origin of circulating microRNAs: a cautionary note for cancer biomarker studies. Cancer Prev Res. 2012;5:492–7.
34. Schott HC, Hodgson DR, Bayly WM. Haematuria, pigmenturia and proteinuria in exercising horses. Equine Vet J. 1995;27:67–72.
35. Hanzawa K, Higara A, Yoshida Y, Hara H, Kai M, Kubo K, Watanabe S. Effects of exercise on plasma haptoglobin composition in control and splenectomized thoroughbred horses. J Equine Sci. 2002;13:89–92.
36. Inoue Y, Matsui A, Asai Y, Aoki F, Matsui T, Yano H. Effect of exercise on iron metabolism in horses. Biol Trace Elem Res. 2005;107:33–42.
37. Hanzawa K, Kai M, Hirag A, Watanabe S. Fragility of red cells during exercise is affected by blood pH and temperature. Equine Vet J. 1999;31:610–1.
38. Hanzawa K, Watanabe S. Changes in osmotic fragility of erythrocytes during exercise in athletic horses. J Equine Sci. 2000;11:51–61.
39. Smith JA, Telford RD, Kolbuch-Braddon M, Weidermann MJ. Lactate/H+ uptake by red blood cells during exercise alters their physical properties. Eur J Appl Physiol Occup Physiol. 1995;75:54–61.
40. Yang Y, Creer A, Jemiolo B, Trappe S. Time course of myogenic and metabolic gene expression in response to acute exercise in human skeletal muscle. J Appl Physiol. 2005;98:1745–52.
41. Mahoney DJ, Safdar A, Parise G, Melov S, Fu M, MacNeil L, Kaczor J, Payne ET, Tarnopolsky MA. Gene expression profiling in human skeletal muscle during recovery from eccentric exercise. Am J Physiol Regul Integr Comp Physiol. 2008;294:R1901–10.
42. Nader GA, von Walden F, Liu C, Lindvall J, Gutmann L, Pistilli EE, Gordon PM. Resistance exercise training modulates acute gene expression during human skeletal muscle hypertrophy. J Appl Physiol. 2014;116:693–702.
43. Frost RJ, Olson EN. Control of glucose homeostasis and insulin sensitivity by the Let-7 family of microRNAs. Proc Natl Acad Sci. 2011;108:21075–80.
44. Ardite E, Perdiguero E, Vidal B, Gutarra S, Serrano AL, Munoz-Canoves P. PAI-1-regulated miR-21 defines a novel age-associated fibrogenic pathway in muscular dystrophy. J Cell Biol. 2012;196:163–75.
45. Guess MG, Barthel KK, Harrison BC, Leinwand LA. miR-30 family microRNAs regulate myogenic differentiation and provide negative feedback on the microRNA pathway. PLoS One. 2015;10:e0118229.

8

The effect of alphacypermethrin-treated mesh protection against African horse sickness virus vectors on jet stall microclimate, clinical variables and faecal glucocorticoid metabolites of horses

Patrick Page[1*], Andre Ganswindt[2], Johan Schoeman[1], Gert Venter[3] and Alan Guthrie[4]

Abstract

Background: African horse sickness (AHS) is of importance to health and international trade in horses worldwide. During export from and transit through AHS endemic countries or zones, physical and chemical measures to protect horses from the vectors of AHS virus (AHSV) are recommended by the World Organization for Animal Health. Protection of containerized air transport systems for horses (jet stalls) with alphacypermethrin insecticide-treated high density polyethylene mesh is effective in reducing the *Culicoides* midge vector attack rate. In order to determine the effect of this mesh on jet stall ventilation and horse welfare under temperate climatic conditions, jet stall microclimate, clinical variables and faecal glucocorticoid metabolite (FGM) levels of 12 horses were monitored during overnight housing in either a treated or untreated stall in two blocks of a 2 × 3 randomized crossover design.

Results: Temperature difference between the treated stall and outside was significantly higher than the difference between the untreated stall and outside at 1/15 time points only ($P = 0.045$, $r = 0.70$). Relative humidity (RH) difference between the treated stall and outside did not differ from the untreated stall and outside. Temperature and RH in the treated stall were highly and significantly correlated with outside temperature ($r = 0.96$, $P < 0.001$) and RH ($r = 0.95$, $P < 0.001$), respectively. No significant differences were detected between rectal temperatures, pulse and respiratory rates of horses in the treated stall compared to the untreated stall. Mean FGM concentrations for horses housed in the treated stall peaked earlier (24 h) and at a higher concentration than horses housed in the untreated stall (48 h), but were not significantly different from baseline. No significant difference was detected in FGM concentrations when the treated and untreated stall groups were compared at individual time points up to 72 h after exiting the jet stall.

Conclusions: Alphacypermethrin-treated HDPE mesh could be used under temperate climatic conditions to protect horses in jet stalls against AHSV vectors, without compromising jet stall microclimate and horse welfare.

Keywords: Horse, Jet stall, Alphacypermethrin, Mesh, Climate, Faecal glucocorticoid metabolites

* Correspondence: patrick.page@bayer.com
[1]Department of Companion Animal Clinical Studies, Faculty of Veterinary Science, University of Pretoria, Private Bag X04, Onderstepoort 0110, South Africa
Full list of author information is available at the end of the article

Background

African horse sickness (AHS) is an infectious, non-contagious, arthropod-borne viral disease that is of importance to health and international trade in equids [1, 2]. Intercontinental trade is a potential route whereby viruses such as AHS virus (AHSV) may be introduced into equid populations, either via movement of infected hosts or *Culicoides* midge vectors [2–6]. In order to reduce risk of AHSV transmission during export from or transit through AHS endemic countries or zones, measures of a physical and chemical nature have been recommended by the World Organisation for Animal Health to protect horses against AHSV vectors [7]. Alphacypermethrin insecticide-treated high density polyethylene (HDPE) mesh has a rapid insecticidal effect against *Culicoides* midges [8] and has recently been shown to significantly reduce the midge attack rate on horses housed in containerised air transport systems (jet stalls) [9].

While horses are frequently transported by air in jet stalls, there is limited published data on jet stall microclimate, stress indicators, or blood parameters related to the welfare of horses during air transport [10–14]. Stall environment and microclimate affects equine respiratory health in particular during air transport [15]. There are currently no published reports on the effects of physical or chemical vector protection measures, such as alphacypermethrin insecticide-treated HDPE mesh, applied to jet stalls on stall microclimate or stress indicators of horses.

Non-invasive means of assessing transport-associated stress in horses include monitoring of behavioural indices, heart rate and heart rate variability, salivary cortisol and faecal glucocorticoid metabolite (FGM) concentrations [11, 12, 14, 16–18]. Glucocorticoid metabolites in faeces increase approximately one day after an increase in blood cortisol concentrations in ponies [19, 20] and mainly reflect prolonged stress [16, 18, 21]. FGM concentrations have been reported for monitoring adrenocortical response to road transport [16–18] and sales consignment [22, 23], but not in response to jet stall housing or air transport of horses.

The aims of the study were to determine the effect of alphacypermethrin insecticide-treated HDPE mesh applied to commercial jet stalls on jet stall microclimate, clinical variables and FGM concentrations of horses housed under stationary jet stall, temperate climatic conditions.

Methods

The study was approved by the Animal Ethics Committee of the University of Pretoria (Study V011–14).

Animals

Twelve clinically healthy, adult horses (six geldings and six mares) of mixed breed (eight Thoroughbred, two Basuto, two Boerperd) with mean (range) age 11 (5–20) years, and body mass 482 (404–584) kg were included in the study. The horses were resident at the study site as part of the research herd. Other than being led into the stalls for subjective behaviour assessment one week prior to the start of the study, horses were not acclimatised to the stalls. Grass and alfalfa hay was fed ad libitum during data collection, and water was provided in buckets every 4 h. Wood shavings were used as bedding in the stalls. During overnight data collection herd mates were kept in adjacent paddocks in direct view of the front of the jet stalls to reduce group separation stress. The study horses were kept grouped with their herd mates in an adjacent grassed paddock during the day. Only routine activities were conducted with the horses from 1 week before until study completion.

Study design

A randomised, crossover experimental study was performed from 28 to 30 April 2014 and from 5 to 7 May 2014 (late summer in the southern hemisphere). Horses were housed between 16 h00 and 06 h00 in two jet stalls, located 8.5 m apart in a grass paddock (58 m × 69 m), at the Faculty of Veterinary Science, Onderstepoort (25°38′51.42″S, 28°10′45.96″E, 1238 m above sea level).

The horses were grouped according to gender and ranked according to body weight, then assigned to same gender pairs to ensure comparable horse body weight housed in each stall each night. One of each gender pair of horses was randomly assigned to either a treated or untreated stall and monitored overnight in two experimental blocks of a 2 × 3 design. The first block consisted of three consecutive nights followed by a five day rest period. Treatments were then crossed over for the stalls and three consecutive nights of data collection for the second block conducted in the same sequence. Horses were therefore housed in the same gender pair and stall compartment for each block, but with the treatment crossed over.

Jets stalls

Two commercial, non-collapsible, Federal Aviation Administration approved, 15.5 m^3 (length 3.18 m, width 2.44 m, height 2.44 m) jet stalls[1] were used. The inside of the stall had 3 adjacent compartments for housing horses, with a separate grooms' compartment in the front for monitoring, feeding and providing water. During data collection horses were housed in the outer compartment of each stall with the middle compartment left unoccupied to facilitate access for clinical monitoring. When closed each stall had a 1.7 square meter rectangular opening above the front and rear ramps for ventilation.

Jet stall treatment

One stall was treated with a black, 400 denier, knitted monofilament HDPE mesh[2] with 0.3 mm hole size, impregnated with 20–40 mg/square meter alphacypermethrin[3] for protection against *Culicoides* biting midges, as previously described [9]. The mesh was custom-made to fit over the stall in a tent-like fashion, with zip connectors for access located at the end panels. When fitted, the mesh covered the ventilation openings of the stall. No mesh was applied to the untreated stall.

Data collection and analyses

Clinical variables

The horses' habitus, appetite and vital signs (rectal temperature,[4] pulse and respiratory rates) were recorded before entering the jet stall (16 h00), and every 4 h while housed inside the stall.

Climatic variables

Microclimate [temperature and relative humidity (RH)] inside each stall was monitored hourly with data loggers[5] secured 1 m above the floor in the grooms' compartment. Outside temperature and RH were monitored on a logger located 10 m away from the stalls. Data were downloaded with commercial software[6] at the end of each treatment block. Additional outside climatic variables (wind speed, rainfall) were recorded hourly using a weather station and data logger[7] located in an adjacent paddock.

Faecal sample collection and analysis

Faecal samples were collected before entry into the jet stall (Baseline), 24, 48 and 72 h after exiting the jet stall. Faecal samples were collected by manual extraction from the rectum using a lubricated, plastic rectal glove. The faecal material was transferred into a 25 ml plastic specimen container, frozen within 4 h of collection, and kept at −20 °C until hormone extraction and assay.

Faecal samples were lyophilized, pulverized, and sifted [24]. Thereafter, 0.10–0.11 g of faecal powder was extracted using 3 ml of 80% ethanol in water. After vortexing for 15 min, the mixtures were centrifuged for 10 min at 1500 *g*, and the supernatants transferred into microcentrifuge tubes and stored at −20 °C until steroid analysis. FGM analysis was performed as previously described using a group-specific 11-oxoaetiocholanolone enzyme immunoassay, measuring 11,17-dioxoandrostanes [20, 25], shown to provide valid information on adrenocortical function in horses [21–23]. Serial dilutions of faecal extracts produced displacement curves parallel to the standard curve of the assay. The sensitivity of the assay determined at 90% binding was 2 ng/g dry faeces. Intra- and inter-assay coefficients of variation, determined by repeated measurement of high- and low-concentration quality controls, ranged between 1.9% - 6.6% and 6.2% - 10.2%, respectively. Cross-reactivity of the antibody used has been previously reported [25].

Statistical analyses

Statistical analyses were performed with SPSS® Statistics.[8] Data were assessed for normality by evaluating descriptive statistics, plotting histograms and performing the Kolmogorov-Smirnov test. All statistical tests were two-tailed at the 5% level of significance.

Differences between treated and untreated jet stall and outside climatic variables were computed and compared at hourly time points by Kruskal Wallis test. Where the test statistic was significant pairwise comparisons were conducted with *P*-values adjusted for multiple comparisons. Effect sizes were calculated for pairwise comparisons. Pearson's correlation coefficient was calculated for the relationship between jet stall microclimate and outside climatic variables. Clinical variables were compared within each treatment group with Friedman's ANOVA. Where the test statistic was significant, pairwise comparisons were conducted with *P*-values adjusted for multiple comparisons. Wilcoxon signed-rank tests were used to compare clinical variables between horses housed in the treated stall versus the untreated stall. Natural-log-transformed FGM concentrations were used for data analysis. FGM data within each treatment group were compared with one-way repeated measures ANOVA with post hoc Bonferroni adjustment of *P*-values for pairwise comparisons. The assumption of sphericity was confirmed with Mauchly's test. Comparisons of FGM data between treatment groups were performed using paired samples t-tests.

Results

Climatic variables

Temperature and RH (median [interquartile range]) recorded in the treated stall, untreated stall and outside were 16.1 °C (12.1–20.3 °C), 14.1 °C (9.5–17.8 °C), 9.8 °C (5.6–14.7 °C) and 73.0% (63.4–77.4%), 77.8% (60.7–83.3%) and 86.6% (67.2–97.8%), respectively (Additional files 1 and 2). Mean (range) outside wind speed during the data collection period was 0.2 km/h (0–0.3 km/h) and no rain was recorded.

Temperature difference between the treated stall and outside was significantly higher than the difference between the untreated stall and outside at the 18 h00 time point only ($P = 0.045$, $r = 0.70$), while temperature difference between the treated stall and outside was significantly higher than the difference between the treated stall and untreated stall at the majority of the time points ($P = 0.001–0.041$, $r = 0.71–1.06$) (Fig. 1). Relative humidity difference between the treated stall and outside

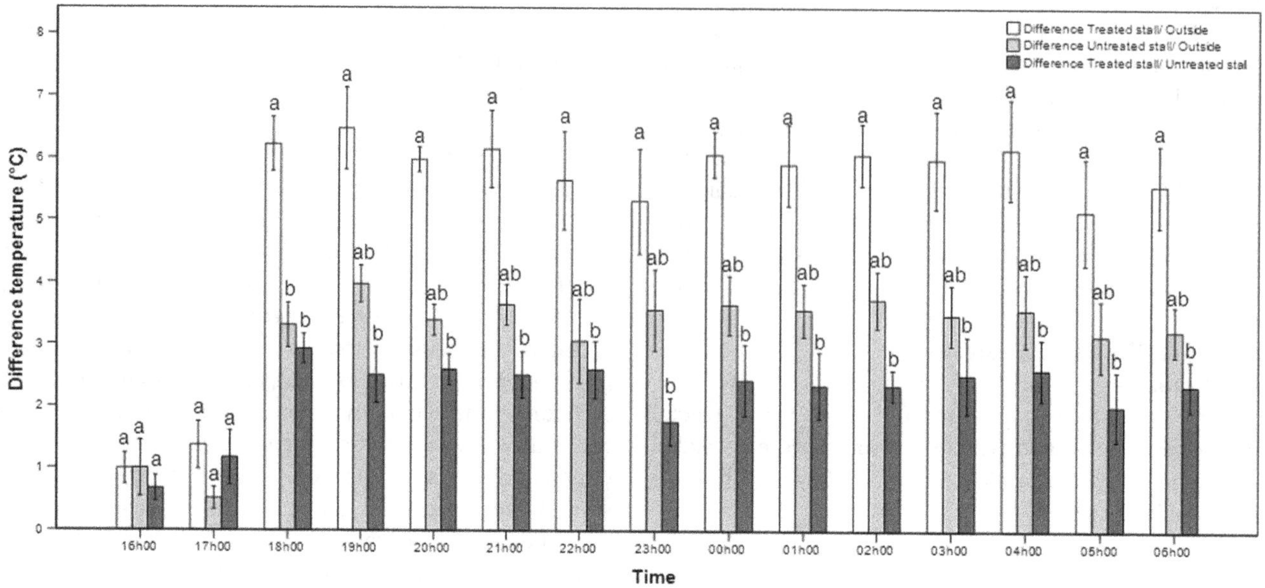

Fig. 1 Hourly differences in temperature. Hourly differences (mean ± SEM) in temperature (°C) between a treated jet stall and outside, an untreated jet stall and outside, and a treated jet stall and an untreated jet stall recorded over 6 nights under temperate climatic conditions. Within each time point bars with a different lower case letter differ significantly ($P < 0.05$)

did not differ from the difference between the untreated stall and outside at any time point, while RH difference between the treated stall and outside was significantly higher than the difference between the treated stall and untreated stall at few time points (P = 0.005–0.033, r = 0.73–0.91) (Fig. 2).

Temperature in the treated stall (r = 0.96, n = 90, $P < 0.001$) and untreated stall (r = 0.99, n = 90, $P < 0.001$) were highly and significantly correlated with outside temperature. RH in the treated stall (r = 0.95, n = 90, $P < 0.001$) and untreated stall (r = 0.97, n = 90, $P < 0.001$) were highly and significantly correlated with outside RH.

Clinical variables

No adverse effects of housing in the treated or untreated stalls were recorded in any of the horses. All horses remained alert and responsive with subjectively normal appetite, water intake, regular faecal output and urination. Vital signs recorded in the treated and untreated groups before entering the stall and during overnight housing are summarised in Table 1 and Additional files 3, 4 and 5.

No significant differences were detected between the 4-hourly rectal temperatures, pulse and respiratory rates for the horses in the untreated stall. For the horses in the treated stall rectal temperature differed significantly for the 20 h00 compared to the 04 h00 time point only (X^2_F = 11.283, df = 3, P = 0.01), while pulse and respiratory rates did not differ significantly between time points. There was no significant difference between rectal temperature, pulse and respiratory rates of horses in the treated stall compared to the untreated stall at individual time points.

FGM concentrations

An increase in mean FGM concentrations from baseline levels was detected in both treatment groups after overnight housing in the jet stalls (Fig. 3). Mean FGM concentrations for horses housed in the treated stall peaked earlier (24 h) and at a higher concentration than horses housed in the untreated stall (48 h). No significant difference was detected in FGM concentrations between baseline samples and samples obtained up to 72 h after exiting the stall for both the treated and untreated stall groups. No significant difference was detected in mean FGM concentrations when the treated and untreated stall groups were compared at individual time points.

Discussion

Alphacypermethrin-treated HDPE mesh applied to commercial jet stalls as a physical and chemical protection barrier against AHSV vectors did not compromise jet stall microclimate, clinical variables or indicators of physiological stress in horses housed under stationary stall, temperate climatic conditions.

Closed top HMA-type jet stalls are commonly used to transport horses internationally. These stalls avoid potential fire alarm concerns associated with air conditioning units of climate-controlled stalls, however ventilation and microclimate could be affected by application of mesh around the stalls for protection against

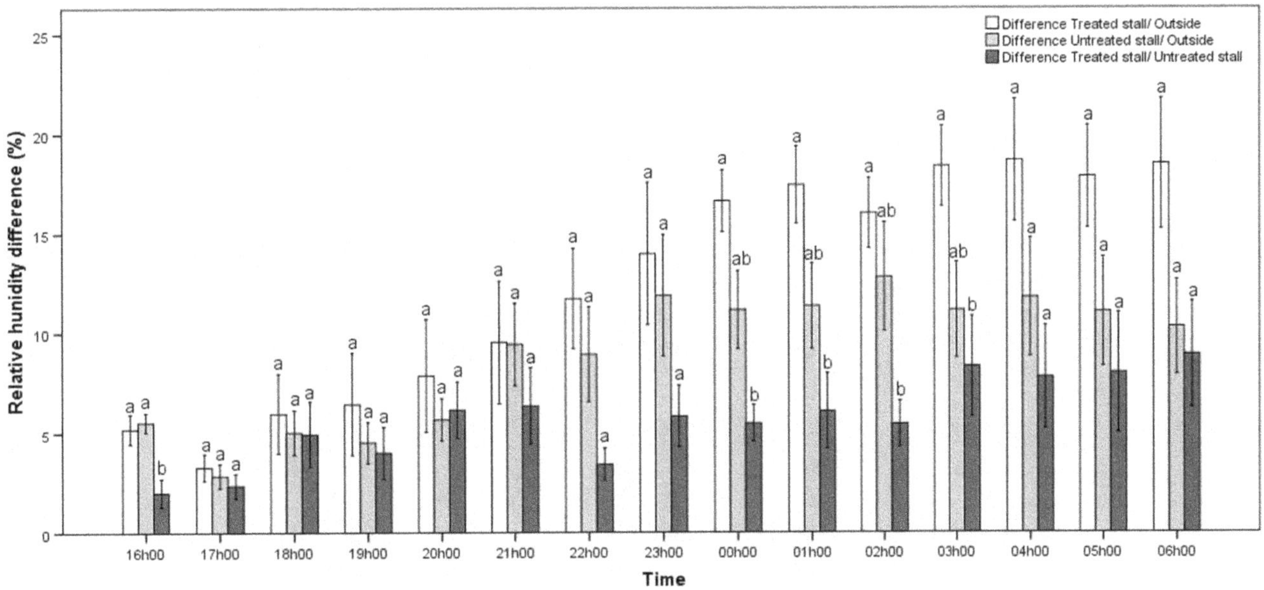

Fig. 2 Hourly differences in relative humidity. Hourly differences (mean ± SEM) in relative humidity (%)between a treated jet stall and outside, an untreated jet stall and outside, and a treated jet stall and an untreated jet stall recorded over 6 nights under temperate climatic conditions. Within each time point bars with a different lower case letter differ significantly ($P < 0.05$)

vectors. The outside temperatures in the present study were within or lower than a guideline range for transport of horses (10–21 °C), while the RH was higher than the recommended range (45–50%) [26], as expected for the overnight study conditions. Similarly, the outside and jet stall temperatures in the present study were within or lower than corresponding cargo hold and jet stall temperature ranges reported during air transit of horses, and the outside and jet stall RH was similar or higher than reported [10–14]. Marked differences in study conditions and the type of jet stall utilised limit direct comparison of microclimate between the present and the cited studies, however.

In order to better assess the impact of the mesh on microclimate, the differences computed between treated and untreated jet stall microclimate and outside climatic variables were analysed as outside conditions, which were highly correlated with those inside the jet stalls, varied daily making comparisons of differences more appropriate than actual values [27]. In the present study, while the temperature in the treated stall was consistently higher than the outside temperature, likely associated with retention of metabolic heat produced by the horses [28] and low overnight outside temperatures, the treated stall/ outside temperature difference was only significantly higher than untreated stall/ outside difference at one time point. The difference between the treated stall/ outside RH also did not differ significantly from the untreated stall/ outside RH. In fact, the treated stall RH was consistently lower than the outside RH despite anticipated evaporative heat loss which would be expected to increase RH [28]. These findings support no increased risk to thermoregulation with application of the HDPE mesh to a jet stall as compared to an untreated stall under similar climatic conditions.

While a thermal index limit of 28 °C is specified for equine competition there is currently no defined value to

Table 1 Clinical variables (mean ± SD) of horses in the treated and untreated jet stall groups before entering the stall (16 h00) and during overnight housing (20 h00, 0 h00 and 04 h00)

	Group	Time point			
		16 h00	20 h00	0 h00	04 h00
Rectal temperature (°C)	Treated stall	37.8 ± 0.7	38.1 ± 0.7	37.8 ± 0.6	37.5 ± 0.7
	Untreated stall	37.7 ± 0.6	37.8 ± 0.6	37.6 ± 0.3	37.5 ± 0.3
Pulse (beats/min)	Treated stall	37 ± 9	40 ± 11	37 ± 7	37 ± 4
	Untreated stall	44 ± 11	38 ± 7	39 ± 9	35 ± 11
Respiration (breaths/min)	Treated stall	16 ± 7	21 ± 12	16 ± 5	14 ± 4
	Untreated stall	14 ± 3	15 ± 5	16 ± 6	14 ± 3

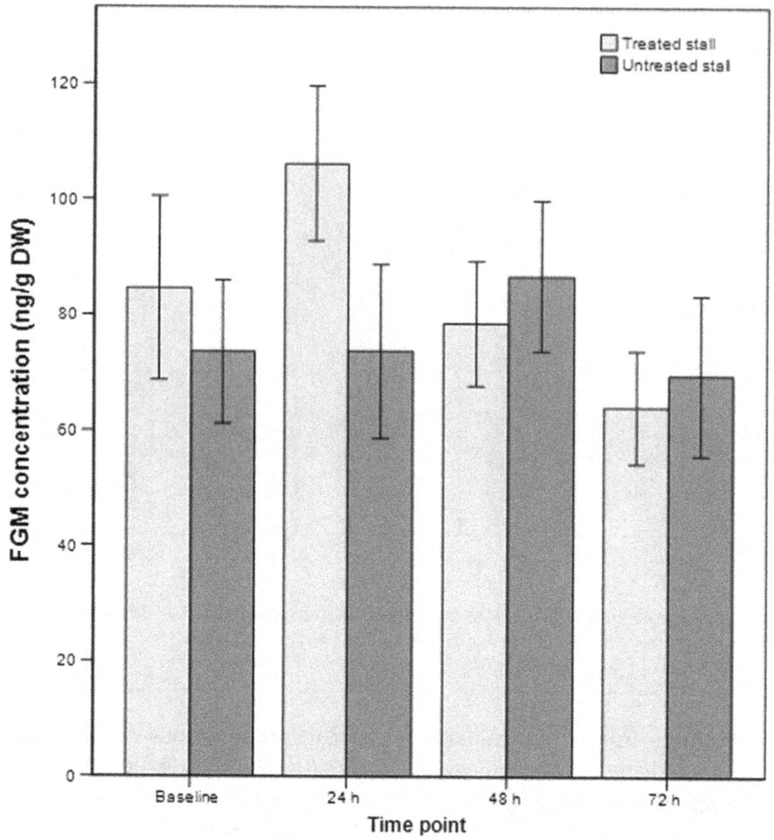

Fig. 3 Faecal glucocorticoid metabolite concentrations. Faecal glucocorticoid metabolite concentrations (mean ± SEM) from horses housed in a treated and untreated jet stall, between 16 h00 and 06 h00 for 6 nights, before entrance into the stall (Baseline), 24, 48, and 72 h after exiting the stall.

prevent equine thermal stress during equine transport [27] and further research has been recommended to improve thermal environment and ventilation of equine transport systems [29]. In the absence of data under more extreme environmental conditions for similar jet stalls protected with HDPE mesh, opening of the mesh flaps adjacent to stall ventilation points (e.g. above the front and back ramps) to promote ventilation is recommended as a precautionary measure if hot or humid environmental conditions arise during the transport process, such as during stopovers with exposure to ambient air [11]. Opening the mesh of stalls located at the rear of an aircraft first is recommended based on the temperature and RH gradient in the cargo hold whereby the stalls at the rear experience warmer, moister conditions, especially when the aircraft is stationary [10]. Furthermore, it is recommended that jet stall microclimate be monitored regularly during the transport process, particularly under more extreme environmental conditions when mesh protection is used. As emergency opening of the mesh to promote ventilation could increase risk of exposure to AHSV vectors, additional methods of protection such as insecticides or repellents applied to horses in the stalls or insecticidal aerosols sprayed in the cargo hold is advised.

Overnight housing in the treated jet stall had no significant effect on clinical variables compared to housing in an untreated stall. Horses were assessed under stationary jet stall field conditions in the present study which precluded confounding factors associated with air transport, such as loading into the aircraft, take off, turbulence, landing and unloading. Increased heart rates have been reported during these transitional events with return to resting values during level flight [11, 12, 14]. In the present study, respiratory rate also did not differ significantly between time points monitored in the treated stall, further supporting a lack of thermal stress as respiratory rate would be expected to increase [28] as a heat loss mechanism if the treated mesh compromised ventilation.

Though the effects of road transport [16–18] on cortisol release, heart rate and HRV have been reported for horses, there is limited information on the effect of air transport on stress indicators [11, 12, 14], and none have reported on the effect of jet stall transport on FGM levels. In contrast to monitoring of adrenocortical function by measurement of plasma and salivary cortisol, which reflect acute changes in cortisol release [30], FGM concentrations reflect only marked or prolonged increases in cortisol release with a lag time of about 24 h related to species-specific intestinal passage time in horses [17, 20, 21]. In the present study, which was limited to investigating the effects of stationary housing in a jet stall, no significant difference from baseline was detected in FGM concentrations, neither was there a significant difference between treatment groups. These findings, which are supported by the clinical variable data, indicate that stationary housing in an untreated jet stall or one protected with alphacypermethrin-treated HDPE mesh under temperate climate conditions is not associated with a significant stress response in horses. The earlier and higher peak in FGM concentrations for horses housed in the treated stall warrants further investigation in a larger cohort, however, but may be associated with other factors, e.g. mesh-associated impaired visual contact with herd mates compounding a herd group disruption effect [22].

Although caution is advised in practical application of the study findings based on the recognised study limitations including a stationary jet stall investigated under temperate field conditions, relatively low number of horses of varying breed, age, gender and temperament enrolled, and lack of a control group not housed in a jet stall, the findings support the safety of the HDPE mesh applied to comparable jet stalls under similar climatic conditions. Other meshes shown to protect housed horses against biting midges [31] could be investigated in a similar fashion.

Conclusions

Alphacypermethrin-treated HDPE mesh applied to jet stalls housing horses had no adverse effect on jet stall microclimate, clinical variables or stress indicators of horses housed in the stalls under temperate climatic conditions. While this mesh could be used as a safe and effective physical and chemical method for protection of horses in jet stalls against *Culicoides* midges under similar temperate climatic conditions, further investigation is required under more extreme climatic conditions as well as during air transport.

Endnotes

[1]KLM HMA jet stall, European Horse Services, Belgium

[2]RK02 70% Shade Cloth, Alnet, South Africa

[3]Fendona®6, BASF Agro BV Arnhem, Switzerland

[4]Thermoval® rapid digital thermometer, Paul Hartmann AG, Heidenheim, Germany

[5]iButton® DS1923, Fairbridge Technologies CC, Wendywood, South Africa

[6]Coldchain Thermo Dynamics Software, Fairbridge Technologies CC, Wendywood, South Africa

[7]Vantage Pro2 and Weatherlink, Davis, USA

[8]SPSS® version 23, IBM, USA

Additional files

Additional file 1: Temperature (°C; mean ± SEM) recorded at hourly time points in a treated jet stall, an untreated jet stall and outside over 6 nights under temperate climatic conditions. (BMP 1953 kb)

Additional file 2: Relative humidity (%; mean ± SEM) recorded at hourly time points in a treated jet stall, an untreated jet stall and outside over 6 nights under temperate climatic conditions. (BMP 1953 kb)

Additional file 3: Rectal temperature (°C; mean ± SEM) of horses in the treated and untreated jet stall groups before entering the stall (16 h00) and during overnight housing (20 h00, 0 h00 and 04 h00). (BMP 952 kb)

Additional file 4: Pulse rate (beats/ min; mean ± SEM) of horses in the treated and untreated jet stall groups before entering the stall (16 h00) and during overnight housing (20 h00, 0 h00 and 04 h00). (BMP 952 kb)

Additional file 5: Respiratory rate (breaths/ min; mean ± SEM) of horses in the treated and untreated jet stall groups before entering the stall (16 h00) and during overnight housing (20 h00, 0 h00 and 04 h00). (BMP 952 kb)

Abbreviations

AHS: African horse sickness; AHSV: African horse sickness virus; ANOVA: Analysis of variance; FGM: Faecal glucocorticoid metabolite; HDPE: High density polyethylene; RH: Relative humidity

Acknowledgements

The authors thank T. Thovokale, A. Schantz, W. Mbethe, L. Mlisa, M. Badenhorst, C. Matjiane and S. Makhubela for assistance with data collection. European Horse Services and Hobday Equestrian Enterprises International Horse Transport are acknowledged for providing KLM Cargo jet stalls.

Funding

The Equine Research Centre, Mary Slack and Daughters Foundation, National Research Foundation (Grant 89,686) and the Equine Health Fund funded the study.

Author's contributions

PP conceived and participated in the design of the study, organised and participated in data collection and interpretation, performed the statistical analysis and drafted the manuscript. AGanswindt participated in the FGM analysis, data interpretation and drafting of the manuscript. JS and GV participated in design of the study, data interpretation and drafting of the manuscript. AGuthrie conceived and participated in the design of the study, data interpretation, statistical analysis and drafting of the manuscript. All authors read and approved the final manuscript.

Competing interests

The authors declare that they have no competing interests.

Author details

[1]Department of Companion Animal Clinical Studies, Faculty of Veterinary Science, University of Pretoria, Private Bag X04, Onderstepoort 0110, South Africa. [2]Endocrine Research Laboratory, Department of Anatomy and Physiology, Faculty of Veterinary Science, University of Pretoria, Private Bag X04, Onderstepoort 0110, South Africa. [3]PVVD, ARC-Onderstepoort Veterinary Institute, Private Bag X05, Onderstepoort 0110, South Africa. [4]Equine Research Centre, Faculty of Veterinary Science, University of Pretoria, Private Bag X04, Onderstepoort 0110, South Africa.

References

1. Coetzer JAW, Guthrie AJ. African horse sickness. In: Coetzer JAW, Tustin RC, editors. Infectious diseases of livestock. 2nd ed. Cape Town: Oxford University Press; 2004. p. 1231–46.
2. MacLachlan NJ, Guthrie AJ. Re-emergence of bluetongue, African horse sickness, and other orbivirus diseases. Vet Res. 2010;41:35.
3. Carpenter S, Wilson A, Mellor PS. *Culicoides* and the emergence of bluetongue virus in northern Europe. Trends Microbiol. 2009;17:172–8.
4. Reiter P. The standardised freight container: vector of vectors and vector-borne diseases. Rev Sci Tech. 2010;29:57–64.
5. de Vos CJ, Hoek CA, Nodelijk G. Risk of introducing African horse sickness virus into the Netherlands by international equine movements. Prev Vet Med. 2012;106:108–22.
6. Napp S, García-Bocanegra I, Pagès N, Allepuz A, Alba A, Casal J. Assessment of the risk of a bluetongue outbreak in Europe caused by *Culicoides* midges introduced through intracontinental transport and trade networks. Med Vet Entomol. 2013;27:19–28.
7. Anon. Infection with African horse sickness virus. In: Terrestrial Animal Health Code, OIE, Paris. 2013. http://www.oie.int/index.php?id=169&L=0&htmfile= chapitre_ahs.htm. Accessed 20 Nov 2015.
8. Page PC, Labuschagne K, Venter GJ, Schoeman JP, Guthrie AJ. Field and *in vitro* insecticidal efficacy of alphacypermethrin-treated high density polyethylene mesh against *Culicoides* biting midges in South Africa. Vet Parasitol. 2014;203:184–8.
9. Page PC, Labuschagne K, Venter GJ, Schoeman JP, Guthrie AJ. Efficacy of alphacypermethrin-treated high density polyethylene mesh applied to jet stalls housing horses against *Culicoides* biting midges in South Africa. Vet Parasitol. 2015;210:84–90.
10. Leadon D, Daykin J, Backhouse W, Frank C, Attoui H. Environmental, haematological and blood biochemistry changes in equine transit stress. Proc Amer Assoc Equine Prac. 1990:485–90.
11. Thornton J. Effect of the microclimate on horses during international air transportation in an enclosed container. Aust Vet J. 2000;78:472–7.
12. Stewart M, Foster TM, Waas JR. The effects of air transport on the behaviour and heart rate of horses. Appl Anim Behav Sci. 2003;80:143–60.
13. Maaskant A, de Gooijer J, Tilburg R, Sloet van Oldruitenborgh-Oosterbaan MM. The effects of ambient temperature and relative humidity on blood parameters in horses during long distance flights. Equine Vet J. 2013;45:10.
14. Munsters CC, de Gooijer JW, van den Broek J, Sloet van Oldruitenborgh-Oosterbaan MM. Heart rate, heart rate variability and behaviour of horses during air transport. Vet Rec. 2013; doi:10.1136/vr.100952.
15. Leadon D, Waran N, Herholz C, Klay M. Veterinary management of horse transport. Vet Ital. 2008;44:149–63.
16. Schmidt A, Biau S, Möstl E, Becker-Birck M, Morillon B, Aurich J, et al. Changes in cortisol release and heart rate variability in sport horses during long-distance road transport. Domest Anim Endocrinol. 2010;38:179–89.
17. Schmidt A, Möstl E, Wehnert C, Aurich J, Muller J, Aurich C. Cortisol release and heart rate variability in horses during road transport. Horm Behav. 2010; 57:209–15.
18. Schmidt A, Hodl S, Möstl E, Aurich J, Muller J, Aurich C. Cortisol release, heart rate, and heart rate variability in transport-naive horses during repeated road transport. Domest Anim Endocrinol. 2010;39:205–13.
19. Palme R, Fischer P, Schildorfer H, Ismail MN. Excretion of infused ^{14}C-steroid hormones via faeces and urine in domestic livestock. Anim Reprod Sci. 1996;43:43–63.
20. Möstl E, Messmann S, Bagu E, Robia C, Palme R. Measurement of glucocorticoid metabolite concentrations in faeces of domestic livestock. J Vet Med A. 1999;46:621–31.
21. Merl S, Scherzer S, Palme R, Möstl E. Pain causes increased concentrations of glucocorticoid metabolites in horse feces. J Eq Vet Sci. 2000;20:586–90.
22. Schulman M, Becker A, Ganswindt S, Guthrie A, Stout T, Ganswindt A. The effect of consignment to broodmare sales on physiological stress measured by faecal glucocorticoid metabolites in pregnant thoroughbred mares. BMC Vet Res. 2014; doi:10.1186/1746-6148-10-25.
23. Badenhorst M, Page P, Ganswindt A, Laver P, Guthrie A, Schulman M. Detection of equine herpesvirus-4 and physiological stress patterns in young thoroughbreds consigned to a south African auction sale. BMC Vet Res. 2015;11:126. doi:10.1186/s12917-015-0443-4.
24. Ganswindt A, Muenscher S, Henley M, Palme R, Thompson P, Bertschinger H. Concentrations of faecal glucocorticoid metabolites in physically injured free-ranging African elephants *Loxodonta africana*. Wildlife Biol. 2010;16:323–32.
25. Palme R, Möstl E. Measurement of cortisol metabolites in faeces of sheep as a parameter of cortisol concentration in blood. Int J Mammal Biol. 1997;62:192–7.
26. International Air Transport Association. Live animals regulations. 25th ed. 1998. Montreal. International Air Transport Association.
27. Purswell JL, Gates RS, Lawrence LM, Davis JD. Thermal environment in a four-horse slant-load trailer. T Am Soc Agric Biol Eng. 2010;53:1885–94.
28. McCutcheon LJ, Geor RJ. Thermoregulation and exercise-associated heat stress. In: Hinchcliff KW, Geor RJ, Kaneps AJ, editors. Equine Exercise Physiology. Philadelphia: Saunders; 2008. p382–396.
29. Padalino B. Effects of the different transport phases on equine health status, behavior, and welfare: a review. J Vet Behav. 2015;10:272–82.
30. Schmidt A, Möstl E, Aurich J, Neuhauser S, Aurich C. Comparison of cortisol and cortisone levels in blood plasma and saliva and cortisol metabolite concentrations in faeces for stress analysis in horses. In: proceedings 5th international conference of the International Society for Equitation Science, Sydney, Australia 2009. p53.
31. Lincoln VJ, Page PC, Kopp C, Mathis A, von Niederhäusern R, Burger D, et al. Protection of horses against *Culicoides* biting midges in different housing systems in Switzerland. Vet Parasitol. 2015;210:206–14.

9

Prospective pre- and post-race evaluation of biochemical, electrophysiologic, and echocardiographic indices in 30 racing thoroughbred horses that received furosemide

Catherine T. Gunther-Harrington[1], Rick Arthur[2], Krista Estell[3,6], Beatriz Martinez Lopez[4], Alexandra Sinnott[1], Eric Ontiveros[1], Anita Varga[3,5] and Joshua A. Stern[1*]

Abstract

Background: Exercise induced cardiac fatigue (EICF) and cardiac dysrhythmias are well described conditions identified in high-level human athletes that increase in frequency with intensity and duration of exercise. Identification of these conditions requires an understanding of normal pre- and post-race cardiac assessment values. The objectives of this study were to (1) characterize selected indices of cardiac function, electrophysiologic parameters, and biochemical markers of heart dysfunction prior to and immediately after high level racing in Thoroughbred horses receiving furosemide; and (2) create pre- and post-race reference values in order to make recommendations on possible screening practices for this population in the future.

Results: Thirty Thoroughbred horses were enrolled in the study with an age range of 3–6 years. All horses received furosemide prior to racing. Physical exams, ECGs, and echocardiograms were performed prior to racing (T0) and within 30–60 min following the race (T1). Blood samples were obtained at T0, T1, 4 h post-race (T4) and 24 h after the race (T24). Electrolytes, hematocrit, cardiac troponin I, and partial pressure CO2 values were obtained at all time points. Heart rate was significantly increased post-race compared to baseline value with a median difference of 49 bpm, 95% CI [31,58],($P < 0.0001$). No dysrhythmias were noted during ECG assessment. Following the race, an increase in number of horses demonstrating regurgitation through the aorta and AV valves was noted. Systolic function measured by fractional shortening increased significantly with a mean difference of 7.9%, 95% CI [4.8, 10.9], ($P < 0.0001$). Cardiac troponin I was not different at pre- and immediately post-race time points, but was significantly increased at T4 ($P < 0.001$). Troponin returned to baseline value by T24.

Conclusions: This study utilized a before and after study design where each horse served as its own control, as such the possible effect of regression to the mean cannot be ruled out. The reference intervals generated in this study may be used to identify selected echocardiographic and electrocardiographic abnormalities in racing horses receiving furosemide.

Keywords: Troponin, Cardiology, Sudden death, Cardiac ultrasound, Exercise

* Correspondence: jstern@ucdavis.edu
[1]Department of Medicine & Epidemiology, School of Veterinary Medicine, University of California Davis, Davis, CA 95616, USA
Full list of author information is available at the end of the article

Background

Exercise induced cardiac fatigue (EICF) and cardiac dysrhythmias are well described conditions identified in high-level human athletes that increase in frequency with intensity and duration of exercise [1–3]. Characterization of cardiovascular abnormalities including EICF and dysrhythmias in equine athletes are limited, however changes consistent with EICF and significant cardiac arrhythmias have been identified in endurance horses [4–6]. Although racing Thoroughbred horses are not subjected to long duration of exercise, the intensity is unmatched in the performance horse industry. For this reason, there is increased attention to cardiac assessment in race horses [7–14].

EICF is identified by echocardiographic evidence of ventricular systolic and/or diastolic dysfunction. Additionally, post-exercise cardiac arrhythmias, changes to electrophysiologic intervals such as the QT interval and cardiac biomarker elevation are all identified to varying degrees in athletes with EICF [1, 2, 6]. The occurrence of EICF has not been evaluated in Thoroughbred racehorses. To date, there has not been a comprehensive assessment of pre- and post-race parameters in Thoroughbred racing horses, therefore there is a need to establish normal reference intervals so outliers may be identified.

Unexplained sudden cardiac death is of great interest for the race horse industry. Thoroughbred racehorse cases of sudden death after racing have increased, particularly in California over the past 5 years.[1] Arrhythmic or cardiac causes of these incidences is speculated and warrants further attention [7, 15]. Understanding the normal electrophysiologic, echocardiographic and biochemical values in this population is important if any meaningful cardiac screening practices are to be proposed.

The objectives of this study were to (1) characterize selected indices of cardiac function, electrophysiologic parameters, and biochemical markers of heart dysfunction prior to and immediately after high level racing in Thoroughbred horses receiving furosemide; and (2) create pre- and post-race reference values in order to make recommendations on the best screening practices for race horses.

Methods

Animals

Thirty-eight Thoroughbred racehorses were recruited for participation in the study during 2 different race weekends at the Santa Anita Park race track between 2/19/2015 and 3/8/2015. Horses were selected based on availability and owner consent. Consent for participation was obtained from all horse owners. This study was performed in accordance with the institutional animal care and use committee at the University of California Davis (IACUC # 18285). All race horses enrolled had a cardiovascular physical examination performed by one investigator (JAS) and were deemed healthy for racing by the attending track veterinarians in accordance with the racing guidelines and practices. Thorough evaluation of the cardiovascular system and any abnormal heart sounds were recorded [16]. Sex, age, race length (in furlongs), race substrate (dirt or turf), and place at finish were recorded. Horses that were claimed and transferred to a new owner and trainer following the race were excluded as no post-race data could be obtained. All horses were noted to receive furosemide after T0 and prior to T1 in keeping with standard pre-race practices in this racing jurisdiction.

Electrocardiography

Electrocardiography studies were performed on all horses 24 to 48 h prior to the race (T0) and within 30–60 min following the race (T1). The ECG recordings were performed using an AliveCor device and application software.[2] The device was placed over the left cardiac apex (Fig. 1). ECGs were recorded for 3–5 min with a paper speed of 50 mm/s and a calibration of 20 mm equal to 1 mV. All AliveCor tracings were reviewed for quality and discarded if they were poor quality or there was excessive artifact. ECGs were printed, randomized and the observer was blinded. ECGs were evaluated for rhythm and abnormalities of conduction. Heart rate (HR), P wave duration, PR interval, QRS duration, ST segment deviation from baseline, and QT interval were measured offline using manual calipers by a single operator (AS) under the direct supervision of the attending cardiologist (JS). QT intervals were corrected for HR using the Bazett's formula and reported as QTc [17].

Echocardiography

All horses were scanned standing and unsedated at 2 time points (T0 and T1) as described [18]. Standard 2-dimensional and M-mode echocardiography from the right side and left sides of the thorax were performed using a the Acuson P300 portable echocardiogram[3] equipped with a nominal 3 MHz frequency transducer [18]. All measurements were performed blinded in random order, by one board-certified cardiologist (JS), using an offline work station[4] as previously described [18, 19]. All measurements were the mean for 3 consecutive cardiac cycles. The following dimensions were measured from the M-mode recordings of the left ventricle, imaged from a right parasternal short axis view at the level of the *chordae tendineae*: the interventricular septum in end-diastole (IVSd), the left ventricular freewall at end-diastole (LVFWd), the left ventricular diameter at end--diastole (LVIDd), and at peak-systole (LVIDs). Left-ventricular systolic function was assessed by calculating

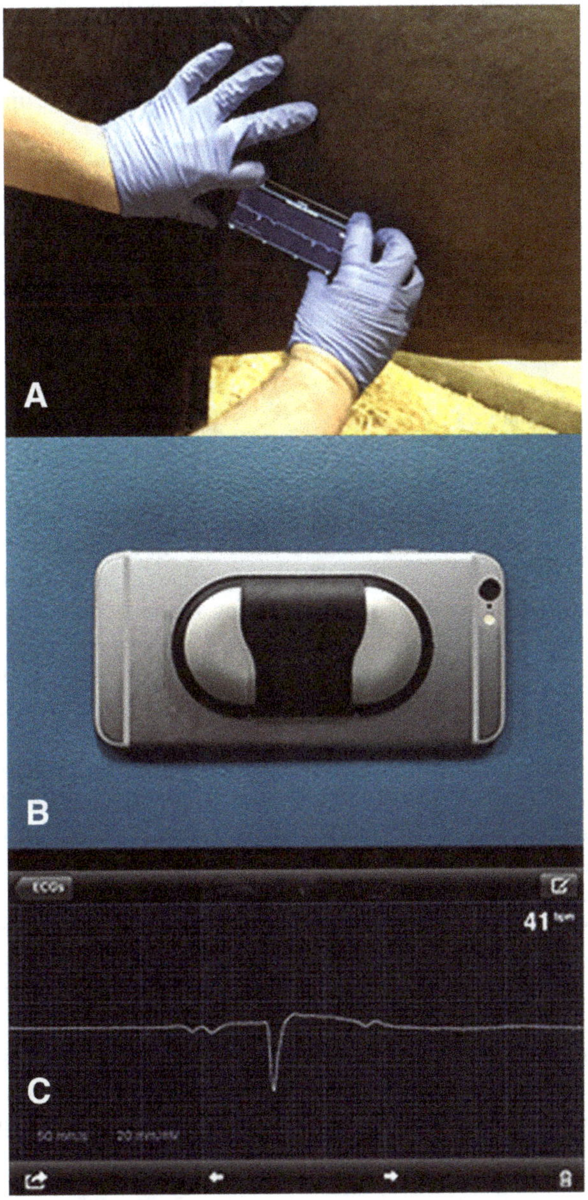

Fig. 1 Acquisition of an AliveCor tracing with device placed over the palpated apex beat (**a**), the AliveCor device (**b**), and the ECG tracing obtained at 50 mm/s and 20 mm/mV (**c**)

left ventricular fractional shortening (FS) in the following way: FS% = (LVIDd-LVIDs)/LVIDd × 100%. The maximal left atrial diameter in systole was measured from the right (LADsax) left hemithorax (LADlax). Color Doppler examination of the mitral, tricuspid, and aortic valves were recorded and scored for presence and severity of regurgitation by the subjective color Doppler surface area method [20].

Blood samples

Twelve milliliters of blood were obtained by jugular vein puncture at time points T0, T1, 4 h after the race (T4) and 24 h post-race (T24). The blood samples were placed into a heparinized blood collection tube and tested within 30 min of collection. Samples were analyzed with an i-STAT point of care analyzer.[5] Detection of cardiac troponin I (cTnI) with this point-of-care analyzer is based on a 2-site ELISA, which uses 2 independent antibodies, a caprine polyclonal and a murine monoclonal antibody, that recognize independent epitopes of human cTnI, with a lower limit of detection of 0.01 ng/ml [Kraus, 2010 #789]. The analytic sensitivity, based on the manufacturer insert is 0.02 ng/ml and a reportable range of 0.0–50 ng/ml, with any value above this range reported as >50 ng/ml. Values ≤0.02 ng/ml cannot be discriminated; however, the analyzer provides a specific point estimate of either 0.00, 0.01 or 0.02 mg/l. This analyzer has been previously reported to have good agreement with a similar equine bench-top immunoassay [21]. At all time points an i-STAT EC8+ cartridge[5] was also used to obtain the following values: pH, pCO_2, bicarbonate (HCO_3), sodium (Na), potassium (K), ionized calcium (iCa), glucose (Gluc), and hematocrit (Hct%).

Statistical analysis

Statistical analysis was performed with commercially available software Prism 7.0 and SPSS 22.0.[6] The difference between echocardiographic measures and electrocardiographic measures pre- and post-race were compared by either a paired t-test if both data sets were normally distributed or by Wilcoxon matched-pairs signed rank test if one or both failed D'Agostino & Pearson normality testing. A value of $P < 0.05$ was considered significant. One-way repeated measures ANOVA with Greenhouse-Geisser correction followed by Tukey's multiple comparisons test with individual variances computed for each comparison was performed for blood values at all time points if they were normally distributed. Repeated cTnI and electrolyte measures were compared using a Friedmans test and Dunn's multiple comparisons test if they were not normally distributed. Mean +/− standard deviation is reported for all normally distributed data and median and interquartile range reported for non-normally distributed data. Where significant differences are identified between time points, the mean or median difference is reported followed by the 95% confidence interval to demonstrate the effect size. Reference ranges for ECG and echocardiographic data were computed using a non-parametric approach (ie. without any distributional assumptions) using percentiles 0.025 and 0.975 to report 95% reference range [22]. Computations were performed using the reference interval package in R language version 3.3.1.[7] Reference ranges for cTnI, electrolytes, and other biochemical date were computed using the Robust method and reported as 90% confidence intervals in accordance with the

American Society for Veterinary Clinical Pathology Guidelines [23, 24].

Results

Thirty-eight Thoroughbred race horses were evaluated from 23 races, with 1–4 horses evaluated per race. Eight horses were excluded because they were claimed and were unavailable for post-race evaluation. Of the 30 horses evaluated pre- and post-race, there were 13 fillies (<5 yrs. of age), 5 mares (>5 yrs. of age), 8 geldings, and 4 colts (<5 yrs. of age). Ages ranged from 3 to 6 years with a mean of 3.8 (+/− 0.9) years. Horses placed 1st through 12th in their races. Length of race ranged from 5.5 furlongs [1106 m] to 9 furlongs [1810 m] with the most common distance being 6.5 furlongs [1308 m] raced by 12 horses. Eighteen horses raced on a dirt track while the remaining 12 horses raced on turf. Furosemide doses were available for 27 horses; 23 horses received 250 mg. The remaining 4 horses received 150 mg, 350 mg, 400 mg, and 500 mg respectively. For the 3 horses for which specific doses were not available the trainer reported a dose range of 150-350 mg given. Given the lack of variability in this data, no statistical testing was performed on the impact of furosemide dose administered.

Electrocardiogram

ECGs were available for all 30 horses at T0 and T1. All AliveCor tracings were readable and clear. No dysrhythmias were recorded. Reference ranges for pre- and post--race values are listed in Table 1. Heart rate was significantly increased at the post-race time point with a median HR of 39 bpm at T0 and 86 bpm at T1 yielding a median difference of 39 bpm, 95% CI [31, 58], ($P <$ 0.0001). The QT interval was shorter post-race with an increase in HR. Once corrected for HR mean QTc was significantly shorter at T1 when compared to T0 with a mean difference of -91 msec, 95% CI [−108, −72], ($P <$ 0.0001). PR interval also decreased post-race with a mean difference of -85 msec, 95% CI [−105, −66], ($P <$ 0.001). There was no significant change in ST segment deviation between T1 and T0 with a median difference of 0.3 mV, 95% CI [−0.2, −0.5], (P 0.11).

Echocardiogram

An increase in number of horses with valvular regurgitation was noted across all valves interrogated on echocardiogram after the race (Table 2). Prior to the race 15 horses (50.0%) had no identifiable aortic regurgitation (AR). Following the race only 4 horses had no AR, 12 had trace, and 14 had mild AR. Tricuspid regurgitation (TR) was noted to be absent in 12 horses (40.4%), trace in 13 (43.3%), and mild in 5 horses (16.7%) prior to racing. On Doppler interrogation after the race TR was noted to be mild in 16 horses (53.3%) and moderate in 8 horses (26.7%). No mitral regurgitation (MR) was appreciated in any horses on echocardiogram prior to racing. Mild MR ($n = 3$) and trace MR ($n = 5$) were noted in 8 horses post-race.

Left atrial dimension and left ventricular internal dimensions decreased significantly with mean differences of −1.2 cm, 95% CI [−1.6, −0.8] and −1.2 cm, 95% CI [−1.5, −0.9] respectively following the race ($P < 0.0001$; Table 1). Fractional shortening % significantly increased after the race when compared to pre-race values with a mean difference of 7.9%, 95% CI [4.8, 10.9], ($P < 0.0001$).

Blood analysis

Blood gas values at all time points and reference ranges are noted in Table 3. Pair-wise comparison of cTnI was significantly different between T0 and T4 with a median difference of 0.02 ng/ml, 95% CI [0.01–0.03], ($P < 0.0001$, Fig. 2). Hematocrit significantly increased between T0 and T1 with a mean difference of 10.2%, 95% CI [7.2, 13.3], ($P < 0.0001$), but returned to T0 values by 24 h post-race. Sodium significantly decreased between T0 and T1 with a mean difference of −2.6 mmol/L, 95% CI [−3.8, −1.4], ($P < 0.0001$). Bicarbonate (HCO3) significantly decreased between T0 and T1 with a mean difference of −13.6 mmol/L, 95% CI [−15.6, −11.6], ($P < 0.0001$). Ionized calcium (iCa) significantly decreased between T0 and T1 with a mean difference of −0.30 mmol/L, 95% CI [−0.33, −0.26], ($P < 0.0001$).

Sodium was significantly decreased at T4 with a mean difference of −2.6 mmol/L, 95% CI [−3.4, −1.9], ($P <$ 0.0001). Potassium was significantly decreased at T4 with a median difference of −0.4 mmol/L, 95% CI [−0.5, −0.1], ($P = 0.0307$). Both sodium and potassium returned to baseline by T24. Serum pH decreased during the time immediately following the race (T1) with a mean difference of −0.14, 95% CI [−0.18, −0.10], ($P < 0.0001$), but returned to baseline value by T4. Graphical representations of biochemical data are presented in Fig. 3.

No single horse was a consistent outlier across the parameters measured on ECG, echocardiogram, or blood values obtained.

Discussion

This study describes normal pre- and post-race values for selected ECG, echocardiogram, and blood parameters in competing Thoroughbred racehorses. This study is unique because it represents acquisition and assessment of these values in competitive racing horses and not in the laboratory or after exercise on a treadmill. No consistent outliers were appreciated and there was no suggestion of EICF at the time points studied, based on the measures employed. There was also no incidence of sudden death observed in this study. This finding does

Table 1 Selected ECG and echocardiogram parameters recorded prior to race and within 30–60 min after the race start time are listed

	Pre-race (T0)	RI (pre-race)	Post-race (T1)	RI (post-race)	*P* value
ECG					
PR interval (sec)	0.279 (+/−0.049)	0.211–0.381	0.193 (+/−0.035)	0.146–0.259	**<0.0001**
QRS duration (sec)	0.098 (+/−0.013)	0.075–0.118	0.093 (+/−0.012)	0.073–0.113	.0789
QT interval (sec)	0.445 (+/− 0.053)	0.355–0.567	0.353 (+/− 0.047)	0.271–0.436	**<0.0001**
QTc interval (sec)	0.507 (+/− 0.051)	0.438–0.591	0.417 (+/− 0.024)	0.371–0.454	**<0.0001**
ST segment (mV)	1.3 (0.6,2.3)	0.2–2.9	1.8 (+/−1.0)	0.4–3.6	0.1115
HR (bpm)	39 (32,45)	26–63	86 (69,100)	58–126	**<0.0001**
Echocardiogram					
LAD Sax (cm)	10.9 (+/−0.7)	9.8–12.2	10.1 (+/−0.9)	8.4–11.4	**<0.0001**
LAD Lax (cm)	13.0 (+/−0.7)	11.8–14.7	11.8 (+/− 1.1)	10.1–13.5	**<0.0001**
Ao (cm)	7.5 (+/−0.6)	6.6–8.6	7.3 (+/−0.5)	7.4–8.4	0.1547
IVSd (cm)	3.3 (+/−0.4)	2.7–4.0	3.5 (+/−0.4)	2.8–4.2	**0.0117**
LVIDd (cm)	12.1 (+/−1.0)	10.5–13.7	10.9 (+/−1.2)	8.5–13.0	**<0.0001**
LVIDs (cm)	6.9 (+/− 1.1)	5.0–8.7	5.5 (+/−1.2)	3.3–7.4	**<0.0001**
LVFWd (cm)	2.8 (+/−0.3)	2.2–3.4	2.8 (+/−0.5)	2.2–3.7	0.7321
FS (%)	42.2 (+/−7.6)	30.8–58.0	50.0 (+/−8.2)	38.4–67.1	**<0.0001**

Pre- (T0) and post-race values (T1) were compared and the *P* value is reported. The *P* value is bolded when a significant difference between T0 and T1 was present. The QT interval was corrected for HR (QTc) using Bazett's formula. Normally distributed data is reported in mean +/− standard deviation. Non-parametric data is reported in median with interquartile range in parenthesis. Reported with reference intervals (RI) computed using a non-parametric approach (ie. without any distributional assumptions) using percentiles 0.025 and 0.975 to report 95% reference range

not preclude the development of either condition in the future or with subsequent exercise or evaluations. It is important to remember that all horses of this study were trained and actively racing during the season, thus T0 evaluations are not representative of the general non-racing Thoroughbred population.

Table 2 Echocardiographic determination of valvular regurgitation at pre- and post-race time points in 30 Thoroughbred horses

	Pre-Race (T0)	Post-Race (T1)
AoV Regurgitation	Number of Horses (%)	Number of Horses (%)
None	15 (50.0%)	4 (13.3%)
Trace	11 (36.6%)	12 (40.0%)
Mild	4 (13.3%)	14 (46.6%)
Moderate	0	0
TV Regurgitation		
None	12 (40.4%)	4 (13.3%)
Trace	13 (43.3%)	2 (6.7%)
Mild	5 (16.7%)	16 (53.3%)
Moderate	0	8 (26.7%)
MV Regurgitation		
None	30 (100%)	22 (73.3%)
Trace	0	5 (16.7%)
Mild	0	3 (10.0%)
Moderate	0	0

Electrocardiograms were easily and effectively collected with the AliveCor device. The AliveCor is smartphone-based handheld ECG that delivered readable and interpretable data without the necessity of a cumbersome machine and electrode clips. AliveCor has been validated for rhythm evaluation in humans, dogs, cats, and water buffalo calves [25–28]. Measurement of QT and QTc in using the AliveCor device has reported to have good agreement with 12-lead ECG in humans [29]. This is a viable option for rhythm and QT assessment immediately after exercise on the race track or in the clinic. There was no gold-standard that this device was compared to as this study did not specially aim to validate this method. Further investigation is needed to determine if the values created in this study can be applied to standard base-apex lead measures although given the results from the human and canine studies with the AliveCor device it is likely similar.

Racing ameliorates vagal tone that is dominant at rest [30]. Increased HR recorded at T1 relative to is likely due to increased sympathetic tone after exercise and decreased vagal influence [16]. This also explains the decrease in PR interval recorded after racing (T1) because sympathetic tone can increase conduction velocity through the atrial myocardium.

Alterations in QT interval can place patients at increased risk of sudden death by extending the vulnerable period for inciting severe cardiac arrhythmias or ventricular fibrillation [16]. No dysrhythmias or prolongation in

Table 3 Bloodwork performed via iSTAT cartridges and sampled across all time points (T0 = pre-race, T1 = post-race, T4 = 4 h post-race, and T24 = 24 h post-race), in 30 Thoroughbred race horses

Blood Parameters	T0	T0 RI	T1	T1 RI	T4	T4 RI	T24	T24 RI
cTnI (ng/ml)	0.01 (0.0,0.01)	<0.01	0.01 (0.0,0.03)	0.0–0.05	0.03 (+/−0.02)[a],+	0.0–0.07	0.01 (0.0,0.02)	0.0–0.05
pH	7.47 (+/−0.03)	7.41–7.52	7.33 (+/−0.11)[a]	7.17–7.56	7.48 (+/−0.05)+	7.40–7.56	7.46 (7.44,7.49)+	7.36–7.57
HCO3 (mmol/L)	29.2 (+/−1.6)	26.4–32.0	15.6 (+/−5.4)[a]	6.0–25.4	28.7 (27.1,30.3)+	24.3–33.3	29.9 (+/−1.5)+	27.3–32.4
pCO2 (mmHg)	40.2 (+/−3.3)	34.4–45.8	27.9 (+/−4.3)[a]	20.5–35.5	37.9 (+/−6.0)+	28.4–49.3	41.5 (40.1–44.7)+	32.3–51.6
Na + (mmol/L)	138 (+/−1.2)	136–140	135 (+/−2.8)[a]	131–141	136 (+/−1.7)+	133–139	139 (+/−1.3)+,[b]	136–140
K+ (mmol/L)	3.7 (+/−0.4)	3.0–4.4	3.5 (+/−0.3)[a]	3.0–4.1	3.5 (3.1,3.7)	2.1–4.9	3.6 (3.4,3.8)	2.8–4.4
iCa++ (mmol/L)	1.63 (+/−0.06)	1.52–1.73	1.34 (+/−0.06)[a]	1.23–1.45	1.56 (+/−0.07)[a],+	1.44–1.68	1.59 (+/−0.05)+	1.51–1.67
Glucose (mg/dL)	102 (92,108)	78–122	161 (145,195)[a]	94–229	107 (91,127)+	52–159	110 (+/−13)+	85–131
Hct (%)	41.6 (+/−5.7)	31.9–51.7	51.8 (+/−6.8)[a]	40.2–63.8	45.0 (+/−5.7)[a]	34.4–54.1	40.5 (33,43)+,[b]	23.3–57.3

Normally distributed data is reported in mean +/− standard deviation. Non-parametric data is reported in median with interquartile range in parenthesis. Reported with reference intervals (RI) calculated using the Robust method reported as 90% confidence interval in accordance with American Society for Veterinary Clinical Pathology guidelines. All values were compared to each other. Values that are significantly different (adjusted $P < 0.05$) than all other time points are marked as follows: [a]denotes significance when compared to T0, + denotes significance when compared to T1, [b]denotes significance when compared to T4

QT or QTc were noted in this study. Sudden cardiac death is of increasing concern post-race and theorized to be due to arrhythmia [9, 10]. However, the low prevalence of sudden death in the racehorse population may have rendered this study underpowered to identify it.[8] Alternatively, previous reports have noted that vagal rebound is a more important factor in post-race dysrhythmias [9]. Thus the sampling time-point of 30–60 min post-race may have been too early to identify recovery associated dysrhythmias. Additionally, some studies have indicated that prolonged ECG monitoring is necessary to identify the true frequency of cardiac arrhythmias in equine athletes. This may implicate that the short duration ECG used in our study is an underestimate of cardiac dysrhythmias in this population [4, 31]. While this represents a limitation, the use of a 3-5 min duration ECG remains a clinically accessible option for racehorses on the track, while ambulatory ECG monitoring is generally unavailable in this setting.

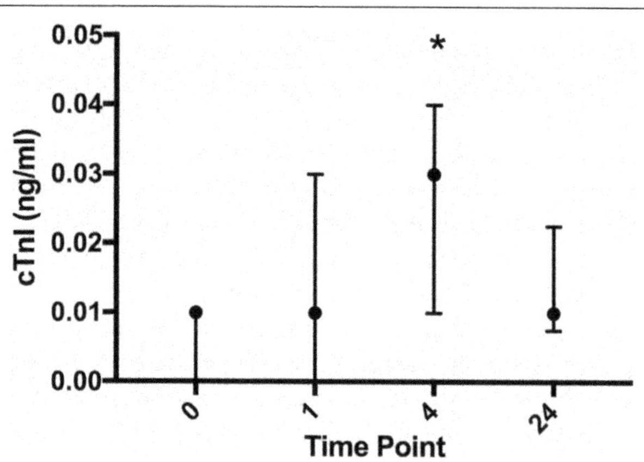

Fig. 2 Graphical representation of serum cTnI levels for each horse over time which demonstrates the delayed release pattern peaking at T4 and returning to baseline by T24. Time points are labeled as T0, T1, T4, and T24 which correspond to measurements obtained before the race, 30–60 min after the race, 4 h post-race, and 24 h post-race respectively. Circles represent the median with lines indicating the interquartile range. Significance ($P < 0.05$) is denoted by *

ST segment alterations suggest changes to cardiac repolarization. The cause of ST segment elevation or depression has not been specifically evaluated in the horse. However, across many other species it serves as an indicator of left ventricular ischemia or hypoxemia [32–34]. The lack of ST segment alteration in this study may be due to the AliveCor's inability to measure minor electrophysiologic alterations or may indicate that our population did not experience this. Further evaluation comparing AliveCor to standard base apex lead measurements in horse is needed.

The echocardiographic changes in LA and LV dimensions are consistent with what has been previously reported in endurance horses [6]. The noted decrease in LA and LV size may be secondary reduction in preload or due to an increase in HR and thus more forward flow and less diastolic filling. Decrease in these chamber sizes could also be secondary to furosemide administration and the resultant volume reduction.

The increase in FS% may be secondary to sympathetic activation and its positive inotropic effect. Alternatively increase in HR may have contributed to an increased in measured systolic function as a result of the Bowditch effect. The impact of alterations in LV volume secondary to furosemide administration may also impact this observation. Previous studies have noted reported variable valvular regurgitation in athletic horses that has not been associated with deleterious effects on athletic performance [35]. A post-exercise increase in valvular regurgitation was noted in our study. Progressive regurgitation may be in-part due to an increase in systolic function post-race and a resultant increase in the velocity of regurgitation.

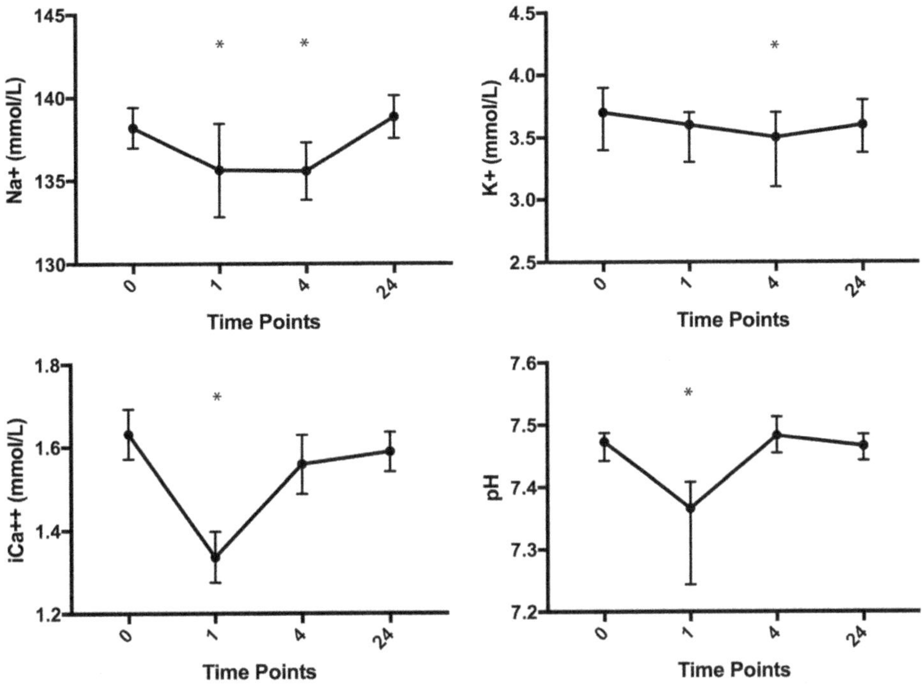

Fig. 3 Graphical representation of biochemical values at Time Points T0, T1, T4, and T24 which correspond to measurements obtained before the race, 30–60 min after the race, 4 h post-race, and 24 h post-race respectively. Significant differences relative to T0 are labeled *

Serum cTnI was no different at all time points except T4 (Fig. 2). Cardiac troponin has a delayed release pattern in mice, humans, dogs, and horses [36, 37]. Previous studies in equine athletes did not note a significant elevation when sampled 1–2 h following a race [37]. Our data supported this finding as there was not significant change in cTnI when sampled shortly after the race (T1). There was however an increase in cTnI at T4 which is consistent with troponin's known delayed release pattern and clearance curves already established [36]. In equine medicine it is assumed but not proven that the magnitude of cardiac damage is correlated with the magnitude of cTnI release. If this is the case, the horses in this study had minor cTnI change and all returned to baseline values by the 24 h time point. This would indicate that a transient release of troponin from the cytosol occurred and permanent or more long-lasting damage to the myocyte did not occur. Theories about transient myocardial hypoxemia have been offered to explain mild increase in cTnI following races [11, 37–39]. Our study would support this notion and suggest that identification of ischemic changes secondary to racing would be best evaluated by measurement of cTnI at 4 h and 24 h post-race, rather than immediately after the race. Alternatively, an undetectable amount of troponin may be released earlier than measured, however this value may not reach detectable levels until at least 4 h after the race. Further investigation using a high- or ultra-sensitivity assay may be considered to evaluate this possibility.

As expected with anaerobic exertion, pH decreased after the race likely due to lactic acidosis from anaerobic metabolism [40]. This is a tightly regulated value and was observed to return to baseline by T4. Partial pressure of CO2 decreased immediately after the race consistent with previous reports [40]. This is hypothesized to be due to either post-race hyperventilation in an effort to recover from this extreme exercise and/or respiratory compensation of metabolic acidosis from anaerobic metabolism and increased lactic acid [40].

While there was a statically significant alteration in Na + values in our study at T1 and T4, however given the overlap in the ranges of these values the clinical significance of this finding is unclear. Previous studies have identified hyperkalemia immediately after exercise likely secondary to transmembrane fluxes from exercising muscles [41]. In contrast, in our study the K values measured were not significantly decreased immediately following the race (at T1) and became significantly decreased at 4 h post-race. The lack of change at T1 could be due the slight delay in sampling time or due to a balance between loss and increase. For instance, loss secondary to furosemide administration together with an increase due to efflux from the intracellular space during extreme exercise may have resulted in a net negligible change in this value. The reduction in K at T4 is most likely due ion loss secondary to furosemide administration [42]. The glucose increase noted is thought to be due to increased sympathetic stimulation [43].

There was a notable increase in Hct consistent with previous studies which could be due to splenic contraction following excitement and exercise known to occur in horses [5, 44]. Increase in Hct could also be due to plasma volume depletion from furosemide administration and post-race dehydration [42]. Hematocrit returned to pre-race values by 4 h after the race. This supports the notion that the increase is transient with a rapid recovery.

There are a number of limitations for this study inherent in performing a field based study. A principal limitation is that all horses were treated with furosemide between T0 and T1. Separating if the observed effects of this study are secondary to exercise, furosemide or a combination of both is not possible using the present study design and may represent a future aim for a study to be completed in horses where furosemide may be withheld. The trainers whose horses were enrolled in this study were unwilling to alter their racing practices to exclude furosemide.

Sample size is a common limitation in veterinary studies and this study is no exception. The access to high-level competing horses immediately post-race is challenging and the enrollment of 38 horses and study completion of 30 horses generated a significant dataset for generation of reference intervals. It is possible that with a larger sampling of horses, more outliers could have been identified and more narrow reference intervals created.

The working nature of these horses significantly limited the extent of echocardiographic and electrocardiographic evaluations that could be performed, as time for evaluation was brief. The authors selected a small number of study variables that may be readily accessible for screening horses in this environment. More robust systolic and diastolic function assessments may have elucidated subtle alterations in function post-race however many diastolic assessments have proven to be technically difficult and unreliable post-exercise [19]. For this reason, horses with EICF could have been overlooked. Fractional shortening, like many systolic function assessments, is both preload and afterload dependent thus the alternations noted to this value may reflect alterations in these factors. The assessment of valvular regurgitation was subjective in nature and thus may be prone to error. Currently there is no accepted gold standard quantitative assessment of valve regurgitation in horses or human athletes and many varieties of assessment rely on subjective qualitative assessment. This assessment was performed by a single investigator to decrease this variability and has been used for evaluation of regurgitation in previous studies [20, 45].

No horses in our study had detectable evidence of EICF and no sudden death events were noted. Identification of horses that demonstrated EICF or sudden death would provide highly valuable information in these conditions. However, the low incidence of EICF or sudden death suggests that designing a study to identify this condition would require massive sample size which was not feasible within the scope of this work. The use of the reference ranges established in this study can however be used to help to early detect horses at high risk of EICF in future races and studies.

Another limitation was in the precise timing that the measurement for ECG and echocardiogram were gathered. Inherent to the nature of racing and the number of animals included, ECGs and echocardiogram evaluations, were performed at a variable time within the first hour post-race. This may have allowed for some cardiovascular recovery and subsequently increased variability in the reference intervals obtained.

Additionally, the ECG measurements were obtained using an AliveCor device which has not been previously validated in horses. In humans, dogs, and cats this device has been used to assess for arrhythmias and ECG wave-form duration but its value in assessment of complex height is limited given the variation that is associated with placement of electrodes on the animal. Complex height was not measured in this study for this reason. It is highly likely that given the nature of ECG duration measure, the values obtained with the AliveCor reflect those that would be obtained with a standard base-apex lead. This however was not a goal of this study and further investigation is needed to confirm this association.

It is also important to note that the reference intervals generated were determined for the iSTAT Chem 8 and cTnI assay and may not necessarily be extrapolated to other devices as there is known variability in cTnI assays [37].

Finally, this study utilized a before and after study design where each horse served as its own control. While this approach is commonly employed and results in greater statistical power with a smaller number of animals, it is subject to a phenomenon called regression to the mean [46]. The impact of possible regression to the mean on this data set cannot be determined.

Further areas of study include the screening of more animals with the protocol established in this study to help identify outliers particularly if there is a suggestion of EICF or decreased athletic performance. Further evaluation in order to correlate the parameters measured in this study with performance outcomes of success on the track is an area of future investigation. Finally following a number of individual horses and their trends over time and subsequent races may help to better identify animals that are at risk of fatigue.

Conclusion

The reference intervals generated in this study may be used to identify racing Thoroughbred horses with inappropriate electrophysiological, biochemical or echocardiographic responses to racing.

Endnotes

[1]California Horse Racing Board (2013) 43rd Annual Report. www.chrb.ca.gov (Publications). Sacramento, CA.

[2]AliveCor, Inc. San Francisco, CA 94108, USA.

[3]Siemens Medical Solutions USA, Inc. Malvern, PA 19355, USA.

[4]syngo Dynamics, Siemens Medical Solutions, Malvern, PA.

[5]Abbott Point of Care Inc., Princeton, NJ 08540, USA.

[6]GraphPad Software, Inc. La Jolla, CA 92037, USA.

[7]R Core Team. 2016. R: A Language and Environment for Statistical Computing. Utilizing R Reference Interval Package (referenceInterval" package in R (https://cran.r-project.org/web/packages/referenceIntervals/referenceIntervals.pdf) R Foundation for Statistical Computing. Vienna, Austria.

[8]California Racing Board (2014) Baffert Sudden Death Report. www.chrb.ca.gov/veterinary_reports/baffert_sudden_death_report_final_1121.pdf

Abbreviations

AR: Aortic regurgitation; cTnI: Cardiac troponin I; ECG: Electrocardiogram; EICF: Exercise induced cardiac fatigue; FS: Shortening fraction; Gluc: Glucose; HCO3: Bicarbonate; Hct: Hematocrit; HR: Heart rate; iCa: Ionized calcium; IVSd: Interventricular septum in end-diastole; K: Potassium; LADlax: Left atrial dimension long-axis; LADsax: Left atrial dimension short-axis; LVFWd: The left ventricular freewall at end-diastole; LVIDd: The left ventricular diameter at end-diastole; LVIDs: The left ventricular diameter at peak-systole; MR: Mitral regurgitation; Na: Sodium; T0: Pre-race time point; T1: 30–60 min post-race time point; T24: 24-h post-race time point; T4: Four-hours post-race time point; TR: Tricuspid regurgitation

Acknowledgements

We are grateful to the California Horse Racing Board, the Santa Anita Race track, as well as all the horse owners and trainers for their support and help during the study.

Funding

Supported by funds from the University of California Davis Center for Equine Health Marcia MacDonald Rivas Grant # 14–04.

Authors' contributions

CGH Data analysis and interpretation, manuscript draft and revision. RA Data acquisition, analysis and interpretation. KE Data acquisition, analysis and interpretation. BM Data analysis and interpretation. AS Data acquisition, analysis and interpretation. EO Data acquisition, analysis and interpretation. AV Conception & design, data acquisition and interpretation. JS Principal Investigator, conception & design, data acquisition, analysis and interpretation, manuscript draft and revision. All authors read and approved the final manuscript.

Consent for publication

Not applicable.

Competing interests

The authors declare that they have no competing interests.

Author details

[1]Department of Medicine & Epidemiology, School of Veterinary Medicine, University of California Davis, Davis, CA 95616, USA. [2]School of Veterinary Medicine, University of California Davis, Davis, CA 95616, USA. [3]William R. Pritchard Veterinary Medical Teaching Hospital (VMTH), University of California Davis, Davis, CA 95616, USA. [4]Center for Animal Disease Modeling And Surveillance (CADMS), Department of Medicine & Epidemiology, School of Veterinary Medicine, University of California Davis, Davis, CA 95616, USA. [5]Present Address: Gold Coast Veterinary Service & Consulting, Esparto, CA 95627, USA. [6]Present Address: Marion duPont Scott Equine Medical Center, Virginia-Maryland College of Veterinary Medicine, Leesburg, VA 20176, USA.

References

1. Oxborough D, Birch K, Shave R, George K. "Exercise-induced cardiac fatigue"–a review of the echocardiographic literature. Echocardiography. 2010;27:1130–40.
2. McGavock JM, Warburton DE, Taylor D, Welsh RC, Quinney HA, Haykowsky MJ. The effects of prolonged strenuous exercise on left ventricular function: a brief review. Heart Lung. 2002;31:279–92. quiz 93-4
3. Wijnberg ID, Franklin SH. The heart remains the core: cardiac causes of poor performance in horses compared to human athletes. Comparative exercise. Physiology. 2017;13:149–74.
4. Flethoj M, Kanters JK, Haugaard MM, Pedersen PJ, Carstensen H, Balling JD, Olsen LH, Buhl R. Changes in heart rate, arrhythmia frequency, and cardiac biomarker values in horses during recovery after a long-distance endurance ride. J Am Vet Med Assoc. 2016;248:1034–42.
5. Flethoj M, Schwarzwald CC, Haugaard MM, Carstensen H, Kanters JK, Olsen LH, Buhl R. Left ventricular function after prolonged exercise in equine endurance athletes. J Vet Intern Med. 2016;30:1260–9.
6. Amory H, Votion DM, Fraipont A, Goachet AG, Robert C, Farnir F, Van Erck E. Altered systolic left ventricular function in horses completing a long distance endurance race. Equine Vet J Suppl. 2010:216–9.
7. Ryan N, Marr CM, McGladdery AJ. Survey of cardiac arrhythmias during submaximal and maximal exercise in thoroughbred racehorses. Equine Vet J. 2005;37:265–8.
8. Boden LA, Charles JA, Slocombe RF, Sandy JR, Finnin PJ, Morton JM, Clarke AF. Sudden death in racing thoroughbreds in Victoria, Australia. Equine Vet J. 2005;37:269–71.
9. Navas de Solis C. Exercising arrhythmias and sudden cardiac death in horses: review of the literature and comparative aspects. Equine Vet J. 2016;48:406–13.
10. Pedersen PJ, Kanters JK, Buhl R, Klaerke DA. Normal electrocardiographic QT interval in race-fit Standardbred horses at rest and its rate dependence during exercise. J Vet Cardiol. 2013;15:23–31.
11. Nostell K, Haggstrom J. Resting concentrations of cardiac troponin I in fit horses and effect of racing. J Vet Cardiol. 2008;10:105–9.
12. Begg LM, Hoffmann KL, Begg AP. Serum and plasma cardiac troponin I concentrations in clinically normal thoroughbreds in training in Australia. Aust Vet J. 2006;84:336–7.
13. Phillips W, Giguere S, Franklin RP, Hernandez J, Adin D, Peloso JG. Cardiac troponin I in pastured and race-training thoroughbred horses. J Vet Intern Med. 2003;17:597–9.
14. Buhl R, Petersen EE, Lindholm M, Bak L, Nostell K. Cardiac arrhythmias in Standardbreds during and after racing—possible association between heart size, Valvular regurgitations, and arrhythmias. Journal of Equine Veterinary Science. 2013;33:590–6.
15. Lyle CH, Uzal FA, McGorum BC, Aida H, Blissitt KJ, Case JT, Charles JT, Gardner I, Horadagoda N, Kusano K, et al. Sudden death in racing thoroughbred horses: an international multicentre study of post mortem findings. Equine Vet J. 2011;43:324–31.

16. Bonagura JD, Reef VB, Schwarzwald CC. Cardiovascular diseases. In: Equine Internal Medicine. 3rd ed; 2010. p. 455–71.
17. Luo S, Michler K, Johnston P, Macfarlane PW. A comparison of commonly used QT correction formulae: the effect of heart rate on the QTc of normal ECGs. J Electrocardiol. 2004;37(Suppl):81–90.
18. Marr CM, Patteson M. Echocardiography. In: Marr CM, editor. Cardiology of the Horse. 2nd ed. Edinburgh, Saunders Elsevier; 2010. p. 105–26.
19. Schefer KD, Bitschnau C, Weishaupt MA, Schwarzwald CC. Quantitative analysis of stress echocardiograms in healthy horses with 2-dimensional (2D) echocardiography, anatomical M-mode, tissue Doppler imaging, and 2D speckle tracking. J Vet Intern Med. 2010;24:918–31.
20. Young LE, Rogers K, Wood JL. Heart murmurs and valvular regurgitation in thoroughbred racehorses: epidemiology and associations with athletic performance. J Vet Intern Med. 2008;22:418–26.
21. Kraus MS, Jesty SA, Gelzer AR, Ducharme NG, Mohammed HO, Mitchell LM, Soderholm LV, Divers TJ. Measurement of plasma cardiac troponin I concentration by use of a point-of-care analyzer in clinically normal horses and horses with experimentally induced cardiac disease. Am J Vet Res. 2010;71:55–9.
22. Bland M. An introduction to medical statistics. 4th ed. Oxford: Oxford University Press; 2015.
23. Friedrichs KR, Harr KE, Freeman KP, Szladovits B, Walton RM, Barnhart KF, Blanco-Chavez J. American Society for Veterinary Clinical P: ASVCP reference interval guidelines: determination of de novo reference intervals in veterinary species and other related topics. Vet Clin Pathol. 2012;41:441–53.
24. Horowitz GL. Defining, establishing, and verifying reference intervals in the clinical laboratory: approved guideline. Wayne, PA: Clinical and Laboratory Standards Institute; 2008.
25. Kraus MS, Gelzer AR, Rishniw M. Detection of heart rate and rhythm with a smartphone-based electrocardiograph versus a reference standard electrocardiograph in dogs and cats. J Am Vet Med Assoc. 2016;249:189–94.
26. Nguyen HH, Silva JN. Use of smartphone technology in cardiology. Trends Cardiovasc Med. 2016;26:376–86.
27. Smith J, Ward JL, Urbano T, Mueller MS. Use of AliveCor heart monitor for heart rate and rhythm evaluation in dairy water buffalo calves (Bubalis Bubalis). J dairy vet Anim Res. 2016;4(2):00113.
28. Vezzosi T, Buralli C, Marchesotti F, Porporato F, Tognetti R, Zini E, Domenech O. Diagnostic accuracy of a smartphone electrocardiograph in dogs: comparison with standard 6-lead electrocardiography. Vet J. 2016;216:33–7.
29. Garabelli P, Stavrakis S, Albert M, Koomson E, Parwani P, Chohan J, Smith L, Albert D, Xie R, Xie Q, et al. Comparison of QT interval readings in normal sinus rhythm between a smartphone heart monitor and a 12-lead ECG for healthy volunteers and inpatients receiving Sotalol or Dofetilide. J Cardiovasc Electrophysiol. 2016;27:827–32.
30. Hamlin RL, Klepinger WL, Gilpin KW, Smith CR. Autonomic control of heart rate in the horse. Am J Phys. 1972;222:976–8.
31. Physick-Sheard PW, McGurrin MK. Ventricular arrhythmias during race recovery in Standardbred racehorses and associations with autonomic activity. J Vet Intern Med. 2010;24:1158–66.
32. Hanna EB, Glancy DL. ST-segment elevation: Differential diagnosis, caveats. Cleve Clin J Med. 2015;82:373–84.
33. Zwanenburg A, Hermans BJ, Andriessen P, Niemarkt HJ, Jellema RK, Ophelders DR, Vullings R, Wolfs TG, Kramer BW, Delhaas T. Comparison of ECG-based physiological markers for hypoxia in a preterm ovine model. Pediatr Res. 2016;79:907–15.
34. Tilley LP. In: Tilley LP, editor. Analysis of canine P-QRS-T deflections. In: Essentials of canine and feline electrocardiographs: interpretation and treatment. 3rd ed. Malvern, PA, Lea & Febiger; 1992. p. 59–99.
35. Reef VB, Bonagura J, Buhl R, McGurrin MK, Schwarzwald CC, van Loon G, Young LE. Recommendations for management of equine athletes with cardiovascular abnormalities. J Vet Intern Med. 2014;28:749–61.
36. Kraus MS, Kaufer BB, Damiani A, Osterrieder N, Rishniw M, Schwark W, Gelzer AR, Divers TJ. Elimination half-life of intravenously administered equine cardiac troponin I in healthy ponies. Equine Vet J. 2013;45:56–9.
37. Rossi TM, Pyle WG, Maxie MG, Pearl DL, Physick-Sheard PW. Troponin assays in the assessment of the equine myocardium. Equine Vet J. 2014;46:270–5.
38. Slack J, Boston RC, Soma L, Reef VB. Cardiac troponin I in racing standardbreds. J Vet Intern Med. 2012;26:1202–8.
39. Holbrook TC, Birks EK, Sleeper MM, Durando M. Endurance exercise is associated with increased plasma cardiac troponin I in horses. Equine Vet J Suppl. 2006:27–31.
40. Snow DH, Mason DK, Ricketts SW, Douglas TA: Post-race blood biochemistry in thoroughbreds. In: Equine exercise physiology. Edited by Snow DH, Persson SGB, Rose RJ. Cambridge: Granta; 1983. p. 389–99.
41. Hyyppa S, Poso AR. Fluid, electrolyte, and acid-base responses to exercise in racehorses. Vet Clin North Am Equine Pract. 1998;14:121–36.
42. Soma LR, Uboh CE. Review of furosemide in horse racing: its effects and regulation. J Vet Pharmacol Ther. 1998;21:228–40.
43. Tyler-McGowan CM, Golland LC, Evans DL, Hodgson DR, Rose RJ. Haematological and biochemical responses to training and overtraining. Equine Vet J Suppl. 1999;30:621–5.
44. McGowan C. Clinical pathology in the racing horse: the role of clinical pathology in assessing fitness and performance in the racehorse. Vet Clin North Am Equine Pract. 2008;24:405–21. vii
45. Reef VB. Heart murmurs in horses: determining their significance with echocardiography. Equine Vet J Suppl. 1995;19:71–80.
46. Davis CE. The effect of regression to the mean in epidemiologic and clinical studies. Am J Epidemiol. 1976;104:493–8.

Modulatory role of regulatory T cells in a murine model of severe equine asthma

Claudio Henríquez[1], Gabriel Morán[1*], Cristian Carrasco[3], José Sarmiento[4], Miguel Barría[2], Hugo Folch[2] and Benjamin Uberti[5]

Abstract

Background: It is accepted that T regulatory cells (Treg) control different types of immune responses. In connection with this role, we have recently described an important increase in CD4+, CD25^{high}, Foxp3+ lymphocytes in the airway system of horses coursing with an exacerbation of severe equine asthma (EA). To explore the potential role of this population in the resolution of EA inflammation, we used a murine experimental model in which airway neutrophilic inflammation, which is similar to that observed in EA, is induced in mice by continual exposure to *Aspergillus fumigatus* contaminated hay. This model has the advantage that in mice we may induce a reduction of the Treg population using low doses of cyclophosphamide (Cy).

Results: The results indicated that the percentage of Treg cells increased with allergen exposure, as in horses; and animals partially depleted of Treg cells by treatment with Cy showed increased airway inflammation, demonstrated by an increased percentage of neutrophils and specific immunoglobulins in bronchoalveolar lavage fluid (BALF). Furthermore, a histopathologic study of animals that were pretreated with Cy before antigenic challenge showed higher cellular infiltration in the lung and deeper remodeling changes in the bronchi, including epithelial and goblet cell hyperplasia as well as airway smooth muscle hypertrophy.

Conclusion: In this murine model of EA, the reduced number and function of Treg induced by low doses of Cy, which directly correlates with increased airway inflammation and lung infiltration, indicates that Treg may play a major role in the regulation and resolution of EA.

Keywords: Equine asthma, Recurrent airway obstruction, Regulatory T cells, Airway inflammation

Background

Equine asthma (EA) [1–3] formerly called inflammatory airway disease (mild asthma) and recurrent airway obstruction (severe asthma) is characterized by periods of acute bronchoconstriction, bronchial hyper-responsiveness, pulmonary neutrophilia, decreased lung compliance and an increase in total lung resistance. Acute episodes of exacerbation are commonly triggered by inhalation of pollutants such as *Faenia rectivirgula*, *Thermoactinomyces vulgaris* and *Aspergillus fumigatus* [4, 5]. Resolution of airways inflammation is likely mediated via multiple mechanisms, with Tregs potentially playing a major contributory role.

It is generally accepted that regulatory T cells play an important role in tumor growth [6], control of autoimmunity [7] and allergic-mediated processes [8]. Since the publication of the seminal paper by Shimon Sakaguchi [9] pointing out the role of CD4+, CD25+ as the T lymphocytes responsible for suppression of the immune response, and because of the important contribution of Fontenot [10], who described the role of transcription factor Foxp3 as a second marker for this lymphoid population, CD4+, CD25+, Foxp3+ cells have been the most studied Treg subpopulation, and their relevance has been evaluated in mice and humans in the context of different immune-mediated diseases [11–18]. However, in domestic animals, information about the role of these cells in immune regulation is scarce. In this context, we have recently demonstrated that in horses with severe EA exacerbation after challenge with moldy hay contaminated with *Aspergillus fumigatus*, the number of Treg cells is greatly

* Correspondence: gmoran@uach.cl
[1]Pharmacology and Morphophysiology Department, Faculty of Veterinary Sciences, Universidad Austral de Chile, Valdivia, Chile
Full list of author information is available at the end of the article

increased in lymphocytes recovered from BALF [19]. This increase occurs in parallel with airway inflammation, but, currently, we may only speculate about the importance of Treg in the control and resolution of the acute severe EA process. An approach to answer this question may be attempted through the use of a recently described murine EA model that we have set up in our laboratory [20]. The essence of this model is the use of hay contaminated with *Aspergillus fumigatus* as bedding for experimental mice. After being housed in this condition, Rockefeller (RK) mice show an increase in the percentage of neutrophils in BALF, higher levels of specific antibodies against the fungus in the respiratory tract, and histology that demonstrates intense polymorphonuclear infiltration of the airway: these are important features that also appear in EA [1]. Moreover, in our experimental model, the disease is induced in animals over 5 months of age because younger mice are less sensitive or refractory to the induction of airway inflammation; the same age dependence occurs in the equine species, where the disease is usually observed in horses older than 8 years. In the mice of this experimental model, as also occurs in horses with exacerbation of severe EA, airway inflammation is resolved when animals return to a non-contaminated environment. It is worthy of note that the murine strain used here does not have increased individual susceptibility to airway inflammation, as does occur in EA-susceptible horses [21]. Despite this limitation of the experimental model, the description of immunological processes could be applicable to EA-susceptible and non-susceptible individuals. This murine model of severe EA presented us with the opportunity to modulate the Treg population using low doses of cyclophosphamide (Cy), as described earlier by Barbon [22]. In this context, Askenase's work [23] showed that Cy given at doses that do not suppress the immune response may increase delayed-type hypersensitivity reactions in mice; our laboratory also reported -in 1980- that low doses of Cy abrogate the phenomenon of antigenic competition [24]; at that time, this effect was attributed to the activation of a T suppressor cell. It since became evident that low doses of Cy potentiate the immune response in several animal models of cancer [25–27].

Methods

Animals

RK female mice, aged 2 months (young) or 8 months (old), were used in all experiments. All animals were obtained and maintained at the Animal Facility of the Universidad Austral de Chile. During exposure to *A. fumigatus* contaminated hay, the animals were placed in an isolation room with appropriate ventilation and filtering systems. This study was approved by the Bioethics Committee for the Use of Animals in Biomedical Research of the Universidad Austral de Chile.

The effect of exposure to the fungus was evaluated in 4 groups of animals: non-exposed young animals (n = 8), exposed young animals (n = 8), non-exposed old animals (n = 8), exposed old animals (n = 8). The measured outcome for fungus exposure was relative Treg content (CD4+, CD25+, Foxp3+) in spleen.

The effect of cyclophosphamide on airway inflammation was evaluated on three groups of 2 month old animals: not exposed to fungus and not treated with cyclophosphamide (n = 6), exposed to fungus but not treated with cyclophosphamide (n = 6), and treated with cyclophosphamide and exposed to fungus (n = 6).

Aspergillus fumigatus culture, protein extraction and hay contamination

Culture of *Aspergillus fumigatus* was carried out in two steps. The fungus was first cultured in peptone agar for 7 days at 37 °C and then in malt broth for 7 additional days. The resulting fungi were used for soluble protein extraction and to contaminate the mouse bedding. For protein extraction, fungi were blended and subsequently sonicated (Ultrasonic Homogenizer, series 4710 Cole Parmer, USA). The resulting suspension was centrifuged at 12.500×g for 10 min, and the supernatant containing soluble proteins was stored at −20 °C for later use. To expose mice to *Aspergillus fumigatus*, hay was sterilized and sprinkled with water containing fungus spores. The contaminated hay was then introduced into plastic bags and incubated for 48 h or more at 37 °C until mold contamination became visible. At this point, the contaminated hay was used as mice bedding. During the experiment, animals were maintained under these conditions according to the design of each study protocol.

Cyclophosphamide administration and induction of bronchial inflammation

Groups of mice were intraperitoneally treated with Cy at a dose of 20 mg/kg of body weight, for three consecutive days immediately before starting the antigenic challenge. As controls, groups of mice were injected with saline and exposed or not exposed to *Aspergillus fumigatus* contaminated hay. Experimental groups were maintained in this condition for different lengths of time, and were then euthanized with an overdose of pentobarbital at days 5, 11 and 17. In each case, blood samples, BALF, spleen and lung tissue were obtained for analysis.

Obtention, processing and analysis of samples

Samples of blood, BALF, spleen and lung were obtained 5, 11 and 17 days after the challenge conditions began. Blood (200 μl) was obtained each time from the treated and control mice and allowed to clot; the collected sera were stored at −20 °C until use. BALF was obtained from previously euthanatized mice; for this purpose, the trachea was exposed and cannulated with a 24G Teflon I.V. catheter. BALF was collected with saline solution (3 × 0.5 ml), and cells were centrifuged once at 500 g for 7 min. Pelleted BALF cells were resuspended in PBS and the total number of leucocytes was counted using a Neubauer chamber. A total of 100.000 cells in a cyto-centrifuged preparation of BALF stained with May-Grünwald's – Giemsa were differentiated under light microscopy, according to classical cell morphology. Lung and spleen were obtained after sacrifice with no previous intervention. Lungs were fixed in 4% formalin and processed for histology, while spleen was teased in cold-culture medium, and the cell suspension was filtered through gauze and adjusted to the desired concentration for flow cytometry.

Flow cytometry analysis

To determine the impact of exposure to *Aspergillus fumigatus* contaminated hay, age and Cy treatment on the Treg cell population, a suspension of splenocytes adjusted to a concentration of 1 × 10^6 cells per ml was washed with PBS (pH 7.2) and then resuspended in flow cytometry staining buffer (eBioscience). For the detection of different markers, cells were incubated with the following eBioscience monoclonal antibodies: APC- eFluorTM 780-labeled anti mouse CD45, PE-Cy5-labeled anti mouse CD3 (145-2C11), FITC-labeled anti mouse CD4 (RM4–5), APC-labeled anti mouse CD25 (PC61.5) and PE-labeled anti mouse Foxp3 (FJK16s), according to the manufacturer's recommendations. At least 30.000 events were assayed using a Beckman Coulter, CyAn™ ADP Analyzer, and data were analyzed using Summit v4.3 software. To determine different cell populations, lymphocytes were gated using SSC and the CD45 marker; then, the CD4 population was visualized and the CD25 positive-cell content was analyzed. Later, Foxp3-positive cells were determined within the total CD4 subpopulation, and the co-expression of CD25 and Foxp3 was determined (Fig. 1).

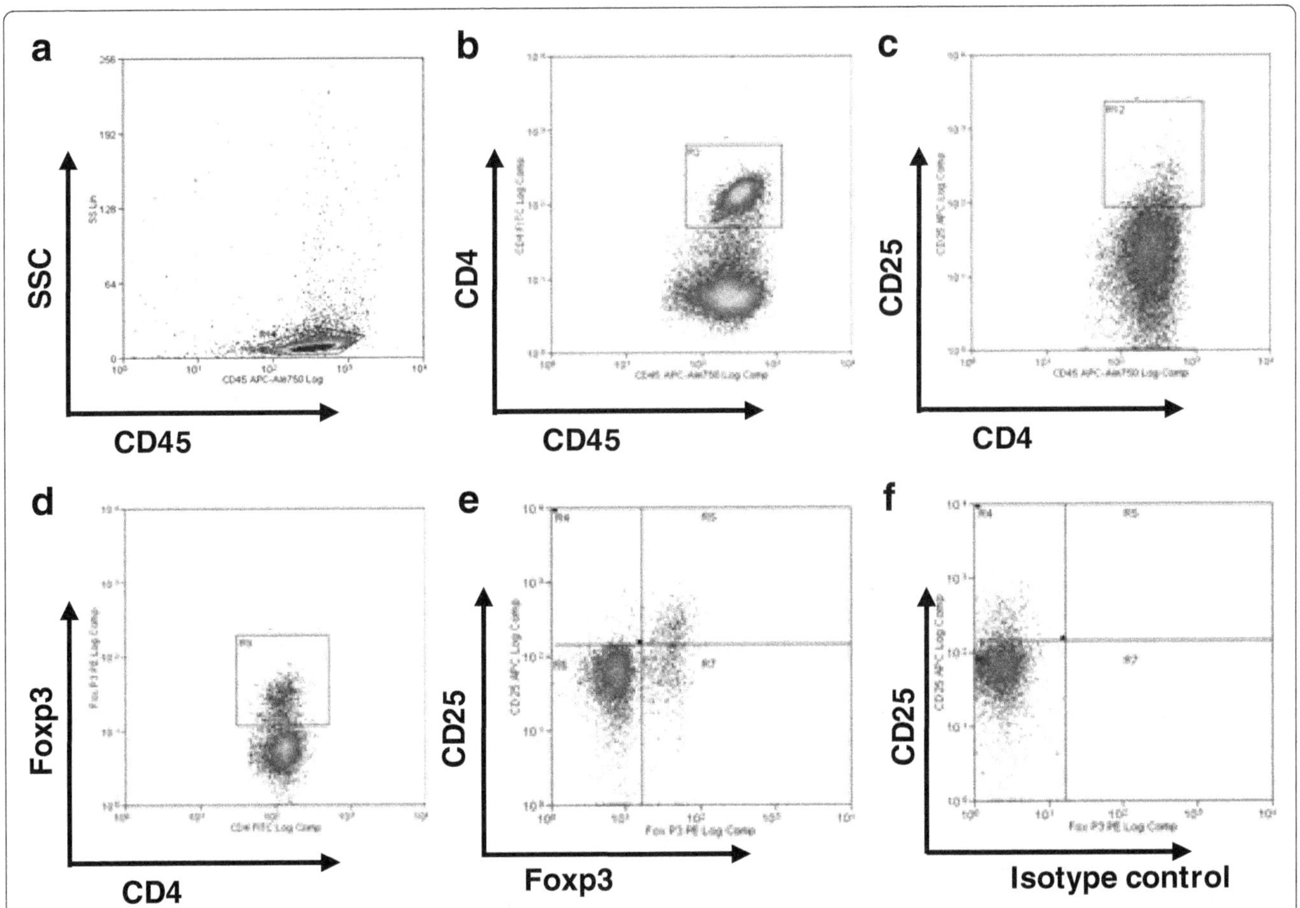

Fig. 1 Representative figures of gating strategy for Treg determination in mice spleen. For this purpose a gate was positioned around lymphocytes (**a**), and the CD4+ population was gated (**b**) in order to determinate the percentage of CD4+ cells that express markers CD25 (**c**) and Foxp3 (**d**) within the CD4 subset. Finally, co-expression of CD25 and Foxp3 were measured within CD4 cells (**e**); isotype control for Foxp3 was used as control (**f**)

Analysis of antibody production

The levels of *Aspergillus*-specific immunoglobulins in BALF and serum were determined by ELISA. Briefly, 96-well polystyrene microplates (Sarstedt, USA) were coated with 10 µg/ml of *Aspergillus fumigatus* total protein that was dissolved in carbonate buffer (pH 9) and incubated overnight. The plates were blocked with a solution of 5% non-fat milk followed by the addition of 100 µl of the appropriate dilution of BALF (1:1) or serum (1:100) into each well. The plates were incubated at 37 °C for 2 h, washed three times and incubated with peroxidase-conjugated anti-mouse IgE, IgG1 or IgG2a antibodies (Santa Cruz, Inc., USA) for an additional 2 h at 37 °C. After incubation, the plates were thoroughly washed, and the reaction was revealed with o-phenylenediamine (OPD; Sigma, USA). The colorimetric reaction was evaluated at 450 nm using a microplate reader (ELx800, Bio-Tek Instruments, USA).

Histological analysis

For histological sections study, control or experimental lung tissues were fixed in 4% formaldehyde, embedded in Paraplast, cut into 5-µm sections and stained with hematoxylin & eosin.

Statistical analysis

SigmaPlot 11.0 was used for statistical analyses. Descriptive statistics by group were run on the data, and the Kolmogorov–Smirnov test showed that the data were normally distributed. ANOVA was performed to compare the differences in CD4+, CD25+, Foxp3+ subpopulation percentages, and this was followed by a Tukey test. Overall, p values <0.05 were regarded as significant.

Results

Splenic Treg cell percentages increase in mice as a function of age and exposition to *Aspergillus fumigatus* contaminated hay

As a first approach, we determined the relative percentage of CD4+, CD25+, Foxp3+ cells in the spleens of two and 8 month old mice by flow cytometry. The results indicated that younger mice had significantly less Treg (5.19% ± 0.45) than older mice (6.77% ± 0.89) prior to Aspergillus exposure, and that the percentage of Treg cells significantly increases only in young mice upon 5 days of exposure to *Aspergillus fumigatus* (from 5.56% ± 0.53 to 6,91% ± 0,94 after mold challenge) (Fig. 2).

Low doses of cy induce a reduction of splenic Treg in mice exposed to *Aspergillus fumigatus* contaminated hay

Knowing that exposure to *Aspergillus fumigatus* contaminated hay induces an increase of the CD4+, CD25+, Foxp3+ population in mice, as a next step, we tested the

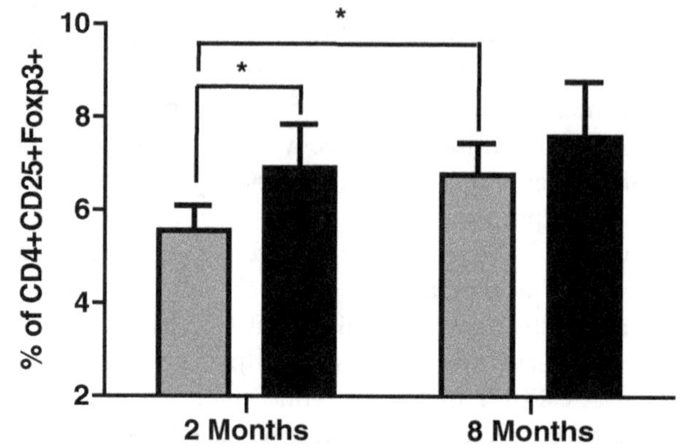

Fig. 2 Percentage of CD4, CD25, Foxp3 positive cells in spleen of 2 and 8 month old mice exposed (■) or non-exposed (□) to *Aspergillus fumigatus*. Data are presented as Median ± SD. $p < 0.05$ ($n = 8$)

effect of low doses of Cy in partially reducing the splenic Treg population, following Barbon et al.'s protocol [22]. In short, before antigenic challenge, the mice were injected daily three times with 20 mg/kg, and the results, which are shown in Fig. 3, indicate that Cy reduced the percentage of CD4+ cells that carried the regulatory markers Foxp3 and CD25. In this experiment, the Treg population was reduced from 7.59% ± 1.17 to 5.90% ± 1.11 5 days after the last dose of the cytostatic drug, indicating that Cy does not induce changes in the percentage of total CD4+ cells compared to the CD3+ population, in total accordance with the results reported previously by Barbon et al. [22].

The reduction of Treg population -induced by low doses of cy- showed a positive correlation with an increased airway inflammatory response in mice exposed to *Aspergillus fumigatus* contaminated hay

Next, to evaluate if the reduction of Treg induced by Cy influenced the inflammatory allergic airway response in mice exposed to *Aspergillus fumigatus* contaminated hay, and knowing that the challenge in this murine experimental model could replicate many clinical findings of horses with acute exacerbation of severe asthma, we evaluated neutrophil percentages in BALF and specific antibodies levels against *Aspergillus fumigatus* in BALF. As observed in Fig. 4, BALF neutrophil percentage was greatly increased in mice pretreated with Cy before exposure to *Aspergillus fumigatus* contaminated hay, compared to animals that were only exposed to the mold. This increase of neutrophils in the Cy-treated group was evident and statistically significant at days 5 and 11 post antigenic challenge. Since the airway inflammatory response to *Aspergillus fumigatus* in horses and in the animals of our murine model is mediated at least in part by the onset of hypersensitivity type I and III, it was interesting to determine specific antibodies against the

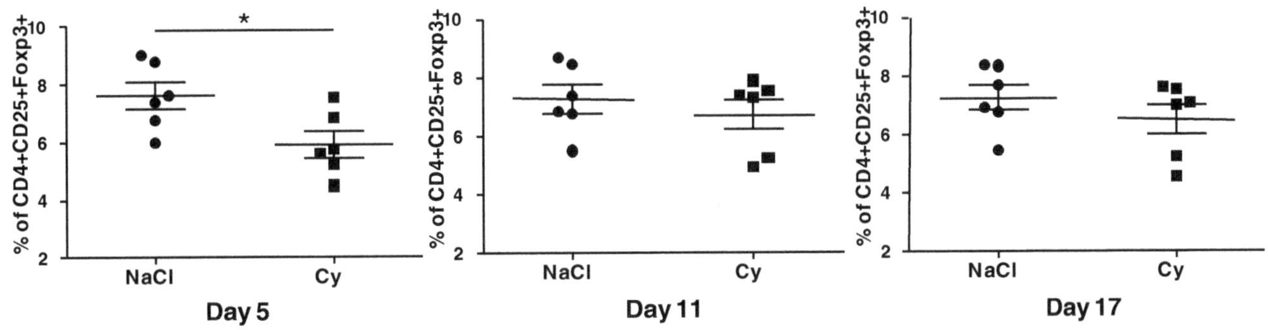

Fig. 3 Effect of treatment with low doses of cyclophosphamide on the relative percentage of CD4+, CD25+, Foxp3+ positive cells in the spleens of mice exposed to *Aspergillus fumigatus*, compared to animals injected with the same volume of isotonic saline solution and exposed to the fungus, 5, 11 and 17 days after treatment. $p < 0.05$ ($n = 6$)

allergen in BALF obtained from animals challenged with the mold, either treated or not treated with the cytostatic drug.

Figure 5 shows *Aspergillus fumigatus*-specific IgE, IgG1 and IgG2a levels in mice that were not exposed and in mice exposed to contaminated hay and either treated or not treated with Cy. IgE levels were significantly higher in the Cy-treated and *Aspergillus*-exposed group only on day 5 (Fig. 5a). IgG1 levels were significantly different between all three experimental groups on day 5 (i.e. control group, *Aspergillus*-exposed group, and Cy-treated and *Aspergillus*-exposed group); on day 11, IgG1 levels were only significantly higher in the Cy-treated and *Aspergillus*-exposed group; by day 17, there were no significant differences between groups (Fig. 5b). IgG2a levels were significantly higher only in the Cy-treated and *Aspergillus*-exposed group on day 5; on day 11 and 17, IgG2a levels were significantly higher in both *Aspergillus*-exposed groups than in the control group (Fig. 5c).

Lastly, lung histopathology of animals challenged with *Aspergillus fumigatus* (Fig. 6) showed that the group of animals pretreated with Cy presented significant peribronchiolar and perivascular mononuclear and neutrophilic infiltration, accumulation of intraluminal bronchiolar mucus and serofibrinous exudates. Moreover, there was extensive folding of the airway epithelia, which is a sign of airway smooth muscle contraction and smooth muscle hypertrophy. This inflammatory response was observed predominantly in the peribronchiolar interstitial tissues and often extended into the lamina propria and luminal surface epithelium of the affected airways. We also observed infiltration of inflammatory cells into the alveolar space.

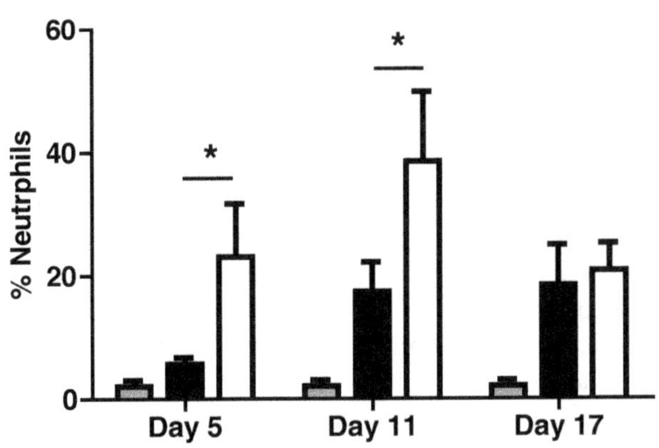

Fig. 4 Effect of treatment with low doses of cyclophosphamide on the relative percentage of neutrophils obtained from BALF in non-exposed controls (▭), compared with animals treated with isotonic saline solution and exposed to *Aspergillus fumigatus* (■), and animals that were pretreated with cyclophosphamide and exposed to *Aspergillus fumigatus* (□). Data are presented as Median ± SD. $p < 0.05$ ($n = 8$)

Discussion

In this paper, we describe that the transient decrease of CD4+, CD25+, Foxp3+ splenic T regulatory cells, induced by Cy, correlates with increased airway inflammation in mice exposed to hay contaminated with *Aspergillus fumigatus*.

The results presented here demonstrate that, in our experimental model, older animals (8 months old) showed a higher percentage of CD4+, CD25+, Foxp3+ cells in the spleen when compared to younger mice (2 months old). Similar findings were reported by Zhao [28], who also compared the capacity of CD4+, CD25+ cells from older and younger mice to inhibit delayed hypersensitivity, mixed lymphocyte reaction or cytokine production. From their results, they concluded that CD4+, CD25+ cells present in the older mice, were less effective in suppressing the above-mentioned assays. These facts may explain why aging produces a progressive decline in immune regulation, and in the case of horses and in the mice of our experimental model [20],

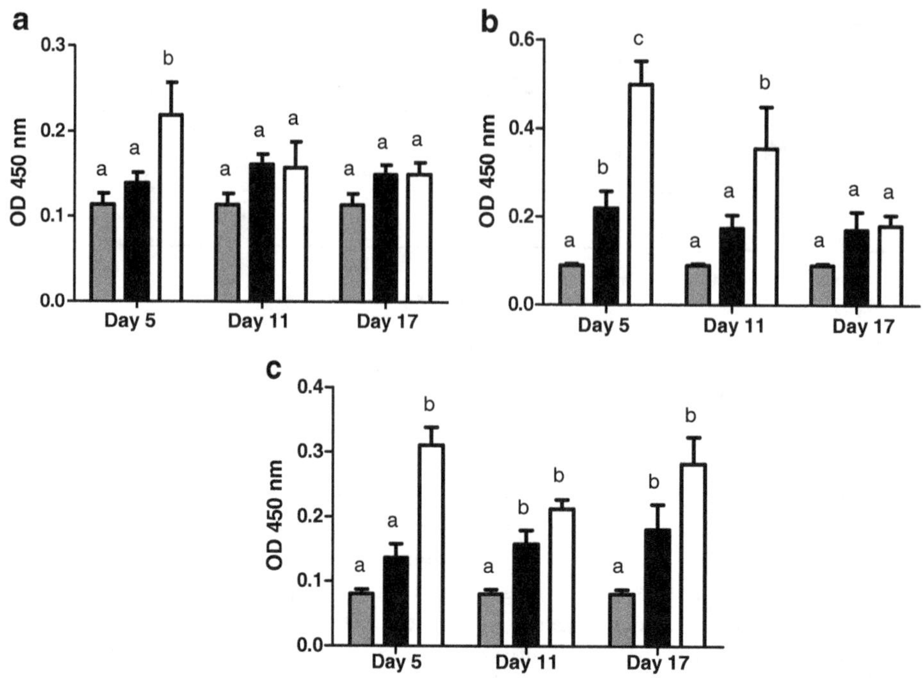

Fig. 5 IgE (**a**), IgG1 (**b**) and IgG2a (**c**) levels in control animals (grey), animals challenged with *Aspergillus fumigatus* and injected with saline (black) and animals pretreated with cyclophosphamide and challenged with *Aspergillus fumigatus* (white). Data are presented as Median ± SD. $p < 0.05$ ($n = 8$)

why age facilitates the occurrence of airway immune-mediated inflammation. On the other hand, our results indicate that upon stimulation only young mice show a significant increase of CD4+, CD25+, Foxp3+ cells percentage in the spleen, allowing us to propose that aging makes these cells less prone to proliferate or be recruited in response to antigenic challenge.

In addition, we demonstrate that Cy at low doses induces a statistically significant decrease in CD4+, CD25+, Foxp3+ cells in the spleens of mice challenged with *Aspergillus fumigatus,* as described in normal mice by Barbon et al. [22]. This treatment does not affect the relative percentages of other T subpopulations, and this effect has been explained by the presence of lower ATP levels in Treg cells than in conventional T cells. This low ATP content, in turn, attenuates the synthesis of glutathione, which results in a lower capacity for Cy detoxification [28, 29]. Moreover, Lutsiak et al. [30] reported that Cy decreased Treg cell numbers and led to decreased functionality by decreasing GITR and Foxp3 expression, a fact that added to the percentage diminution of Treg and could account for the exaggerated airway immune response observed in animals that received Cy. The fact that a low dose of Cy treatment prior to challenge with *Aspergillus fumigatus* correlated with augmented inflammation and an increase in specific immunoglobulins against the fungus in BALF, may indicate the regulatory role of Treg in this process. In this respect, IgE and IgG1 isotypes are especially important because both have the ability to bind to the high-affinity IgE Fc receptors on mast cells and basophils; therefore, their enhanced production correlates with increased sensitization of the airways and a more aggravated hypersensitivity type I reaction. On the other hand, the IgG2a isotype, which is the only IgG subclass that fixes complement in mice, appears to be responsible for type III hypersensitivity because, upon forming immunocomplexes with the antigen, complement is activated and pro-inflammatory factors such as C3a and C5a are released. Therefore, we may conclude that the increase in immunoglobulins that are responsible for type I and III hypersensitivity, could directly influence the pathogenesis of airway immune-mediated inflammation. As a consequence of antigen-antibody complex formation in the airways, complement activation and the production of other chemoattractants by resident cells in our experimental model mice and in severe equine asthma, neutrophils migrate to the airways, producing an increase of these cells in BALF, which serves as an important diagnostic finding for this disease. Our results show that there is an important increase in BALF neutrophils of mice exposed to *Aspergillus fumigatus*, and this phenomenon is even greater in mice pretreated with low doses of Cy, which indicates that the airway immune-mediated inflammation process induced by the fungus is aggravated by Cy. This conclusion is corroborated by the histopathological study that showed that the highest degree of lung infiltration was found in animals exposed to the antigen and pretreated with Cy

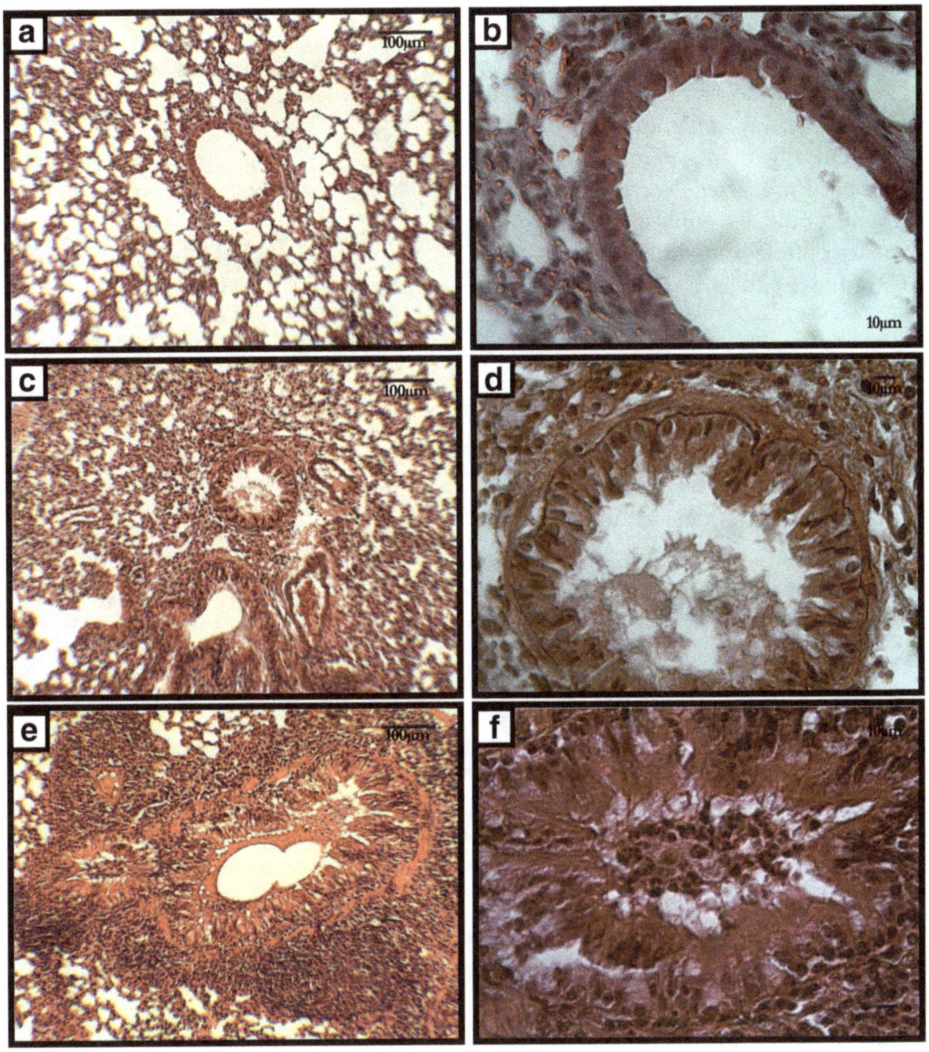

Fig. 6 Representative histological features of normal mice lung (**a**) and a normal bronchus (**b**) compared with micrographs of lungs obtained from mice 17 days after the initial challenge with *Aspergillus fumigatus* (**c** & **d**) and of lungs from animals pretreated with cyclophosphamide and exposed to *Aspergillus fumigatus* (**e** & **f**)

before challenge. Finally, considering that the natural thymus-derived, or peripherally induced adaptive Treg cell populations have been associated with the outcome of processes such as autoimmunity, transplantation rejection, cancer and mucosal tolerance [31]; it is not surprising that local airway-induced inflammation correlates with an increase of splenic Treg cells, and a regulatory role of this population as was described here. One of this study's limitations is the lack of information about specific Treg changes at the site of inflammation (the airways); Treg subpopulations should ideally be evaluated in the lungs and in BALF. However, these results do reveal the systemic effect of Cy on Treg populations, and strongly suggest participation of this cell subset in inflammatory processes. Another limitation of this study is that Cy has been shown to induce lung inflammation at high doses in rats [32]. While in our experience this is not noticeable through the parameters evaluated in this study (histology or BALF relative cellular content, data not shown), this does not exclude the possibility that potential damage induced by Cy may have influenced the inflammatory response against *Aspergillus fumigatus*.

Our study group has previously reported a similar Treg cell subpopulation in horses with exacerbated severe EA [19]. Treg subpopulations may well play a regulatory role in inflammatory processes in different tissues, and our findings here certainly show that inhibition of Treg (through pre-treatment with Cy) coincides with severe airway inflammation after inhalatory challenge. However, translation of these results to the equine species is limited by horses′ individual susceptibility to EA. Multiple factors may affect horses′ susceptibility to inhalatory allergens, including heritable or genetic traits. Familial traits have been proven in said species, and the same has been shown in humans [21, 33]. The murine strain used in this study doesn't have an increased individual susceptibility to airway inflammation, and as such does not relate specifically to EA-susceptible horses; however, the immunological processes described here are valid across species, and could be applicable to equine susceptible and non-susceptible individuals, albeit the necessary limitations inherent to any research model.

Conclusion

In this murine model of asthma, the reduced number and function of Treg induced by low doses of Cy and which directly correlates with increased airway inflammation and lung infiltration, indicates that Treg may play a role in the regulation and resolution of severe equine asthma.

Abbreviations

BALF: Bronchoalveolar Lavage Fluid; Cy: Cyclophosphamide; EA: Equine asthma; OPD: O-phenylenediamine; RK: Rockefeller; Treg: T regulatory cells

Acknowledgements

Not applicable.

Funding

This work was partially supported by FONDECYT grant 1160352 Doctoral Scholarship MESECUP AUS-601, and Graduate School Faculty of Veterinary Sciences, Universidad Austral de Chile.

Authors' contributions

CH conceived the study, participated in the design of the study, sample obtaining and processing. GM participated in the design of the study and cooperates with the animal model. CC carried out the flow cytometry analysis. JS participated in the design of the study and helped to draft the manuscript. MB participated in the design of the study and helped to draft the manuscript. HF participated in design and coordination of the study and helped to draft the manuscript. BU helped to draft the manuscript and data interpretation. All authors read and approved the final manuscript.

Authors' information

Not applicable.

Competing interests

The authors declare that they have no competing interests.

Consent for publication

Not applicable.

Author details

[1]Pharmacology and Morphophysiology Department, Faculty of Veterinary Sciences, Universidad Austral de Chile, Valdivia, Chile. [2]Immunology Department, Faculty of Medicine, Universidad Austral de Chile, Valdivia, Chile. [3]Pathology Department, Regional Hospital of Valdivia, Valdivia, Chile. [4]Physiology Department, Faculty of Medicine, Universidad Austral de Chile, Valdivia, Chile. [5]Veterinary Clinical Sciences Department, Faculty of Veterinary Sciences, Universidad Austral de Chile, Valdivia, Chile.

References

1. Bullone M, Lavoie J-P. Asthma, "of horses and men"–how can equine heaves help us better understand human asthma immunopathology and its functional consequences? Mol Immunol. 2015;66:97–105.
2. Couetil LL, Cardwell JM, Gerber V, Lavoie JP, Leguillette R, Richard EA. Inflammatory airway disease of horses – revised consensus statement. J Vet Intern Med. 2016;30:503–15.
3. Pirie RS, Couetil LL, Robinson NE, Lavoie JP. Equine asthma: an appropriate, translational and comprehendible terminology? Equine Vet J. 2016;48:403–5.
4. Leclere M, Lavoie-Lamoureux A, Lavoie JP. Heaves, an asthma-like disease of horses. Respirology. 2011;16:1027–46.
5. Leguillette R. Recurrent airway obstruction–heaves. Vet Clin North Am Equine Pract. 2003;19:63–86.
6. Ha TY. The role of regulatory T cells in cancer. Immune Netw. 2009;9:209–35.
7. Shevach EM. Regulatory T cells in autoimmmunity*. Annu Rev Immunol. 2000;18:423–49.
8. Akdis M, Blaser K, Akdis CA. T regulatory cells in allergy: novel concepts in the pathogenesis, prevention, and treatment of allergic diseases. J Allergy Clin Immunol. 2005;116:961–8.
9. Sakaguchi S, Sakaguchi N, Asano M, Itoh M, Toda M. Immunologic self-tolerance maintained by activated T cells expressing IL-2 receptor alpha-chains (CD25). Breakdown of a single mechanism of self-tolerance causes various autoimmune diseases. J Immunol. 1995;155:1151–64.
10. Fontenot JD, Gavin MA, Rudensky AY. Foxp3 programs the development and function of CD4+CD25+ regulatory T cells. Nat Immunol. 2003;4:330–6.
11. Bacchetta R, Gambineri E, Roncarolo MG. Role of regulatory T cells and FOXP3 in human diseases. J Allergy Clin Immunol. 2007;120:227–35. quiz 236-227
12. Banerjee A, Vasanthakumar A, Grigoriadis G. Modulating T regulatory cells in cancer: how close are we? Immunol Cell Biol. 2013;91:340–9.
13. Beres AJ, Drobyski WR. The role of regulatory T cells in the biology of graft versus host disease. Front Immunol. 2013;4:163.
14. Cao T, Wenzel SE, Faubion WA, Harriman G, Li L. Enhanced suppressive function of regulatory T cells from patients with immune-mediated diseases following successful ex vivo expansion. Clin Immunol. 2010;136:329–37.
15. Nishimoto T, Kuwana M. CD4+CD25+Foxp3+ regulatory T cells in the pathophysiology of immune thrombocytopenia. Semin Hematol. 2013; 50(Suppl 1):S43–9.
16. Palomares O, Yaman G, Azkur AK, Akkoc T, Akdis M, Akdis CA. Role of Treg in immune regulation of allergic diseases. Eur J Immunol. 2010;40:1232–40.
17. Wainwright DA, Dey M, Chang A, Lesniak MS. Targeting Tregs in malignant brain cancer: overcoming IDO. Front Immunol. 2013;4:116.
18. Wing K, Sakaguchi S. Regulatory T cells exert checks and balances on self tolerance and autoimmunity. Nat Immunol. 2010;11:7–13.
19. Henríquez C, Perez B, Morales N, Carrasco C, Sarmiento J, Morán G, Folch H. Participation of T regulatory cells in equine recurrent airway obstruction. Vet Immunol Immunophatol. 2014;158:128–34.
20. Moran G, Ojeda G, Diedrichs K, Ortloff A, Barria M, Folch H. Inhalation of Aspergillus fumigatus spores induces airway inflammation in mice in a similar manner as observed in recurrent airway obstruction in horses. Arch Med Vet. 2011;43:163–71.
21. Gerber V, Tessier C, Marti E. Genetics of upper and lower airway diseases in the horse. Equine Vet J. 2015;47(4):390–7.
22. Barbon CM, Yang M, Wands GD, Ramesh R, Slusher BS, Hedley ML, Luby TM. Consecutive low doses of cyclophosphamide preferentially target Tregs and potentiate T cell responses induced by DNA PLG microparticle immunization. Cell Immunol. 2010;262:150–61.
23. Askenase PW, Hayden BJ, Gershon RK. Augmentation of delayed-type hypersensitivity by doses of cyclophosphamide which do not affect antibody responses. J Exp Med. 1975;141:697–702.
24. Folch H, Lopetegui F, Stegmeier E. Abrogation of antigenic competition phenomenon by a low dose of cyclophosphamide. Zentralbl Veterinarmed B. 1980;27:139–43.
25. Audia S, Nicolas A, Cathelin D, Larmonier N, Ferrand C, Foucher P, Fanton A, Bergoin E, Maynadie M, Arnould L, Bateman A, Lorcerie B, Solary E, Chauffert B, Bonnotte B. Increase of CD4+ CD25+ regulatory T cells in the peripheral blood of patients with metastatic carcinoma: a phase I clinical trial using cyclophosphamide and immunotherapy to eliminate CD4+ CD25+ T lymphocytes. Clin Exp Immunol. 2007;150:523–30.

26. Rech AJ, Vonderheide RH. Clinical use of anti-CD25 antibody daclizumab to enhance immune responses to tumor antigen vaccination by targeting regulatory T cells. Ann N Y Acad Sci. 2009;1174:99–106.
27. Schabowsky RH, Madireddi S, Sharma R, Yolcu ES, Shirwan H. Targeting CD4 +CD25+FoxP3+ regulatory T-cells for the augmentation of cancer immunotherapy. Curr Opin Investig Drugs. 2007;8:1002–8.
28. Zhao L, Sun L, Wang H, Ma H, Liu G, Zhao Y. Changes of CD4+CD25+Foxp3 + regulatory T cells in aged Balb/c mice. J Leukoc Biol. 2007;81:1386–94.
29. Schenk U, Frascoli M, Proietti M, Geffers R, Traggiai E, Buer J, Ricordi C, Westendorf AM, Grassi F. ATP inhibits the generation and function of regulatory T cells through the activation of purinergic P2X receptors. Science Signaling 4. Sci Signal. 2011;4(162):ra12.
30. Lutsiak ME, Semnani RT, De Pascalis R, Kashmiri SV, Schlom J, Sabzevari H. Inhibition of CD4(+)25+ T regulatory cell function implicated in enhanced immune response by low-dose cyclophosphamide. Blood. 2005;105:2862–8.
31. Curotto de Lafaille MA, Lafaille JJ. CD4(+) regulatory T cells in autoimmunity and allergy. Curr Opin Immunol. 2002;14:771–8.
32. Cooper JA Jr, Merrill WW, Reynolds HY. Cyclophosphamide modulation of bronchoalveolar cellular populations and macrophage oxidative metabolism. Possible mechanisms of pulmonary pharmacotoxicity. Am Rev Respir Dis. 1986;134(1):108–14.
33. Pirie RS. Recurrent airway obstruction: a review. Equine Vet J. 2014;46(3):276–88.

11

Reliability of breath by breath spirometry and relative flow-time indices for pulmonary function testing in horses

K. Burnheim, K. J. Hughes, D. L. Evans and S. L. Raidal*

Abstract

Background: Respiratory problems are common in horses, and are often diagnosed as a cause of poor athletic performance. Reliable, accurate and sensitive spirometric tests of airway function in resting horses would assist with the diagnosis of limitations to breathing and facilitate investigations of the effects of various treatments on breathing capacity. The evaluation of respiratory function in horses is challenging and suitable procedures are not widely available to equine practitioners. The determination of relative flow or flow-time measures is used in paediatric patients where compliance may limit conventional pulmonary function techniques. The aim of the current study was to characterise absolute and relative indices of respiratory function in healthy horses during eupnoea (tidal breathing) and carbon dioxide (CO_2)-induced hyperpnoea (rebreathing) using a modified mask pneumotrachographic technique well suited to equine practice, and to evaluate the reliability of this technique over three consecutive days. Coefficients of variation, intra-class correlations, mean differences and 95% confidence intervals across all days of testing were established for each parameter.

Results: The technique provided absolute measures of respiratory function (respiratory rate, tidal volume, peak inspiratory and expiratory flows, time to peak flow) consistent with previous studies and there was no significant effect of day on any measure of respiratory function. Variability of measurements was decreased during hyperpnea caused by rebreathing CO_2, but a number of relative flow-time variables demonstrated good agreement during eupnoeic respiration.

Conclusions: The technique was well tolerated by horses and study findings suggest the technique is suitable for evaluation of respiratory function in horses. The use of relative flow-time variables provided reproducible (consistent) results, suggesting the technique may be of use for repeated measures studies in horses during tidal breathing or rebreathing.

Keywords: Lung function, Respiratory disease, Horse, Pneumotachography, Variability

Background

Horses are affected by a number of discrete, non-infectious conditions causing reversible airway obstruction similar in many respects to asthma [1]. Recurrent airway obstruction (RAO) is a potentially debilitating condition affecting mature stabled horses in the northern hemisphere. Clinical signs of RAO are readily identified in affected horses, and include coughing, respiratory distress and increased respiratory effort [2]. Pulmonary function testing (PFT) has been used to characterise the condition, including acute exacerbations, and to demonstrate response to treatment. Inflammatory airway disease (IAD), a more subtle but very common condition worldwide, has been associated with poor performance, delayed respiratory recovery following exercise, and more severe exercise-induced hypoxaemia than in healthy, fit controls [3, 4]. As clinical signs of IAD may be subtle or inapparent in resting horses, recognition of the condition is more challenging and usually requires demonstration of altered bronchoalveolar lavage cytology, accumulation of tracheal exudate, and/or changes in respiratory function [1, 5].

* Correspondence: sraidal@csu.edu.au
School of Animal and Veterinary Sciences, Charles Sturt University, Wagga Wagga 2650, NSW, Australia

Non-invasive PFT is the cornerstone of diagnosis for obstructive respiratory conditions in people, however PFT is challenging in horses due to high airflows, large pulmonary reserve and the inability of equine patients to follow instructions. Techniques adapted for evaluation of lung function in horses include measures of 'conventional' lung mechanics by simultaneous determination of transpulmonary pressure (estimated by oesophageal manometry) and airflow at the nostrils [6, 7], forced or impulse oscillation techniques [8, 9], flowmetric plethysmography [10] and forced expiratory techniques [11]. The ideal pulmonary function test is objective, repeatable, reproducible, accurate, valid, sensitive and specific [12]. In addition, in equine practice, the test would be non-invasive, acceptable to the horse and owner, and readily implemented in a field setting. Instruments should be robust and easily calibrated under field conditions.

Passage of an oesophageal pressure manometer may be unacceptable in a clinical setting, and conventional flow mechanics may lack sensitivity for the detection of IAD [13], although more recently the use of rebreathing techniques has improved the sensitivity of this technique [14]. Forced oscillation techniques require heavy sedation and specialised equipment ill-suited to a field setting. Open plethysmography, which uses inductance bands around the horse's thorax and abdomen combined with penuemotachographic measurement airflow [10] is better suited to field conditions, and has been used to evaluate respiratory function in horses [5, 10, 15]. Forced expiration studies are common in human subjects, but in horses have been performed only in anaesthetised or heavily sedated patients [4, 11]. Increased tidal volumes and airflows have been elicited in conscious horses following exercise, by increased inspired CO_2 concentration, or by administration of lobeline [14, 16–20].

In pediatric patients, where patient compliance is similarly limiting, relative flow indices have been developed to permit assessment of respiratory function at rest or during increased ventilatory manoeuvres. The ratio of time to reach peak expiratory flow to expiratory time (Tpef/Te) has been used to differentiate and characterise airflow obstruction in children and infants during forced expiratory breaths [21, 22] and tidal breathing [23]. As biphasic respiration, characteristic of healthy horses, is lost with obstructive conditions [24, 25], characterisation of relative flow values may prove helpful in equine patients. It has been proposed that relative flow-time relationships can indicate lower airway disease and negate the need to use maximal forced inspirations and expirations in horses [18], and the assessment of relative flow-time relationships has been used to demonstrate potential airflow limitations in horses with increased tracheal wash neutrophil percentages [26].

The current study was designed as a pilot study to characterise a novel pneumotachographic system for determination of absolute and relative flow-time indices of respiratory function in healthy horses during eupnoea (tidal breathing) and carbon dioxide induced hyperpnoea. In the context of PFT, Cotes et al. [12] have defined *repeatability* as the extent to which a result varies when it is repeated within a session, and *reproducibility* as the extent to which a result varies when it is repeated with changed condition, such as repeated measurements over a longer period of time. In the absence of an agreed 'gold standard' permitting assessment of accuracy, both concepts relate to measurement precision or reliability. Hence the aims of this study were to compare absolute indices of respiratory function derived using the mask pneumotachographic system with published results, and to determine the reliability of absolute and relative flow-time measures in healthy horses. We hypothesised that this approach would generate reproducible results in healthy, unsedated horses during eupnoeic breathing and hyperpnoea.

Methods

Horses

Eight healthy Standardbred mares, 3–13 years old (6.2 ± 3.3 years, mean ± standard deviation) and mean bodyweight 518 ± 29.8 kg, were used for this study. All horses were resident on site for at least 6 months prior to commencing the study, and none was routinely engaged in strenuous exercise. No abnormalities were evident in any horse following full clinical examination, including examination of body temperature, heart rate, respiratory rate and thoracic auscultation of left and right lung fields. Blood was collected for routine haematology and serum biochemistry to exclude systemic disease. For the duration of the study, no mare was coughing or had nasal discharge, and no horse had evidence of upper airway disease during endoscopic evaluation conducted subsequent to spirometry testing. Tracheal mucus was graded as previously described [27], and tracheal wash (TW) and broncholalveolar lavage (BAL) were performed at this time.

Horses were accustomed to the stocks, testing area and a modified face mask (Aeromask, Trudell Medical International, distributed via Ranvet Banksmeadow NSW Australia) prior to commencement of the study. All pulmonary airflow analysis occurred between 11:00 and 15:00 h and horses were tested in the same order on experiment days, to reduce the effects of circadian rhythm on pulmonary function. An elevated head position was maintained throughout all spirometry procedures (Fig. 1). The daily temperature and relative humidity during measurements were, respectively, 16.7–20.3 °C and 41–76%.

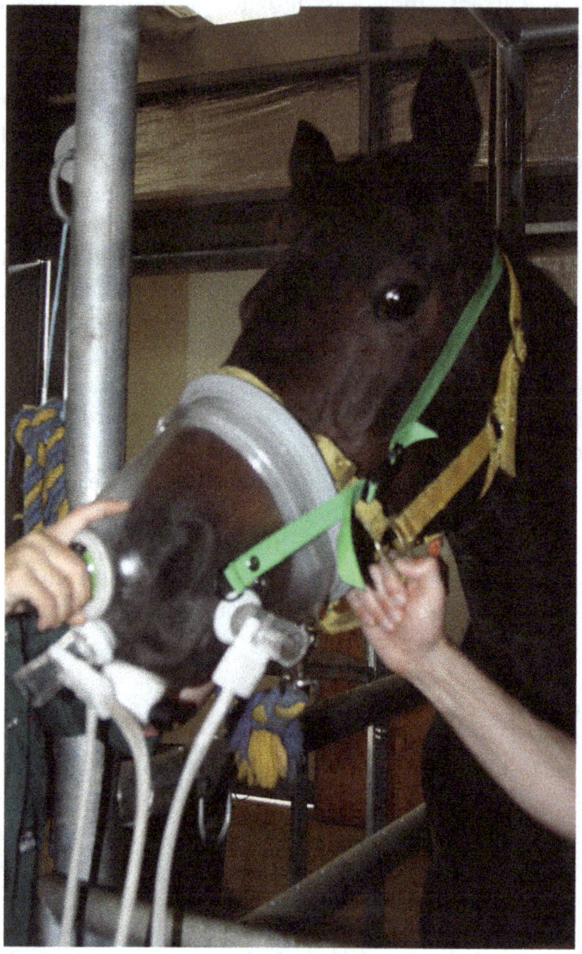

Fig. 1 Facemask in position with three bi-directional pitot flow meters attached. Flow data was collected simultaneously from each sensor and summed to provide volume and flow results. Gas analysis was performed on samples aspirated continuously from the middle sensor. The horses head was maintained in the position shown throughout testing

The horses were kept in a one hectare paddock for the duration of the experiment with access to summer grass pasture, and were fed lucerne hay once daily. Horses were in a holding yard at for at least 30 min prior to testing to prevent increased respiratory rate due to exercise and excitement. Study design was approved by the Animal Care and Ethics Committee of Charles Sturt University, Wagga Wagga (ACEC approval number 10/077).

Spirometry

A face mask (Aeromask, Trudell Medical International, distributed via Ranvet Banksmeadow NSW Australia) was modified to accommodate three bi-directional pitot flow meters (preVent Flow Sensor, MGC Diagnostics Corporation, St Paul, Minnesota) as described previously for breath-by-breath analysis of airflow [18, 28] and attached over the horse's muzzle covering the nose and mouth (Fig. 1). Three pitot tubes were placed in 18 mm circular holes in the face mask: two tubes were positioned laterally and one was placed centrally. Each pitot sensor measured air flow to a maximum of 18 L/s, and the outputs from each tube were summed and recorded with a CPFS/D Laboratory Spirometer (MGC Diagnostics Corporation, St Paul, Minnesota). Gas flow was measured to 0.1 L/s resolution every 10 milliseconds, and tubes were calibrated using a seven litre certified calibration syringe (Hans Rudolph Incorporated, Shawnee, Kansas) prior to pulmonary function testing. Calibration was successful if the total flow in the tubes differed from the reference by less than two percent (range 0.20–1.90%, mean 0.74%). Flow rates were calibrated to body temperature and pressure, saturated with water vapour (BTPS) based on daily measurement of barometric pressure, ambient temperature and relative humidity. Oxygen and carbon dioxide concentrations were determined (ML206 Gas Analyser, ADInstruments, Bella Vista, NSW) in expired gas via a sensor incorporated into the central flow tube and following a two-step calibration procedure utilising room air and Carbogen (5% carbon dioxide, 95% oxygen; Carbogen, BOC, North Ryde, NSW). A rubber seal and stoppers were used to ensure the face mask was airtight and mask fit was assessed visually before and during every recording to ensure it was airtight.

Spirometry studies were conducted over consecutive days. Temperature, relative humidity and ambient pressure were recorded immediately prior to each spirometry test. Horses were loaded into familiar stocks and fitted with the face mask. Once settled, the three pitot tubes (each with umbilicus attached) were connected to the mask and five minutes of eupnoeic breathing was recorded. After completing spirometry on horses during eupnoeic breathing, a plastic bag (capacity 60 L) was placed over the mask and pitot tubes. The bag was held in place by one or two assistants who ensured an airtight seal was maintained between the bag and mask and that the bag was not interfering with airflow through the pitot tubes. Recording started once the bag was in place and rebreathing continued until carbon dioxide levels reached a plateau or exceeded 4.5% end tidal CO_2, tidal volume was greater than 15 L or the horse no longer tolerated the rebreathing bag (typically two to three minutes, mean 4.8 ± 0.54% end tidal CO_2). The bag was then removed and recording of spirometry measurements was continued until the horse's tidal volume and flow measurements returned to resting values, at which time the mask was removed.

Spirometry measurements

Spirometry recordings were evaluated from 5 min of eupnoeic breathing and from the final 2 to 3 min of carbon dioxide induced hyperpnoeic respiration. Three breaths were chosen for analysis from each recording that were free of artefacts such as swallowing or head movement, evidenced less than 10% difference in inspiratory and expiratory volume, and had the same flow curve with peak inspiratory and expiratory flow at similar locations for the three breaths (that is, all breaths evidenced early or late flow peaks and were considered representative of tidal breathing throughout the trace) (Additional file 1: Figure S1). Representative breaths during rebreathing were selected from the final 30 s of rebreathing when respiratory excursions were greatest. Where possible, three consecutive breaths were selected, however as ventilation during both eupnoea and rebreathing was labile, analysis of consecutive breaths was not always possible.

Respiratory frequency (Rf), tidal volume (V_T), total breath period (Tt), inspiratory and expiratory periods (Ti and Te), peak inspiratory and expiratory flows (PIF and PEF), time to PIF (Tpif) and time to PEF (Tpef) were measured for each selected breath. Minute ventilation (MVe), and ratios of Te to Tt, Te to Ti, Tpef to Te and Tpif to Ti were calculated for each selected breath (Additional file 1: Table S1). Relative flow-time variables were calculated as described by [18] for each breath to determine the percentage of peak expiratory flow (PEF) at 25, 50 and 75% of the time from commencement of expiration to peak expiratory flow (Tpef) and were identified as $ezp_{25\%}$, $ezp_{50\%}$ and $ezp_{75\%}$, respectively. Similar relative flow-time measurements were made for 25, 50 and 75% of the time from Tpef to end of expiration ($epz_{25\%}$, $epz_{50\%}$ and $epz_{75\%}$). Analogous zero to peak ($zp_{\%}$) and peak to zero ($pz_{\%}$) measurements were determined for inspiratory phases of each breath (Fig. 2). Definitions of all relative flow-time indices are provided in Additional file 1: Table S2.

Statistical methods

The repeatability and reproducibility of PFT methodology was assessed during eupnoeic breathing and rebreathing induced hyperpnoea by comparison of results for six indices of respiratory function (Rf, Vt, MVe, PEF, PIF, Tpef), two relative flow measures (Tpef/Te and Te/Tt) and 12 relative flow values (izp25%, izp50%, izp75%, ipz25%, ipz50%, ipz75%, ezp25%, ezp50%, ezp75%, epz25%, epz50%, epz75%) on each of the three days tested. Repeatability was assessed by determination of the coefficient of variation (CV) for the three breaths selected for analysis on each day. Reproducibility was assessed by comparison of mean results (average of three selected breaths) obtained on each of three days. Descriptive data is reported as the mean ± standard deviation for each the three days, and the CV across all days. The effect of repeated sampling (day) on indices of respiratory function was compared by one-way repeated measures analysis of variance, with separate analyses for eupneoic and hyperpnoeic ventilation. Data were checked for normality, equal variance and sphericity (equal variability of differences), and the Geisser-Greenhouse correction was applied as required. Where a significant replicate (day) or individual horse effect was

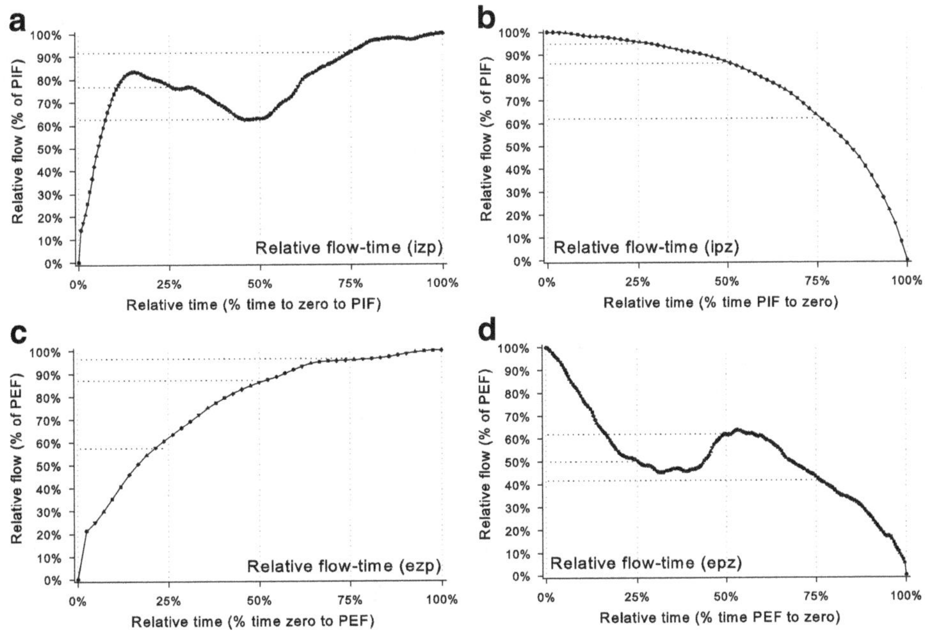

Fig 2 Relative flow-time graphs during a representative breath. Airflow is plotted as a percentage of peak inspiratory (**a** and **b**) or expiratory (**c** and **d**) flow. Figures **a** and **c** show flow between zero and peak, Figures **b** and **d** show flow from peak to zero. Relative flows are shown at 25, 50, and 75% of each phase of the respiratory cycle. Biphasic respiration is evident in Figures **a** and **d**

observed, multiple pair-wise comparisons were performed using the Tukey test. Attempts were made to transform data that did not conform to a normal distribution or, if unsuccessful, such data was analysed by non-parametric analysis (Friedman one-way RM-ANOVA on ranks with post-hoc testing using Dunn's multiple comparisons test). Intra-class correlation co-efficients (ICC) were calculated [29] for each measurement on each day tested using the F statistic derived from analysis of variance [30], with the 90% confidence interval calculated as previously described [31].

Possible associations between tracheal secretions and airway cytology were evaluated by graphing the endoscopic grade for tracheal secretions, percentage of neutrophils in tracheal wash cytology (TW % PMN), and the percentage of neutrophils (BAL % PMN), mast cells (BAL % mast cells) and eosinophils (BAL % eosinophils) in BAL fluid against measured or derived indices of pulmonary function. In addition, results were compared for horses that exhibited endoscopic (grade 2 tracheal secretions) or cytological evidence (BAL % PMN >10%, BAL % mast cells >5% or BAL % eosinophils >5%) of IAD [1] ($n = 4$) against the remaining horses with normal endoscopic and airway cytology findings. Spearman or Pearson correlations were calculated for categorical or continuous data (respectively) where a possible effect was evident graphically. All analyses were performed using GraphPad Prism version 6.0 for Windows (GraphPad Software, San Diego, California, USA, www.graphpad.com).

Results

Endoscopic evaluation of the upper airway was unremarkable for each horse. Tracheal mucus scores and cytological results of TW and BAL samples are shown in Table 1. Whilst no horse demonstrated clinical signs suggestive of respiratory disease, five of the eight horses had increased tracheal secretions (grade 2), increased neutrophils in tracheal wash cytology, or fulfilled cytological definitions of IAD (increased BAL neutrophils, mast cells or eosinophils) [1]. The mask and rebreathing apparatus were tolerated well by unsedated horses, although considerable time was invested prior to commencing the study to acclimatise horses to PFT procedures. Ambient temperature (20.2 °C, 19.6 °C, 20.3 °C), humidity (58%, 52%, 76%) and atmospheric pressure (991 millibars, 996 millibars, 960 millibars) varied slightly on the three days of testing untreated horses.

Absolute and relative measurements determined from data obtained during spirometry testing with the modified face mask are shown in Table 2. Respiratory frequency, tidal volume and peak flows are shown in Figs. 3 and 4; differences in means for each pair of tests (Day 1 vs Day 2, Day 2 vs Day 3, Day 1 vs Day 3) are provided (Additional file 1: Figure S2). Repeatability (comparison of the three selected breaths on the same day of testing) was high for most parameters, as within day CV's were less than 10% for all parameters except time to peak expiratory and inspiratory flows. Rebreathing was associated with reduced variation relative to eupnoeic breathing, evidenced by lower within day and between day CVs. During eupnoeic breathing the position of both inspiratory and expiratory peak flow was highly variable for each horse, with peak flow occurring variably and seemingly randomly in early, middle or late inspiration and expiration for all horses. Biphasic respiration was noted during both inspiration and expiration, resulting in non-uniform changes in flow during each stage of the respiratory cycle in some horses. Rebreathing was associated with marked increases in respiratory frequency, airflow, tidal and minute volumes. Whereas PIF was higher than PEF during eupnoeic breathing, rebreathing was associated with higher PEF than PIF, and both PIF and PEF tended to occur closer to the start of inspiration or expiration, evidenced by lower Tpif and Tpef values.

Table 1 Endoscopic tracheal mucus score and cytology results for study horses. Results that fulfil endoscopic or cytological definitions for inflammatory airway disease [1] have been highlighted

Horse	TW mucus score	TW % PMN	BAL % PMN	BAL % mast cells	BAL % eosinophils
A	2	2	0.5	1.3	0
B	1	0	0.6	2.4	0
C	2	3	1.9	2.4	0
D	1	37	2.8	2.8	2.5
E	2	2	2.9	5.7	0
F	1	4	3.0	1.0	0
G	0	0	3.4	1.2	0
H	2	2	6.2	2.1	0

Table 2 Mean ± standard deviation (SD) for absolute and relative spirometry measurements from eight untreated horses at rest (eupnoea) and during rebreathing over three consecutive days

Parameter	Rest					Rebreathing				
	Mean	± SD	Within day CV %	Between day CV %	ICC (90% CI)	Mean	± SD	Within day CV %	Between day CV %	ICC (90% CI)
Rf (bpm)	12.6	2.0	6.2	15.9	0.11 (-0.2-0.6)	20.1	2.8	3.8	13.7	0.67 (0.3-0.9)
Vt (L)	7.89	1.43	8.2	18.2	0.41 (0.0-0.8)	21.16	2.05	3.7	9.7	0.17 (-0.2-0.)
Tt (msec)	5051.7	890.3	6.1	17.6	0.20 (-0.2-0.7)	3049.5	396.3	3.8	13.0	0.05 (-0.3-0.6)
Ti (msec)	2212.5	360.5	8.6	16.3	-0.50 (-0.5- -0.5)	1505.5	186.9	4.3	12.4	-0.02 (-0.3-0.5)
Te (msec)	2812.8	590.7	6.3	21.0	-0.37 (-0.5-0.0)	1543.9	228.7	4.9	14.8	0.07 (-0.3-0.6)
PIF (L/sec)	5.03	0.87	7.2	17.0	0.36 (-0.1-0.8)	16.82	1.14	4.2	6.7	-0.03 (-0.3-0.4)
PEF (L/sec)	4.87	1.02	7.8	20.9	0.44 (0.1-0.8)	18.28	1.69	4.7	9.2	0.44 (0.1-0.8)
MVe (L)	96.1	9.7	8.8	10.1	-0.07 (-0.3-0.4)	420.1	26.7	4.3	6.4	-0.03 (-0.3-0.4)
Tpif (msec)	1433.7	475.5	19.6	33.2	0.40 (0.0-0.8)	786.1	281.3	18.3	35.8	-0.03 (-0.3-0.4)
Tpef (msec)	621.2	1051.2	10.2	169	0.97 (0.9-1.0)	185.6	41.8	19.7	22.5	0.77 (0.5-0.9)
Te/Tt	0.56	0.04	4.0	6.1	0.68 (0.4-0.9)	0.51	0.02	2.7	4.3	0.68 (0.3-0.9)
Te/Ti	1.28	0.17	9.2	13.1	0.65 (0.3-0.9)	1.03	0.09	5.4	8.6	0.67 (0.3-0.9)
Tpef/Te	0.19	0.25	13.6	132	0.97 (0.9-1.0)	0.12	0.03	19.0	23.1	0.61 (0.3-0.9)
Tpif/Ti	0.64	0.20	18.6	31.3	-0.49 (-0.5-0.4)	0.52	0.18	16.3	33.6	-0.49 (-0.5-0.4)

Each parameter was determined by analysis of three breaths on each testing day, and within day coefficients of variation (CV) were calculated across this data as a measure of repeatability (within day variation). Mean values (± SD) reported below, between day CV (reproducibility), and intraclass correlation coefficients (ICC, reported with 90% confidence interval), were determined by analysis of pooled data (mean of three breaths) collected on each day of testing. Ghosted (grey) results for ICC indicate poor or moderate agreement

Abbreviations: Rf respiratory frequency, *bpm* breaths per minute, *Vt* tidal volume, *L* litres, *Tt* total breath period, *msec* milliseconds, *Ti* inspiratory period, *Te* expiratory period, *PIF* peak inspiratory flow, *PEF* peak expiratory flow, *L/sec* litres per second, *MVe* minute ventilation, *Tpif* time to PIF, *Tpef* time to PEF

A significant day effect was observed for the relative flow value Tpef/Te during eupnoeic breathing ($P = 0.010$, determined by Friedman one-way RM-ANOVA on ranks). No significant differences attributable to day of testing were observed for any other parameter. Higher CVs were evident when comparing results across the three days tested, by comparison with repeatability analyses on each day, indicating that variability was greater between days than within traces obtained on a single day. Results calculated for ICC values were consistent with strong agreement across days for Rf (during rebreathing only), and for Tpef, Te/Tt, Te/Ti and Tpef/Te (Table 2), suggesting that values relating to the time of PEF were consistent for individual animals across the three days. Significant differences were evident between individual horses for PEF during eupnoeic respiration and rebreathing ($P = 0.025$ and $P = 0.026$, respectively). Mean differences for relative flow variables are shown in Additional file 1: Figure S3.

Relative flow-time variables (Table 3) did not demonstrate any significant effect attributable to the day on which they were determined. Inspiratory and expiratory relative flow-time variables are shown in Figs. 5 and 6, respectively; differences in means for each pair of tests

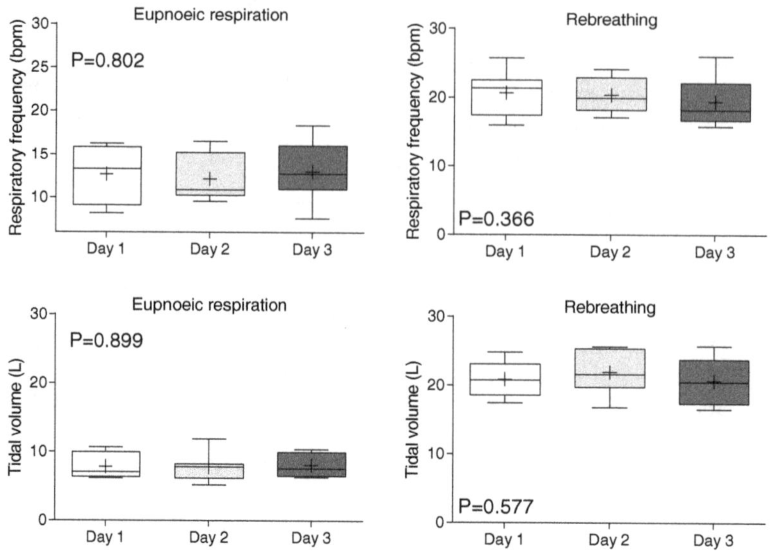

Fig. 3 Respiratory frequency and tidal volume determination on each day of testing (reproducibility). Results are shown as mean (*cross*), median (*horizontal line*), quartiles (*box*) and 10–90th percentile (whiskers). Results from each day of testing represent the mean of three breaths analysed for each horse. P values were determined by one-way RM-ANOVA

(Day 1 vs Day 2, Day 2 vs Day 3, Day 1 vs Day 3) are provided (Additional file 1: Figure S4). Repeatability (comparison of the three selected breaths on the same day of testing) and reproducibility (comparison of results across three days) were more variable during eupneoic respiration than was observed for absolute and relative flow values. Values obtained during rebreathing evidenced substantially less variation, but significant differences were observed between individual horses for all relative flow-time variables during eupnoeic respiration and/or rebreathing. Agreement was strongest, indicated by high ICC values, for expiratory flows around PEF (ezp50%, ezp75% and epz25%) during eupnoeic respiration (Table 3).

Consistent with the equivocal endoscopic and cytological findings from healthy horses in the current study, comparison of absolute and relative flow-time indices against endoscopic and cytological definitions of IAD demonstrated no significant associations between airway cytology and spirometry results in these horses.

Discussion

In the current study, horses averaged a tidal volume of 7.89 ± 1.43 L (mean ± stdev) and respiratory frequency of

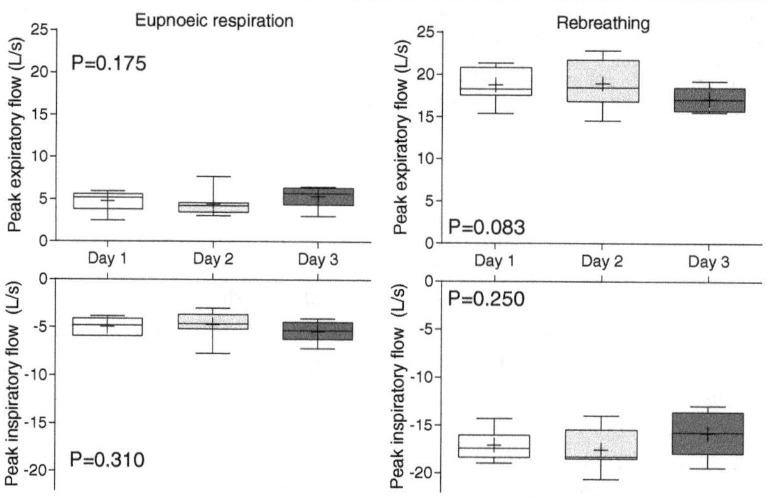

Fig. 4 Peak inspiratory and expiratory flows on each day of testing (reproducibility). Results are shown as mean (*cross*), median (*horizontal line*), quartiles (*box*) and 10-90th percentile (whiskers). Results from each day of testing represent the mean of three breaths analysed for each horse. P values were determined by one-way RM-ANOVA

Table 3 Mean ± standard deviation (SD) for relative flow measurements from eight untreated horses at rest (eupnoea) and during rebreathing over three consecutive days

Parameter	Rest					Rebreathing				
	Mean	± SD	Within day CV %	Between day CV %	ICC (90% CI)	Mean	± SD	Within day CV %	Between day CV %	ICC (90% CI)
izp25%	61.9	11.9	15.0	19.2	0.45 (0.1-0.8)	82.2	7.2	7.9	8.8	0.42 (0.0-0.8)
izp50%	67.5	11.8	14.1	17.5	0.79 (0.5-0.9)	88.7	4.2	4.7	4.8	0.54 (0.2-0.8)
izp75%	85.6	5.2	8.4	6.0	0.37 (0.0-0.7)	93.4	3.2	3.4	3.4	0.48 (0.1-0.8)
ipz25%	89.4	11.9	5.7	13.3	0.55 (0.2-0.8)	93.6	2.3	3.7	2.4	0.25 (-0.1-0.7)
ipz50%	85.1	7.1	7.2	8.4	0.45 (0.1-0.8)	90.3	2.7	5.4	3.0	0.22 (-0.1-0.6)
ipz75%	70.6	6.0	15.1	8.5	0.17 (-0.2-0.6)	82.0	9.1	8.0	11.1	0.77 (0.5-0.9)
ezp25%	57.1	7.0	9.0	12.2	0.38 (0.1-0.7)	66.4	3.9	9.0	5.8	-0.01 (-0.3-0.6)
ezp50%	80.1	9.9	5.3	12.3	0.90 (0.7-1.0)	89.9	1.6	3.4	1.8	-0.14 (-0.4-0.4)
ezp75%	93.2	5.7	2.6	6.2	0.82 (0.6-1.0)	96.9	0.7	1.8	0.7	-0.10 (-0.3-0.4)
epz25%	56.8	18.1	13.7	31.9	0.80 (0.6-0.9)	81.8	5.5	5.5	6.7	0.64 (0.2-0.9)
epz50%	58.5	14.9	14.7	25.5	0.67 (0.3-0.9)	75.1	8.0	5.3	10.7	0.64 (0.2-0.9)
epz75%	61.7	10.1	13.2	16.4	0.29 (-0.1-0.7)	77.0	10.2	7.4	13.3	0.58 (0.2-0.9)

Each parameter represented the percent of peak flow at the appropriate relative time within each breath cycle, and was determined by analysis of three breaths on each testing day. Within day coefficients of variation (CV) were calculated across this data as a measure of repeatability. Mean values (± SD) reported below, between day CV (reproducibility), and intraclass correlation coefficients (ICC, reported with 90% confidence interval), were determined by analysis of pooled data (mean of three breaths) collected on each day of testing. Ghosted (grey) results for ICC indicate poor or moderate agreement
Abbreviations: izp inspiratory flow zero to peak, *ipz* inspiratory flow peak to zero, expiratory flow zero to peak, *epz* expiratory flow peak to zero, *SD* standard deviation, *ICC* intraclass correlation coefficient, *CI* confidence interval

12 bpm during eupnoeic respiration, which is similar to previous studies using ultrasound or Fleisch-type pneumotachometers [32–35], and slightly greater than values determined by respiratory inductance plethysmography and pneumotachography [25, 36]. In addition to differences due to technique, it is possible that equipment differences, such as mask volume and airflow resistance, or physiological differences between horses, such as age [36], use [35] or sub-clinical airway disease [34, 35], may influence values determined during pulmonary function testing. Hyperpnoea induced by carbon dioxide rebreathing was investigated in the current study because previous studies have suggested that PFT during tidal breathing is insensitive for detection of subtle changes, such as those associated with IAD [14, 16, 17]. Bag rebreathing as a respiratory stimulus in the current study resulted in a 1.6 times increase in respiratory frequency and 2.8 times increase in tidal volume compared to eupnoeic breathing. Tidal volumes were consistent with previous results derived from hypercapnia [14, 16], and slightly greater than results reported during or following exercise [16, 18, 20]. Values for PEF (18 L/s) and PIF (17 L/s) during hyperpnoea in this study were lower than results obtained following exercise (80 L/s) [18] or lobeline administration (40 L/s) [19].

During eupnoea in the current study, all horses demonstrated variable breathing patterns within the same day and on a breath to breath basis. Unsurprisingly, given that breaths were selected for analysis partly based on uniformity, the within day variation was much less than that observed between days. Some variability in tidal volumes and respiratory frequency was expected

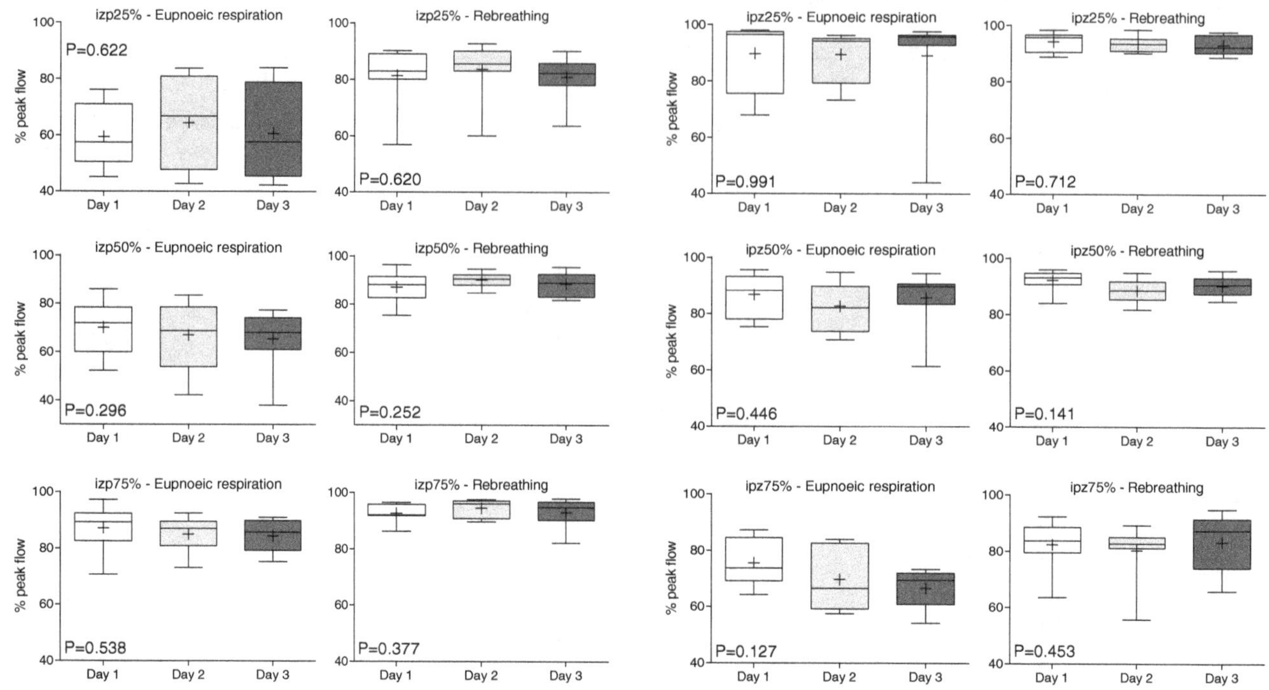

Fig. 5 Inspiratory relative flow-time values on each day of testing (reproducibility). Results are shown as mean (*cross*), median (*horizontal line*), quartiles (*box*) and 10–90th percentile (whiskers). Results from each day of testing represent the mean of three breaths analysed for each horse. P values were determined by one-way RM-ANOVA. Inspiratory zero to peak (izp) values represent the relative percentage of peak inspiratory flow measured at 25, 50 and 75% of the time from zero to peak flow; inspiratory peak to zero (ipz) values represent the relative percentage of peak inspiratory flow measured at 25, 50 and 75% of the time from peak to zero flow

during eupnoea, as horses have significant respiratory reserve, and ventilation is subject to rapid change in response to excitement, fear and other emotional states. Additionally, horses regularly take single large breaths (sighs), which serve to redistribute ventilation within pulmonary fields [37]. Carbon dioxide-induced hyperpnoea attenuated both the within day and between day variability observed in the current study. Rebreathing was expected to reduce variability in respiratory patterns as biphasic breathing is eliminated if respiratory muscles are activated before peak passive flow is obtained [32], as occurs during increased respiratory effort for physiological or pathological reasons. The use of capnography to standardise the degree of rebreathing in this study may have further served to reduce variation in measures obtained during hyperpnoea.

Values obtained in this study for most absolute and relative respiratory indices demonstrated adequate reproducibility during eupnoeic respiration and rebreathing. Time invested acclimatising horses to the test environment and spirometry procedures likely improved the reliability of the findings of the current study, and research methodology based on selection of three consecutive breaths, representative of the available spirometry trace and based on carefully defined inclusion criteria, was also designed to optimise repeatability and precision of PFT procedures. Previous respiratory studies have utilised analysis of three breaths from each epoch [18, 37], however, analysis of a greater number of breaths might increase the accuracy of derived measures of respiratory function [23], and further analyses may be indicated to determine the optimal number of breaths for analysis. Coefficients of variation in the current study were similar to, or less than, analogous results from previous studies [11, 34], and within acceptable limits for PFT [12]. However evaluation of individual variation, mean differences and 95% confidence intervals from repeated measures analysis suggested that the technique might be better suited to repeated studies in the same individual, rather than to the establishment of absolute reference ranges and cross-sectional studies. Results from determination of ICC demonstrated that measures of expiratory time (absolute Tpef, Tpef/Te, Te/Tt and Te/Ti) had the greatest agreement which, in this context, suggests these measures were the most repeatable for individual animals. Similarly, based on ICC results, relative flow-time indices derived during eupnoeic respiration demonstrated slightly better agreement than values obtained during rebreathing.

The time at which PEF occurred within each breath was highly variable between horses in the current study. Unlike humans, dogs and cats, the mechanical equilibrium of respiration for horses is at the midpoint of tidal volume, as opposed to the end of expiration, resulting in active

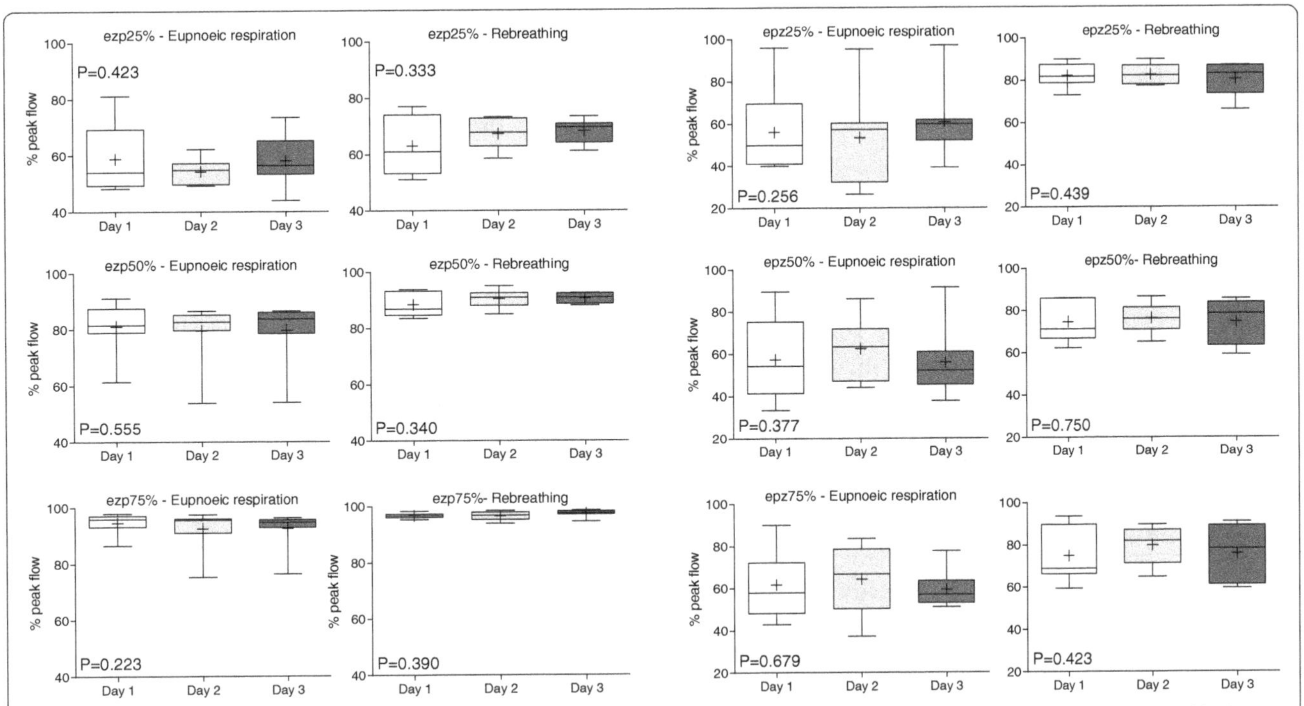

Fig. 6 Expiratory relative flow-time values on each day of testing (reproducibility). Results are shown as mean (*cross*), median (*horizontal line*), quartiles (*box*) and 10-90th percentile (whiskers). Results from each day of testing represent the mean of three breaths analysed for each horse. P values were determined by one-way RM-ANOVA. Expiratory zero to peak (ezp) values represent the relative percentage of peak inspiratory flow measured at 25, 50 and 75% of the time from zero to peak flow; expiratory peak to zero (epz) values represent the relative percentage of peak inspiratory flow measured at 25, 50 and 75% of the time from peak to zero flow

and passive components of both inspiration and expiration [32]. Consequently, horses may exhibit monophasic or biphasic respiratory patterns during eupnoeic breathing, with consequent variation in the position of peak inspiratory and expiratory flows between breaths. In the current study all horses demonstrated biphasic expiration during eupnoea; however inspiration was monophasic, biphasic or both. Study horses exhibited PIF and PEF variably in early, middle and late phases of respiration in apparent random distribution. Although such variability is well documented [17] and previous studies have differed in their conclusions regarding normal resting respiratory patterns in horses [20, 32, 38], it has been suggested that normal horses typically have PEF early in expiration and PIF late in inspiration [25, 32, 33]. Expiratory flows have greater sensitivity and accuracy for the diagnosis of obstructive airway disease in human patients and horses [4], and both human and equine studies have demonstrated that PEF occurs earlier in expiration in individuals with airway obstruction [22, 39, 40].

During hyperpnoea, expiration remained biphasic, whilst inspiration tended to become monophasic in the current study, in agreement with previous findings during lobeline-induced hyperpnoea [16]. Hyperpnoea induced by exercise typically results in loss of both biphasic inspiration and expiration as consequence of earlier and more intense respiratory muscle contraction and locomotion coupling [32, 38]. The current study found both PIF and PEF occurred close to the start of inspiration and expiration during rebreathing; PEF was higher and increased more than PIF, as has been previously reported [16].

There was no apparent variation attributable to day of testing in relative flow-time indices derived from spirometry traces in the current study. Variability was least for relative flow-time values obtained between peak and zero inspiratory flow (ipz) and between zero and peak expiratory flow (ezp), suggesting that these measurements might be the most suitable for experimental studies. Between day variability was reduced during hyperpnoea for all derived flow-time values, and higher relative flows were obtained earlier within each phase of the breathing cycle than was evident in eupneoic breathing. Consistent with the variable flow characteristics observed, significant individual variation was identified for most relative flow-time variables during both eupnoeic respiration and rebreathing. As was observed in the current study, relative flow-time values after PEF (epz) had the greatest variation in adult human subjects [41]. In horses in the current study, expiratory flow after PEF typically had a biphasic pattern (as PEF occurs early in expiration), therefore the values of epz25%, epz50% and epz75% may be of similar magnitude and not accurately represent flow limitation (Fig. 2). As horses with airway obstruction have reduced maximal flows in final stages of expiration [11], future experiments might focus on calculations at relative flow-time values later in the expiratory period (eg. epz 75%, 80%, 85%, 90% and 95%). Despite considerable individual horse variation, relative flow-time values derived during expiration in the current study showed the greatest agreement, as indicated by high ICC values. Again this is similar to studies on tidal breathing in adult patients [41], where evaluation of expiratory flows after PEF was useful in identifying obstructive respiratory conditions. Further studies are required to determine whether these relative flow-time indices are useful for characterisation of obstructive lower airway disease in horses. Although the current study was not intended to evaluate the diagnostic utility of breath by breath spirometry or relative flow-time indices for the diagnosis of obstructive airway conditions, and indeed used horses that were clinically healthy, endoscopy and airway cytology suggested minor changes (slight increase in tracheal mucus) were present in four of the eight horses. These changes barely fulfilled inclusion criteria for IAD [1] and had no obvious effect on indices of respiratory function in the present study.

Conclusions

Individual horse variation observed in all relative flow-time parameters in the current study may prove a limitation in determining reference ranges for use in a diagnostic setting. However, the current study demonstrated that the mask spirometry system used was able to provide reliable (repeatable and reproducible) absolute and relative indices of respiratory function in healthy horses. Further evaluation of the technique as a tool in the diagnosis or monitoring of respiratory disease in horses is required. The reliability of the technique suggests its utility in the evaluation of repeated measures of airway function, such as would be required for bronchoprovocation tests or the assessment of the response to treatment.

Additional files

Additional file 1: Figure S1. Representative volume (green) and flow (pink) traces obtained during spontaneous respiration showing uniform volume and flow traces which would satisfy inclusion criteria for analysis. Note biphasic expiratory and inspiratory respiration. **Table S1.** Respiratory parameters measured for each of three selected breaths. Data from each breath was evaluated to ensure inclusion criteria were met (≤10% difference in inspiratory and expiratory volumes, ≤10% difference in time to peak inspiratory and expiratory flow (Tpif, Tpef) for the three breaths). **Table S2.** Definition of relative flow-time variables calculated for each of three selected breaths. **Figure S2.** Mean difference and 95% confidence intervals between days for absolute measures (respiratory frequency, Rf; tidal volume, Vt; peak inspiratory and expiratory flows, PIF and PEF; time to PEF, Tpef) determined during pulmonary function testing over three consecutive days. **Figure S3.** Mean difference and 95% confidence intervals between days for relative expiratory flow indices (ratio of time to PEF to expiratory time; Tpef/Te; ratio of time to PEF to total breath duration; Tpef/Tt) determined during pulmonary function testing over three consecutive days. **Figure S4.** Mean difference and 95% confidence intervals between days for relative flow-time indices determined during pulmonary function testing over. (PDF 525 kb)

Additional file 2: Raw data. (XLS 414 kb)

Abbreviations

ANOVA: Analysis of variance; BAL: Bronchoalveolar lavage; CO_2: Carbon dioxide; CV: Coefficient of variation; $epz_{25\%}$, $epz_{50\%}$, $epz_{75\%}$: 25%, 50%, 75% time from PEF to zero flow; $ezp_{25\%}$, $ezp_{50\%}$, $ezp_{75\%}$: 25%, 50%, 75% time from zero to PEF; IAD: Inflammatory airway disease; $ipz_{25\%}$, $ipz_{50\%}$, $ipz_{75\%}$: 25%, 50%, 75% time from PIF to zero flow; $izp_{25\%}$, $izp_{50\%}$, $izp_{75\%}$: 25%, 50%, 75% time from zero to PIF; MVe: Minute ventilation; PEF: Peak expiratory flow; PFT: Pulmonary function testing; PIF: Peak inspiratory flow; PMN: Polymorphonuclear cells (neutrophils); RAO: Recurrent airway obstruction; Rf: Respiratory frequency; Te: Expiratory period; Ti: Inspiratory period; Tpef: Time to peak expiratory flow; Tpif: Time to peak inspiratory flow; Tt: Total breath period; TW: Tracheal wash; V_T: Tidal volume

Acknowledgements

Peter Taylor and staff at Mortara Pty Ltd provided vital assistance with construction of the manifold that enabled summing of the outputs from the three Prevents, and with implementation of the CPFS/D software used in this study. This manuscript includes information presented as a dissertation submitted by Dr Burnheim to the Charles Sturt University Faculty of Science as partial fulfilment of the requirements for Honours in Veterinary Science.

Funding

The study was partly funded by Honours operating funds from the School of Animal and Veterinary Sciences, Charles Sturt University.

Authors' contributions

KB contributed to study conception and design, data acquisition, analysis and interpretation, drafting and critical revision of manuscript. KH contributed to study conception and design, data acquisition, analysis and interpretation, and critical revision of manuscript. DE contributed to study conception and design, data analysis and interpretation, and critical revision of manuscript. SLR contributed to study conception and design, data acquisition, analysis and interpretation, drafting and critical revision of manuscript. All authors contributed to experimental design and manuscript preparation; all have read and approved the final version of the manuscript. SLR, KB and KH performed pulmonary function testing; SLR and KB completed data analysis.

Competing interests

The authors declare that they have no competing interests.

Consent for publication

Not applicable.

References

1. Couetil LL, Cardwell JM, Gerber V, Lavoie JP, Leguillette R, Richard EA. Inflammatory airway disease of horses-revised consensus statement. J Vet Int Med. 2016;30(2):503–15.
2. Leclere M, Lavoie-Lamoureux A, Lavoie JP. Heaves, an asthma-like disease of horses. Respirology. 2011;16(7):1027–46.

3. Couetil L, DeNicola DB. Blood gas, plasma lactate, and bronchoalveolar lavage cytology analyses in racehorses with respiratory disease. Equine Vet J. 1999;30:77–82.
4. Couetil LL, Rosenthal FS, DeNicola DB, Chilcoat CD. Clinical signs, evaluation of bronchoalveolar lavage fluid, and assessment of pulmonary function in horses with inflammatory respiratory disease. Am J Vet Res. 2001;62(4):538–46.
5. Wichtel M, Gomez D, Burton S, Wichtel J, Hoffman A. Relationships between equine airway reactivity measured by flowmetric plethysmography and specific indicators of airway inflammation in horses with suspected inflammatory airway disease. Equine Vet J. 2015. doi:10.1111/evj.12482.
6. Derksen FJ, Scott D, Robinson NE, Slocombe RF, Armstrong PJ. Intravenous histamine administration in ponies with recurrent airway obstruction (heaves). Am J Vet Res. 1985;46(4):774–7.
7. Stadler P, Deegen E. Diurnal variation of dynamic compliance, resistance and viscous work of breathing in normal horses and horses with lung disorders. Equine Vet J. 1986;18(3):171–8.
8. Mazan MR, Hoffman AM, Manjerovic N. Comparison of forced oscillation with the conventional method for histamine bronchoprovocation in horses. Am J Vet Res. 1999;60:174–80.
9. Young SS, Tesarowski D. Respiratory mechanics of horses measured by conventional and forced oscillation techniques. J Appl Phys. 1994;76(6):2467–72.
10. Hoffman AM, Kuehn H, Reidelberger K, Kupcinskas R, Miskovic M. Flowmetric comparison of respiratory inductance plethysmography and pneumotachography in horses. J Appl Phys. 2001;91:2767–75.
11. Couetil L, Rosenthal FS, Simpson CM. Forced expiration: a test for airflow obstruction in horses. J Appl Phys. 2000;88(5):1870–9.
12. Cotes JE, Chinn DJ, Miller MR. Basic equipment and measurement techniques. In: Cotes JE, Chinn DJ, Miller MR, editors. Lung Function: Physiology, Measurement and Application in Medicine. 6 edn. Massachusetts,: Blackwell Publishing Ltd; 2006. p. 59-81.
13. Woolcock AJ, Vincent NJ, Macklem PT. Frequency dependence of compliance as a test for obstruction in the small airways. J Clinical Invest. 1969;48(6):1097–106.
14. Pirrone F, Albertini M, Clement MG, Lafortuna CL. Respiratory mechanics in Standardbred horses with sub-clinical inflammatory airway disease and poor athletic performance. Vet J. 2007;173(1):144–50.
15. Mazan MR, Lascola K, Bruns SJ, Hoffman AM. Use of a novel one-nostril mask-spacer device to evaluate airway hyperresponsiveness (AHR) in horses after chronic administration of albuterol. Can J Vet Res. 2014;78(3):214–20.
16. Art T, Desmecht D, Amory H, Lekeux P. Lobeline-induced hyperpnea in equids. Comparison with rebreathing bag and exercise. Zentralbl Veterinarmed A. 1991;38(2):148–52.
17. Herholz C, Tschudi P, Gerber H, Moens Y, Straub R. Ultrasound spirometry in the horse: a preliminary report on the method and the effects of xylazine and lobeline hydrochloride medication. Schweiz Arch Tierheilkd. 1997; 139(12):558–63.
18. Kusano K, Curtis RA, Goldman CA, Evans DL. Relative flow-time relationships in single breaths recorded after treadmill exercise in Thoroughbred horses. J Equine Vet Sci. 2007;27(8):362–8.
19. Kästner SB, Marlin DJ, Roberts CA, Auer JA, Lekeux P. Comparison of the performance of linear resistance and ultrasonic pneumotachometers at rest and during lobeline-induced hyperpnoea. Res Vet Sci. 2000;68(2):153–9.
20. Lafortuna CE, Saibene F. Mechanics of breathing in horses at rest and during exericse. Journal of Exp Biol. 1991;155(1):245–59.
21. Morris MJ, Lane DJ. Tidal expiratory flow patterns in airflow obstruction. Thorax. 1981;36(2):135–42.
22. Morris MJ, Madgwick RG, Collyer I, Denby F, Lane DJ. Analysis of expiratory tidal flow patterns as a diagnostic tool in airflow obstruction. Euro Resp J. 1998;12(5):1113–7.
23. Stocks J, Dezateux CA, Jackson EA, Hoo AF, Costeloe KL, Wade AM. Analysis of tidal breathing parameters in infancy: how variable is TPTEF:TE? Am J Respir Crit Care Med. 1994;150(5 Pt 1):1347–54.
24. Behan AL, Hauptman JG, Robinson NE. Telemetric analysis of breathing pattern variability in recurrent airway obstruction (heaves)-affected horses. Am J Vet Res. 2013;74(6):925–33.
25. Hoffman AM, Oura TJ, Reidelberger KJ, Mazan MR. Plethysmographic comparison of breathing pattern in heaves (recurrent airway obstruction) versus exprimental bronchoconstriction or hyperpnea in horses. J Vet Int Med. 2007;21:184–92.
26. Evans DL, Kiddell L, Smith CL. Pulmonary funciton measurements immediately after exercise are correlated with neutrophil percentage in tracheal aspirates in horses with poor racing performance. Res Vet Sci. 2011;90:510–5.
27. Gerber V, Straub EA. Endoscopic scoring of mucus quantity and quality: observer and horse variance and relationship to inflammation, mucus viscoelasticity and volume. Equine Vet J. 2004;36(7):576–82.
28. Curtis RA, Kusano K, Evans DL, Lovell NH, Hodgson DR. Reliability of cardiorespiratory measurements with a new ergospirometer during intense treadmill exercise in Thoroughbred horses. Vet J. 2005;169(2):223–31.
29. Hopkins WG. Calculating the reliability intraclass correlation coefficient and its confidence limits. 2009. newstats.org/xICC.xls.
30. Bartko JJ. The intraclass correlation coefficient as a measure of reliability. Psychol Rep. 1966;19:3–11.
31. McGraw KO, Wong SP. Forming inferences about some intraclass correlation coefficients. Psychol Meth. 1996;1:30–46.
32. Koterba AM, Kosch PC, Beech J, Whitlock T. Breathing strategy of the adult horse (Equus caballus) at rest. J Appl Phys. 1988;64(1):337–46.
33. Guthrie AJ, Beadle RE, Bateman RD, White CE. Characterization of normal tidal breathing flow-volume loops for thoroughbred horses. Vet Res Commun. 1995;19(4):331–42.
34. Herholz C, Straub R, Busato A. Ultrasound-spirometry and capnography in horses: analysis of measurement reliability. Vet Res Commun. 2001; 25(2):137–47.
35. Herholz C, Straub R, Braendlin C, Imhof A, Lüthi S, Busato A. Measurement of tidal breathing flow-volume loop indices in horses used for different sporting purposes with and without recurrent airway obstruction. Vet Rec. 2003;152:288–92.
36. Pacheco AP, Paradis MR, Hoffman AM, Hermida P, Sanchez A, Nadeau JA, Tufts M, Mazan MR. Age effects on blood gas, spirometry, airway reactivity and bronchoalveolar lavage fluid cytology in clinically healhy horses. J Vet Intern Med. 2014;28:603–8.
37. Ambrisko TD, Schramel JP, Adler A, Kutasi O, Makra Z, Moens YP. Assessment of distribution of ventilation by electrical impedance tomography in standing horses. Physiol Meas. 2016;37(2):175–86.
38. Art T, Lekeux P. Respiratory airflow patterns in ponies at rest and during exercise. Can J Vet Res. 1988;52(3):299–303.
39. Carlsen KH, Lodrup Carlsen KC. Tidal breathing analysis and response to salbutamol in awake young children with and without asthma. Euro Resp J. 1994;7(12):2154–9.
40. Pollmann U, Hörnicke H. Characteristics of respiratory airflow during exercise in horses with reduced performance due to pulmonary emphysema or bronchitis. In: Gillespie JR, Robinson NE, editors. International conference on equine exercise physiology 2. Davis, California: ICEEP Publications; 1987. p. 760–77.
41. Williams EM, Madgwick RG, Morris MJ. Tidal expired airflow patterns in adults with airway obstruction. Euro Resp J. 1998;12(5):1118–23.

12

Effects of stanozolol on normal and IL-1β-stimulated equine chondrocytes in vitro

Mariana Castro Martins[1*], Mandy J. Peffers[2], Katie Lee[2] and Luis M. Rubio-Martinez[1]

Abstract

Background: Intra-articular administration of stanozolol has shown promising results by improving the clinical management of lameness associated with naturally-occurring osteoarthritis (OA) in horses, and by decreasing osteophyte formation and subchondral bone reaction in sheep following surgically induced OA. However, there is limited evidence on the anti-inflammatory and modulatory properties of stanozolol on articular tissues. The objective of the current study was to evaluate the effects of stanozolol on chondrocyte viability and gene expression in normal equine chondrocytes and an inflammatory in vitro system of OA (interleukin-1β (IL-1β) treated chondrocytes).

Results: Chondrocytes from normal metacarpophalangeal joints of skeletally mature horses were exposed to four treatment groups: (1) media only (2) media+IL-1β (3) media+IL-1β + stanozolol (4) media+stanozolol. Following exposure, chondrocyte viability and the expression of catabolic, anabolic and structural genes were determined. General linear models with Dunnet's comparisons with Bonferroni's adjustment were performed. Cell viability was similar in all groups. Stanozolol treatment reduced gene expression of MMP-13, MMP-1, IL-6 and COX-2 in both normal and IL-1β treated chondrocytes. Stanozolol treatment reduced ADAMTS4 gene expression in normal chondrocytes. Stanozolol reduced the expression of COL2A1.

Conclusions: The current study demonstrates stanozolol has chondroprotective effects through downregulation of genes for pro-inflammatory/catabolic cytokines and enzymes associated with OA. However, there is no evidence of increased cartilage stimulation through upregulation of the anabolic and structural genes tested.

Keywords: Osteoarthritis, Stanozolol, Chondrocyte, Equine, Gene expression, In vitro

Background

Osteoarthritis (OA) is caused by a combination of biomechanical and biochemical changes in the joint that include synovium and subchondral bone abnormalities, ultimately resulting in cartilage degeneration [1]. In the past decade, major advances have been made in molecular biology and OA research in both human and veterinary medicine. Equine models have been used extensively providing invaluable insights into the molecular pathogenesis during disease establishment and in response to treatment [2, 3].

* Correspondence: mcm@liverpool.ac.uk
[1]Department of Equine Clinical Studies, Institute of Veterinary Science, University of Liverpool, Leahurst Campus, Chester High Road, Neston CH64 7TE, UK
Full list of author information is available at the end of the article

One of the main goals in the treatment of OA is to inhibit further progression of cartilage degeneration and to restore a functional synovial environment with the potential to promote cartilage repair. Cartilage repair is mediated by the balance between chondrocyte gene expression of catabolic and anabolic genes [4, 5]. The most important mediator of cartilage degeneration is interleukin-1 (IL-1) [5, 6] and it has been reported that low innate production of IL-1β and IL-6 is associated with the absence of OA in old age [7]. IL-1 enhances the expression of pro-inflammatory mediators including matrix metalloproteinases (MMP-3 and -13), inflammatory cytokines (IL-6), a disintegrin and metalloproteinase with thrombospondin motifs (ADAMTS-4 and -5), cyclooxygenase 2 (COX-2), prostaglandin E2 (PGE2) and free radicals [1]. Cartilage repair is mediated by anabolic growth factors including the transforming growth factor β (TGF-β), insulin-like growth factor 1 (IGF-1), bone morphogenetic proteins (BMPs) and fibroblast growth factors (FGF) [8]. The IGF-1, TGF-β and BMPs act in part by induction of the transcription factor SOX-9, a key regulator of mesenchymal chondrogenesis during embryologic development [9, 10]. No therapy is currently available to prevent the onset or progression of OA, and latest research has focused on disease-modifying drugs with the capacity not only to counteract the effects of pro-inflammatory cytokines but also to promote articular cartilage repair.

Anabolic-androgenic steroids (AAS) are synthetic derivatives of testosterone and were first introduced in the early 1930s. Since then, an attempt has been made to minimize the androgenic side effects by increasing their anabolic: androgenic ratio. Stanozolol has one of the highest anabolic: androgenic ratios, suggesting it has anabolic activity with minimal androgenic side effects [11]. Stanozolol has a wide range of applications in human medicine and has been used to treat rheumatoid arthritis [12, 13], hereditary angioedema [14], idiopathic osteonecrosis [15], postmenopausal osteoporosis [16, 17], muscle wastage and age-related sarcopenia [11], amongst others [18]. The main claims for stanozolol's therapeutic effects are based on its anabolic activity on the musculoskeletal system and its potential to influence lean body mass, tissue repair, fibrinolysis, collagen synthesis and bone metabolism [11]. To our knowledge there are no human studies evaluating the effects of AAS on articular cartilage and there are no reports on the intra-articular use of stanozolol in human patients.

Intra-articular administration of stanozolol has recently been postulated as a treatment for OA. Studies investigating the clinical effects of the intra-articular use of stanozolol in horses have shown promising results in the ability of this drug to effectively manage lameness associated with OA and have suggested that stanozolol has the potential to stimulate cartilage repair [19, 20]. There is also anecdotal evidence of positive results obtained in equine clinical practice, including cases refractory to intra-articular glucocorticoids [21] and in the management of subchondral bone pain [22]. Furthermore, stanozolol has been used in an experimental animal model (sheep meniscectomy), demonstrating decreased osteophyte formation, subchondral bone reaction and synovial fibrosis, and articular cartilage regeneration [23]. However, there is limited evidence of the anti-inflammatory properties of stanozolol and how it affects articular chondrocytes in vitro. Previous data suggests that it reduces chondrocyte apoptosis by decreasing the production of nitric oxide in equine chondrocytes [24], enhances collagen synthesis though the upregulation of TGF-β in adult human dermal fibroblasts [25] and enhances the proliferation of cultured growth plate chondrocytes from pubertal female rats treated with GnRHa [26].

The objective of the current study is to evaluate the effect of stanozolol on chondrocyte viability and gene expression in normal chondrocytes and an in vitro inflammatory system of OA. We hypothesise that stanozolol will not have an effect on chondrocyte viability; will have a chondroprotective effect by reducing the expression of pro-inflammatory/catabolic genes (MMP-13, MMP-1, IL-6, ADAMTS4 and COX-2) in both normal and IL-1β treated chondrocytes; and will have an anabolic effect by increasing the expression of SOX9, COL2A1 and aggrecan in both normal and IL-1β treated chondrocytes.

Methods

Sample collection

Articular cartilage was aseptically harvested from the entire articular surface of macroscopically normal metacarpophalangeal joints of seven skeletally mature horses euthanized for reasons unrelated to this study, ages ranging from five to eleven years (mean 7.7 +/− SD 2.1). Samples were collected from an abattoir as a by-product of the agricultural industry and processed within 12 h of euthanasia. The Animals (Scientific Procedures) Act 1986, Schedule 2, does not define collection from these sources as scientific procedures and ethical approval was therefore not required.

Tissue culture and cell viability

The chondrocytes were isolated as previously described [27] and the cell viability was determined by trypan blue exclusion test [28] for each horse. The chondrocytes were then plated as monolayers in Dulbecco's modified eagles medium (DMEM) (Sigma-Aldrich, Dorset, UK), supplemented with 10% foetal calf serum (FCS), 100 units/ml penicillin, 100 mg/ml streptomycin (all from Invitrogen, Paisley, UK) and 500 ng/ml amphotericin B (BioWhittaker, Lonza, USA), at a concentration of 100,000 live cells/cm^2 (total of 16 wells of a 24-well plate used per horse). The chondrocytes were incubated in a 5% CO_2 humidified atmosphere at 37 °C for 48 h. The medium was changed and replaced with serum-free DMEM 24 h prior to exposure. Each horse was exposed to 4 different treatment groups (4 wells per group): (1) media only (negative control) (2) media + IL-1β (Recombinant Equine IL-1β, R&D Systems, Abingdon, UK) (10 ng/ml) (positive control) (3) media + IL-1β (10 ng/ml) + stanozolol (Sungate, ACME, Cavriago, Italy) (0.4 mg/ml) 4) media + stanozolol (0.4 mg/ml). The stanozolol concentration was extrapolated by using the clinically recommended dose of 5 mg per joint [20] and assuming the volume of a non-distended metacarpalphalangeal joint to be 12.5 ml [29]. After 24 h in culture conditions, cell viability was performed on one well per group.

Real-time PCR

Total RNA was isolated separately from 3 wells per group using 0.5 ml of Tri Reagent (Sigma-Aldrich, Dorset, UK) per well and stored at -80 °C for later analysis. The RNA isolated from each well was processed individually and was purified by the acid guanidinium thiocyanate-phenol-chloroform extraction technique as previously described [30]. Total RNA concentrations and purity were determined spectrophotometrically (NanoDrop™ 1000 Spectrophotometer, Thermo Fisher Scientific, Waltham, US) and all the samples used presented a ratio of absorbance at 260 nm and 280 nm (A_{260}/A_{280}) between 1.8 and 2.0. cDNA was synthetized from 500 ng of RNA in a 29 μL reaction using Moloney Murine Leukemia Virus Reverse Transcriptase (M-MLV RT) and random hexamer oligonucleotides (both Promega, Southampton, UK). cDNA samples were individually diluted to a final concentration of 5 ng/μL and 5 μL aliquots of cDNA were amplified by reverse transcription polymerase chain reaction (RT-PCR) (ABI PRISM® 7500 Sequence Detection System, Applied Biosystems, Warrington, UK) in a 20 μL reaction volume using a SYBR Green PCR mastermix (Applied Biosystems, Warrington, UK). Glyceraldehyde 3-phosphate dehydrogenase (GAPDH) was used as the housekeeping gene and the relative expression of catabolic, anabolic and structural genes was analysed using the $2_T^{-\Delta\Delta C}$ method [31]. The fitness of GAPDH as a valid normalisation factor has been previously identified by us [32, 33]. All primers used were designed by Applied Biosystems Assays-by-Design and have been previously validated by our group. Primers for equine IL-6 and COX-2 had the following sequences: IL-6 Forward: CTG-CTC-CTG-GTG-ATG-G CT-AC, Reverse: CCG-AGG-ATG-TGT-ACT-TAA-T GT-GCT-G; COX-2 Forward: CAG-CAT-AAA-CTG-C GC-CTT-TTC, Reverse: AGG-CGG-GTA-GAT-CAT-T TC-CA. The primer sequences for GAPDH, SOX9, COL2A1, aggrecan, MMP-13 and -1, and ADAMTS4 have been previously reported [32, 34].

Statistical analysis

Statistical analysis was performed using SPSS (IBM, Portsmouth, UK). Normality of the data was analysed using a Shapiro-Wilk test, and non-parametric data was LOG_{10} transformed prior to analysis. A general linear model was used for all analyses with Dunnet's comparisons against the control group and pairwise comparisons with Bonferroni's adjustment. Statistical significance was defined as $P < 0.05$.

Results

Stanozolol does not affect chondrocyte viability

There were no significant differences in cell viability between the different treatment groups.

Stanozolol reduces catabolic gene expression

There was a statistically significant increase in the expression of MMP-13, MMP-1, IL-6, ADAMTS4 and COX-2 mRNA expression in chondrocytes treated with IL-1β only (group 2- positive control) compared to media only (group 1- negative control) ($P < 0.001$). Conversely, chondrocytes exposed to stanozolol only (group 4) had a significantly decreased expression of all the above catabolic genes compared to the negative control (group 1) ($P < 0.001$) (Fig. 1).

When comparing both groups with IL-1β treated chondrocytes, there was a significant downregulation of MMP-13 ($P < 0.001$), MMP-1 ($P < 0.03$), IL-6 ($P < 0.001$) and COX-2 ($P < 0.001$) expression in chondrocytes exposed to IL-1β and stanozolol (group 3) compared to chondrocytes exposed to IL-1β alone (group 2). ADAMTS4 gene expression was not significantly supressed in chondrocytes exposed to IL-1β and stanozolol (group 3) compared to chondrocytes exposed to IL-1β only (group 2) (Fig. 1).

Stanazolol reduces COL2A1 gene expression

There was no statistically significant difference in SOX9 gene expression between treatment groups. COL2A1 gene expression was significantly supressed in both groups treated with stanozolol (groups 3 and 4) compared to both groups not treated with stanozolol (groups 1 and 2). Aggrecan gene expression was significantly supressed in both groups treated with IL-1β (groups 2 and 3) compared to both groups not treated with IL-1β (groups 1 and 4). No statistically significant difference was seen on COL2A1 gene expression between groups 1 and 2 or 3 and 4, or on aggrecan expression between groups 1 and 4 or 2 and 3 (Fig. 2).

Discussion

In OA the balance between anabolic and catabolic activities is compromised and cartilage degeneration prevails over the capacity of repair. In the present study, treatment with stanozolol was investigated in both normal and IL-1β stimulated chondrocytes. In accordance with previous reports [35–37] exposure to IL-1β induced a catabolic response on equine articular chondrocytes and increased the gene expression of MMP-13, MMP-1, IL-6, ADAMTS4 and COX-2. Addition of stanozolol to IL-1β stimulated chondrocytes counteracted the catabolic effects of IL-1β and downregulated the expression of MMP-13, MMP-1, IL-6, and COX-2. Similarly, corticosteroids have been demonstrated to inhibit MMP transcription [38–42] and downregulate the expression of COX-2 [40–42] in cytokine-treated chondrocytes. In the present study, stanozolol supressed ADAMTS4 gene expression in normal chondrocytes compared to control but did not counteract the upregulation induced by IL-1β. This is in contrast with observations in corticosteroids studies [39, 40].

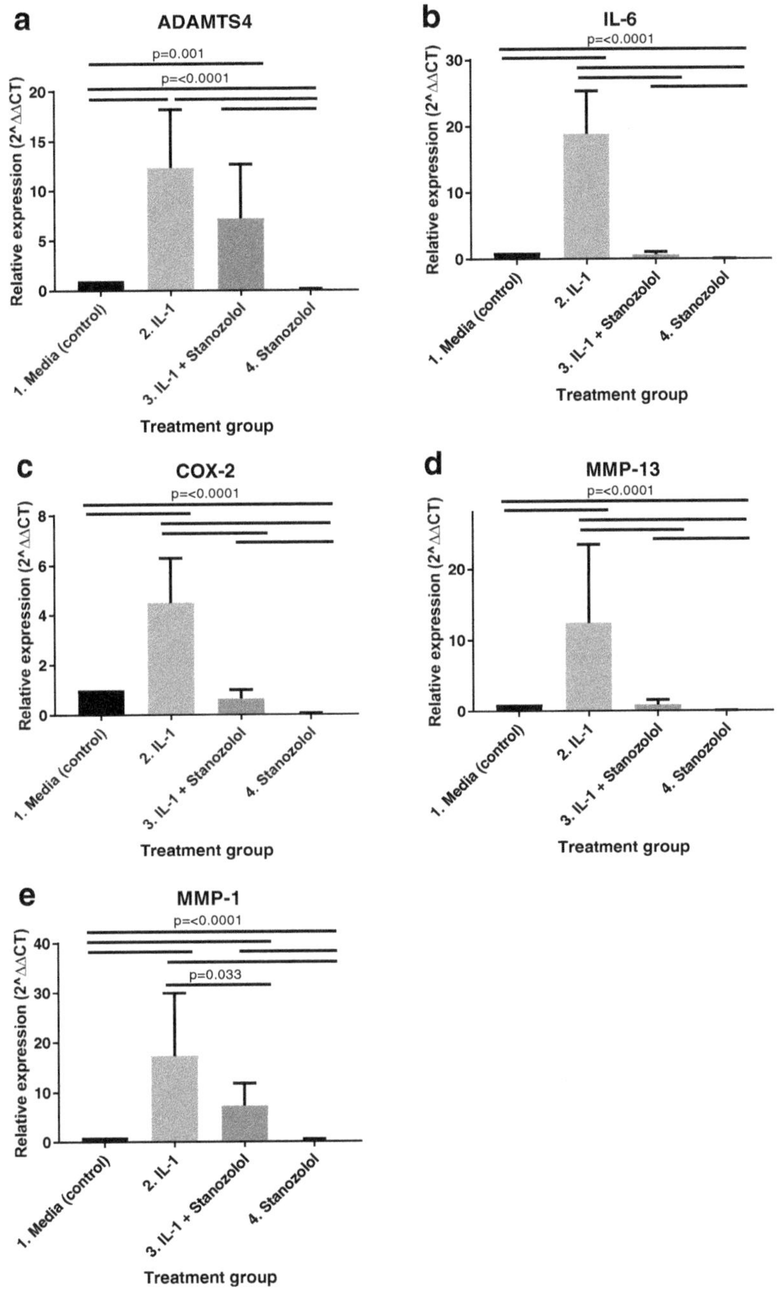

Fig. 1 Effects of stanozolol on (**a**) ADAMTS4, (**b**) IL-6, (**c**) COX-2, (**d**) MMP-13 and (**e**) MMP-1 gene expression in normal and IL-1β-treated equine articular chondrocytes. Real-time-PCR analysis of the above genes mRNA in monolayer cultures exposed to media, IL-1β, IL-1β + stanozolol and stanozolol. GAPDH was used as the housekeeping gene and data are represented as relative expression using the $2_T^{-\Delta\Delta C}$ method. Data were evaluated using a general linear model with Dunnet's comparisons against the control group and pairwise comparisons with Bonferroni's adjustment ($n = 7$, three technical replicates per treatment group)

Further analysis of our results showed that when normal chondrocytes were treated with stanozolol there was a significant decrease in the expression of all the catabolic genes tested (MMP-13, MMP-1, IL-6, ADAMTS4 and COX-2) compared to control. Again, similar results have been obtained in in vitro models studying the effects of corticosteroids on articular cartilage [38, 39]. Knych et al. [43] recently evaluated changes in synovial fluid gene expression following in vivo administration of triamcinolone in healthy horses undergoing a standardized exercise programme. In this study they found no significant differences in COX-2 and MMP-3 gene expression between baseline and the triamcinolone treatment group. These results suggest a protective and stronger anti-inflammatory

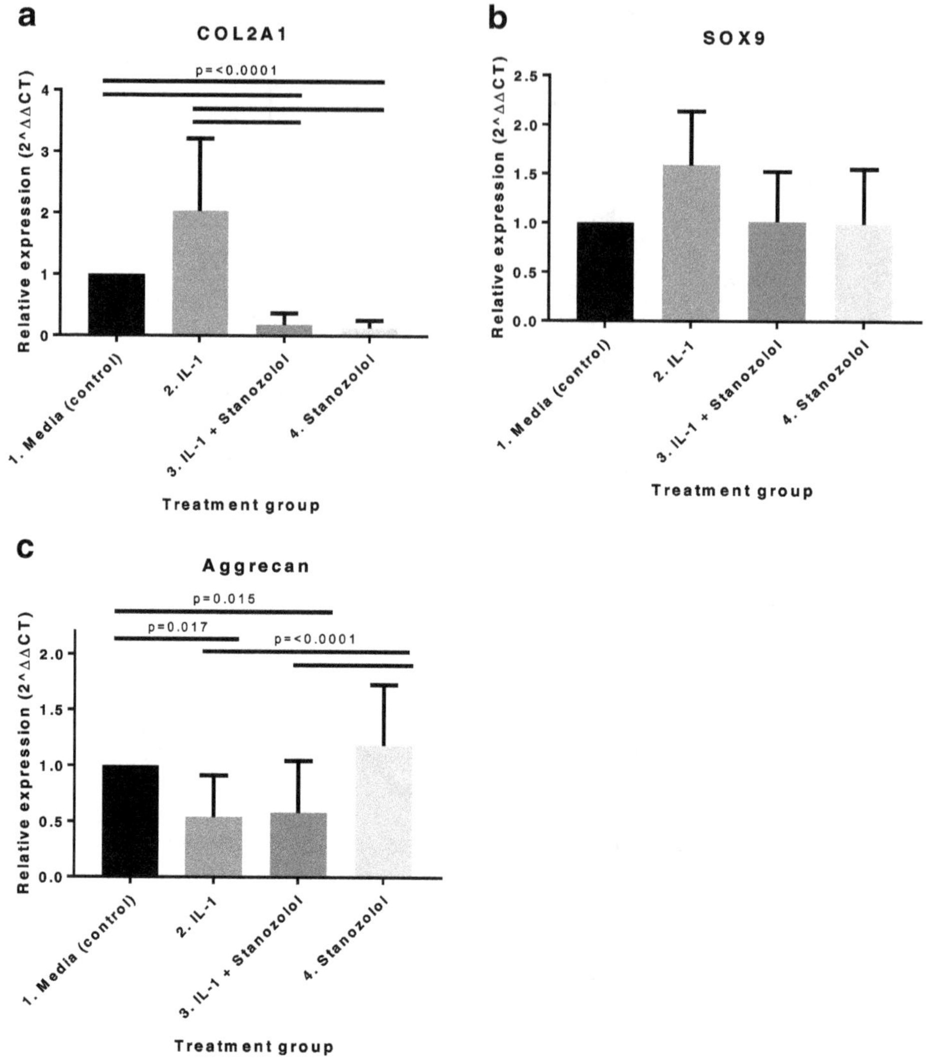

Fig. 2 Effect of stanozolol on (**a**) COL2A1, (**b**) SOX-9 and (**c**) aggrecan gene expression in normal and IL-1β-treated equine articular chondrocytes. Real-time-PCR analysis of the above genes mRNA in monolayer cultures exposed to media, IL-1β, IL-1β + stanozolol and stanozolol. GAPDH was used as the housekeeping gene and data are represented as relative expression using the $2_T^{-\Delta\Delta C}$ method. Data were evaluated using a general linear model with Dunnet's comparisons against the control group and pairwise comparisons with Bonferroni's adjustment (*n* = 7, three technical replicates per treatment group)

response after intra-articular administration of stanozolol compared to triamcinolone; however, different experimental models limit direct comparisons between studies.

Contrary to our hypothesis, stanozolol did not enhance the expression of SOX-9, COL2A1 or aggrecan. The pathway through which anabolic growth factors promote upregulation of chondrocyte specific genes remains largely unclear. The transcription factor SOX9 has elicited much interest as it is co-expressed with type II collagen in mouse fetal chondrocytes and is thought to be involved in chondrocyte differentiation and cartilage formation during development [44]. SOX9 has been shown to mediate the expression of many genes encoding cartilage extracellular matrix proteins, including COL2A1 and aggrecan [9, 45, 46]. Kolettas et al. [9] investigated the effects of IGF-1 and IL-1 on chondrocyte survival and phenotype and reported an antagonist effect. IL-1 supressed the expression of chondrocyte-specific genes (collagen types II and IX, aggrecan, biglycan and link protein) and downregulated SOX-9; and IGF-1 upregulated SOX-9, relieved the IL-1 induced inhibition of chondrocyte-specific genes and enhanced chondrocyte survival. The authors therefore suggested that IGF-1 and IL-1 modulate chondrocyte survival and differentiation through changes in SOX-9 gene expression. Further studies have challenged this concept and showed a negative correlation between COL2A1 and SOX9 gene expression. In human adult articular chondrocytes, IL-1 had no significant influence on SOX9 mRNA expression whereas COL2A1 was significantly downregulated. The same experiment also demonstrated that IGF-I up-regulated COL2A1 expression, but not SOX9 [47]. In our study, treatment with IL-1 and stanozolol, alone or in combination, did not alter SOX-9 gene expression in comparison to control. IL-1 did not downregulate SOX-9 as previously reported, had no effect on COL2A1 and downregulated aggrecan expression. Furthermore, treatment with stanozolol supressed COL2A1 without affecting SOX-9 gene expression. Our results suggest that COL2A1 and aggrecan gene expression are not correlated with the expression of SOX9 in equine articular chondrocytes and that treatment with stanozolol does not elicit an anabolic response through the upregulation of SOX-9, COL2A1 or aggrecan.

Both COL2A1 and aggrecan are important structural genes essential for cartilage integrity and formation. Stanozolol has been shown to increase collagen synthesis in cultures of human dermal fibroblasts [25]. The decrease in COL2A1 levels, which we have observed when chondrocytes were treated with stanozolol, goes against what has been reported in human dermal fibroblasts, and is similar to that reported by Knych et al. [43] in synovial fluid and Richardson and Dodge [38] in articular chondrocytes following treatment with corticosteroids. In the present study, aggrecan expression was downregulated by IL-1β and treatment with stanozolol did not ameliorate the IL-1 inhibition of aggrecan, which is also in accordance with what has been reported with corticosteroids [38]. Furthermore, the downregulation of COL2A1 induced by stanozolol in this study warrants careful consideration of its intra-articular use as it may suggest deleterious effects on cartilage. A limitation of our study is the use of a short-term in vitro system and different results may have been obtained with longer exposure times or with repeat exposures mimicking what has been described in clinical trials. Additionally, this study used chondrocytes and not cartilage explants. However, we used freshly isolated chondrocytes plated at high density in order to reduce dedifferentiation of chondrocytes in cell culture which can results in an altered phenotype. Future studies using cartilage explants are needed.

The similarities between the anti-catabolic effects of stanozolol and corticosteroids might be associated with the previously reported affinity of AAS for the glucocorticoid receptors [48]. Alternative pathways through which AAS might be able to exert an anabolic effect on articular tissues merit further investigation; and a plausible explanation for the lack of anabolic activity in our in vitro system might be related to a single and short-lived exposure time. Further studies investigating the systemic effects of a low intra-articular dose of stanozolol and its local effects on articular tissues with naturally-occurring OA are warranted. The use of AAS is banned by the main organizations overseeing drug regulation in sport, therefore its use should only be considered in non-competing individuals.

Conclusions

Stanozolol has been described as having disease-modifying activity by attenuating the degenerative response in osteoarthritic cartilage in in vivo studies. The results of our in vitro study support the hypothesis that stanozolol has an anti-inflammatory effect and is effective at inhibiting the production of pro-inflammatory mediators in both normal and IL-1 treated chondrocytes. However, in our in vitro system there is no evidence of stanozolol having an anabolic effect through upregulation of SOX-9, COL2A1 and aggrecan gene expression.

Abbreviations

AAS: Anabolic-androgenic steroids; ADAMTS: Disintegrin and metalloproteinase with thrombospondin motifs; BMPs: Bone morphogenetic proteins; cDNA: Complimentary deoxyribonucleic acid; CO_2: Carbon dioxide; COL2A1: Collagen type 2 alpha 1; COX-2: Cyclooxygenase-2; DMEM: Dulbecco's modified eagles medium; FCS: Foetal calf serum; FGF: Fibroblast growth factor; GAPDH: Glyceraldehyde 3-phosphate dehydrogenase; GnRHa: Gonadotropin-releasing hormone agonist; IGF-1: Insulin-like growth factor 1; IL-1β: Interleukin-1β; IL-6: Interleukin 6; M-MLV RT: Moloney Murine Leukemia Virus Reverse Transcriptase; MMP: Matrix metalloproteinase; mRNA: Messenger ribonucleic acid; OA: Osteoarthritis; PGE2: Prostaglandin E2; RT-PCR: Reverse transcription polymerase chain reaction; SOX-9: Transcripton gactor SOX-9; TGF-β: Transforming growth factor β

Acknowledgements

The authors would like to thank Maria M. Torres for her assistance in the acquisition of data.

Funding

This study was funded by the Institute of Veterinary Science, University of Liverpool (VET039-VSRP). Mandy Peffers is funded through a Wellcome Trust Intermediate Clinical Fellowship (107471/Z/15/Z).

Authors' contributions

MCM, LRM and MJP were involved in the conception, design of the study and experiments, and the analysis and interpretation of data. MCM was involved in organizing this research, the acquisition of data and drafting the manuscript. KL was involved in the statistical analysis and interpretation of data. All authors read and approved the final manuscript.

Consent for publication

Not applicable.

Competing interests

The authors declare that they have no competing interests.

Author details

[1]Department of Equine Clinical Studies, Institute of Veterinary Science, University of Liverpool, Leahurst Campus, Chester High Road, Neston CH64 7TE, UK. [2]Department of Musculoskeletal Biology, Institute of Ageing and Chronic Disease, University of Liverpool, Liverpool, UK.

References

1. McIlwraith CW. Traumatic arthritis and posttraumatic osteoarthritis in the horse. In: CW MI, Frisbie DD, Kawcak C, van Weeren R, editors. Joint disease in the horse. 2nd ed. Missouri: Elsevier; 2016. p. 33–48.
2. Little CB, Smith MM. Animal models of osteoarthritis. Cur Rheumatol Rev. 2008;4(3):175–82.
3. McIlwraith CW, Frisbie DD, Kawcak CE. The horse as a model of naturally occurring osteoarthritis. Bone Joint Res. 2012;1(11):297–309.
4. Goldring MB, Otero M, Tsuchimochi K, et al. Defining the roles of inflammatory and anabolic cytokines in cartilage metabolism. Ann Rheum Dis. 2008;67(Suppl 3):iii75–82.
5. Mueller MB, Tuan RS. Anabolic/catabolic balance in pathogenesis of osteoarthritis: identifying molecular targets. PM&R. 2011;3(6):S3–11.
6. Blom AB, Van Der Kraan PM, Van Den Berg WB. Cytokine targeting in osteoarthritis. Curr Drug Targets. 2007;8(2):283–92.
7. Goekoop RJ, Kloppenburg M, Kroon HM, et al. Low innate production of interleukin-1β and interleukin-6 is associated with the absence of osteoarthritis in old age. Osteoarthr Cartil. 2010;18(7):942–7.
8. Fortier LA, Barker JU, Strauss EJ, et al. The role of growth factors in cartilage repair. Clin Orthop Relat Res. 2011;469(10):2706–15.
9. Kolettas E, Muir HI, Barrett JC, Hardingham TE. Chondrocyte phenotype and cell survival are regulated by culture conditions and by specific cytokines through the expression of sox-9 transcription factor. Rheumatology. 2001; 40(10):1146–56.
10. Wagner T, Wirth J, Meyer J, et al. Autosomal sex reversal and campomelic dysplasia are caused by mutations in and around the SRY-related gene SOX9. Cell. 1994;79(6):1111–20.
11. Evans NA. Current concepts in anabolic-androgenic steroids. Am J Sports Med. 2004;32(2):534–42.
12. Belch JJ, Madhok R, McArdle B, et al. The effect of increasing fibrinolysis in patients with rheumatoid arthritis: a double blind study of stanozolol. Q J Med. 1986;58(1):19–27.
13. Pullar T. Disease modifying drugs for rheumatoid arthritis: yesterday's treatment today or today's treatment tomorrow? Br J Clin Pharmacol. 1990;30(4):501–10.
14. Sloane DE, Lee CW, Sheffer AL. Hereditary angioedema: safety of long-term stanozolol therapy. J Allergy Clin Immunol. 2007;120(3):654–8.
15. Glueck CJ, Freiberg R, Glueck HI, et al. Idiopathic osteonecrosis, hypofibrinolysis, high plasminogen activator inhibitor, high lipoprotein (a), and therapy with Stanozolol. Am J Hematol. 1995;48(4):213–20.
16. Chesnut CH, Ivey JL, Gruber HE, et al. Stanozolol in postmenopausal osteoporosis: therapeutic efficacy and possible mechanisms of action. Metabolism. 1983;32(6):571–80.
17. El-Ganzuri MA, Ahmed RR, Bastawy EM. Osteoporosis and its treatments. Int. J Adv Res. 2015;3(9):303–18.
18. Helfman T, Falanga V. Stanozolol as a novel therapeutic agent in dermatology. J Am Acad Dermatol. 1995;33(2):254–8.
19. Spadari A, Rinnovati R, Babbini S, Romagnoli N. Clinical evaluation of intra-articular administration of stanozolol to manage lameness associated with acute and chronic osteoarthritis in horses. J Equine Vet Sci. 2015;35(2):105–10.
20. Rinnovati R, Romagnoli N, Spadari A. Dose-finding study for intraarticular treatment with Stanozolol in horses. J Equine Vet Sci. 2015;35(10):860–4.
21. Ramzan P, Somerville G, Shepherd M, et al. Preliminary clinical impressions on the use of stanozolol as a novel intra-articular therapy for athletic horses: 60 cases (abstract). In: Abstracts European veterinary conference Voorjaarsdagen; 2012. file:///C:/Users/mcm/Downloads/CH08-Ramzan-PreliminaryClinical%20(1).pdf. Accessed 4 Apr 2012.
22. Bladon B. Managing subchondral bone pain in thoroughbreds. Birmingham: Beva Congress Proceedings; 2012. p. 170.
23. Spadari A, Romagnoli N, Predieri PG, et al. Effects of intraarticular treatment with stanozolol on synovial membrane and cartilage in an ovine model of osteoarthritis. Res Vet Sci. 2013;94(3):379–87.
24. Saleri R, Dondi M, Bianchi E, et al. Stanozolol inhibits nitric oxide production by horse chondrocyte cell cultures (abstract). Abstracts from the workshop: Frontiers of skeletal biology. Bone. 2004;34:S38–9.
25. Falanga V, Greenberg AS, Zhou L, et al. Stimulation of collagen synthesis by the anabolic steroid stanozolol. J Invest Dermatol. 1998;111(6):1193 7.
26. Shun-ye ZH, Hua-mei MA, Yan-hong LI, et al. Effects of Stanozolol on proliferation and differentiation of cultured growth plate chondrocytes from pubertal female rat treated with GnRHa in vitro. J Sun Yat-Sen Univ (Med Sci). 2009;4:018.
27. Tew SR, Murdoch AD, Rauchenberg RP, Hardingham TE. Cellular methods in cartilage research: primary human chondrocytes in culture and chondrogenesis in human bone marrow stem cells. Methods. 2008;45(1):2–9.
28. Strober W. Trypan blue exclusion test of cell viability. Curr Protoc Immunol. 2001; Appendix 3B. http://dx.doi.org/10.1002/0471142735.ima03bs21
29. Ekman L, Nilsson G, Persson L, Lumsdan JH. Volume of the synovia in certain joint cavities in the horse. Acta Vet Scand (Denmark). 1981;22:23–31.
30. Chomczynski P, Sacchi N. The single-step method of RNA isolation by acid guanidinium thiocyanate–phenol–chloroform extraction: twenty-something years on. Nature. 2006;1(2):581–5.
31. Livak KJ, Schmittgen TD. Analysis of relative gene expression data using real-time quantitative PCR and the 2– ΔΔCT method. Methods. 2001;25(4):402–8.
32. Peffers MJ, Milner PI, Tew SR, Clegg PD. Regulation of SOX9 in normal and osteoarthritic equine articular chondrocytes by hyperosmotic loading. Osteoarthr Cartil. 2010;18(11):1502–8.
33. Tew SR, Peffers MJ, McKay TR, Lowe ET, Khan WS, Hardingham TE, Clegg PD. Hyperosmolarity regulates SOX9 mRNA posttranscriptionally in human articular chondrocytes. Am J Physiol Cell Physiol. 2009;297(4):C898–906.
34. Peffers MJ, Liu X, Clegg PD. Transcriptomic signatures in cartilage ageing. Arthritis Res Ther. 2013;15(4):R98.
35. Richardson DW, Dodge GR. Effects of interleukin-1β and tumor necrosis factor-α on expression of matrix-related genes by cultured equine articular chondrocytes. Am J Vet Res. 2000;61(6):624–30.
36. Tung JT, Fenton JI, Arnold C, et al. Recombinant equine interleukin-1ß induces putative mediators of articular cartilage degradation in equine chondrocytes. Can J Vet Res. 2002;66:19–25.
37. Ross TN, Kisiday JD, Hess T, McIlwraith CW. Evaluation of the inflammatory response in experimentally induced synovitis in the horse: a comparison of recombinant equine interleukin 1 beta and lipopolysaccharide. Osteoarthr Cartil. 2012;20(12):1583–90.
38. Richardson DW, Dodge GR. Dose-dependent effects of corticosteroids on the expression of matrix-related genes in normal and cytokine-treated articular chondrocytes. Inflamm Res. 2003;52(1):39–49.
39. Busschers E, Holt JP, Richardson DW. Effects of glucocorticoids and interleukin-1β on expression and activity of aggrecanases in equine chondrocytes. Am J Vet Res. 2010;71(2):176–85.
40. Caron JP, Gandy JC, Schmidt M, et al. Influence of corticosteroids on interleukin-1β-stimulated equine chondrocyte gene expression. Vet Surg. 2013;42(3):231–7.
41. Schaefer EC, Stewart AA, Durgam SS, et al. Effects of sodium hyaluronate and triamcinolone acetonide on glucosaminoglycan metabolism in equine articular chondrocytes treated with interleukin-1. Am J Vet Res. 2009;70(12):1494–501.
42. Yates AC, Stewart AA, Byron CR, et al. Effects of sodium hyaluronate and methylprednisolone acetate on proteoglycan metabolism in equine articular chondrocytes treated with interleukin-1. Am J Vet Res. 2006;67(12):1980–6.
43. Knych HK, Vidal MA, Chouicha N, et al. Cytokine, catabolic enzyme and structural matrix gene expression in synovial fluid following intraarticular administration of triamcinolone acetonide in exercised horses. Equine Vet J. 2017;49(1):107–15.
44. Ng LJ, Wheatley S, Muscat GE, et al. SOX9 binds DNA, activates transcription, and coexpresses with type II collagen during chondrogenesis in the mouse. Dev Biol. 1997;183(1):108–21.
45. Bell DM, Leung KK, Wheatley SC, et al. SOX9 directly regulates the type 2 collagen gene. Nat Genet. 1997;16(2):174–8.
46. Bi W, Deng JM, Zhang Z, Behringer RR, de Crombrugghe B. Sox9 is required for cartilage formation. Nat Genet. 1999;22(1):85–9.
47. Aigner T, Gebhard PM, Schmid E, et al. SOX9 expression does not correlate with type II collagen expression in adult articular chondrocytes. Matrix Biol. 2003;22(4):363–72.
48. Basaria S, Wahlstrom JT, Dobs AS. Anabolic-androgenic steroid therapy in the treatment of chronic diseases. J Clin Endocrinol Metab. 2001;86(11): 5108–17.

13

The refractive state of the eye in Icelandic horses with the *Silver* mutation

Maria K. Johansson[1*], Kim Jäderkvist Fegraeus[1], Gabriella Lindgren[1†] and Björn Ekesten[2†]

Abstract

Background: The syndrome Multiple Congenital Ocular Anomalies (MCOA) is a congenital eye disorder in horses. Both the MCOA syndrome and the Silver coat colour in horses are caused by the same missense mutation in the *premelanosome protein* (*PMEL)* gene. Horses homozygous for the *Silver* mutation (TT) are affected by multiple ocular defects causing visual impairment or blindness. Horses heterozygous for the *Silver* mutation (CT) have less severe clinical signs, usually cysts arising from the ciliary body iris or retina temporally. It is still unknown if the vision is impaired in horses heterozygous for the *Silver* mutation. A recent study reported that Comtois horses carrying the *Silver* mutation had significantly deeper anterior chambers of the eye compared to wild-type horses. This could potentially cause refractive errors. The purpose of the present study was to investigate if Icelandic horses with the *Silver* mutation have refractive errors compared to wild-type horses. One hundred and fifty-two Icelandic horses were included in the study, 71 CT horses and five TT horses. All horses were genotyped for the missense mutation in *PMEL*. Each CT and TT horse was matched by a wild-type (CC) horse of the same age ± 1 year. Skiascopy and a brief ophthalmic examination were performed in all horses. Association between refraction and age, eye, genotype and sex was tested by linear mixed-effect model analysis. TT horses with controls were not included in the statistical analyses as they were too few.

Results: The interaction between age and genotype had a significant impact on the refractive state ($P = 0.0001$). CT horses older than 16 years were on average more myopic than wild-type horses of the same age. No difference in the refractive state could be observed between genotypes (CT and CC) in horses younger than 16 years. TT horses were myopic (−2 D or more) in one or both eyes regardless of age.

Conclusion: Our results indicate that an elderly Icelandic horse (older than 16 years) carrying the *Silver* mutation is more likely to be myopic than a wild-type horse of the same age.

Keywords: Multiple Congenital Ocular Anomalies, MCOA, Refraction, Myopia, Skiascopy, Horse -Icelandic horses

Background

The syndrome Multiple Congenital Ocular Anomalies (MCOA) is a congenital eye disorder in horses. It was first described in Rocky Mountain Horses in 1999 [1]. Previous studies have shown that both the Silver coat colour and the MCOA syndrome in horses are caused by the same missense mutation in the *premelanosome protein* (*PMEL)* gene [2, 3]. The mutation, a change from cytosine (C) to thymine (T), causes a dilution of the eumelanin pigment especially in the mane and tail [2].

* Correspondence: mariakjoh@hotmail.com
[†]Equal contributors
[1]Department of Animal Breeding and Genetics, Swedish University of Agricultural Sciences, -750 07 Uppsala, SE, Sweden
Full list of author information is available at the end of the article

PMEL encodes the transmembrane glycoprotein PMEL also known as PMEL17, which is essential for the biogenesis of eumelanin in the melanosomes. PMEL forms fibrillary structures where melanin is deposited during melanogenesis [4, 5]. Post translational and proteolytic processing of PMEL are required for a correct formation of the fibrillar matrix. It is not clear how these processes are regulated [6, 7]. In a study from 2011 a knock-out mouse line where *PMEL* had been inactivated was created [8]. It was shown that PMEL was important for eumelanin production in skin, choroid and retinal pigment epithelium. However, full-field electroretinogram did not show any impaired function of the retina [8].

Clinically, Silver coloured horses can be subdivided into two different groups, the Cyst phenotype and the

MCOA phenotype, according to the severity of the ocular defects. Horses with the Cyst phenotype are known to be heterozygous for the *Silver* mutation (CT). They have less severe ocular signs predominantly iridociliary cysts, usually in the temporal quadrant of the eye. The cysts are translucent and can be up to a centimetre in size. Horses with the MCOA phenotype are known to be homozygous for the *Silver* mutation (TT). They have more severe clinical signs including iridal stromal hypoplasia, miotic pupils, retinal dysplasia, cataract, cornea globosa and iridociliary cysts occasionally extending subretinally [1, 9–11]. An incomplete dominant mode of inheritance has been suggested [10, 12, 13].

The ocular defects that are present in horses homozygous for the *Silver* mutation cause visual impairment or blindness [1, 9–11]. It is still unknown if vision is impaired in horses heterozygous for the *Silver* mutation. Hence, more information is needed to investigate how the MCOA syndrome affects the vision in horses heterozygous for the *Silver* mutation. A recent study in Comtois and Rocky Mountain horses reported that horses with the *Silver* mutation, both heterozygotes and homozygotes, had deeper anterior chambers of the eye compared to wild-type horses. A significant difference in the depth of the chamber was also detected between heterozygous and homozygous horses [11]. An abnormal distance between the refractive surfaces of the eye is likely to cause refractive errors. The purpose of the present study was to investigate if Icelandic horses with the *Silver* mutation have refractive errors compared to wild-type horses of the same breed.

Methods

Animals

In total 152 Icelandic horses were included in the study, 71 were heterozygous and five homozygous for the *Silver* mutation. Each CT and TT horse was matched by a control (wild-type) horse of the same breed and age ± 1 year. Control horses were confirmed being wild-type (CC) for both disease-alleles. In the CT group was the median age of both CT and controls 10.3 years, ranging from 1 to 27 years in CT and from 1 to 28 years in control horses (Figs. 1 and 2). The median age of the TT horses was 11.4 years and 11.8 years in their age-matched controls with a range from 1 to 22 years in both TT and control horses. The sex distribution in the CT horse group was 33 males and 38 females in CT horses and 24 males and 47 females in controls. In the TT group one male and four females were compared to four males and one female controls. All horses in the study were enrolled after posting information on social media and by contacting horse farms near Uppsala, Sweden.

Phenotypic assessment

Phenotypic data on all horses in the study were obtained from a brief ophthalmic examination and skiascopy without dilation of the pupil. The ophthalmic examination was performed in the stable under dim-light conditions. The examination included testing of direct and indirect pupillary light reflexes, dazzle reflex and menace response to crudely assess the function of the retina and the optic nerve. Palpebral and corneal reflexes were tested to control the function of the sensory innervation

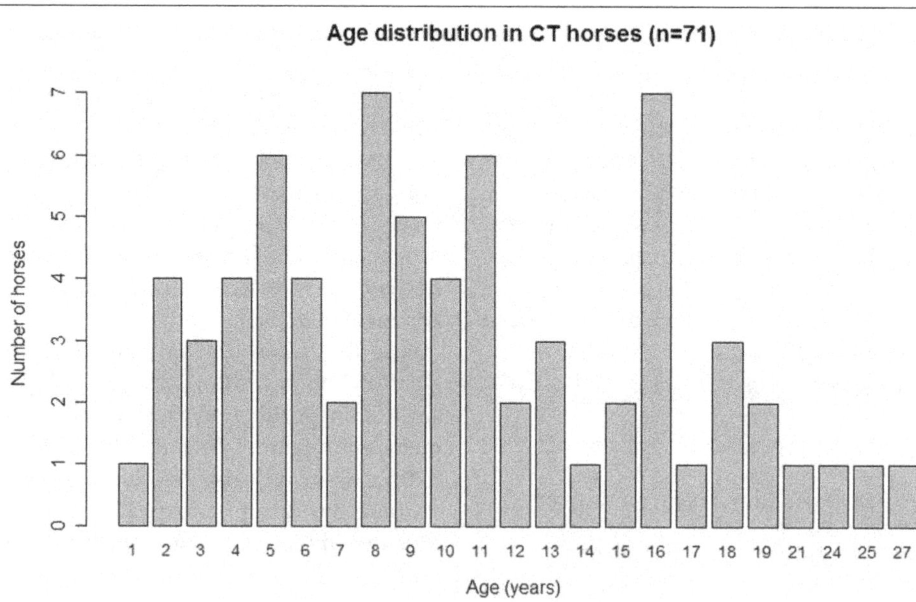

Fig. 1 The age distribution of CT horses (n = 71)

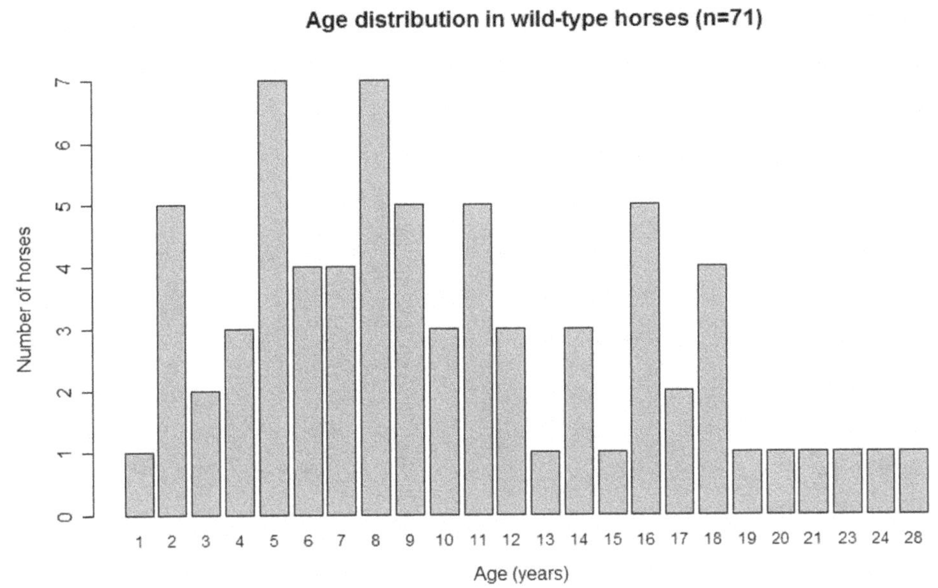

Fig. 2 The age distribution in controls (wild-type) horses (n = 71)

of the eye. The reflexes were all graded as normal, decreased or absent. If the reflex was decreased it was described as being either slow or incomplete. All eyes were scanned for opacities in the ocular media visible to the examiner's naked eye with the retinoscope as a light source. Opacities, if present, were graded based on extension and location. The cornea was observed to find signs of obvious cornea globosa. Iridociliary cysts or other anomalies were also noted. The exam record used in this study can be found in Additional file 1.

Skiascopy was performed with a streak retinoscope (Heine Beta 200) and Trousseau racks without dilation of the pupils. Lenses in steps of 0.5 D were used to reach the neutralization point and the working distance was subtracted. The refractive power was measured both horizontally and vertically in both eyes. Astigmatism was defined as a difference of more than 0.5 D between the horizontal and vertical meridians.

DNA isolation and genotyping

Genomic DNA was isolated from hair samples by the standard hair-preparation method as previously described [14]. All horses in the study were genotyped for the missense mutation in *PMEL* previously shown to be associated with both the Silver coat colour and the MCOA syndrome [2, 3]. The genotyping was performed by using custom designed TaqMan SNP Genotyping Assays (Applied Biosystems StepOnePlus™ Instrument by Life Technologies) for SNP g.73665304 on chromosome 6 [3]. Horses were classified according to the genotype into three groups; wild-type (CC), heterozygous (CT) and homozygous (TT) for the *PMEL* missense mutation.

Statistical analysis

All statistical analyses were performed in the software environment R-3.1.2 (R Development Core Team, 2014) and significance was defined as $P \leq 0.05$. TT horses were not included in the statistical analyses because of very small sample size.

Association between refraction and age, eye, genotype and sex was tested by linear mixed-effect model analysis with the function lmer and the packages lme4 and car. There were two observations per horse, one for each eye (right and left) and the model used in lme4 was:

lmer(refraction ~ (age + eye + genotype + sex)^2 + (1| horse), data = data.

The fixed factors in the model; age (age of the horse at the examination in years), eye (right or left), genotype (CT or CC) and sex (male or female) were defined as factor variables. Pairwise interactions between each fixed factor were included in the model. The identity of the horse was used as a random factor. The dependent variable refraction (the horizontal refractive value determined by skiascopy) was defined as a continuous numeric variable. A Wald chi-square test was used in the post hoc test with Anova type 3 to estimate P-values. Differences in refraction related to genotype and age were further tested in a post hoc test with the function least-square means (lsmeans). Horses were divided into two-year age-classes and pairwise comparisons were calculated.

Table 1 The refractive state of all 152 horses for right and left eye respectively

Right eye	Number of CT horses	Number of TT horses[a]	Number of CC horses
Emmetropic (normal sighted) 0 D	37 (52.1%)	0 (0%)	32 (42.1%)
Hyperopic (farsighted)			
Slightly (+0,5–1 D)	24 (33.8%)	0 (0%)	41 (53.9%)
Moderate (+1,5–2,5 D)	0 (0%)	0 (0%)	0 (0%)
Severe > +3 D	0 (0%)	0 (0%)	0 (0%)
Myopic (nearsighted)			
Slightly (−0,5–1 D)	3 (4.2%)	0 (0%)	3 (3.9%)
Moderate (−1,5–2,5 D)	5 (7.0%)	3 (75%)	0 (0%)
Severe (−3 D or more)	2 (2.8%)	1 (25%)	0 (0%)
Left eye	Number of CT horses	Number of TT horses[a]	Number of CC horses
Emmetropic (normal sighted) 0 D	37 (52.1%)	1 (25%)	29 (38.2%)
Hyperopic (farsighted)			
Slightly (+0,5–1 D)	25 (35.2%)	0 (0%)	44 (57.9%)
Moderate (+1,5–2,5 D)	0 (0%)	0 (0%)	0 (0%)
Severe > +3 D	0 (0%)	0 (0%)	0 (0%)
Myopic (nearsighted)			
Slightly (−0,5–1 D)	3 (4.2%)	0 (0%)	3 (3.9%)
Moderate (−1,5–2,5 D)	5 (7.0%)	3 (75%)	0 (0%)
Severe (−3 D or more)	1 (1.4%)	0 (0%)	0 (0%)

[a]Notice that sciascopy could not be performed in one of the TT horses because of miotic pupils and dense cataract on both eyes

Results

Heterozygous (CT) horses

The mean refractive value ± SE was −0.09 ± 0.10 D for the right eye and 0.0 ± 0.09 D for the left eye in CT horses compared to 0.26 ± 0.04 D for right and 0.28 ± 0.04D for left eye in wild-type horses. The refractive state of the majority of both CT and wild-type horses was close to 0 D, although the average wild-type Icelandic horse was slightly hyperopic (farsighted) (Table 1). None of the horses were astigmatic according to the definition used in the study. Two CT horses, 18 and 21 years old, had severe refractive errors (−3 D or more) in one or both eyes (Fig. 3). The interaction between age and genotype had a significant impact on the refractive state (P = 0.0001). No other interactions tested were statistically significant. The refractive state was significantly different between genotypes (CT and CC) in ages 16–21 years. CT horses older than 16 years were on average more myopic compared to CC horses of

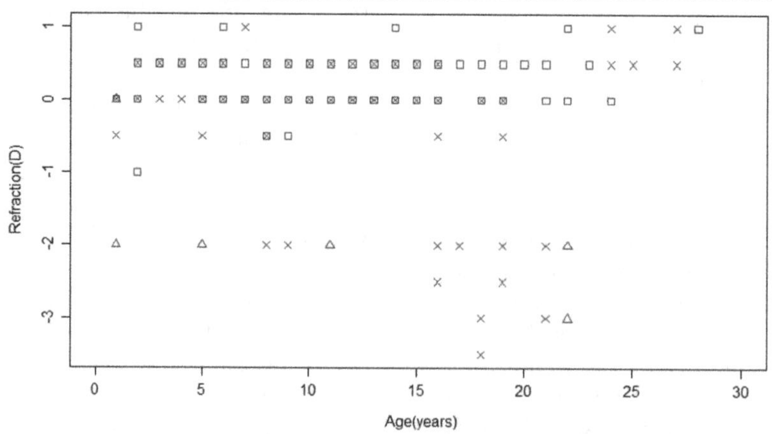

Fig. 3 The refraction values according to age in all 152 Icelandic horses. *Blue* squares indicate wild-type horses, *red crosses* CT horses and *red* triangles TT horses. (Notice that some horses of the same age have the same refraction value and therefore some data points are superimposed on each other). Refraction values for both right and left eye are presented for each of the 152 horses

the same age. The P value was 0.003 for age group 16–17 years, 0.0001 for age group 18–19 years and <0.0001 for age group 20–21 years. Horses 22 years and older could not be analysed because they were too few.

Only one CT horse in the study had an immature cataract visible to the naked eye. It affected about 25% of the area of the lens in the coronal plane in the right eye. This horse was also myopic (−3 D in the right eye and −2 D in the left eye). Eight CT horses had mild cornea globosa and two CT horses had moderate cornea globosa in one or both eyes. A 25 year old CT horse had moderately miotic pupils and the pupillary reflexes were abnormal in both eyes. All CT horses in the study, except the horse with miotic pupils, had normal reflexes. Twenty-three CT horses of different ages had temporal cysts in one or both eyes that were visible to the naked eye. The cysts ranged in diameter up to a centimetre. No correlation between age and presence of cysts was observed.

Homozygous (TT) horses

The mean refractive value ± SE was −2.25 ± 0.22 D for the right eye and −1.50 ± 0.43 D for the left eye in TT horses compared to 0.40 ± 0.17 D for right and 0.20 ± 0.11 D for left eye in wild-type horses. One 18 years old TT horse had dense cataract, severely miotic pupils and absent pupillary light reflexes in both eyes. Skiascopy could not be performed in this horse. All the other TT horses in the study had mild to moderate cornea globosa and moderately miotic pupils with a decreased and incomplete pupillary light reflexes in both eyes. All four TT horses were myopic (−2 D or more) in one or both eyes (Table 1). The presence of cysts and minor, peripheral cataracts was difficult to assess in the TT horses because of their miotic pupils.

Discussion

This study was performed to provide additional insight into how the MCOA syndrome affects the vision in horses heterozygous for the *Silver* mutation. Our results indicate that horses older than 16 years carrying the *Silver* mutation are more likely to be myopic than wild-type horses of the same age. In the present study CT horses older than 16 years on average were more myopic than wild-type horses of the same age. No difference in the refractive state could be observed between genotypes (CT and CC) in horses younger than 16 years.

A myopic shift in elderly individuals has also been observed in human beings and dogs [15–17]. Although humans experience a hyperopic shift with age as they develop presbyopia, a long-term study has shown that this trend reverses in the direction of myopia in the oldest group (70 years and older) [15]. To our knowledge, there are few studies on how the refractive state changes with age in horses. A degree project at the Swedish University of Agricultural Sciences by Löf from 2007, where 116 Standardbred trotters were included in a cross-sectional study, showed that elderly horses had a progression towards myopia. In the current study we observed a significant difference in the refractive state between CT and CC horses in ages 16–21 years. Horses older than 21 years could not be further analysed because of small sample size. Seven of the CT horses had moderate or severe myopia (−1.5 D or more) and five of these were 16 years or older. These horses were not closely related and they came from different stables.

The observed shift towards myopia in elderly CT horses may also suggest that the *Silver* mutation exerts a slowly progressive effect on the optics of the eye. However, one important limitation is that this was a cross-sectional study and we did not have the possibility to follow these horses from when they were foals up to old age. The MCOA syndrome is generally thought to be non-progressive [1], although there are indications that at least some clinical signs may progress [11]. The study by Ségard et al. from 2013, where 59 Comtois and 16 Rocky Mountain horses ranging from 10 days to 18 years of age were included, reported no differences in presence of ocular abnormalities between young, adult and old horses for the majority of the defects detected [11]. However, a possible increase in the number of cystic lesions with age was suggested. Foals with the *Silver* mutation, both homozygotes and heterozygotes, had significantly fewer cysts compared to adult and old horses of the same genotype [11]. The study by Plummer and Ramsey from 2011 [18], where 53 American Miniature horses were included, showed no correlation between age and presence of ocular abnormalities. The median age of the horses in that study was 5.3 years with a range from 1.5 to 219 months (18.25 years). Hence, the median age of the horses was lower in the previous studies [11, 18] compared to our study. In our study, 23 (32%) of the CT horses of different ages had visible cysts in one or both eyes. No correlation between age and presence of cysts or other ocular abnormalities could be observed. Cysts were hard to detect in TT horses because of miotic pupils. Most likely both CT and TT horses had cysts that could not be detected because we neither dilated the pupil, nor used more sensitive methods such as ultrasonography to evaluate the presence of cysts. However, that was beyond the scope of this study.

We found no difference in the refractive state between genotypes (CT and CC) in horses younger than 16 years. One possible reason could be that the refractive errors were minimized by other, compensatory mechanisms. Therefore it would have been interesting to measure other parameters, including anterior chamber depth and axial length that could shed light on the underlying causes of the refractive results of the horses in our study. Unfortunately, the ophthalmic examinations were performed in stables and no equipment for precise measuring of additional ocular biometric parameters was available.

Only five TT horses were included in our study. These horses were difficult to find, probably because of a low frequency of the TT genotype, as horse owners are recommended not to mate two Silver coloured horses. TT horses had more severe ocular signs than CT horses, which is in accordance with previous studies [1, 9–11]. These horses also represented a special challenge to refract because of their miotic pupils. Skiascopy could not be performed in one of the TT horses because of cataractous lenses in combination with very miotic pupils, two clinical signs already described as being part of the MCOA phenotype [1, 9–11]. TT horses were myopic (−2 D or more) in one or both eyes regardless of age. Only one CT horse in the study had an immature cataract visible to the naked eye. This horse was also myopic (−3 D in the right eye and −2 D in the left eye). Some individuals, both CT and TT, seem to have more severe clinical signs of the MCOA syndrome. Hence, additional genetic factors may be involved. None of the wild-type horses in the study were myopic (−1.5 D or more). The Icelandic horse as a breed seems to be slightly hyperopic on average. This is in accordance with the results from a degree project at the Swedish University of Agricultural Sciences by Östberg in 2007, where 26 Icelandic horses with a median age of 11.5 years were included.

Eye (left or right) did not have a significant impact on the refractive state. This was as expected since the MCOA syndrome is reported to affect the eyes bilaterally [1]. The previous study by Ségard et al. from 2013 reported no significant difference in depth of the anterior chamber between right and left eye [11]. Sex was also not found to affect the refractive state in the present study. This was in accordance with previous studies [19, 20].

The horses in the present study were examined without dilation of the pupils. Previous studies have shown that cycloplegia has no impact on streak retinoscopic evaluation of refraction [19, 21]. Two degree projects at the Swedish University of Agricultural Sciences from 2007 by Östberg and Löf also showed that cycloplegia is not needed before retinoscopy in horses older than 9 months.

We considered the horizontal refractive values most convenient to obtain because of the ellipsoid shape of the pupil in horses and therefore most accurate to assess. Hence, only the horizontal values were used in the statistical analyses. However, the differences between the horizontal and vertical values were less than 0.5 D in all horses and therefore none of the horses were considered to be astigmatic.

One of the major strengths of our study is that we have a large dataset that represents a wide range of ages in a homogenous population with only one breed. Each CT and TT horse was well matched by a wild-type horse of the same breed and age ± 1 year.

This study provides valuable information about the refractive state in Icelandic horses with the *Silver* mutation which can be used in future breeding recommendations. Horse owners should be aware that Silver colored horses older than about 16 years may have an increased risk to become myopic compared with wild-type horses.

Conclusion

Our results indicate that horses older than 16 years carrying the *Silver* mutation are more likely to be myopic than wild-type horses of the same age.

Abbreviations

MCOA: Multiple Congenital Ocular Anomalies; PMEL: Premelanosome protein; SE: Standard error; SNP: Single nucleotide polymorphism

Acknowledgements

The authors would like to thank all horse owners who have contributed with valuable information and allowing us to examine their horses. We are grateful to Ulf Olsson and Mikael Andersson Franko for valuable advice regarding the statistical analyses. We would also like to thank Lisa S Andersson and Brandon D Velie for all valuable advices.

Funding

Financial support was obtained from The Swedish Research Council (VR), The Swedish Research Council for Environment, Agricultural Sciences and Spatial Planning (FORMAS) and the Swedish-Norwegian Foundation for Equine Research.

Authors' contributions

BE and GL planned and advised the study. MJ examined and genotyped the horses and drafted the manuscript. KJF helped to advise the study. All authors read and approved the final manuscript.

Competing interests

The authors declare that they have no competing interests.

Consent for publication

Not applicable.

Author details

[1]Department of Animal Breeding and Genetics, Swedish University of Agricultural Sciences, -750 07 Uppsala, SE, Sweden. [2]Department of Clinical Sciences, Swedish University of Agricultural Sciences, -750 07 Uppsala, SE, Sweden.

References

1. Ramsey DT, Ewart SL, Render JA, Cook CS, Latimer CA. Congenital ocular abnormalities of Rocky Mountain Horses. Vet Ophthalmol. 1999;2:47–59.
2. Brunberg E, Andersson L, Cothran G, Sandberg K, Mikko S, Lindgren G. A missense mutation in PMEL17 is associated with the Silver coat color in the horse. BMC Genet. 2006;7:46.
3. Andersson LS, Wilbe M, Viluma A, Cothran G, Ekesten B, Ewart S, Lindgren G. Equine Multiple Congenital Ocular Anomalies and Silver Coat Colour Result from the Pleiotropic Effects of Mutant *PMEL*. PLoS One 2013; doi: 10.1371/journal.pone.0075639.

4. Berson JF, Harper D, Tenza D, Raposo G, Marks MS. Pmel17 initiates premelanosome morphogenesis within multivesicular bodies. Mol Biol Cell. 2001;12(11):3451–64.
5. Raposo G, Tenza D, Murphy DM, Berson JF, Marks MS. Distinct protein sorting and localization to premelanosomes, melanosomes, and lysosomes in pigmented melanocytic cells. J Cell Biol. 2001;152(4):809–24.
6. Rochin L, Hurbain I, Serneels L, Fort C, Watt B, Leblanc P, Marks MS, De Strooper B, Raposo G, van Niel G. BACE2 processes PMEL to form the melanosome amyloid matrix in pigment cells. Proc Natl Acad Sci U S A. 2013;110(26):10658–63.
7. Kawaguchi M, Hozumi Y, Suzuki T. ADAM protease inhibitors reduce melanogenesis by regulating PMEL17 processing in human melanocytes. J Dermatol Sci. 2015;78(2):133–42.
8. Hellström AR, Watt B, Fard SS, Tenza D, Mannström P, Narfström K, Ekesten B, Ito S, Wakamatsu K, Larsson J, Ulfendahl M, Kullander K, Raposo G, Kerje S, Hallböök F, Marks MS, Andersson L. Inactivation of *Pmel* Alters Melanosome Shape But Has Only a Subtle Effect on Visible Pigmentation. PLoS Genet 2011; doi: 10.1371/journal.pgen.1002285.
9. Andersson LS, Axelsson J, Dubielzig RR, Lindgren G, Ekesten B. Multiple congenital ocular anomalies in Icelandic horses. BMC Vet Res. 2011;7:21.
10. Komáromy AM, Rowlan JS, La Croix NC, Mangan BG. Equine Multiple Congenital Ocular Anomalies (MCOA) syndrome in *PMEL17* (*Silver*) mutant ponies: five cases. Vet Ophthalmol. 2011;14(5):313–20.
11. Ségard EM, Depecker MC, Lang J, Gemperli A, Cadoré J-L. Ultrasonographic features of *PMEL17* (*Silver*) mutant gene-associated multiple congenital ocular anomalies (MCOA) in Comtois and Rocky Mountain horses. Vet Ophthalmol. 2013;16(6):429–35.
12. Andersson LS, Juras R, Ramsey DT, Eason-Butler J, Ewart S, Cothran G, Lindgren G. Equine Multiple Congenital Ocular Anomalies maps to a 4.9 megabase interval on horse chomosome 6. BMC Genet. 2008;9:88.
13. Grahn BH, Pinard C, Archer S, Bellone R, Forsyth G, Sandmeyer LS. Congenital ocular anomalies in purebred and crossbred Rocky and Kentucky Mountain horses in Canada. Can Vet J. 2008;49:675–81.
14. Jäderkvist K, Andersson LS, Johansson AM, Árnason T, Mikko S, Eriksson S, Andersson L, Lindgren G. The DMRT3 'Gait keeper' mutation affects performance of Nordic and Standardbred trotters. J Anim Sci. 2014;92(10):4279–86.
15. Lee KE, Klein BE, Klein R, Wong TY. Changes in refraction over 10 years in an adult population: the Beaver Dam Eye Study. Invest Opthalmol Vis Sci. 2002;43(8):2566–71.
16. Murphy CJ, Zadnik K, Mannis MJ. Myopia and Refractive Error in Dogs. Invest Ophthalmol Vis Sci. 1992;33(8):2459–63.
17. Kubai MA, Bentley E, Miller PE, Mutti DO, Murphy CJ. Refractive states of eyes and association between ametropia and breed in dogs. Am J Vet Res. 2008;69(7):946–51.
18. Plummer CE, Ramsey DT. A Survey of ocular abnormalities in Miniature Horses. Vet Ophthalmol. 2011;14(4):239–43.
19. Rull-Cotrina J, Molleda JM, Gallardo J, Martín-Suárez E. Refractive state of the Spanish Thoroughbred horse: a comparison with the Crossbred horse. Vet Ophthalmol. 2013;16(1):25–8.
20. Bracun A, Ellis AD, Hall C. A retinoscopic survey of 333 horses and ponies in the UK. Vet Opthalmol. 2014;17(Suppl 1):90–6.
21. McMullen RJ Jr, Davidson MG, Gilger BC. The effect of 1% tropicamide-induced mydriasis and cycloplegia on spherical refraction of the adult horse. Vet Ophthalmol. 2014;17(2):120–5.

14

Molecular characterization of *Rhodococcus equi* isolates from horses in Poland: pVapA characteristics and plasmid new variant, 85-kb type V

Lucjan Witkowski[1*], Magdalena Rzewuska[2], Shinji Takai[3], Dorota Chrobak-Chmiel[2], Magdalena Kizerwetter-Świda[2], Małgorzata Feret[2], Marta Gawryś[2], Maciej Witkowski[4] and Jerzy Kita[1]

Abstract

Background: *Rhodococcus equi* is one of the most significant bacterial pathogens affecting foals up to 6 months of age worldwide. Rhodococcosis is present in Poland however information about molecular characterization of *R. equi* isolates is scarce.

This study describes molecular characterization of *Rhodococcus equi* infection on 13 horse breeding farms in Poland between 2001 and 2012. Samples were collected by tracheobronchial aspiration from pneumonic foals or during necropsy. The *R. equi* isolates were genotyped by plasmid profiling and pulsed-field gel electrophoresis.

Results: Totally, 58 *R. equi* isolates were investigated. One isolate lost its plasmid. Among the 57 VapA-positive isolates, 48 contained 85-kb type I plasmid (82.8%), 8 contained 87-kb type I plasmid (13.8%). One isolate (1.7%) had a unique restriction cleavage pattern and the 2nd fragment of *Eco*RI digests of this plasmid DNA was about 2600 bases smaller than that of the 85 kb type I. This new plasmid variant was designated as the "85-kb type V".

Among the 58 isolates typeable with *Vsp*I-PFGE, ten PFGE clusters were detected. The majority of foals were infected mostly with isolates of low genetic diversity.

Conclusions: Most of clinical isolates of *R. equi* from foals in Poland contain pVapA 85-kb type I and 87-kb type I similarly to the other European countries and the United States. However, the new variant of pVapA 85-kb type V was identified.

The chromosomal variability was detected among some of the investigated isolates and the presence of farm-specific isolates might be possible.

Keywords: Rhodococcosis, Epidemiology, PFGE, Horse, Plasmid profile

Background

Rhodococcus equi is one of the most significant bacterial pathogens affecting foals up to six months of age and occasionally can cause diseases in other animal species including humans [1–6]. Typical manifestation of the infection in foals includes pyogranulomatous bronchopneumonia with abscessation. Epidemiology of the disease is similar worldwide: it occurs endemically on some farms and rarely strikes the others. The prevalence and severity of the disease on endemic farms may vary among seasons [1–5]. *R. equi* infection in foals has been recognized and described in Poland [7–9], but without any information about molecular characterization of *R. equi* isolates. Recently, prevalence of *R. equi* in horse carcasses intended for human consumption was investigated in Poland. Single *R. equi* strain carried 85-kb type I plasmid was isolated from 0.5% (1/198) samples of healthy middle tracheo-branchiales lymph nodes while no lymphocentrum retropharyngeum sample was positive (0/198) [10].

* Correspondence: lucjan_witkowski@sggw.pl
[1]Laboratory of Veterinary Epidemiology and Economics, Faculty of Veterinary Medicine, Warsaw University of Life Sciences, Nowoursynowska 159c, 02-776 Warsaw, Poland
Full list of author information is available at the end of the article

The virulence of *R. equi* is determined by genes *vaps* located on virulence-associated plasmids (VAPs). Isolates carrying the *vapA* gene encoding virulence-associated 15–17-kDa protein (VapA) are known as virulent and are capable of causing disease in foals [11, 12]. To date analysis of the restriction enzyme digestion patterns revealed 12 distinct VAPA types and some of them have geographical specificity [13–24].

Epidemiological studies on genetic relations among *R. equi* isolates are usually based on genotyping by the pulsed-field gel electrophoresis (PFGE) method. Some of the studies report that horses from individual regions or farms seem to harbor isolates with low genetic diversity [13, 23, 25]. On the other side, the great diversity in the genotypes of isolates within and among farms or among countries also has been shown [26]. Furthermore, one foal can be infected with various *R. equi* isolates that vary in plasmid type and genotype [17, 27].

The aim of this study was to characterize types of virulence plasmids in isolates originating from Polish farms and to determine the genetic diversity of the isolates.

Results

Totally 58 isolates from 13 horse farms were investigated. The isolate ID (code of the horse farm) and year of isolation are presented in Fig. 1. The *vapA* gene specific for *R. equi* which is virulent for horses was detected in all 58 isolates. However, the virulent VapA-positive isolate 635/05 lost its plasmid during subculturing. Thus, PFGE was performed on 58 whereas plasmid profiling on 57 isolates.

Among 57 VapA-positive isolates, 48 (82.8%) contained 85-kb type I plasmid, 8 (13.8%) contained 87-kb type I plasmid (Table 1). One isolate (1.7%) had a unique restriction cleavage pattern and the 2nd fragment of *Eco*RI digests of this plasmid DNA was about 2600 bases smaller than that of the 85 kb type I (Fig. 2). This new plasmid variant was designated as the "85-kb type V".

All 58 VapA-positive isolates were typeable with *Vsp*I-PFGE, resulting in the detection of ten PFGE clusters (from A to J) (Fig. 1). The major cluster (A) was shared by 29 isolates from 8 horse farms. Cluster B was shared by 13 isolates from 3 farms, cluster C by 6 isolates from 2 farms. Four isolates from 2 farms belonged to cluster D and 2 isolates from one farm belonged to cluster E. The remaining 4 isolates exhibited various pulsed-field patterns. The most of investigated isolates belonged to three main clusters (A. B and C). Part of them were indistinguishable and had the same PFGE pattern despite the fact that they were isolated on various horse farms in various years. PFGE patterns of the isolates were compared with virulence plasmid types and no concordance was observed. Some of the isolates carried pVapA 85-kb type I, 87-kb type I, new variant 85-kb type V, as well as the one had lost the plasmid had the same PFGE pattern.

Discussion

The prevalence of plasmid 85-kb type I and 87-kb type I in Poland is similar to other studies from Europe [13–15] as well as the USA [16], while in the South America 87-kb type I is most often isolated than 85-kb type I [19, 28]. New type of plasmid 85-kb type V might be a local type similar for example to 85-kb type IV in Texas [16] (Table 1).

We were not able to investigate plasmid type in one case because of the plasmid loss [11, 14, 29]. The guidelines for molecular epidemiologic investigation using PFGE assay indicate that the isolate characterization should only be applied to small sets of isolates related to potential outbreaks [30]. In this study, investigated isolates met these criteria as the breeding horse population in Poland is relatively small and mostly concentrated on several breeding farms and most of the isolates used in this study were collected in several years during *R. equi* outbreaks.

The study has several limitations. Firstly, it was a descriptive study: we used the isolates obtained from collaborators as diagnostic material (no random sampling). Secondly, samples were obtained from all of the suspected horses only from a few farms and only during one or a few seasons (farms AA and AB). That's the reason why the isolates from those farms are overrepresented in the analysis. Most of the isolates from the other farms were isolated from individual samples delivered to the laboratory. No data concerning the number of suspected or affected foals on a farm were available. In conclusion, collected isolates and data were not sufficient for the proper statistical analysis and obtained results are only descriptive.

Our results are consistent with some previous data [13, 23, 25] where a particular isolate or isolates with low genetic diversity are associated with the individual farms or regions. We identified the isolates typical for certain farms. For example almost all predominant isolates from the farm AA belonged to two main PFGE clusters (A and B) and most of them were indistinguishable. On the other hand, the same isolates occur on more than one farm, for example on the farms AI and AL as well as BB and AL. The high similarity of isolates on mentioned farms may be explained by the exchange of mares between them. Mares shed *R. equi* with feces in which the pathogen may multiply and inhalation of virulent *R. equi* is the major route of infection of foals in the first few days of life [3, 5]. Furthermore, the infected foals shed a large amount of VapA positive *R. equi* and this may explain why several major pulsotypes were

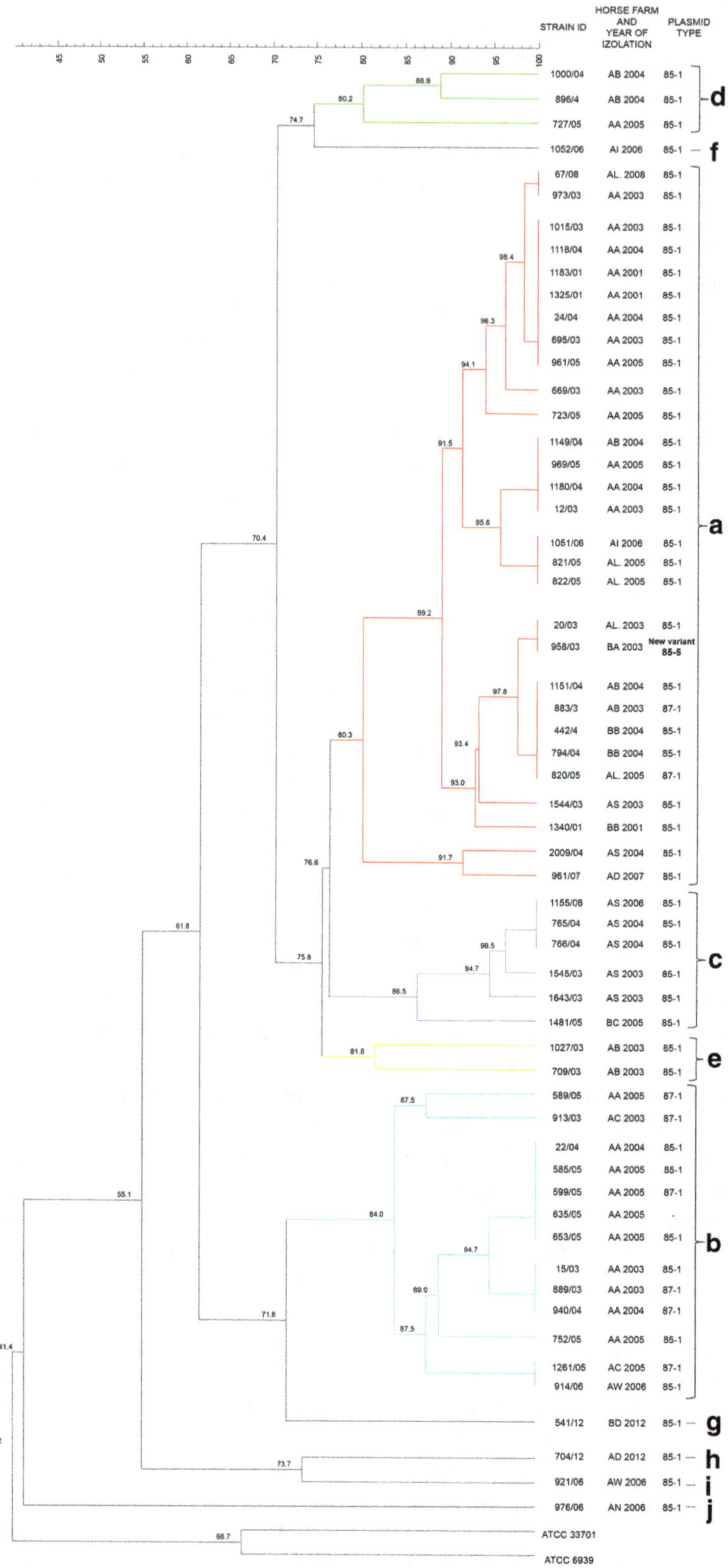

Fig. 1 Dendrogram of 57 virulent and 1 plasmid cured isolates of *R. equi* obtained from foals from Poland genotyped with *Vsp*I-PFGE method. Among the isolates ten PFGE clusters were detected clusters (**a**-**j**)

Table 1 Plasmid profiles of VapA-positive *R. equi*

No.	Plasmid type	Isolation rate (%)	Sample source	Country	Reference
1.	85-kb type I	96.4%	Foal	Germany	[13]
		95.3%	Foal	Hungary	[15]
		82.8%	Foal	Poland	This study
		71.4%	Soil	Hungary	[20]
		69.0%	Foal	France	[14]
		64.5%	Soil	USA	[16]
		54.2%	Soil	Hungary	[15]
		53.1%	Foal	USA	[16]
		41.7%	Soil and feces	France	[14]
		38.5%	Foals	Argentina	[28]
		14.6%	Foal	Brazil	[19]
		14.6%	Foals	Brazil	[19]
		3.6%	Soil	South Africa	[18]
		-	Foals	South Africa	[18]
		100%	Adult horse lymph node	Poland	[10]
2.	85-kb type II	4.9%	Foals	France	[14]
3.	85-kb type III	15,3%	Soil	Hungary	[20]
		8.0%	Soil	USA	[16]
		4.2%	Foals	USA	[16]
4.	85-kb type IV	2.1%	Foals	USA	[16]
		1.1%	Soil	USA	[16]
5.	85-kb type V	1.7%	Foal	Poland	This study
6.	87-kb type I	80.5%	Foals	Brazil	[19]
		80.0%	Foals	Brazil	[19]
		57.7%	Foals	Argentina	[28]
		40.6%	Foals	USA	[16]
		27.8%	Soil and feces	France	[14]
		26.4%	Soil	USA	[16]
		24.6%	Foals	France	[14]
		13.8%	Foal	Poland	This study
		13.3%	Soil	Hungary	[15]
		7.1%	Soil	South Africa	[18]
		4.7%	Foals	Hungary	[15]
		3.6%	Foal	Germany	[13]
7.	87-kb type II	85.2	Foals	Japan	[28]
8.	87-kb type III	4.9%	Foals	Brazil	[19]
9.	90-kb type I	74.5%	Foals and dams	Japan	[22]
10.	90-kb type II	47.1%	Foals, soil and feces	Korea	[23]
		0.8%	Soil and feces	Korea	[24]
11.	90-kb type III	24.7%	Foals and dams feces	Japan	[22]
		-	Foals	Japan	[14]
12.	90-kb type IV	0.9%	Foals and dams feces	Japan	[22]
		-	Foals	Japan	[14]
13.	90-kb type V	52.9%	Foals, soil and feces	Korea	[23]
		1.2%	Soil and feces	Korea	[24]

widespread in the environment of endemic farms. Moreover, the analyzed samples were collected mostly during outbreaks (rhodococcosis morbidity in foals reached even 100%) at relatively close time intervals (year by year).

Comparison of PFGE patterns and plasmid type which was conducted in this study confirms previously indicated observations in horses [13], pigs [31] cattle [32] and wild boars [21]. However, *R. equi* isolates containing the same plasmid type revealed different PFGE patterns and isolates with identical PFGE patterns contained different virulence plasmids or were plasmid-less.

During the study we detected chromosomal variability among some of investigated isolates what had been previously described even among isolates collected from the same farm [26, 33, 34]. However, these studies were

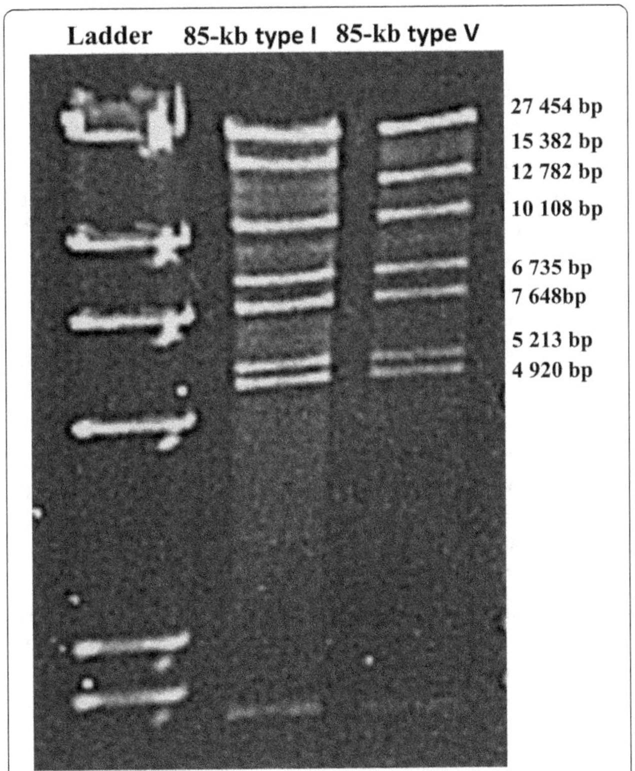

Fig. 2 EcoRI restriction fragments of the plasmids of *R. equi*. Lanes: 1, 85-kb type I; line 2, 85-kb type V (new type)

performed on a high number of isolates from heterogeneous horse populations with numerous clinical cases and soil samples from many farms contrary to our study conducted on smaller farms that stay in contact, for example by exchange of the horses.

Given the limitations of this study we can only speculate that the persistence of farm-specific isolates might be possible on some horse farms with limited movement of horses in Poland. Moreover, our observations are supported by reports from Germany and Australia were particular isolates were associated with individual farms [13, 25].

Conclusions

Most clinical isolates of *R. equi* from foals in Poland contain VapA plasmids 85-kb type I and 87-kb type I similar to the other European countries and the United States. There is a new variant of VapA plasmid identified as 85-kb type V.

The chromosomal variability was detected among some investigated isolates, however farm-specific isolates appear to exist.

Methods

Isolates of *R. equi* were obtained from samples collected by tracheobronchial aspiration from pneumonic foals or during necropsy. Foals originated from 13 horse breeding farms in Poland and were examined between 2001 and 2012.

Bacteria isolation, phenotypic and genotypic identification of isolates were conducted as described previously [35]. Briefly, modified CAZ-NB medium was used for bacteria isolation, API Coryne test (bioMerieux, France) was used for determination of biochemical properties and the presence of "equi factor" was studied in CAMP test. Presence of *R. equi* genes, *choE, traA* and *vapA* was determined by PCR. Alkaline lysis method with some modification was used for plasmid DNA isolation from the *vapA*-positive *R. equi* isolates. Isolated DNA was digested with restriction endonucleases EcoRI, EcoT221, HindIII and BamHI [35–38]. Bacterial DNA extraction and PFGE was performed as previously described [21, 23]. The *VspI* was used as the restriction enzyme. The gel images were analysed by Gel Compar II version 4.6 (Applied Maths, Belgium). Cluster analysis was performed by UPGMA using dice similarity coefficient with optimization set at 1% and position tolerance at 1.5%. The isolates were considered to be closely related and assigned to the same PFGE cluster using an 80% of homology cut-off [30]. The reference *R. equi* strains ATCC 6939 and ATCC 33701 were used as controls.

Abbreviations

PFGE: Pulsed-field gel electrophoresis; VapA: Virulence-associated protein A; VAPs: Virulence-associated plasmids

Acknowledgements

None.

Funding

The study was partially supported by a grant from the National Science Centre in years 2010–2013 as a research project No. N N308 131638 and grant from the Polish State Committee for Scientific Research in years 2004–2006 as a research project No. 2 P06K 006 27.
Publication was funded by KNOW (Leading National Research Centre) Scientific Consortium "Healthy Animal - Safe Food", decision of Ministry of Science and Higher Education No. 05-1/KNOW2/2015.

Authors' contributions

LW acquisition of funding, conceiving, designing and coordination of the study, general supervision of the research group, participation in material and data collection, participation in laboratory analysis, drafting the manuscript. MR participation in acquisition of funding, participation in conceiving and designing the study, participation in laboratory analysis and assistance in drafting the manuscript. ST participation in laboratory analysis and assistance in drafting the manuscript. DCC participation in laboratory analysis and assistance in drafting the manuscript. MKS participation in laboratory analysis and assistance in drafting the manuscript. MF participation in laboratory analysis and assistance in drafting the manuscript. MG participation in laboratory analysis and assistance in drafting the manuscript. MW participation in material and data collection and assistance in drafting the manuscript. JK participation in acquisition of funding, assistance in conceiving and designing the study, assistance in drafting the manuscript. All authors read and approved the final manuscript.

Competing interests

The authors declare that they have no competing interests.

Consent for publication

Not applicable.

Author details

[1]Laboratory of Veterinary Epidemiology and Economics, Faculty of Veterinary Medicine, Warsaw University of Life Sciences, Nowoursynowska 159c, 02-776 Warsaw, Poland. [2]Department of Preclinical Sciences, Faculty of Veterinary Medicine, Warsaw University of Life Sciences, Ciszewskiego 8, 02-786 Warsaw, Poland. [3]Department of Animal Hygiene, School of Veterinary Medicine, Kitasato University, Higashi 23-35-1, Towada, Aomori 034-8628, Japan. [4]University Center of Veterinary Medicine UJ-UR, Mickiewicza 24/28, 30-059 Cracow, Poland.

References

1. Chaffin MK, Cohen ND, Martens RJ, Edwards RF, Nevill M. Foal-related risk factors associated with development of Rhodococcus equi pneumonia on farms with endemic infection. J Am Vet Med Assoc. 2003;223(12):1791–9.
2. Muscatello G, Anderson GA, Gilkerson JR, Browning GF. Associations between the ecology of virulent Rhodococcus equi and the epidemiology of R. equi pneumonia on Australian thoroughbred farms. Appl Environ Microbiol. 2006;72(9):6152–60.
3. Giguere S, Cohen ND, Chaffin MK, Hines SA, Hondalus MK, Prescott JF, Slovis NM. Rhodococcus equi: clinical manifestations, virulence, and immunity. J Vet Intern Med. 2011;25(6):1221–30.
4. Muscatello G. Rhodococcus equi pneumonia in the foal–part 1: pathogenesis and epidemiology. Vet J. 2012;192(1):20–6.

5. Cohen ND. Rhodococcus equi foal pneumonia. Vet Clin North Am Equine Pract. 2014;30(3):609–22.
6. Yamshchikov AV, Schuetz A, Lyon GM. Rhodococcus equi infection. Lancet Infect Dis. 2010;10(5):350–9.
7. Witkowski L, Kaba J, Rzewuska M, Nowicki M, Szalus-Jordanow O, Kita J. Development of ELISA test for determination of the level of antibodies against Rhodococcus equi in equine serum and colostrum. Vet Immunol Immunopathol. 2012;149(3–4):280–5.
8. Gradzki Z, Zietek-Barszcz A. Detection of Rhodococcus equi in tracheobronchial aspirate of foals in enzootic farms depending on age and season. Bull Vet Inst Pulawy. 2011;55(4):619–24.
9. Banbura MW, Witkowski L, Chmielewska A, Tucholska A, Rzewuska M, Ruszczyk A. Isolation of equine herpes viruses type 1 and 2 (EHV-1 and EHV-2) from foals infected with Rhodocaccus equi. Med Weter. 2004;60(12):1333–6.
10. Witkowski L, Rzewuska M, Takai S, Kizerwetter-Swida M, Kita J. Molecular epidemiology of Rhodococcus equi in slaughtered swine, cattle and horses in Poland. BMC Microbiol. 2016;16:98.
11. Vazquez-Boland JA, Giguere S, Hapeshi A, MacArthur I, Anastasi E, Valero-Rello A. Rhodococcus equi: the many facets of a pathogenic actinomycete. Vet Microbiol. 2013;167(1–2):9–33.
12. Ocampo-Sosa AA, Lewis DA, Navas J, Quigley F, Callejo R, Scortti M, Leadon DP, Fogarty U, Vazquez-Boland JA. Molecular epidemiology of Rhodococcus equi based on traA, vapA, and vapB virulence plasmid markers. J Infect Dis. 2007;196(5):763–9.
13. Venner M, Meyer-Hamme B, Verspohl J, Hatori F, Shimizu N, Sasaki Y, Kakuda T, Tsubaki S, Takai S. Genotypic characterization of VapA positive Rhodococcus equi in foals with pulmonary affection and their soil environment on a warmblood horse breeding farm in Germany. Res Vet Sci. 2007;83(3):311–7.
14. Duquesne F, Hebert L, Sevin C, Breuil MF, Tapprest J, Laugier C, Petry S. Analysis of plasmid diversity in 96 Rhodococcus equi strains isolated in Normandy (France) and sequencing of the 87-kb type I virulence plasmid. FEMS Microbiol Lett. 2010;311(1):76–81.
15. Makrai L, Takai S, Tamura M, Tsukamoto A, Sekimoto R, Sasaki Y, Kakuda T, Tsubaki S, Varga J, Fodor L, et al. Characterization of virulence plasmid types in Rhodococcus equi isolates from foals, pigs, humans and soil in Hungary. Vet Microbiol. 2002;88(4):377–84.
16. Takai S, Chaffin MK, Cohen ND, Hara M, Nakamura M, Kakuda T, Sasaki Y, Tsubaki S, Martens RJ. Prevalence of virulent Rhodococcus equi in soil from five R. equi-endemic horse-breeding farms and restriction fragment length polymorphisms of virulence plasmids in isolates from soil and infected foals in Texas. J Vet Diagn Invest. 2001;13(6):489–94.
17. Takai S, Murata N, Kudo R, Narematsu N, Kakuda T, Sasaki Y, Tsubaki S. Two new variants of the Rhodococcus equi virulence plasmid, 90 kb type III and type IV, recovered from a foal in Japan. Vet Microbiol. 2001;82(4):373–81.
18. Takai S, Henton MM, Picard JA, Guthrie AJ, Fukushi H, Sugimoto C. Prevalence of virulent Rhodococcus equi in isolates from soil collected from two horse farms in South Africa and restriction fragment length polymorphisms of virulence plasmids in the isolates from infected foals, a dog and a monkey. Onderstepoort J Vet Res. 2001;68(2):105–10.
19. Ribeiro MG, Seki I, Yasuoka K, Kakuda T, Sasaki Y, Tsubaki S, Takai S. Molecular epidemiology of virulent Rhodococcus equi from foals in Brazil: virulence plasmids of 85-kb type I, 87-kb type I, and a new variant, 87-kb type III. Comp Immunol Microbiol Infect Dis. 2005;28(1):53–61.
20. Makrai L, Kira K, Kono A, Sasaki Y, Kakuda T, Tsubaki S, Fodor L, Varga J, Takai S. Plasmid profiles of virulent Rhodococcus equi isolates from soil environment on horse-breeding farms in Hungary. Acta Vet Hung. 2006;54(1):11–8.
21. Witkowski L, Rzewuska M, Cisek AA, Chrobak-Chmiel D, Kizerwetter-Swida M, Czopowicz M, Welz M, Kita J. Prevalence and genetic diversity of Rhodococcus equi in wild boars (Sus scrofa), roe deer (Capreolus capreolus) and red deer (Cervus elaphus) in Poland. BMC Microbiol. 2015;15(1):110.
22. Yuyama T, Yusa S, Yoshizumi K, Yamano S, Murata S, Hirose T, Osanai R, Onishi Y, Osato S, Sasaki C, et al. Molecular epidemiology of VapA-positive Rhodococcus equi in thoroughbred horses in Kagoshima, Japan. J Vet Med Sci. 2002;64(8):715–8.
23. Son WG, Lee DS, Yamatoda N, Hatori F, Shimizu N, Kakuda T, Sasaki Y, Tsubaki S, Takai S. Molecular typing of VapA-Positive Rhodococcus equi isolates from Jeju native horses, Korea. J Vet Med Sci. 2006;68(3):249–53.
24. Takai S, Son WG, Lee DS, Madarame H, Seki I, Yamatoda N, Kimura A, Kakuda T, Sasaki Y, Tsubaki S, et al. Rhodococcus equi virulence plasmids recovered from horses and their environment in Jeju, Korea: 90-kb type II and a new variant, 90-kb type V. J Vet Med Sci. 2003;65(12):1313–7.
25. Morton AC, Begg AP, Anderson GA, Takai S, Lammler C, Browning GF. Epidemiology of Rhodococcus equi strains on Thoroughbred horse farms. Appl Environ Microbiol. 2001;67(5):2167–75.
26. Cohen ND, Smith KE, Ficht TA, Takai S, Libal MC, West BR, DelRosario LS, Becu T, Leadon DP, Buckley T, et al. Epidemiologic study of results of pulsed-field gel electrophoresis of isolates of Rhodococcus equi obtained from horses and horse farms. Am J Vet Res. 2003;64(2):153–61.
27. Bolton T, Kuskie K, Halbert N, Chaffin K, Healy M, Lawhon S, Jackson A, Cohen N. Detection of strain variation in isolates of Rhodococcus equi from an affected foal using repetitive sequence-based polymerase chain reaction. J Vet Diagn Invest. 2010;22(4):611–5.
28. Takai S, Shoda M, Sasaki Y, Tsubaki S, Fortier G, Pronost S, Rahal K, Becu T, Begg A, Browning G, et al. Restriction fragment length polymorphisms of virulence plasmids in Rhodococcus equi. J Clin Microbiol. 1999;37(10):3417–20.
29. Takai S, Ohbushi S, Koike K, Tsubaki S, Oishi H, Kamada M. Prevalence of virulent Rhodococcus equi in isolates from soil and feces of horses from horse-breeding farms with and without endemic infections. J Clin Microbiol. 1991;29(12):2887–9.
30. Tenover FC, Arbeit RD, Goering RV, Mickelsen PA, Murray BE, Persing DH, Swaminathan B. Interpreting chromosomal DNA restriction patterns produced by pulsed-field gel-electrophoresis - criteria for bacterial strain typing. J Clin Microbiol. 1995;33(9):2233–9.
31. Pate M, Ocepek M, Zdovc I, Minato C, Ohtsu Y, Matsuoka M, Honda Y, Hashimoto L, Sasaki Y, Kakuda T, et al. Intermediately virulent Rhodococcus equi isolates from pigs in Slovenia: discovery of new plasmid types and assessment of genetic diversity by pulsed-field gel electrophoresis. Vet Med (Praha). 2009;54(3):111–7.
32. Soedarmanto I, Zhicai W, Setyamahanani A, Lammler C. Pheno- and genotyping of Rhodococcus equi isolated from faeces of healthy horses and cattle. Res Vet Sci. 1998;64(3):181–5.
33. Morton AC, Baseggio N, Peters MA, Browning GF. Diversity of isolates of Rhodococcus equi from Australian thoroughbred horse farms. Antonie Van Leeuwenhoek. 1998;74(1–3):21–5.
34. Martens RJ, Takai S, Cohen ND, Chaffin MK, Liu H, Sakurai K, Sugimoto H, Lingsweiler SW. Association of disease with isolation and virulence of Rhodococcus equi from farm soil and foals with pneumonia. J Am Vet Med Assoc. 2000;217(2):220–5.
35. Rzewuska M, Witkowski L, Cisek AA, Stefanska I, Chrobak D, Stefaniuk E, Kizerwetter-Swida M, Takai S. Characterization of Rhodococcus equi isolates from submaxillary lymph nodes of wild boars (Sus scrofa), red deer (Cervus elaphus) and roe deer (Capreolus capreolus). Vet Microbiol. 2014;172(1–2):272–8.
36. Takai S, Watanabe Y, Ikeda T, Ozawa T, Matsukura S, Tamada Y, Tsubaki S, Sekizaki T. Virulence-associated plasmids in Rhodococcus equi. J Clin Microbiol. 1993;31(7):1726–9.
37. Birnboim HC, Doly J. A rapid alkaline extraction procedure for screening recombinant plasmid DNA. Nucleic Acids Res. 1979;7(6):1513–23.
38. Takai S, Sekizaki T, Ozawa T, Sugawara T, Watanabe Y, Tsubaki S. Association between a large plasmid and 15-kilodalton to 17-kilodalton antigens in virulent Rhodococcus-equi. Infect Immun. 1991;59(11):4056–60.

15

Local anaesthetics or their combination with morphine and/or magnesium sulphate are toxic for equine chondrocytes and synoviocytes in vitro

L. M. Rubio-Martínez[1*], E. Rioja[1], M. Castro Martins[1], S. Wipawee[2], P. Clegg[3] and M. J. Peffers[3]

Abstract

Background: Chondrotoxic effects of local anaesthetics are well reported in humans and some animal species but knowledge on their toxic effects on synoviocytes or equine chondrocytes or the effects on cellular production of inflammatory cytokines is limited. The purpose of this study was to evaluate the in vitro effects of local anaesthetics, morphine, magnesium sulphate ($MgSO_4$) or their combinations on cell viability and pro-inflammatory cytokine gene expression of equine synoviocytes and chondrocytes.

Equine synoviocytes and cartilage explants harvested from normal joints in a co-culture system were exposed to mepivacaine (4.4 mg/ml), bupivacaine (2.2 mg/ml), morphine (2.85 mg/ml) and $MgSO_4$ (37 mg/ml) alone or each local anaesthetic plus morphine or $MgSO_4$ or both together. Chondrocyte and synoviocyte cell viability was assessed by CellTiter-Glo Luminescent Cell Viability Assay. Synoviocyte gene expression of IL-1β, IL-6 or TNF-α was measured and compared using the ΔΔCT method.

Results: Morphine alone, $MgSO_4$ alone or their combination did not alter cell viability or the expression of IL-1β, IL-6 or TNF-α. However, local anaesthetics alone or in combination with morphine and/or $MgSO_4$ reduced cell viability and increased the gene expression of IL-1β, IL-6 or TNF-α. Single short exposure to local anaesthetics is toxic to both chondrocytes and synoviocytes and their combination with morphine and/or $MgSO_4$ enhanced the cytotoxic effects.

Conclusions: This in vitro study gives further evidence of the absence of cytotoxic effects of morphine alone, $MgSO_4$ alone or their combination on normal articular tissues. However, local anaesthetics alone or in combination with morphine and/or $MgSO_4$ have cytotoxic effects on equine articular tissues.

Keywords: Local anaesthetic, Morphine, Magnesium sulphate, Chondrocyte, Synoviocyte, Equine

Background

Intra-articular injections of local anaesthetics are commonly performed in humans and horses to determine sources of pain and as perioperative pain control [1]. Despite their widespread use, there is growing concern over the potential toxicity of these substances and their long-term effects on articular tissue [2, 3]. Chondrotoxic properties of local anaesthetic agents have been reported in humans and animals [2, 4–6], but knowledge of their effect on equine chondrocytes is limited [7, 8]. The majority of these studies have investigated their effects on chondrocyte viability, but the effects of local anaesthetics on synoviocytes are still largely unknown. The synovium contributes to nociceptive, inflammatory and degradative responses and therefore it is vital that the effects of intra-articular injections are also studied on the synovium. Recent studies on rabbits and dogs suggest that the toxic effects of local anaesthetic on synoviocytes may affect the onset of chondrolysis associated with intra-articular use of local anaesthetics [9–11].

* Correspondence: luis.rubiomartinez@hotmail.com
[1]Institute of Veterinary Science, University of Liverpool, Leahurst Campus, Chester High Road, CH647TE Neston, UK
Full list of author information is available at the end of the article

Because of the local anaesthetic related chondrotoxic effects, alternatives for articular analgesia are being sought in humans [3]. Morphine is an opioid that provides excellent articular analgesic and anti-inflammatory effects when administered intra-articularly in humans [12, 13] with apparently minimal toxic effects on human and canine chondrocytes [2, 14]. Intra-articular administration of morphine causes analgesia, and reduces swelling and synovial inflammatory markers in horses [15–18], although it was associated with release of large molecular weight proteoglycans into the synovial fluid [19]. Magnesium sulphate ($MgSO_4$) is routinely administered intra-articularly to human patients for peri-operative analgesia [20] and does not cause a significant reduction in human chondrocyte viability [21]. Moreover, addition of $MgSO_4$ to local anaesthetics reduced the toxic effects of the latter on human chondrocytes in vitro [22]; and intra-articular administration of $MgSO_4$ attenuated the development of osteoarthritis (OA) in a rat model [23].

We hypothesised that local anaesthetics but not morphine or $MgSO_4$, would produce deleterious effects on chondrocyte and synoviocyte viability and increase the expression of pro-inflammatory cytokines. We further hypothesised that morphine or $MgSO_4$ in combination with a local anaesthetic would prevent the negative effects exerted by local anaesthetics alone.

Methods

The aim of this study was to evaluate the in vitro effects of clinically-relevant doses of local anaesthetics, morphine, $MgSO_4$ or their combinations on equine chondrocyte and synoviocyte viability and gene expression of pro-inflammatory cytokines in a co-culture in vitro model. We hypothesised that local anaesthetics would produce deleterious effects on chondrocyte and synoviocyte viability and increase the expression of pro-inflammatory cytokines. We further hypothesised that morphine and/or $MgSO_4$ in combination with a local anaesthetic would reduce the impact of the negative effects exerted by local anaesthetics alone on cell viability and gene expression of pro-inflammatory cytokines.

Study design

An experimental in vitro study was performed on equine synoviocytes and cartilage explants harvested from normal joints and using a co-culture system.

Tissue sample collection

Tissue samples were obtained from metacarpophalangeal joints of 10 skeletally mature horses (6–10 years old) from an abattoir within 5 h of slaughter. Synoviocytes were obtained from three horses and articular cartilage samples obtained from seven different horses. Only horses with grossly normal joints were included in the study.

Under sterile conditions, synovial membrane was harvested from the entire synovial surface of the joint and synoviocytes isolated as previously described [24]. Synoviocytes were cultured in Dulbecco's Modified Eagle Medium (DMEM) (Sigma-Aldrich, Darmstadt, Germany) supplemented with 10% foetal calf serum (FCS), 100 units/ml penicillin, 100 µg/ml streptomycin, L-glutamine 4 mM (all from Invitrogen, Paisley, UK) and 500 ng/ml amphotericin B (Bio Whittaker, Lonza, San Diego, California, USA), in routine laboratory conditions (37 °C, 5% O_2) until 90% confluent. After treatment with 0.05% w/v trypsin, synoviocytes were passaged and cultured until 90% confluent. Synoviocytes (passage 2) were then frozen in 10% DMSO in DMEM complete (DMEM supplemented as above) and stored in liquid nitrogen. Full thickness cartilage was collected from the entire surface of the distal condylar area of the third metacarpus. Cartilage was diced into explants of approximately 2 mm x 2 mm, mixed and placed in complete DMEM complete at 37 °C, 5% O_2 for 18 h to equilibrate.

Synoviocytes from three horses were thawed in a water bath at 37 °C for 1 min, mixed and suspended in DMEM complete to a final concentration of 50,000 live cells per ml. Synoviocytes were plated in 24-well plates at a concentration of 50,000 cells per well (2 wells per group). After equilibration at 37 °C, 5% O_2 for 24 h, trans-well inserts (0.45 µm pore, 12 mm; Millicell Cell Culture Inserts PIHA01250; Sigma-Aldrich, Darmstadt, Germany) were located into the wells and cartilage explants from 7 horses were placed separately into the inserts (5 explants per insert) in duplicate. The co-culture system was maintained in an incubator at 37 °C, 5% O_2 for 24 h at which time co-cultures were exposed to different treatments for 2 h (Table 1). Drugs were diluted in DMEM complete to a total volume of 2 ml per well to achieve the following final concentrations: mepivacaine 4.4 mg/ml, bupivacaine 2.2 mg/ml, morphine 2.85 mg/ml, magnesium sulphate 37 mg/ml. Concentrations were based on the average volume of synovial fluid in the equine metacarpophalangeal joint (12.5 mL) [25] and the doses commonly used in clinical practice [16, 17, 26–29]. Exposure time (2 h) was based on the reported half-life for the local anaesthetics in horses [26, 30]. After exposure, the medium containing the different treatments was removed and replaced by DMEM complete and cultured for additional 48 h. At this time synoviocytes and explants were harvested. Cartilage explants were snap-frozen in liquid nitrogen and stored at -80 °C. Synoviocytes from the same group were released from the wells using 250 µL Tri-reagent (Sigma-Aldrich, Darmstadt, Germany) per well for 30 min and immediately stored at -80 °C

Table 1 Treatment groups

Group	Treatment
1	Control
2	Mepivacaine only
3	Mepivacaine + morphine
4	Mepivacaine + MgSO4
5	Mepivacaine + morphine + MgSO4
6	Morphine only
7	MgSO4 only
8	Morphine + MgSO4
9	Bupivacaine only
10	Bupivacaine + morphine
11	Bupivacaine + MgSO4
12	Bupivacaine + morphine + MgSO4

Treatment groups to which synoviocyte-articular cartilage explant co-cultures were exposed. Concentrations used were mepivacaine 4.4 mg/ml, bupivacaine 2.2 mg/ml, morphine 2.85 mg/ml and magnesium sulphate 37 mg/ml diluted in DMEM complete to a total volume of 2 ml per well

Cell viability

Cell viability was performed on tissues from one well per group. Chondrocytes were recovered after digesting cartilage explants with 1 mg/ml collagenase II (Worthington Biochemical Corporation, Lakewood, US). Cell viability analysis was performed on synoviocytes and chondrocytes with CellTiter-Glo Luminescent Cell Viability Assay using a Glomax Detection System as per manufacturer instructions (Promega, Wisconsin, US). This assay determines the number of viable cells in culture based on quantification of adenosine triphosphate by luminescence, which signals the presence of metabolically active cells [31, 32].

RNA extraction and Real-time Quantitative Polymerase Chain Reaction (qPCR) analysis

RNA was extracted from cartilage explants and synoviocytes as previously described [33]. Total RNA concentration was determined using a Nanodrop-2000c (Thermo Fisher Scientific). Complimentary DNA (cDNA) was prepared [33]. Real-time qPCR was used to measure relative gene expression for markers of three pro-inflammatory cytokines: Interleukin 1 beta (IL1β), Interleukin 6 (IL6) and Tumour Necrosis Factor alpha (TNFα) compared to the reference gene glyceraldehydes-3-phosphatedhyrogenase (GAPDH) as described previously using SYBR Green technology [33]. Primer sequences are listed in Table 2.

Statistical analysis

Data were analysed using commercially available statistical software (SPSS, version 22.0, 2013, Chicago, USA). Graphical displays and Anderson-Darling test were used to check for departures from assumptions of normality. Log transformations were applied when data were non-normally distributed. Gene expression data were normalised to the reference gene using the ΔΔCT method [34] and statistical analysis applied to the 2^-ΔCT values. General linear models with Dunnet's comparisons with control group were performed. Significance was considered when $p < 0.05$. Gene expression results were normalised to the control group.

Table 2 Primer sequences of the reference gene (GAPDH) and pro-inflammatory cytokines IL1β, IL6 and TNFα used in the study

Gene	GeneBank Accession	Direction	Primer Sequence (5′-3′)
GAPDH	NM_001163856	Forward	GCATCGTGGAGGGACTCA
		Reverse	GCCACATCTTCCCAGAGG
IL-1β	NM_001317261	Forward	GCCTAAGAATACTACATCCAGAGA
		Reverse	GGCATTGATTAGACAACAGTGAA
IL-6	NM_001082496	Forward	CTGCTCCTCGTGATGGCTAC
		Reverse	CCGAGGATGTACTTAATGTGCTG
TNF-α	NM_001081819	Forward	CCTTCCACTCAATCAACCCTCT
		Reverse	CACGCCCACTCAGCCACT

Primer sequences of the reference gene (GAPDH) and proinflammatory cytokines IL1β, IL6 and TNFα used in the study

Results

Cell viability

Raw data of cell vaiability are provided in Additional file 1. The effects of different treatments on synoviocyte and chondrocyte viability are presented in Figs. 1 and 2

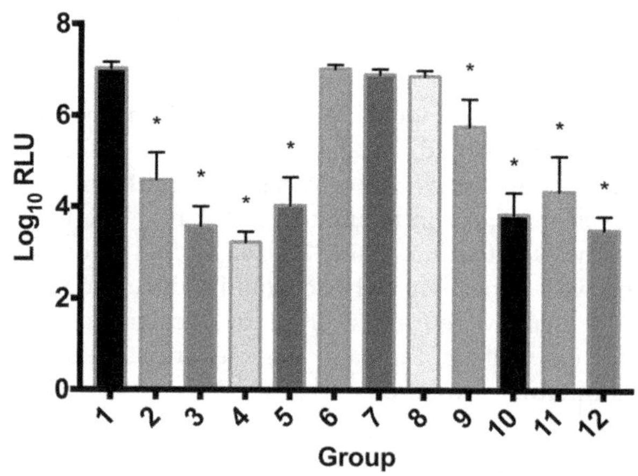

Fig. 1 Synoviocyte viability Cell viability measured as luminescence signal (shown as log10 transformed Relative Light Units [RLU]) for synoviocytes exposed to different treatments (for further information on treatment groups refer to Table 1). Error bars indicate 95% confidence interval. Asterisk (*) indicates significant difference ($p < 0.05$) with group 1 (control). Groups included are: control (group 1); mepivacaine (group 2); mepivacaine + morphine (group 3); mepivacaine + $MgSO_4$ (group 4); mepivacaine + morphine + $MgSO_4$ (group 5); morphine (group 6); $MgSO_4$ (group 7); morphine + $MgSO_4$ (group 8); bupivacaine (group 9); bupivacaine + morphine (group 10); bupivacaine + $MgSO_4$ (group 11); and bupivacaine + morphine + $MgSO_4$ (group 12)

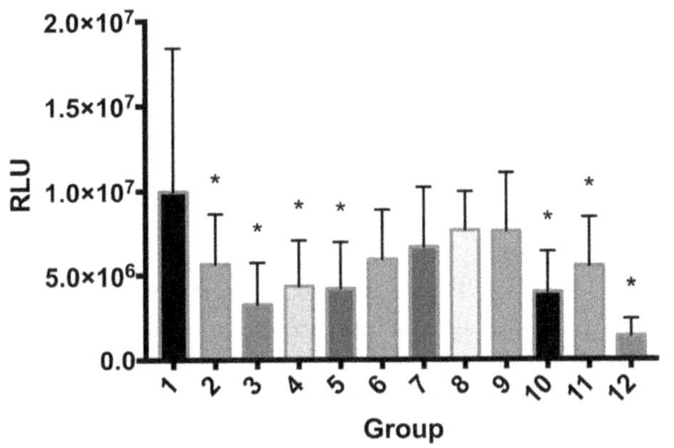

Fig. 2 Chondrocyte viability Cell viability measured as luminescence signal (mean values of Relative Light Units [RLU]) for chondrocytes exposed to different treatment groups (for further information on treatment groups refer to Table 1). Error bars indicate 95% confidence interval. Asterisk (*) indicates significant difference ($p < 0.05$) with group 1 (control). Groups included are: control (group 1); mepivacaine (group 2); mepivacaine + morphine (group 3); mepivacaine + $MgSO_4$ (group 4); mepivacaine + morphine + $MgSO_4$ (group 5); morphine (group 6); $MgSO_4$ (group 7); morphine + $MgSO_4$ (group 8); bupivacaine (group 9); bupivacaine + morphine (group 10); bupivacaine + $MgSO_4$ (group 11); and bupivacaine + morphine + $MgSO_4$ (group 12)

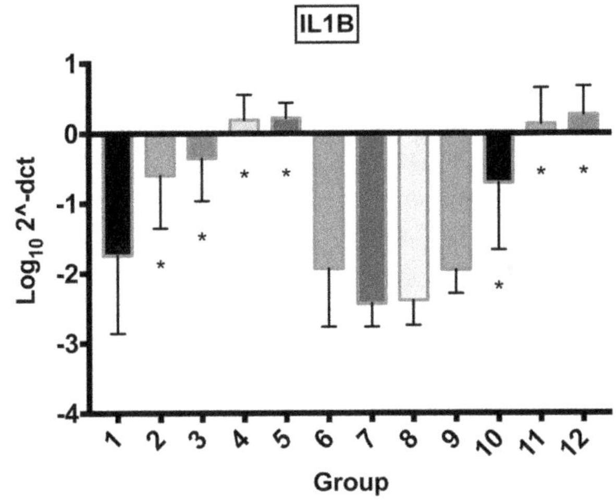

Fig. 3 Synoviocyte IL1β gene expression IL1β gene expression (mean $\log_{10}2^{\wedge}$-ΔCT) for synoviocytes exposed to different treatment groups (for further information on treatment groups refer to Table 1). Error bars indicate 95% confidence interval. Asterisk (*) indicates significant difference ($p < 0.05$) with group 1 (control). Groups included are: control (group 1); mepivacaine (group 2); mepivacaine + morphine (group 3); mepivacaine + $MgSO_4$ (group 4); mepivacaine + morphine + $MgSO_4$ (group 5); morphine (group 6); $MgSO_4$ (group 7); morphine + $MgSO_4$ (group 8); bupivacaine (group 9); bupivacaine + morphine (group 10); bupivacaine + $MgSO_4$ (group 11); and bupivacaine + morphine + $MgSO_4$ (group 12).

respectively. Compared with control group, chondrocyte or synoviocyte viability did not change in groups exposed to morphine alone, $MgSO_4$ alone or morphine and $MgSO_4$ in combination. Chondrocyte viability was significantly reduced in chondrocytes exposed mepivacaine alone or in combination with morphine and/or $MgSO_4$ (groups 2, 3, 4 and 5). Exposure to bupivacaine alone did not reduce chondrocyte viability in comparison with control group; however, chondrocyte viability was significantly reduced in groups exposed to combinations of bupivacaine with either morphine or $MgSO_4$ or both combines (groups 10, 11 and 12). Synoviocyte viability was reduced in all groups exposed to either local anaesthetic (mepivacaine or bupivacaine), and any of their combinations with morphine and/or $MgSO_4$. (groups 2, 3, 4, 5, 9, 10, 11 and 12).

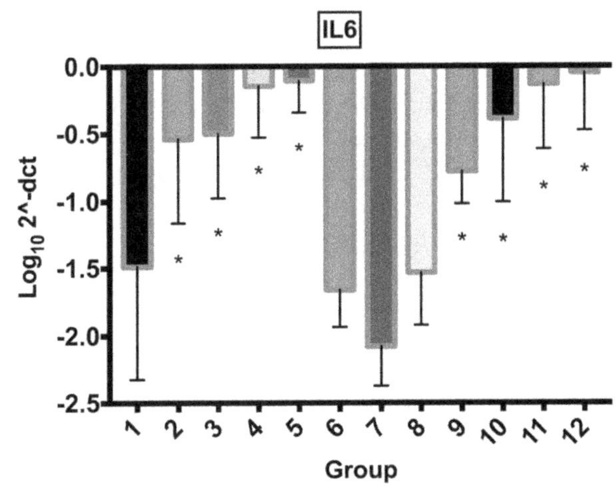

Fig. 4 Synoviocyte IL6 gene expression IL6 gene expression (mean $\log_{10}2^{\wedge}$-ΔCT) for synoviocytes exposed to different treatment groups (for further information on treatment groups refer to Table 1). Error bars indicate 95% confidence interval. Asterisk (*) indicates significant difference ($p < 0.05$) with group 1 (control). Groups included are: control (group 1); mepivacaine (group 2); mepivacaine + morphine (group 3); mepivacaine + $MgSO_4$ (group 4); mepivacaine + morphine + $MgSO_4$ (group 5); morphine (group 6); $MgSO_4$ (group 7); morphine + $MgSO_4$ (group 8); bupivacaine (group 9); bupivacaine + morphine (group 10); bupivacaine + $MgSO_4$ (group 11); and bupivacaine + morphine + $MgSO_4$ (group 12).

Real-time qPCR

Raw data on gene expression are provided in Additional file 1. Treatment with morphine, $MgSO_4$ or their combination did not have an effect on synoviocyte gene expression of IL-1β, IL-6 or TNF-α. Exposure to mepivacaine alone (group 2) increased expression of IL-1 β, IL6 and TNF-α, while exposure to bupivacaine alone (group 9) only significantly increased expression of IL6. Combination of either mepivacaine or bupivacaine with morphine, $MgSO_4$, or both (groups 3, 4, 5, 10, 11 and 12) increased expression of IL-1β, IL-6 and TNF-α (Figs.

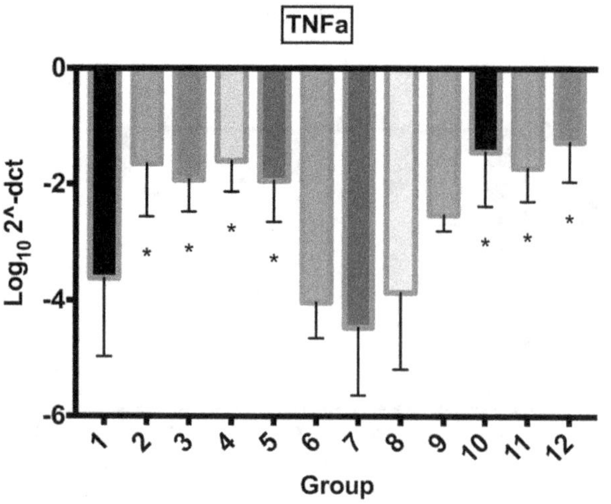

Fig. 5 Synoviocyte TNFα gene expression (mean $\log_{10}2^{\wedge}$-ΔCT) for synoviocytes exposed to different treatment groups (for further information on treatment groups refer to Table 1). Error bars indicate 95% confidence interval. Asterisk (*) indicates significant difference ($p < 0.05$) with group 1 (control). Groups included are: control (group 1); mepivacaine (group 2); mepivacaine + morphine (group 3); mepivacaine + $MgSO_4$ (group 4); mepivacaine + morphine + $MgSO_4$ (group 5); morphine (group 6); $MgSO_4$ (group 7); morphine + $MgSO_4$ (group 8); bupivacaine (group 9); bupivacaine + morphine (group 10); bupivacaine + $MgSO_4$ (group 11); and bupivacaine + morphine + $MgSO_4$ (group 12)

3, 4, 5). Gene expression from cartilage explants did not yield consistent amount of RNA for downstream qRT-PCR.

Discussion

Chondrotoxic effects of local anaesthetics are reported in the literature and results of this study confirm that a single short exposure to local anaesthetics causes significant articular cytotoxic effects characterised by decreased viability of both equine synoviocytes and chondrocytes. These effects were not counteracted by the addition of morphine and/or $MgSO_4$. Except for the mepivacaine effect on TNF-α expression, local anaesthetics alone, as well as morphine alone, $MgSO_4$ alone, or morphine and $MgSO_4$ combined, did not increase the expression of pro-inflammatory cytokines by synoviocytes; however, the pro-inflammatory cytokines expression were increased when local anaesthetics were combined with morphine and/or $MgSO_4$.

The present study demonstrates that bupivacaine at a concentration of 0.22% is harmful for articular equine synoviocytes but its negative effects are less pronounced on chondrocytes. A protective effect from the existence of intact extracellular matrix on chondrocytes from the cartilage explant has been previously suggested [6, 14], although this was recently questioned on an experimental canine model [10]. Local anaesthetics have drug-, dose- and time-dependent cytotoxic effects [5, 10, 35–37]. Bupivacaine 0.0625% did not cause cell death in canine cartilage and synovium explants [10] and varying toxicity has been observed for bupivacaine concentrations in the range of 0.125–0.25% [2, 5, 10, 35]. Bupivacaine concentrations ≥0.5% have consistently been reported to exert toxic effects on human and animal chondrocytes [5, 35], including horses [7] but interestingly did not affect the viability of rabbit type B synoviocytes in monolayer [11]. Different species sensitivities, methodologies or cell lines may explain different results between studies. Mepivacaine is less frequently administered as an intra-articular analgesic in people and there are fewer studies investigating its effects on articular cells. In contrast to our study, mepivacaine was less toxic than bupivacaine on human [35] and equine [7] chondrocytes on monolayer cultures. However, the bupivacaine concentration used in the present study was lower than in previous studies and has been previously associated with chondrotoxic effects on human cartilage [35] and equine chondrocytes [38]. Mepivacaine is commonly administered intra-articularly in horses at doses similar to that in the present study and temporary synovitis has occasionally been reported [27].

Few studies have investigated the effects of local anaesthetics on the production of inflammatory molecules by articular tissues. Following exposure to bupivacaine a decrease in nitric oxide and PGE_2 concentrations was observed in an IL-1-treated co-culture explant model; and that was suggested to be the result of the lack of viable cells remaining after the exposure [2]. However, in our study increased expression of IL1-β, IL6 or TNF-α was observed despite decreased viability

Intra-articular administration of morphine or $MgSO_4$ produces analgesia without clinical evidence of adverse effects in people [12, 13, 20, 39–41]. The present study corroborates the absence of deleterious effects of morphine or $MgSO_4$ on canine human and canine chondrocyte viability in vitro [2, 14, 21, 22], and extends this absence of toxicity to synoviocytes. Furthermore, the combination of morphine and $MgSO_4$ did not have negative effects on cell viability, which warrants investigation of the potential analgesic effect of the combination *in vivo*. In addition, no effects on expression of pro-inflammatory cytokines were observed when tissues were exposed to morphine and/or $MgSO_4$. Anti-inflammatory effects of opioids have been reported after systemic or local administration. Morphine exposure of IL-1-treated cartilage explants decreased nitric oxide and PGE_2 production [2]. Intra-articular administration of morphine reduced nucleated cell count in synovial fluid of chronic arthritis patients [42] and serum amyloid A and total protein levels in horses with experimentally-induced synovitis [15]. Anti-inflammatory effects of magnesium have also been recognised. Low magnesium promotes inflammation and up-regulates IL1α and IL6 production in endothelial cells [43] while magnesium supplementation attenuated the development of OA [23] and rheumatoid arthritis (RA) [44]. $MgSO_4$ acts on *N*-methyl-D-aspartate receptors and although the present study did not include an OA or RA model, *N*-methyl-D-aspartate receptors involved in the development of OA and RA are also present in normal human and mouse articular chondrocytes [45]. Results of this study support the clinical use of morphine and warrant further investigation on $MgSO_4$ as intra-articular analgesic drugs in horses and other species.

Addition of $MgSO_4$ to local anaesthetics counteracted harmful effects on human chondrocyte viability in vitro [22] and we aimed to determine if the same was true in a synoviocyte and cartilage explant co-culture model. However, the addition of morphine, $MgSO_4$ or both to mepivacaine or bupivacaine did not counteract cell death caused by mepivacaine and furthermore, decreased chondrocyte viability in comparison with the control group when combined with bupivacaine. Combination of either local anaesthetic with morphine and/or $MgSO_4$ also enhanced the synoviocyte expression of IL1β, IL6 and TNFα. The reasons for the enhanced toxicity of the drug combinations are unclear. The mechanisms of action of local anaesthetics, morphine and $MgSO_4$ differ. The cytotoxic effects of local anaesthetics are related to a concentration-dependent mitochondrial depolarization with subsequent alteration in transmembrane potential and cell death [46]. Osmolality-related cytotoxicity has been observed with high concentrations of magnesium (500 mg/ml) [22] but the concentration used in the present study was 37 mg/ml. Interaction between molecules or their combination with the culture medium or changes in the pH of the environment may be involved [47]. A time-dependent increased chondrotoxicity has been observed for the combination of corticosteroid and local anaesthetics [48]. The pH of the treatment solutions in the present study were nor determined and buffer solutions were not used; however, low pH was not the cause for decreased viability of bovine chondrocytes [1, 49] and addition of buffering solution can increase chondrotoxicity [47]. Chemical incompatibility between the anaesthetic solution and culture medium leading to crystal formation and high cell death rates has been suggested by some authors [1, 7]; however, precipitation was not observed in the present or other studies [2, 10, 38]. Although combination of local anaesthetics and $MgSO_4$ are being administered clinically into joints without reported clinical side effects [20, 50] further research into the chemical compatibility or interactions between drugs is warranted.

The present study has a number of limitations. A co-culture equine model was used to allow evaluations of both cartilage and synovium components as many inflammatory mediators and analgesic receptors are found in the synovium, and synoviocytes have important roles in maintaining articular health and participating in pathophysiological processes [51, 52]. However, results from this in vitro study may not be the same *in vivo*. Use of synovial explants [2, 10] could have enhanced the system although recent studies support the comparability of explants and monolayer cultures to assess cytotoxicity [2, 10]. The preferential type of synoviocyte present in the culture is uncertain and a mixture of both macrophage-like and fibroblast-like synoviocytes is suspected in this study as they were frozen at passage 2 [52]. Drug concentrations and duration of exposure were based on clinically used doses, joint volume and pharmacokinetics in horses. However, the drug concentrations remained constant during the 2 h exposure, which could be interpreted as a relative overdose as clearance of the drug is expected to occur already within this time in the live animal. The horse is an accepted translational models of naturally-occurring osteoarthritis [53] but drug effects can differ between species. Normal articular tissues were used and more severe chondrotoxic effects are expected on degenerative versus normal cartilage [35]. The reasons for the poor RNA extraction from cartilage explants are uncertain. This methodology has been used successfully in other studies but equine mature articular cartilage is relatively acellular and we used small size explants. Previous studies in our lab have yielded 1 μg of RNA from the cartilage harvested from both third metacarpal condyles in adult horses (Peffers M.J. Unpublished data). The use of isolated chondrocytes, larger size or higher number of cartilage explants, or use of a different methodology may have yielded gene expression data from the cartilage explants. Quantification of adenosine triphosphate by luminescence has been shown reliable method to assess cell viability [14, 31].

Conclusions

The present study corroborate the toxic effects of single short exposure to local anaesthetics on both equine chondrocytes and synoviocytes using an in vitro co-culture model, with more severe effects observed for mepivacaine than bupivacaine. It also provides evidence that synoviocytes respond to drugs commonly administered intra-articularly, which warrants further investigation. The present study indicates that morphine and $MgSO_4$ are not toxic to synoviocytes when exposed either alone or in combination, which supports the clinical use of morphine and warrants further investigation of $MgSO_4$ as intra-articular analgesic drugs in horses and other species. However, further investigation into drug incompatibilities is required as combinations of either mepivacaine or bupivacaine with morphine, $MgSO_4$ or both did not alleviate any detrimental effects from the local anaesthetics, but actually caused cell death and increased expression of pro-inflammatory enzymes.

Abbreviations

cDNA: Complimentary deoxyribonucleic acid; DMSO: Dimethyl sulfoxide; FCS: Foetal calf Serum; GAPDH: Glyceraldehyde-3-phosphatedhyrogenase; IL-1β: Interleukin 1β; IL-6: Interleukin 6; $MgSO_4$: Magnesium sulphate; OA: Osteoarthritis; qRT-PCR: Real-time quantitative polymerase chain reaction; TNF-α: Tumour necrosis factor α

Acknowledgements

We wish to thank Ian Richards for his contribution in the acquisition of data. None of the authors have conflicts of interests.

Funding

This study was funded by the Horserace Betting Levy Board (SPrj015). Mandy Peffers is funded through a Wellcome Trust Clinical Intermediate Fellowship (107471). Funding bodies did not take part in the study design or conclusion of the study.

Authors' contributions

LMRM, MJP, ER and PC participated in the design of the study and the experiments and interpretation of the data. LRM, MCM and SW participated in the design of the study, performing the majority of the experiments and interpretation of data. LRM and ER performed statistical analysis and interpretation of the data. MJP and PC supervised all the experiments. All authors read and approved the final manuscript.

Consent for publication

Not applicable.

Competing interests

All authors declare that they have no competing interests.

Author details

[1]Institute of Veterinary Science, University of Liverpool, Leahurst Campus, Chester High Road, CH647TE Neston, UK. [2]Faculty of Veterinary Science, Rajamangala University of Technology Srivijaya (Thailand) and Institute of Aging and Chronic Disease, University of Liverpool, Liverpool, UK. [3]Institute of Aging and Chronic Disease, University of Liverpool, Liverpool, UK.

References

1. Bogatch MT, Ferachi DG, Kyle B, Popinchalk S, Howell MH, Ge D, You Z, Savoie FH. Is chemical incompatibility responsible for chondrocyte death induced by local anesthetics? Am J Sports Med. 2010;38(3):520–6.
2. Anz A, Smith MJ, Stoker A, Linville C, Markway H, Branson K, Cook JL. The effect of bupivacaine and morphine in a coculture model of diarthrodial joints. Arthroscopy. 2009;25(3):225–31.
3. Gulihar A, Robati S, Twaij H, Salih A, Taylor GJ. Articular cartilage and local anaesthetic: A systematic review of the current literature. J Orthop. 2015; 12(Suppl 2):S200–10.
4. Dragoo JL, Braun HJ, Kim HJ, Phan HD, Golish SR. The in vitro chondrotoxicity of single-dose local anesthetics. Am J Sports Med. 2012;40(4):794–9.
5. Chu CR, Izzo NJ, Coyle CH, Papas NE, Logar A. The in vitro effects of bupivacaine on articular chondrocytes. J Bone Joint Surg Br. 2008;90(6): 814–20.
6. Chu CR, Izzo NJ, Papas NE, Fu FH. In vitro exposure to 0.5% bupivacaine is cytotoxic to bovine articular chondrocytes. Arthroscopy. 2006;22(7):693–9.
7. Park J, Sutradhar BC, Hong G, Choi SH, Kim G. Comparison of the cytotoxic effects of bupivacaine, lidocaine, and mepivacaine in equine articular chondrocytes. Vet Anaesth Analg. 2011;38(2):127–33.
8. Piat P, Richard H, Beauchamp G, Laverty S. In vivo effects of a single intra-articular injection of 2% lidocaine or 0.5% bupivacaine on articular cartilage of normal horses. Vet Surg. 2012;41(8):1002–10.
9. Sherman SL, James C, Stoker AM, Cook CR, Khazai RS, Flood DL, Cook JL. In Vivo Toxicity of Local Anesthetics and Corticosteroids on Chondrocyte and Synoviocyte Viability and Metabolism. Cartilage. 2015;6(2):106–12.
10. Sherman SL, Khazai RS, James CH, Stoker AM, Flood DL, Cook JL. In Vitro Toxicity of Local Anesthetics and Corticosteroids on Chondrocyte and Synoviocyte Viability and Metabolism. Cartilage. 2015;6(4):233–40.
11. Braun HJ, Busfield BT, Kim HJ, Scuderi GJ, Dragoo JL. The effect of local anaesthetics on synoviocytes: a possible indirect mechanism of chondrolysis. Knee Surg Sports Traumatol Arthrosc. 2013;21(6):1468–74.
12. Grabowska-Gawel A, Gawel K, Hagner W, Bilinski PJ. Morphine or bupivacaine in controlling postoperative pain in patients subjected to knee joint arthroscopy. Ortop Traumatol Rehabil. 2003;5(6):758–62.
13. Kalso E, Smith L, McQuay HJ, Andrew Moore R. No pain, no gain: clinical excellence and scientific rigour–lessons learned from IA morphine. Pain. 2002;98(3):269–75.
14. Ickert I, Herten M, Vogl M, Ziskoven C, Zilkens C, Krauspe R, Kircher J. Opioids as an alternative to amide-type local anaesthetics for intra-articular application. Knee Surg Sports Traumatol Arthrosc. 2015;23(9):2674–81.
15. Lindegaard C, Gleerup KB, Thomsen MH, Martinussen T, Jacobsen S, Andersen PH. Anti-inflammatory effects of intra-articular administration of morphine in horses with experimentally induced synovitis. Am J Vet Res. 2010;71(1):69–75.
16. Lindegaard C, Thomsen MH, Larsen S, Andersen PH. Analgesic efficacy of intra-articular morphine in experimentally induced radiocarpal synovitis in horses. Vet Anaesth Analg. 2010;37(2):171–85.
17. Santos LC, de Moraes AN, Saito ME. Effects of intraarticular ropivacaine and morphine on lipopolysaccharide-induced synovitis in horses. Vet Anaesth Analg. 2009;36(3):280–6.
18. van Loon JP, de Grauw JC, van Dierendonck M, L'Ami JJ, Back W, van Weeren PR. Intra-articular opioid analgesia is effective in reducing pain and inflammation in an equine LPS induced synovitis model. Equine Vet J. 2010; 42(5):412–9.
19. Tulamo RM, Raekallio M, Taylor P, Johnson CB, Salonen M. Intra-articular morphine and saline injections induce release of large molecular weight proteoglycans into equine synovial fluid. Zentralbl Veterinarmed A. 1996; 43(3):147–53.
20. Elsharnouby NM, Eid HE, Abou Elezz NF, Moharram AN: Intraarticular injection of magnesium sulphate and/or bupivacaine for postoperative analgesia after arthroscopic knee surgery. Anesth Analg 2008, 106(5): 1548–1552, table of contents.
21. Baker JF, Walsh PM, Byrne DP, Mulhall KJ. In vitro assessment of human chondrocyte viability after treatment with local anaesthetic, magnesium sulphate or normal saline. Knee Surg Sports Traumatol Arthrosc. 2011; 19(6):1043–6.
22. Baker JF, Byrne DP, Walsh PM, Mulhall KJ. Human chondrocyte viability after treatment with local anesthetic and/or magnesium: results from an in vitro study. Arthroscopy. 2011;27(2):213–7.
23. Lee CH, Wen ZH, Chang YC, Huang SY, Tang CC, Chen WF, Hsieh SP, Hsieh CS, Jean YH. Intra-articular magnesium sulfate (MgSO4) reduces experimental osteoarthritis and nociception: association with attenuation of N-methyl-D-aspartate (NMDA) receptor subunit 1 phosphorylation and apoptosis in rat chondrocytes. Osteoarthritis Cartilage. 2009;17(11):1485–93.
24. Rosengren S, Boyle DL, Firestein GS. Acquisition, culture, and phenotyping of synovial fibroblasts. Methods Mol Med. 2007;135:365–75.
25. Ekman L, Nilsson G, Persson L, Lumsden JH. Volume of the synovia in certain joint cavities in the horse. Acta Vet Scand. 1981;22(1):23–31.
26. Lindegaard C, Frost AB, Thomsen MH, Larsen C, Hansen SH, Andersen PH. Pharmacokinetics of intra-articular morphine in horses with lipopolysaccharide-induced synovitis. Vet Anaesth Analg.

2010;37(2):186–95.

27. Bassage LH, Ross MW. Diagnostic analgesia. In: Ross MW, Dyson SJ, editors. Diagnosis and management of lameness in the horse. 2nd ed. St. Louis, Missouri: Elsevier Saunders; 2011. p. 100–34.
28. Koltka K, Koknel-Talu G, Asik M, Ozyalcin S. Comparison of efficacy of intraarticular application of magnesium, levobupivacaine and lornoxicam with placebo in arthroscopic surgery. Knee Surg Sports Traumatol Arthrosc. 2011;19(11):1884–9.
29. Zeng C, Gao SG, Cheng L, Luo W, Li YS, Tu M, Tian J, Xu M, Zhang FJ, Jiang W, et al. Single-Dose Intra-Articular Morphine After Arthroscopic Knee Surgery: A Meta-Analysis of Randomized Placebo-Controlled Studies. Arthroscopy. 2013;29(8):1450–8.
30. Wintzer HJ, Fitzek A, Frey HH. Pharmacokinetics of procaine injected into the hock joint of the horse. Equine Vet J. 1981;13(1):68–9.
31. Niles AL, Moravec RA, Riss TL. In vitro viability and cytotoxicity testing and same-well multi-parametric combinations for high throughput screening. Curr Chem Genomics. 2009;3:33–41.
32. Riss TL, Moravec RA, Niles AL, Benink HA, Worzella TJ, Minor L: Cell Viability Assays. In: *Assay Guidance Manual.* edn. Edited by Sittampalam GS, Coussens NP, Nelson H, Arkin M, Auld D, Austin C, Bejcek B, Glicksman M, Inglese J, Iversen PW et al. Bethesda (MD); 2004.
33. Peffers M, Liu X, Clegg P. Transcriptomic signatures in cartilage ageing. Arthritis Res Ther. 2013;15(4):R98.
34. Livak KJ, Schmittgen TD. Analysis of relative gene expression data using real-time quantitative PCR and the 2(–Delta Delta C(T)) Method. Methods. 2001;25(4):402–8.
35. Breu A, Rosenmeier K, Kujat R, Angele P, Zink W. The cytotoxicity of bupivacaine, ropivacaine, and mepivacaine on human chondrocytes and cartilage. Anesth Analg. 2013;117(2):514–22.
36. Grishko V, Xu M, Wilson G, Pearsall AW. Apoptosis and mitochondrial dysfunction in human chondrocytes following exposure to lidocaine, bupivacaine, and ropivacaine. J Bone Joint Surg Am. 2010;92(3):609–18.
37. Miyazaki T, Kobayashi S, Takeno K, Yayama T, Meir A, Baba H. Lidocaine cytotoxicity to the bovine articular chondrocytes in vitro: changes in cell viability and proteoglycan metabolism. Knee Surg Sports Traumatol Arthrosc. 2011;19(7):1198–205.
38. Bolt DM, Ishihara A, Weisbrode SE, Bertone AL. Effects of triamcinolone acetonide, sodium hyaluronate, amikacin sulfate, and mepivacaine hydrochloride, alone and in combination, on morphology and matrix composition of lipopolysaccharide-challenged and unchallenged equine articular cartilage explants. Am J Vet Res. 2008;69(7):861–7.
39. Eroglu A, Saracoglu S, Erturk E, Kosucu M, Kerimoglu S. A comparison of intraarticular morphine and bupivacaine for pain control and outpatient status after an arthroscopic knee surgery under a low dose of spinal anaesthesia. Knee Surg Sports Traumatol Arthrosc. 2010;18(11):1487–95.
40. Elkousy H, Kannan V, Calder CT, Zumwalt J, O'Connor DP, Woods GW. Intra-articular morphine versus bupivacaine for postoperative pain management. Orthopedics. 2013;36(9):e1121–7.
41. Bondok RS, Abd El-Hady AM. Intra-articular magnesium is effective for postoperative analgesia in arthroscopic knee surgery. Br J Anaesth. 2006; 97(3):389–92.
42. Stein A, Yassouridis A, Szopko C, Helmke K, Stein C. Intraarticular morphine versus dexamethasone in chronic arthritis. Pain. 1999;83(3):525–32.
43. Bernardini D, Nasulewic A, Mazur A, Maier JA. Magnesium and microvascular endothelial cells: a role in inflammation and angiogenesis. Front Biosci. 2005;10:1177–82.
44. Nagai N, Fukuhata T, Ito Y, Tai H, Hataguchi Y, Nakagawa K. Preventive effect of water containing magnesium ion on paw edema in adjuvant-induced arthritis rat. Biol Pharm Bull. 2007;30(10):1934–7.
45. Salter DM, Wright MO, Millward-Sadler SJ. NMDA receptor expression and roles in human articular chondrocyte mechanotransduction. Biorheology. 2004;41(3–4):273–81.
46. Irwin W, Fontaine E, Agnolucci L, Penzo D, Betto R, Bortolotto S, Reggiani C, Salviati G, Bernardi P. Bupivacaine myotoxicity is mediated by mitochondria. J Biol Chem. 2002;277(14):12221–7.
47. Syed HM, Green L, Bianski B, Jobe CM, Wongworawat MD. Bupivacaine and triamcinolone may be toxic to human chondrocytes: a pilot study. Clin Orthop Relat Res. 2011;469(10):2941–7.
48. Farkas B, Kvell K, Czompoly T, Illes T, Bardos T. Increased chondrocyte death after steroid and local anesthetic combination. Clin Orthop Relat Res. 2010; 468(11):3112–20.
49. Karpie JC, Chu CR. Lidocaine exhibits dose- and time-dependent cytotoxic effects on bovine articular chondrocytes in vitro. Am J Sports Med. 2007; 35(10):1621–7.
50. Chen Y, Zhang Y, Zhu YL, Fu PL. Efficacy and safety of an intra-operative intra-articular magnesium/ropivacaine injection for pain control following total knee arthroplasty. J Int Med Res. 2012;40(5):2032–40.
51. Chang X, Shen J, Yang H, Xu Y, Gao W, Wang J, Zhang H, He S. Upregulated expression of CCR3 in osteoarthritis and CCR3 mediated activation of fibroblast-like synoviocytes. Cytokine. 2016;77:211–9.
52. Bartok B, Firestein GS. Fibroblast-like synoviocytes: key effector cells in rheumatoid arthritis. Immunol Rev. 2010;233(1):233–55.
53. Gregory MH, Capito N, Kuroki K, Stoker AM, Cook JL, Sherman SL. A review of translational animal models for knee osteoarthritis. Arthritis. 2012;2012:764621.

16

Algometry to measure pain threshold in the horse's back – An in vivo and in vitro study

Una Pongratz[1] and Theresia Licka[1,2*]

Abstract

Background: The aim of this study was to provide information on algometric transmission of pressure through the dorsal thoracolumbar tissues of the equine back. Using a commercially available algometer, measurements were carried out with six different tips (hemispheric and cylindrical surfaces, contact areas 0.5 cm^2, 1 cm^2, and 2 cm^2). In nine live horses the threshold of pressure that lead to any reaction was documented. In postmortem specimens of five euthanized horses the transmission of algometer pressure onto a pressure sensor placed underneath the dorsal thoracolumbar tissues at the level of the ribs or the transverse lumbar processes respectively was measured.

Results: Algometer tips with a contact area of 1 cm^2 led to widely similar results irrespective of the surface shape; these measurements also had the lowest variance. Contact areas of 0.5 cm^2 resulted in a lower pressure threshold, and those of 2 cm^2 resulted in a higher pressure threshold. The hemispheric shape of the contact area resulted in a higher pressure threshold, than the cylindrical contact area.
Compared to the thoracic region, a significantly higher pressure threshold was found in the lumbar region in the live horses. This result corresponds to the increased tissue thickness in the lumbar region compared to the thoracic region, also documented as less pressure transmission in the lumbar region on the in vitro specimens.

Conclusions: Algometry is an easily practicable and well tolerated method to quantify pain but it is important to consider the many factors influencing the results obtained.

Keywords: Thoracolumbar pain, Horse, Algometry

Background

Musculoskeletal disorders of the horse are one of the most common reasons for veterinary intervention, and associated clinical, economic, and ethical aspects are increasingly important [1, 2]. The diagnosis of pain in the thoracolumbar area can be challenging due to the variety of possible clinical signs and the lack of objective parameters [3–8].

Even though a large number of diagnostic aids are available for the investigation of thoracolumbar pain, palpation remains one of the most important methods; this is even described as the most valuable part of the clinical assessment [7]. A standardized manual and digital palpation is recommended [7, 9], however this is limited by a large degree of subjectivity [9]. Algometry has been shown to be an objective method to quantify pressure sensitivity or pain on pressure; it is easy to use and it has been successful in a number of studies in veterinary and human medicine [3–5, 9–11]. The pressure exerted via the algometer at which a first reaction of the subject of the examination is noted is known as the mechanical nociceptive threshold. This pressure is then documented as N (Newton) or kg/cm^2, and – obviously larger values indicate a higher threshold than smaller values [2]. Even though algometry is a quantitative measure for pain thresholds, it is also influenced by factors of the examiner and the subject examined [12]. Some degree of variation between examiners is to be expected [3], and the consistency of results is increased notably if a single examiner is carrying out all measurements [13]. In veterinary medicine the nature of the animals investigated

* Correspondence: theresia.licka@vetmeduni.ac.at
[1]Equine Clinic, University of Veterinary Medicine Vienna (Vetmeduni Vienna), Veterinaerplatz 1, 1210 Vienna, Austria
[2]Department of Veterinary Clinical Science, Royal (Dick) School of Veterinary Studies, University of Edinburgh, Easter Bush, Edinburgh EH25 9RG, UK

is also an important factor. While the short term repeatability of algometric examinations is good overall, even these can vary within an individual [14]. Within an individual, an increase of the nocicpetive threshold has been noted from cranial to caudal along the back [4, 5]. Between individuals, factors such as sex, age and breed have been noted to influence algometry results, with a higher threshold described in young, heavy, non-Thoroughbred horses and geldings [4, 5].

A variety of algometer tips have been used in human and veterinary medicine. In human medicine algometer tips above the size of 1.6 mm are thought to measure the summation of sensation of deeper tissues [14–17], while algometer tips 0.2 mm diameter are thought to measure intraepidermal nerve endings [17], while larger algometer tips with surfaces of up to 2.1 cm2 are used to imitate the area of two finger tips [18]. The majority of studies in human and veterinary medicine are using tip sizes of 0.5 cm2 and 1 cm2 [4, 5, 11], but they have not yet been compared in the back of the horse.

The aim of the present study was to document the influence of tissue thickness on the penetration of algometric pressure and to compare these results using hemispherical and cylindrical algometer tips of different diameters.

Methods

Animals

Nine horses (seven geldings, two mares, 9–22 years, Standardbred Trotters and Warmblood horses) without a history of muscular problems, thoracolumbar pain, surgery, wounds or trauma of the back were used for this study. None of the horses was used for ridden exercise in the year prior to the data collection.

For the post mortem part of the study, six trunks of horses (three mares, three geldings, Warmbloods, Standarbred Trotters, Coldblood, 3–10 years) were obtained; in these cases euthanasia was carried out for reasons other than musculoskeletal problems; also these horses had no known history of, thoracolumbar pain, surgery, wounds or trauma of the back.

Equipment

Measurements were carried out using a Pain Test FDX 100 Algometer (Wagner Instruments) (Fig. 1) and results were noted in Newton (N). Six aluminium tips were specifically made for this study (ADT Anker Datentechnik GesmbH) three hemispherical and three cylindrical tips with surface areas of 0.5cm^2, 1cm^2, and 2 cm^2 (Fig. 2).

For the investigation of the post mortem specimens, a pressure sensor (FSR-152 NS) and a multimeter (Multikraft Multimeter VC 666) were used to translate the pressure exerted to the bottom of the into electrical resistance. In order to position the specimens in a standardized way, they were introduced into a Plexiglas cylinder (Fig. 3). The readings of the multimeter were documented using continuous video recording.

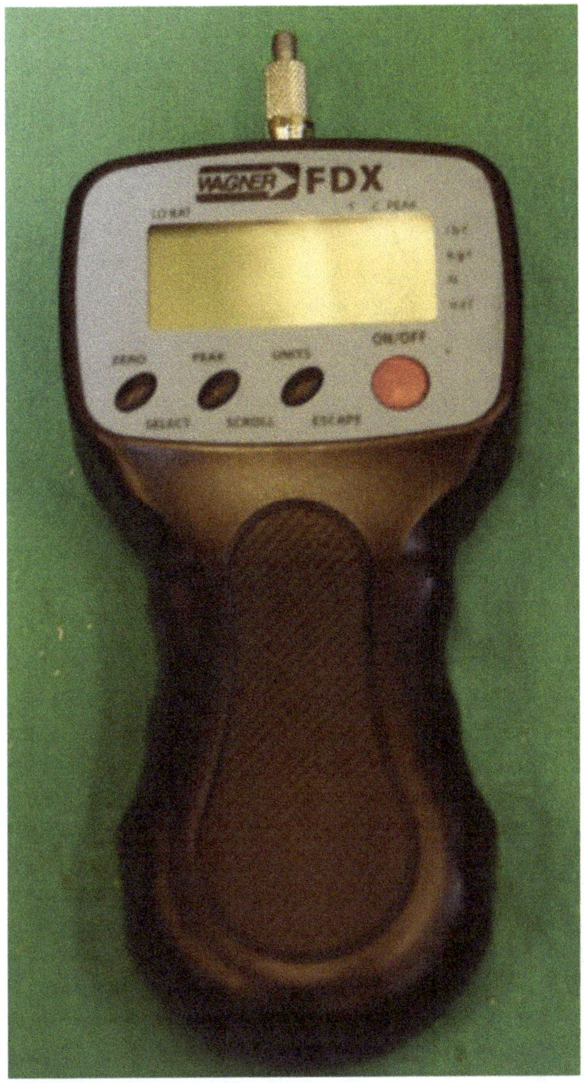

Fig. 1 The Algometer used in this study (Pain Test FDX 100, Wagner Instruments Inc., Greenwich, Conn., USA)

All algometric measurements were carried out by one investigator (UP), and the pressure threshold was measured. This represents the nociceptive threshold in the live horses, and the pressure transfer threshold in the post mortem specimens. At the start of the in vivo measurements horses were accustomed to manipulations in their back area, and a back examination was carried out. The ensuing algometric measurements were carried out in such an order, that the algometer tips as well as the localizations of the thoracolumbar region were always changing, in order to avoid habituation effects as much as possible. A

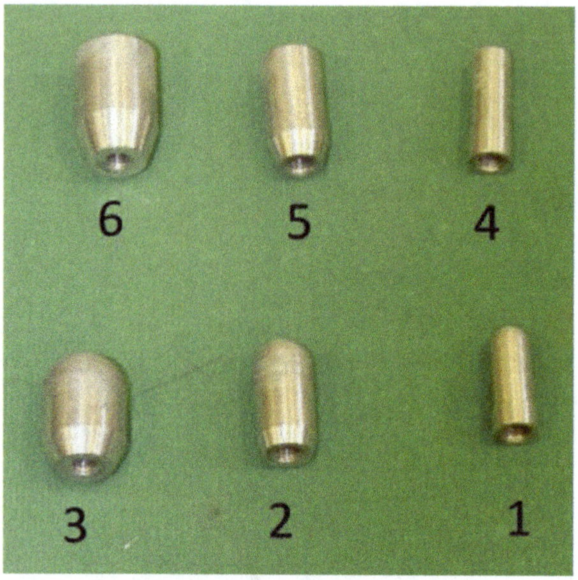

Fig. 2 The algometer tips used in this study, tips 1–3 with semisperical and tips 4–6 with cylindrical shape

total of 216 measurements were carried out in each individual horse, with six localizations on each side of the back examined with each of the six algometer tips. The localizations examined were marked with a chalk about 5 cm paramedian at the level of T14, T16, and T18, as well as at the level of L1, L3, and L5, based on detailed palpation of the dorsal spinous processes during induced arching of the back The algometer was used in a perpendicular orientation (Fig. 4), and at first was held light contact with the skin for about 3 s, to reduce any reaction due to startle effects. Afterwards the pressure was gradually increased in 2 s–3 s intervals based on the studies of Haussler and Erb [4, 5] as well as Buthe and Hertsch [3] in order to create smooth transitions without abrupt pressure changes. As a positive reaction indicative of reaching nociceptive threshold behaviors such as turning of the ears, looking back at the examiner, stepping away from the examiner, hollowing the back away from the pressure as well as the sudden lifting of a limb with a stamping the foot to the ground or kicking. After the algometric measurements the examined localization were assessed ultrasonographically. This was done after the algometry measurements to avoid effects of habituation and/or skin irritation.

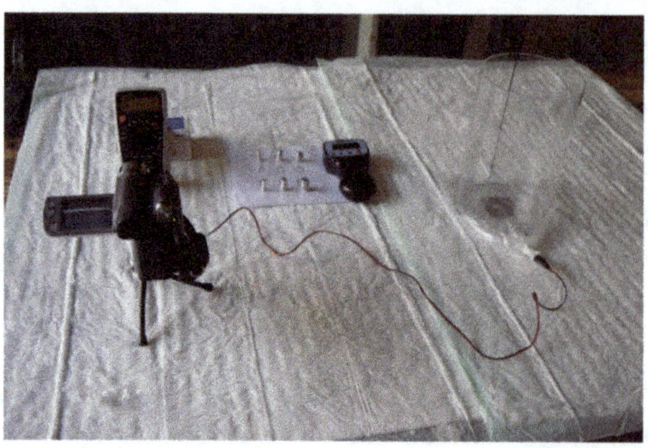

Fig. 3 Measurement set-up for the post mortem specimens. On the *left* there is multimeter and the video camera, in the *middle* is the algometer with the tips used and on the *right* is the pressure sensor below the plexiglass cylinder later containing the tissue section

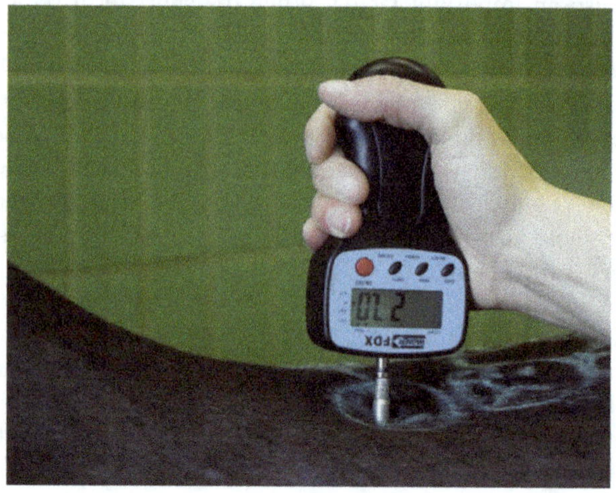

Fig. 4 Algometry measurement at the level of the 14th thoracic vertebra (Pain Test FDX 100 Algometer)

The postmortem specimens of the thoracolumbar region were prepared as follows: At the level of T14/T15, T18/L1, and L5/L6 transverse sections of all the tissues including the skin lateral to the dorsal spinous processes and dorsal to the ribs and the transverse processes respectively were carefully isolated. The resulting six sections with a diameter of about 20 cm were placed in the Plexiglas cylinder to avoid spreading of the tissues with the application of pressure. Prior to the measurement, the tissues were also assessed ultrasonographically. The different algometer tips were first applied at full tissue thickness, after removing the ventral half of the tissue at half the original tissue thickness and lastly with only the skin and the subcutaneous layers. The algometer was placed in the middle of the Plexiglas cylinder and pressure was exerted perpendicularly (Fig. 5). Results of the reduction in the electrical resistance of the pressure sensor placed below the tissue were noted at 5 N, 10 N, 15 N, 20 N, and 25 N.

In order to allow the calculation of the pressure sensor readings in ohm (Ω) of this setup into N, measurements of the algometer perpendicularly direct onto the pressure sensor were carried out.

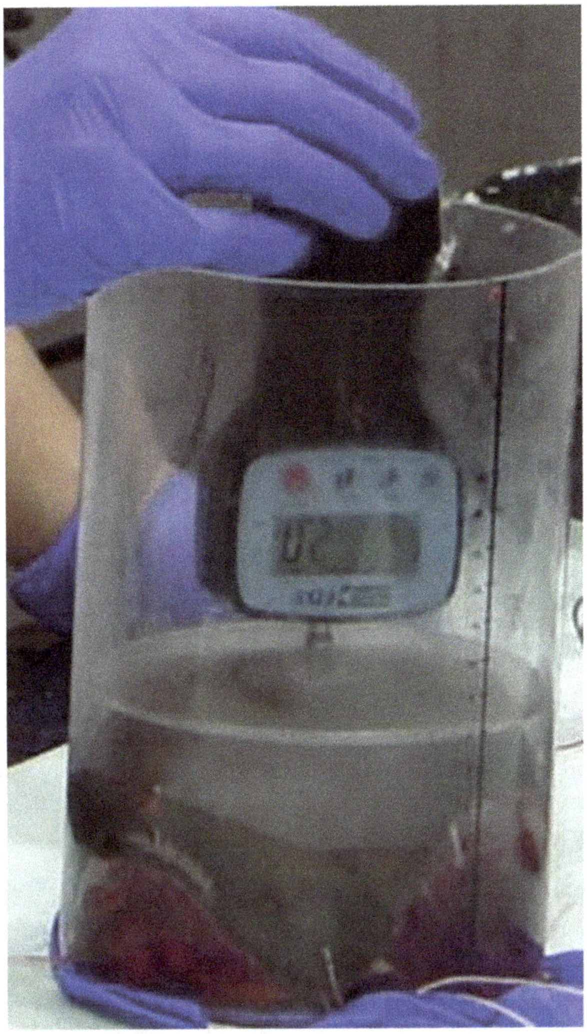

Fig. 5 Pressure application with the algometer to the middle of a back tissue section

Statistical analyses

For statistical analyses, the software R (R Version 3.1.2 (2014–10-31)) was used. Levels of significance were set at $p < 0.05$. Medians and quartiles were calculated and presented. Mean values and standard errors were calculated.

Results

There was no significant difference between body sides ($F(df = 1;1941) = 0.11$; $P = 736$), therefore the results were pooled.

In vivo

Influence of the surface area and shape of the algometer tips

Both the surface area (0.5 cm2/1 cm2/2cm^2; Chi^2(df = 2) = 1147.08, $p < 0.001$) as well as the shape of the tips (hemispherical vs cylindrical; Chi^2(df = 1) = 43.64, $p < 0.001$) showed an effect on the pressure threshold. The cylindrical tip with a surface of 0.5cm^2 resulted in the lowest pressure threshold (median = 19.6 N [16.6, 23.9]), while the hemispherical tip with 2cm^2 surface resulted in the highest pressure threshold (median = 34.0 N [30.0, 40.0]). The tips with a surface of 1cm^2 lead to very similar results (hemispherical median 25.9 N [23.6, 31.7], cylindrical median = 25.1 N [23.0, 29.8]). The regression analysis showed the differences comparing the shape (hemispherical vs cylindrical) with a coefficient of B = 2.31 (SE = 0.35), while the regression analysis of the surface areas resulted in an increase of B = 6.51 (SE = 0.35) between 0.5cm^2 and 1cm^2, as well as B = 11.83 (SE = 0.35) between 1cm^2 and 2cm^2. Using the tips with the 2 cm2 surface, the widest distribution of results was obtained (Fig. 6).

The effect of anatomical location and tissue thickness

Tissue thickness had a noticeable effect on the pressure threshold as well as on the spread of the results. With increasing tissue thickness (measured sonographically) the pressure pain threshold increased (Chi^2(df = 1) = 2.94, $p = 0.086$), as well as the variability of the results. A larger effect was found for the influence of the anatomical location (Chi^2(df = 5) = 119.63, $p < 0.001$) with an increase of the pressure threshold at a tissue thickness of 7 cm (mean 27.59 N 95%Ci = [23.19, 31.99]) and at a tissue thickness of 11 cm (mean 29.04 N 95%Ci = [24.65, 33.42]). With a regression coefficient of B = 0.04 (SE = 0.02) pressure threshold increased with increasing tissue thickness, as is the case from cranial to caudal

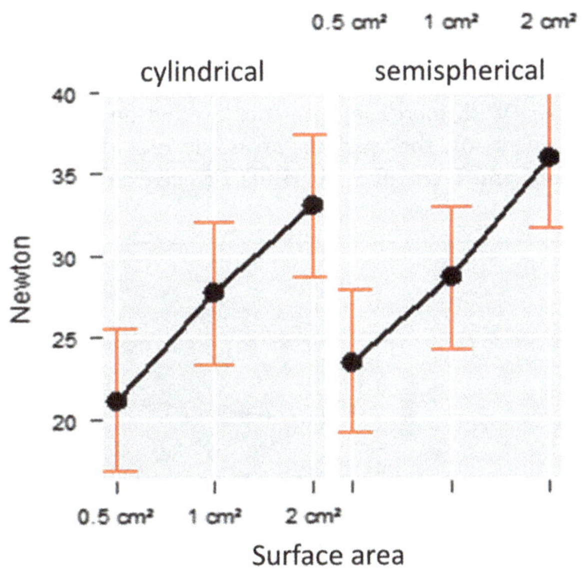

Fig. 6 Linear regression of the pressure pain threshold of the thoracolumbar region of horses using 6 different algometer tips (cylindrical, hemispherical; surface area 0.5 cm2, 1 cm2, 2 cm2) The mean values and the confidence intervals are given

along the thoracolumbar region. The largest increase in pressure threshold was found between L3 and L5, with a regression coefficient of B = 5.08 (SE = 0.66) (Fig. 7).

In vitro

There was a linear relationship ($Chi^2(df = 1) = 27{,}428.25$, $p < 0.001$) between the pressure exerted onto the pressure sensor and the resulting decrease in electrical resistance with a regression coefficient B = −0.12 (SE = 0.00). Pressure of 5 N directly onto the pressure sensor created 3.90 kΩ 95%Ci = [3.63, 4.18], 10 N 2.14 kΩ 95%Ci = [1.99, 2.29], 15 N 1.16 kΩ 95%Ci = [1.08, 1.25], 20 N 0.64 kΩ 95%Ci = [0.59, 0.68] and 25 N 0.35 kΩ 95%Ci = [0.32, 0.38]. Based on the manufacturer's description of an inverted exponential function characteristic for the sensor the results in kΩ were transformed logarithmically.

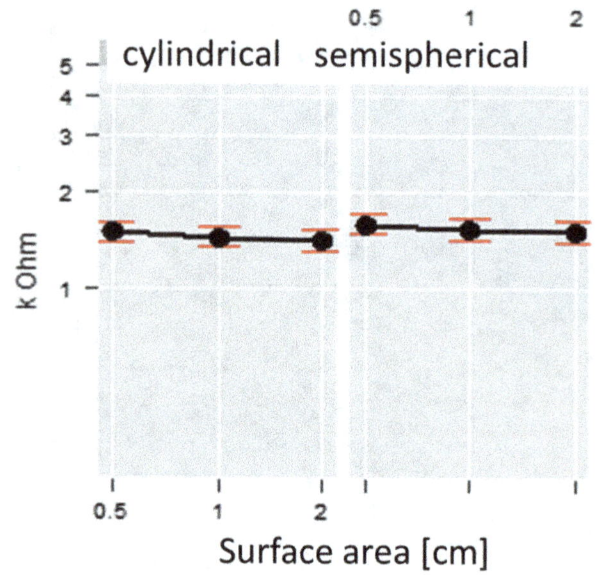

Fig. 8 Linear regression of the effects of surface area and shape of the algometer tips on tissue pressure transmission

The effect of tip surface area and tip shape

The first recording of pressure below the tissue specimen shows a marked influence of the size of the tip surface, with smaller surface areas transmitting pressure at much lower levels than larger surface areas. This effect is significantly independent of tissue thickness ($Chi^2(df = 2) = 1836.90$, $p < 0.001$). The shape of the tip only created small differences ($p = 0.015$ ($Chi^2(df = 1) = 5.97$)) in pressure transmission through the tissue (Fig. 8), with differences of 0.1 N–0.15 N between cylindrical and semispherical tips. During the measurements of the skin and subcutaneous tissues only the smallest variation of results was obtained, with results of median 0.6 N [0.5, 0.7] at 0.5 cm^2, 0.9 N [0.7, 1.0] at 1 cm^2 and 1.1 N [1.0, 1.2] at 2cm^2. The difference between cylindrical tips (median 0.9 N [0.7, 1.1]) and hemispherical tips (median 0.8 N [0.6, 1.0]) was much smaller. With increasing pressure exerted on the tissues the effect of the surface areas decreased (between 0.5 cm^2 and 1 cm^2 B = −0.04 (0.02); between 1 cm^2 and 2 cm^2 B = −0.06 (0.02); $Chi^2(df = 2) = 8.31$, $p = 0.016$), and the effect of the shape decreased as well, with a tendency of cylindrical tips transmitting more pressure than hemispherical tips (B = 0.06 (SE = 0.02); $p = 0.003$, $Chi^2(df = 1) = 8.81$).

Effect of anatomical location and tissue thickness

There was a linear relationship between the pressure transmission and the thickness of the tissue ($Chi^2(df = 2) = 4171.13$, $p < 0.001$) with a regression coefficient of the effect of tissue thickness on the pressure transmission of B = −0.48 (SE = 0.01) between full and half thickness tissue samples, and B = −1.92 (SE = 0.01) between half thickness and skin/subcutaneous samples (Fig. 9). The marked effect of the anatomical location ($Chi^2(df = 2) = 25.46$, $p < 0.001$) was again

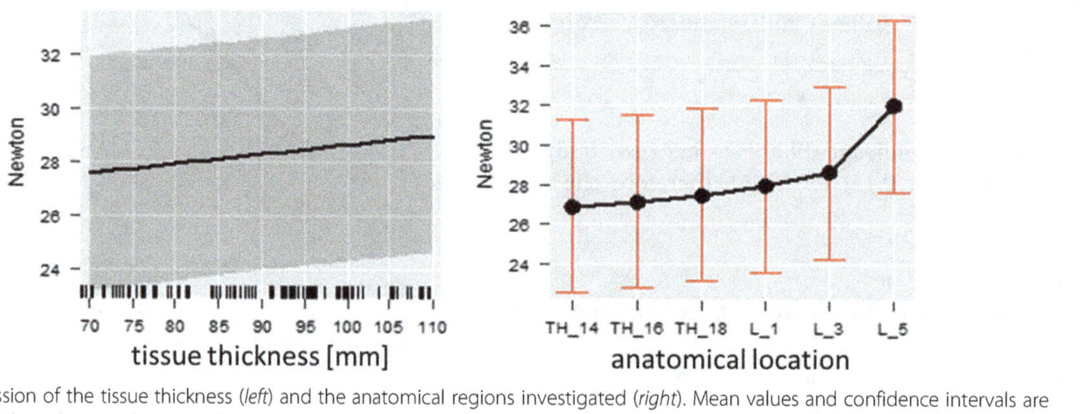

Fig. 7 Linear regression of the tissue thickness (*left*) and the anatomical regions investigated (*right*). Mean values and confidence intervals are given. A clear parallel can be seen between the two

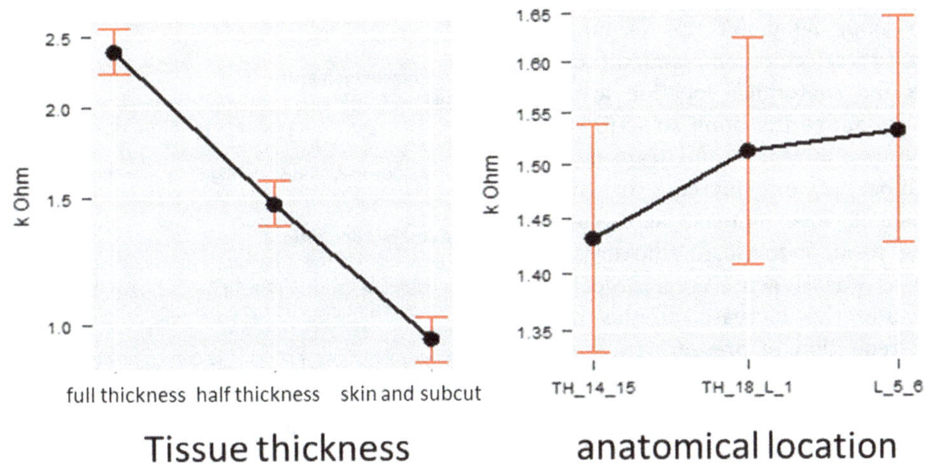

Fig. 9 Linear regression of the effects of tissue thickness (*left*) and anatomical location (*right*) on the pressure transmission from an algometer through thoracolumbar tissues of horses. The reduction of kΩ values indicates an increase in pressure measured below the tissue

noted, with pressure transmission decreasing from cranial to caudal, both between T14/T15 and T18/L1 (B = 0.05; SE = 0.01) and between T18/L1 and L5/L6 (B = 0.07; SE = 0.01).

Discussion

In the present study we have sought to carry out the algometry in a standardized fashion, based on the current literature [19]. However, we did not repeat the measurements even though this might have increased the value of our findings. The high number of measurements in each live horse (36 times 6) did not allow a full measurement repetition, but, as an indication of repeatability of results single measurements might have been repeated without creating undue stress to the horses. This should be seen as a limitation of the study.

Algometry is a non invasive method to quantify pain sensation in horses quantitatively and easily [9, 20]. However, algometry is not absolutely objective, as it depends on the pain reaction of the subject studied [12] and therefore the different reactivity individuals will create different results even though the pain experienced might be the same. The individuality of sensation as well as the individuality of reaction to sensation has been discussed repeatedly in humans [21], as well as in animals [12, 20, 22, 23]. Breed differences might be explained by a genetic selection for the coding of neurotransmitters and neuromodulators [24] or by a selection for placid demeanor. In the present study, the live horses were Warmbloods and Standardbred Trotters, and the results showed relatively small variations, indicating that these breeds might not be too different in their sensation as well as in their reactivity. The time of day also appears to influence the pain sensation of horses [22], and there is the possibility that horses might learn to avoid pressure by showing an earlier reaction. In the present study horses were measured during daylight hours over two consecutive days, but no standardized time was used, as this would not have been logistically possible.

It is not surprising that the results of the present study showed smaller algometer tips to lead to lower pressure thresholds than larger tips, similar to round surfaces being tolerated better than surfaces with an edge. Parallel results were found in the post mortem study, where the pressure transmission was similarly affected by surface area and shape. The results of present study using the 1 cm2 surface tips are comparable to other studies also using tips of this surface area [2, 4, 5, 9, 20, 22, 25, 26]. However, no other study used aluminium tips similar to the ones used in the present study, but all of them used a rubber surface, the mechanical qualities of which have not been reported. As the rubber is expected to have some elasticity, and this elasticity might potentially be variable in different temperatures, we elected to use the hard and stable material of aluminium for our investigation. Other algometry investigations have used tips of 2 mm to 14 mm in diameter [3, 10, 11, 23], and these results cannot be directly compared with the results of the present study, as the effect of surface area could be clearly shown. Smaller tips reduced the pressure threshold in the present study as well as in previously published studies [23, 27] and they also created the most consistent results.

In human algometry, surface areas of 0.5 cm^2 or 1 cm^2 have been used successfully for quantification of pain in the deeper layers of muscles [12, 15]. Small algometer tips (e.g. 0,2 mm diameter) deform the skin surface and activate intraepidermal nerve endings before relevant pressure is achieved in the deeper tissues, whereas surface areas of 1cm^2 create a skin deformation as well as pressure in the deeper tissues, allowing also the evaluation of these deeper tissues [17]. For the measurement of muscular pain, algometer tips of more than 1.6 mm diameter are therefore recommended [16].

Tissue thickness and anatomical location are closely related as the tissues above the bony structures of the back (ribs in the thoracic region and transverse processes in the lumbar region) increase in thickness from cranial to caudal. This increase in tissue thickness is mainly due to an increase in thickness of the long back muscle as was shown sonographically [28]. In the present study the increase of the pressure threshold (i.e. the reduction of pressure transmission) from cranial to caudal was clearly documented in vivo as well as in vitro. The effect of an increase in the pressure threshold in the present study was most obvious in the lumbar region; this is similar to other studies [11, 20, 22, 29]. This marked increase in pressure threshold the lumbar region is not the consequence of a marked increase in tissue thickness at this level. For humans, where a similar increase was found, a variation in the density of neurovascular structures at this level is discussed [29, 30].

The tissue quality in addition to the tissue thickness is of relevance for the transmission of pressure exerted by an algometer. In the present study, all of the measurements in vivo were carried out over muscled areas of the back, while the pressure threshold over bony areas was found to be much smaller in a human study [14], as well as in a study on the pressure threshold in horses over the dorsal spinous processes [3]. This is reflected in the results of the in vitro part of the present study, where the skin and subcutaneous tissue samples showed direct, nearly unattenuated pressure transmission. In this context it is important though, that the reduction in muscle mass commonly present in horses with prolonged thoracolumbar pain and the reduction of the pressure pain threshold due to the reduction of muscle volume are not interpreted as two independent indications of thoracolumbar pain and dysfunction.

Conclusions

Based on the results of this study, tissue thickness and tissue character as well as anatomical location should be considered for the interpretation of algometry results of the equine back, with cranial thoracolumbar areas, as well as areas with less tissue thickness, especially less muscle, creating lower pressure thresholds even in horses without any clinical signs of back pain. The algometer tip used should also be carefully chosen regarding its shape and surface area, with smaller tips creating lower pressure thresholds, and rounded tips creating higher pressure thresholds.

Abbreviations

L: Lumbar vertebra; T: Thoracic vertebra

Acknowledgements

We would like to acknowledge the personnel of the Institute of Pathology and the Clinic for Horses at the University of Veterinary Medicine Vienna for their cooperation during the course of this study.
The study was funded through in house funding.

Authors' contibutions

UP developed the study protocol, carried out the data acquisition, and interpreted the data together with TL and wrote the manuscript draft. TL conceived of the study, and participated in its design and coordination, interpreted the data together with UP and revised and finalized the manuscript. Both authors read and approved the final manuscript.

Competing interests

The authors declare that they have no competing interests.

References

1. Peloso JG, Mundy GD, Cohen ND. Prevalence of, and factors associated with, musculoskeletal racing injuries of thoroughbreds. J Am Vet Med Assoc. 1994;204:620–6.
2. Haussler KK, Hill AE, Frisbie DD, McIlwraith CW. Determination and use of mechanical nociceptive thresholds of the thoracic limb to assess pain associated with induced osteoarthritis of the middle carpal joint in horses. Am J Vet Res. 2007;68:1167–76.
3. Buthe A, Hertsch B. Objektivierung der Stempelprobe als Bestandteil der klinischen Rückenuntersuchung zur Diagnose des Kissing Spines- Syndroms mittels Algometrie in Korrelation mit Röntgenbefunden. Der Praktische Tierarzt. 2002;83:436–40.
4. Haussler KK, Erb HN. Pressure algometry for the detection of induced back pain in horses: a preliminary study. Equine Vet J. 2006;37:76–81.
5. Haussler KK, Erb HN. Mechanical nociceptive thresholds in the axial skeleton of horses. Equine Vet J. 2006;38:70–5.
6. Jeffcott LB. Historical perspective and clinical indications. Vet Clin N Am Equine Pract. 1999;15:1–11.
7. Ranner W, Gerhards H. Diagnostik bei Verdacht auf Rückenerkrankungen beim Pferd. Pferdeheilkunde. 2001;17:225–32.
8. Veres-Nyeki K. Recognition and assessment of pain in horses. Proceedings of the 13th international congress of the world equine veterinary Association 2013.
9. Varcoe-Cocks K, Sagar KN, Jeffcott LB, McGowan CM. Pressure algometry to quantify muscle pain in racehorses with suspected sacroiliac dysfunction. Equine Vet J. 2006;38:558–62.
10. Kalinowski S, Rohn K, Kreling K, Stadler P. Die Therapie von Pferden mit Rückenproblemen in einer Infrarot- Strahlungskabine. Pferdeheilkunde. 2008;24:313–24.
11. Matzhold U. Untersuchung der Druckschmerzhaftigkeit von myofaszialen Triggerpunkten entlang des Rückens von Lipizzanern. Austria: Diploma Thesis, Veterinary University Vienna; 2008.
12. Ylinen J. Pressure algometry. Aust J Physiother. 2007;53:207.
13. Nussbaum EL, Downes L. Reliability of clinical pressure pain algometric measurements obtained on consecutive days. Phys Ther. 1998;78:160–9.
14. Kosek E, Ekholm J, Hansson P. Pressure pain thresholds in different tissues in one body region. The influence of skin sensitivity in pressure algometry. Scand J Rehabil Med. 1999;31:89–93.
15. Fischer AA. Pressure algometry over normal muscles. Standard values, validity and reproducibility of pressure threshold. Pain. 1987;30:115–26.
16. Takahashi K, Taguchi T, Itoh K, Okada K, Kawakita K, Mizumura K. Influence of surface anesthesia on the pressure pain threshold measured with different-sized probes. Somatosens Mot Res. 2005;22:299–305.
17. Treede R-D, Rolke R, Andrews K, Magerl W. Pain elicited by blunt pressure: neurobiological basis and clinical relevance. Pain. 2002;98:235–40.
18. Stohler CS, Ashton-Miller JA. Servo-controlled stepped and ramped mechanical tissue algometry. J Biomech. 2007;40:1635–40.
19. Haussler KK. Objective measures of somatic pain and the effects of manual therapies in horses. Proc Am Assoc Equine Pract. 2009;235–253.
20. Haussler KK, Erb HN. Pressure algometry: objective assessment of back pain

and effects of chiropractic treatment. 49th annual convention of the American Association of Equine Practitioners 2003.

21. Pöntinen PJ. Reliability, validity, reproducibility of algometry in diagnosis of active and latent tender spots and trigger points. J Musculoskelet Pain. 1998;6:61–71.
22. De Heus P, Van Oossanen G, Van Dierendonck MC. A pressure algometer is a useful tool to objectively monitor the effect of diagnostic palpation by a physiotherapist in warmblood horses. J Equine Vet. 2010;30:310–21.
23. Harris LK, Murrel JC, Van Klink EMG, Whay HR. Influence of experimental protocol on response rate and repeatability of mechanical threshold testing in dogs. Vet J. 2015;204:82–7.
24. Bagshaw CS, Ralston SL, Fischer H. Behavioral and physiological effect of orally administered tryptophan on horses subjected to acute isolation stress. Appl Anim Behav Sci. 1994;40:1–12.
25. Biermann NM, Riedler N, Buchner HHF. The effect of pulsed electromagnetic fields on back pain in polo ponies evaluated by pressure algometry and flexion testing- a randomized, double-blind, placebo-controlled trial. J Equine Vet. 2014;34:500–7.
26. Sullivan K, Hill A, Haussler KK. Effect of different treatment modalities on spinal Nociceptive thresholds in horses. Proceedings of the 53rd annual convention of the American Association of Equine Practitioners 2007.
27. Garell CP, McGillis SLB, Greenspan JD. Mechanical response properties of nociceptors innervating feline hairy skin. J Neurophysiol. 1996;75:1177–89.
28. Frey R. Sonographische Untersuchungen an Strukturen des Pferderückens. Switzerland: Doctoral Thesis of the Veterinary Faculty University Berne; 1999.
29. Vanderween L, Oostendorp RAB, Vaes P, Duquet W. Pressure algometry in manual therapy. Man Ther. 1996;1:258–65.
30. Keating L, Lubke C, Powell V, Young T, Souvlis T, Jull G. Mid- thoracic tenderness: a comparison of pressure pain threshold between spinal regions, in asymptomatic subjects. Man Ther. 2001;6:34–9.

17

Multipulse transcranial electrical stimulation (TES): normative data for motor evoked potentials in healthy horses

Sanne Lotte Journée[1], Henricus Louis Journée[2*], Cornelis Marinus de Bruijn[3] and Cathérine John Ghislaine Delesalle[4]

Abstract

Background: There are indications that transcranial electrical stimulation (TES) assesses the motor function of the spinal cord in horses in a more sensitive and reproducible fashion than transcranial magnetic stimulation (TMS). However, no normative data of TES evoked motor potentials (MEP) is available.

Results: In this prospective study normative data of TES induced MEP wave characteristics (motor latency times (MLT); amplitude and waveform) was obtained from the extensor carpi radialis (ECR) and tibial cranialis (TC) muscles in a group of healthy horses to create a reference frame for functional diagnostic purposes. For the 12 horses involved in the study 95% confidence intervals for MLTs were 16.1–22.6 ms and 31.9–41.1 ms for ECR and TC muscles respectively. Intra-individual coefficients of variation (CV) and mean of MLTs were: ECR: 2.2–8,2% and 4.5% and TC: 1.4–6.3% and 3.5% respectively. Inter-individual CVs for MLTs were higher, though below 10% on all occasions.
The mean ± sd of MEP amplitudes was respectively 3.61 ± 2.55 mV (ECR muscle left) and 4.53 ± 3.1 mV (right) and 2.66 ± 2.22 mV (TC muscle left) and 2.55 ± 1.85 mV (right). MLTs showed no significant left versus right differences.
All MLTs showed significant ($p < 0.05$) voltage dependent decreases with slope coefficients of linear regression for ECR: − 0.049; − 0.061 ms/V and TC: − 0.082; − 0.089 ms/V (left; right). There was a positive correlation found between height at withers and MLTs in all 4 muscle groups. Finally, reliable assessment of MEP characteristics was for all muscle groups restricted to a transcranial time window of approximately 15–19 ms.

Conclusions: TES is a novel and sensitive technique to assess spinal motor function in horses. It is easy applicable and highly reproducible. This study provides normative data in healthy horses on TES induced MEPs in the extensor carpi radialis and tibialis cranialis muscles bilaterally. No significant differences between MLTs of the left and right side could be demonstrated. A significant effect of stimulation voltage on MLTs was found. No significant effect of height at the withers could be found based upon the results of the current study. A study in which both TMS and TES are applied on the same group of horses is needed.

Keywords: Transcranial electric stimulation, TES, TMS, MEP, Neurology, Horses, Spinal cord function

Background

After transcranial magnetic stimulation (TMS) was introduced in equine medicine by Mayhew and Washborn in 1996, the method evolved into a diagnostic tool used to assess the motor function of the spinal cord in horses [1–3]. Lesions of the spinal cord are mostly characterized by a significant increase of motor latency times (MLT) and a decrease of muscular evoked potential (MEP) amplitudes in response to TMS [4]. The TMS technique is based on the induction of electrical currents by a strong magnetic pulse, created by a coil, which is placed on the forehead of the horse with subsequent activation of axons in the motor cortex taking place [5, 6]. The generated action potentials are relayed by upper motor neurons (UMNs) before further conduction takes place along the motor pathway of the corticospinal tract, the lower motor

* Correspondence: hljournee@gmail.com
[2]Department of Neurosurgery, University Groningen, University Medical Center Groningen, Hanzeplein 1, 9713 GZ Groningen, The Netherlands
Full list of author information is available at the end of the article

neurons (LMN) and finally the motor nerves to the skeletal muscles.

Recently, our group has published an alternative stimulation technique: transcranial electrical stimulation (TES) [7].

In contrast to TMS, the TES technique entails direct application of an electrical current to a pair of needle electrodes, which are subcutaneously inserted on the forehead of the horse. In contrast to TMS, the TES technique bypasses predominantly the route via the motor cortex of the brain [8] to the pyramidal tract. This explains why the technique is preferred over TMS to be applied in human patients under generalized anesthesia [9]. Indeed, unlike TMS, TES predominantly targets direct stimulation of the corticospinal tract. Corticospinal axons in humans and primates are oriented perpendicular to the cortical surface. Anodal transcranial stimulation depolarizes corticospinal axons directly and has a lower stimulation threshold than cathodal stimulation [5, 10–12]. These direct action potentials can be recorded as d-waves [7]. Cell bodies of UMNs are predominantly bypassed and less influenced by modulating inputs from the cortex of the brain [8, 13–17]. This is in contrast to the elicited action potentials in the cortex from TMS that are relayed via UMNs and are recorded as indirect waves, i-waves, in the corticospinal tract [18]. In TMS, d-waves are incidentally also generated, however these are less dominant than i-waves [16, 17]. Like in TMS, TES has to be performed in sedated horses [19, 20] while sedation was reported not to affect MLTs [20].

In our previous prospective study, we showed that there are clear indications that the TES technique is less sensitive to cortical function due to direct stimulation of the corticospinal tract [7]. The applied TES multipulse train stimulation protocol helps to overcome hyperpolarization induced by sedation, which is a disadvantage of a single pulse stimulation protocol applied in the TMS technique. Indeed, the multipulse train stimulation protocol is more robust, since each stimulation pulse is able to produce multiple descending volleys of d- and i-waves in the pyramidal tract [11, 12, 21]. These initiate spatial and temporal summations of excitatory postsynaptic potentials (epsp). This summation process from multipulse stimulation results in a powerful depolarization of LMNs.

Normative data on TMS in horses has been published by Nollet et al. [3]. However, no normative data is available for TES in horses. The aim of the current study was 1) to obtain normative data of MLTs, waveform, and amplitudes of TES induced muscular evoked potentials (MEP), as well as earlier reported boundaries of the transcranial time windows [7] in muscle groups of four extremities in a group of healthy horses to create an initial frame of reference for clinical diagnostic purposes and 2) to study the effect of body side (left versus right), stimulation voltage intensity and height at withers of the horses on MEP characterizing parameters.

Methods

Twelve healthy client owned warmblood horses, consisting of 6 gelding and 6 mares, aged: 10.7 ± 5.5 years (mean ± sd) were included in the study. No abnormalities were found during clinical neurological examination. The height at withers was 160.8 ± 10 cm (mean ± sd). The animal ethics committee of the University of Groningen, The Netherlands approved the study protocol (DEC6440A).

Horses were prepared as previously described [7]. Sedation was performed in all horses ($n = 12$), each time by I.V. administration of detomidine (Detosedan, AST Farma B.V., Oudewater, The Netherlands) and butorphanol (Butomidor, AST Farma B.V., Oudewater, The Netherlands) (both 1.5–2.0 µg/kg bwt in total). Two needle electrodes (L 35 mm, Ø 0.45 mm, type RMN35/0.45 Electrocap BV, Nieuwkoop, Netherlands) were inserted subcutaneously parallel to each other and caudo-rostrally on the forehead (Fig. 1). The needle electrodes were separated 5 cm from each other, with their middle points 2.5 cm bilateral from the central location Cz on the forehead. The horses returned to their owners after completion of the procedure and a final clinical examination.

TES was performed using biphasic multipulse trains using a constant voltage of a human intraoperative neurophysiological monitoring system (Neuro-Guard JS Center, Bedum, The Netherlands). A bandpass filter was used with a high pass filter of 50 Hz, and a low pass filter of 2500 Hz (3 dB cut-off level). Muscular evoked potentials (MEPs) were recorded bilaterally from subcutaneously placed needle electrodes over the musculus extensor carpi radialis (ECR) (10 and 20 cm above the os carpi accessorium) and the musculus tibialis cranialis (TC) (10 and 20 cm above the medial malleolus). These electrodes were connected to the differential inputs of the physiological amplifiers of the measuring system. A ground needle electrode was placed subcutaneously in the neck at the right side of the horse. Multipulse TES was performed with 3 biphasic pulses per train (ppt), pulse width (pw) of 0.1 ms/ phase and interpulse interval (ipi) of 1.3 ms. The stimulation voltage was increased using a stepwise protocol: 0, 2, 4, 6, 8, 10, 12, 14, 16, 18, 20, 22, 25, 30, 35, 40, 45, 50, 60, 70, 80, 90, 100, 110, 120, 130, 140, 150, 160, 170, 180, 190, 200 V. At each voltage, transcranial stimulation was performed twice. When transcranial motor thresholds (MT) were reached for both muscle groups, stimulation was continued to MT + 50 V or otherwise stopped at 200 V. At each occasion of stimulation, the motor responses were recorded for later retrieval of MEP amplitudes, MLTs and waveform morphology.

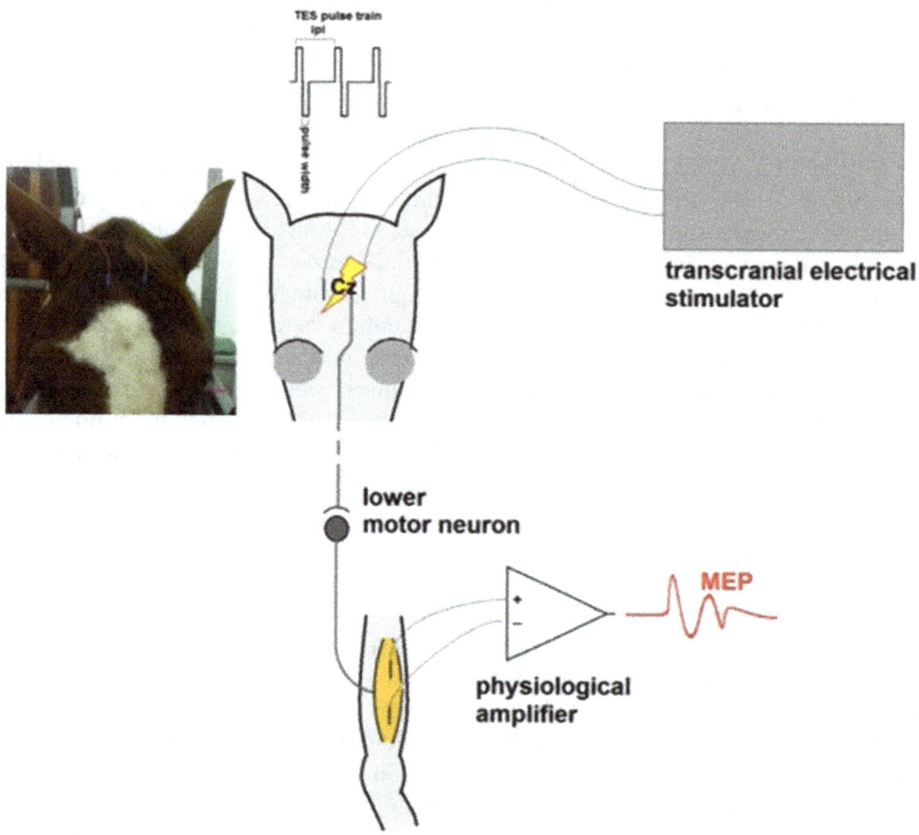

Fig. 1 Schematic drawing of the TES-MEP set-up. A transcranial electrical stimulator is connected to subcutaneously inserted needle electrodes bilaterally from the vertex of the skull. A multipulse stimulation consists of 3 biphasic pulses/train, pulse width 0.1 ms/phase, ipi = 1.3 ms. Elicited action potentials in corticospinal axons cross the midline at the decussatio pyramis and are conveyed to LMNs that relay to peripheral motor axons. After passing the neuromuscular junction muscular motor potentials are generated in muscle fibers and recorded at a pair of needle electrodes that are connected to a physiological amplifier

MEP parameters

Considered parameters were: MLT, MEP amplitude and waveform morphology. The MLTs $MLT_{n,i,m}$ were defined as 'the time lag between the onsets of electrical stimulation and MEP response' when these were unambiguously distinguishable from baseline noise level. Indices n, i and m refer to the n-th MEP, case number and muscle group in one of 4 extremities being ECR or TC. The amplitude $A_{n,i,m}$. is the top-top amplitude of MEPs within the time window, between cessation of the stimulation artefact and onset of extracranially elicited late MEP responses. This time window precludes interference by extracranially elicited late MEP responses when analyzing transcranial MEPs [7]. We established a time delay of 0.7 ms between the trigger pulse and the onset of the stimulator trigger signal and actual start of the TES pulse train by an oscilloscope. The MLT values were subsequently corrected for the trigger delay. The waveforms are characterized by the number of phases.

The transcranial time window (TCW) is defined as 'the time interval between the onsets of the transcranial and extracranial MEP components 'and computed at a TES voltage of MT + 20 V. For an in depth description of the determination of the transcranial time windows for the ECR and TC muscle MEPs we refer to the previously published scouting study [7]. MLTs and MEP amplitudes are analyzed within the TCW.

Statistical analyses

Statistical analysis was performed with SPSS™ software, version 20.0.0, IBM™. A descriptive analysis was performed on the MLTs, amplitude and waveform morphology of the recorded MEPs. The normality of the relevant differences was graphically assessed using qq-plots. The conclusions of the graphical assessment were confirmed with a Shapiro-Wilk test. Overall, the assumption of normality could be accepted. For each case i and muscle group m, mean $MLT_{i,m}$ and standard deviation $SD_{i,m}$ were computed as 6 latency values of the latency data pairs from repeated stimulations at 10, 20 and 30 V above MT respectively. The MLT has its center point at MT + 20 V representing a common stimulation voltage that applies to the averages of 6 MLT values.

The reproducibility of the MLT measurements, expressing their intra- and inter-individual variability, was computed.

The mean MLT_m, standard deviation SD_m and coefficients of variation, CV_m, were computed from $MLT_{i,m}$ and $SD_{i,m}$ for all $N = 12$ cases. $SD_{intra,i,m}$ is the intra-individual standard deviation and was used for computation of the mean intra-individual standard deviation $mSD_{intra,m}$.

Left/right differences of MLTs and amplitudes were tested by a paired t-test with zero difference as a null hypothesis.

The voltage dependency of MLT_m was approximated by linear regression analysis. To exclude inter-individual variations of the MLTs, the $6 \times 12 = 72$ values were subtracted by $MLT_{i,m}$ prior to further processing. Theoretically, the expectation value of zero is at MT + 20 V.

The dependency of MLT_m values on the height at withers was approximated by linear regression analysis.

A significance level of $p \leq 5\%$ and confidence interval of 95% was applied throughout the study.

Results

The measurements were successfully performed in all horses on all four limbs.

Recorded normative values for MEP parameters

Table 1 provides an overview of normative data for MLTs, MEP amplitudes and waveform morphology recorded in ECR and TC muscles on the left and right side. MLTs showed no left versus right differences. Values of MLT were between 16.1–22.6 ms for the ECR and 31.9–41.1 ms for the TC muscles and were statistically equal within 95% confidence intervals. Intra-individual coefficients of variation, CV, for MLTs were low; their range and mean being 2.2–8,2% and 4.5% for the ECR and 1.4–6.3% and 3.5% for the TC. Inter-individual CVs for MLTs were higher, however below 10% on all occasions.

Only in the thoracic limb muscle groups the MEP amplitudes showed a left-right difference ($p < 0.05$) in favor of the right side.

MEP waveforms were 2- or 3-phasic in about 80% of cases, regardless the muscle group. The remaining 20% were polyphasic, while a single MEP in the right TC muscle group was monophasic.

Transcranial time windows

The 95% confidence intervals of the TCW were 15.8–19. 0 ms (left) and 15.7–20.3 ms (right) for the ECR and 14. 9–18.0 ms (left) and 15.1–18.4 ms (right) for the TC.

Analyzed correlations

There was a clear voltage dependent decrease of MLTs, as depicted in Fig. 2 and Table 2.

All correlation factors were significant in the 4 muscle groups and most pronounced for the pelvic limb muscles. The slopes of the regression lines of the thoracic limb latency times were less steep with coefficients of – 0.049 (left) and – 0.061 ms/V (right), compared to those of the pelvic

Table 1 Overview of the MLTs, MEP amplitude and number of phases per muscle group

Muscle group			ECR		TC	
			left	right	left	right
MLT (ms)	m		19.70	19.10	36.17	36.32
	SD | CV		1.48 | 0.075	0.83 | 0.042	2.12 | 0.059	2.40 | 0.066
	SD_{intra} | CV_{intra}		0.83 | 0.042	0.89 | 0.047	1.23 | 0.051	1.21 | 0.033
	m-1.96 SD		16.8	16.1	31.9	31.5
	m + 1.96 SD		22.6	22.1	40.4	41.1
MEP amplitude (mV)	m		3.61	4.53	2.66	2.55
	SD | CV		2.55 | 0.71	3.10 | 0.68	2.22 | 0.83	1.85 | 0.73
	paired difference left-right	m	−0.93		0.11	
		SD	1.15		1.10	
		sig	0.017*		0.75	
Number of phases	biphasic		7	5	3	6
	triphasic		3	6	7	3
	four-phasic		2	1	1	1
	polyphasic (> 4)		–	–	1	1

MLTs are characterized by mean (m), standard deviation (SD), coefficient of variation (CV) mean intra-individual standard deviation (SD_{intra}) being the average of SD_i over 12 cases, where SD_i is the standard deviation belonging to MLT_i, and mean ±1.96 SD delineating 95% probability ranges. MEP amplitudes are given as mean (m), SD and CV together with the mean (m), standard deviation (SD) and significance (sig) of paired MEP amplitude differences between the left and right muscle groups. CV is the coefficient of variation of mean MLTs. CV_{intra} is the coefficient of variation of mean paired MLT differences. *) significant for $p \leq 0.05$
*)significant for $p \leq 0.05$

limb muscles, with coefficients of – 0.082 (left) and – 0. 089 ms/V (right). No left-right differences were found. For a stimulation voltage increase of 20 V, the reduction in MLTs for the ECR was about – 1.5 ms and – 2.5 ms for the TC muscles. The reproducibility of a latency measurement is computed as the average of the standard errors of mean of the 12 cases. This yielded for the ECR: 0.34 ms (left), 0. 36 ms (right) and bilateral mean: 0.35 ms, and for the TC: 0.50 ms, (left), 0.53 (right) and bilateral mean 0.52 ms.

With respect to height at withers, only a significant correlation with MLTs for the left TC muscle was found and none for amplitudes (Fig. 3 and Table 3).

The coefficients of the regression lines are listed in Table 3.

Table 2 Overview of characteristic parameters of the regression lines of the MLT and TES-voltage

Muscle group		ΔMLT = a + b (V_{stim} – MT) a [ms]	b [ms/V]	Correlation	Significance
ECR	left	0.971	−0.049	0.480	.000*
	right	1.271	−0.061	0.559	.000*
TC	left	1.637	−0.082	0.566	.000*
	right	1.788	−0.089	0.563	.000*

ECR extensor carpi radialis, *TC* tibialis cranialis, *ΔMLT* MLT difference as function of V_{stim}–MT. Number of included values: 72 = 12 cases × 6 observations per case
*significant for $p \leq 0.05$

Discussion

The goal of the current study was to provide normative data on TES induced MLTs, amplitudes and waveform morphology in the m. extensor carpi radialis and the *M. tibialis* cranialis bilaterally in a group of healthy horses. Furthermore, TES induced MEPs were checked for their intra-and inter individual reproducibility. The MLTs of the induced MEPs were checked for their stimulation voltage dependency. The influence of body side (left versus right) and height at withers of the horses was studied for both amplitude and MLTs. TES-muscle induced MEP studies have been used in different animal species like pigs, monkeys, cats, dogs and rabbits [5, 16, 22–25]. To our knowledge, this is the first study providing this

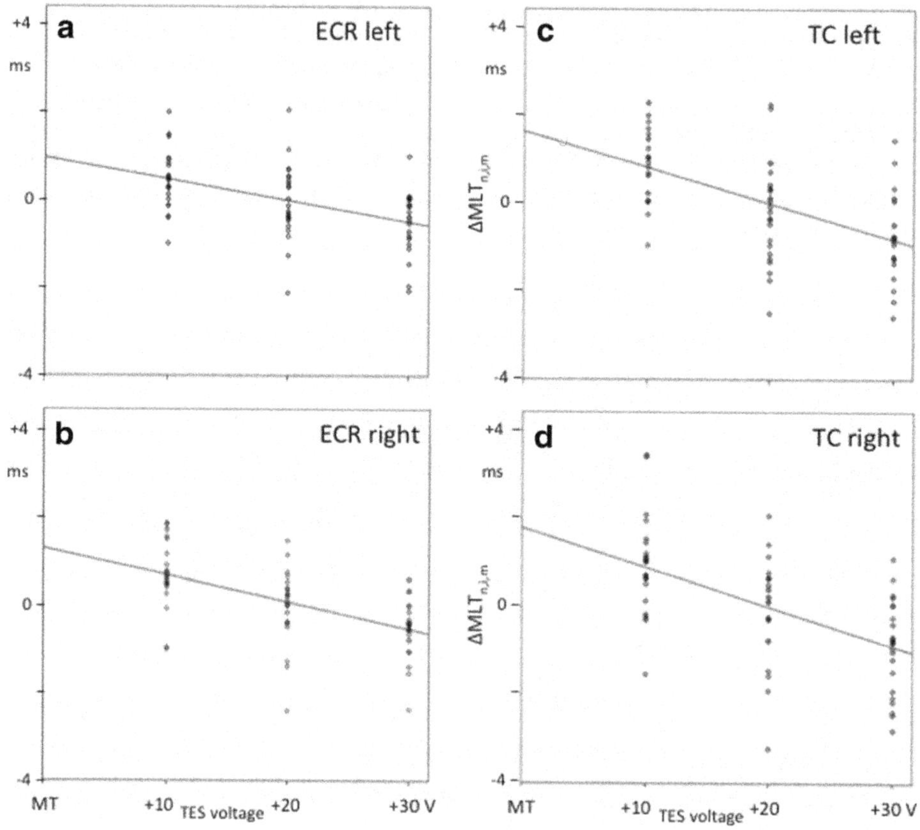

Fig. 2 Scatter plots showing the correlation between motor MLT and TES intensity. Considered are changes of MLT due to increases in TES-voltage. Motor latency differences $\Delta MLT_{n,i,m}$ are plotted vertically and the TES-intensity is related to the motor threshold MT and plotted along the horizontal axis as V_{TES} – MT. $\Delta MLT_{n,i,m}$ is obtained after subtraction of the mean MLT, $MLT_{i,m}$, from $MLT_{n,i,m}$. n denotes case number, i is one of 6 data points per case and m refers to the muscle group. Each plot represents a muscle group: figures (**a**) and (**b**) refer to ECR: extensor carpi radialis muscle, respectively left and right. Figures: (**c**) and (**d**) refer to TC: tibial cranial muscle, respectively left and right. The parameters of the regression line with correlation and significance are specified in Table 2. All regression lines show decreasing courses with significant correlation

data in healthy horses, when using the TES technique [7]. Mayhew et al. [1] published the first normative data on MLTs in ponies, and later Nollet et al. [3] in horses, using the TMS technique.

Our study shows that TES -a method currently used in intra-operative spinal function monitoring to promptly warn of impending damage to the nervous system in human patients subjected to brain or spinal surgery- is a promising technique to assess spinal motor function in horses.

The technique is easily applied. In our previous and current study, we showed that TES is painless, and usually well tolerated, in horses. The technique appears less sensitive to cortical function due to direct stimulation of the corticospinal tract [7]. Like in TMS, horses need to be sedated for reasons of safety.

Table 3 Overview of the characteristic parameters of the regression lines of the MLT and height at withers

Muscle group		MLT = a + b * withers		Correlation	Significance
		a [ms]	b [ms/cm]		
ECR	left	10.708	0.060	0.415	0.181
	right	8.531	0.070	0.465	0.128
TC	left	17.691	0.119	0.579	0.049*
	right	15.993	0.131	0.561	0.058

ECR extensor carpi radialis, *TC* tibialis cranialis, *MLT* is a function of the height at withers where a is the intercept and b the slope expressing increase of MLT per increase of height at withers. 12 cases are included
*Significant for $p \leq 0.05$

Comparison of MEP characteristics between TES and TMS

Mayhew et al. [1] reported mean MLTs of 19.0 ms for the ECR, and 30.2 ms for the TC muscles. Data in our study are quite similar. Therefore, based upon normative values published in literature on TMS, no significant difference between the two techniques can be claimed at this point.

Several factors hamper comparison between reported TMS normative data with the normative data on TES induced MEPs obtained in the current study. One is the dependence of MLTs on the height at withers. The data of Nollet et al. [3] is based on a height at withers of 137.

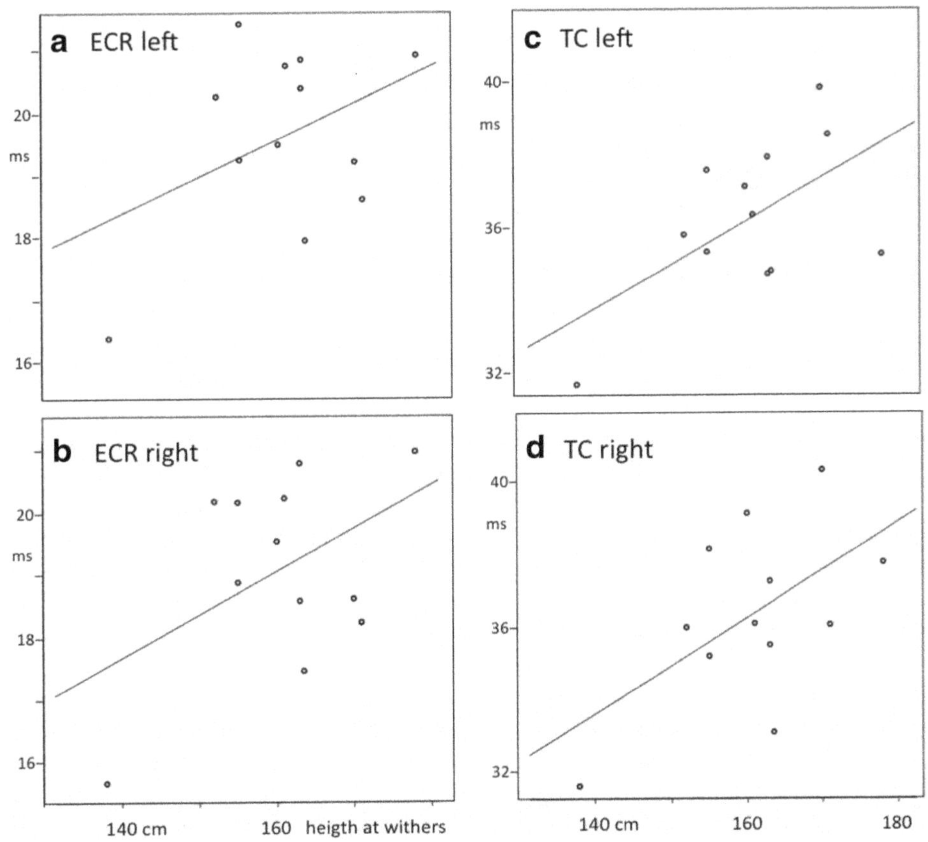

Fig. 3 Scatter plots of MLT_i as a function of the height at withers. Scatter plots of MLT_i as a function of the height at withers where i refers to the case number. MLT_i is the mean MLT of 3 data pairs at stimulation voltages V_{stim} of 10, 20 and 30 V above motor threshold MT. One point represents the mean value of one case. All 12 cases are included. Each plot represents a muscle group. Figures (**a**) and (**b**) refer to ECR: extensor carpi radialis muscle, respectively left and right. Figures (**c**) and (**d**) refer to TC: tibial cranial muscle, respectively left and right. The parameters of the regression lines are specified in Table 3. All regression lines show increasing courses of which the left TC muscle group is significant for $p \leq 0.05$

8 ± 27.07 cm, which is marked lower than in our study. Nollet et al. [3] depict at 160.8 cm (mean height in our study) MLTs of 21.2 ms for the thoracic and 34.1 ms for the pelvic limb muscles. This was in our study 1.8 ms lower for the ECR and 2.1 ms higher for the TC muscles. The mentioned insecurities limit comparisons within 2–3 ms accuracy. This marge is too large to detect the small differences up to 2 ms in MLTs from TES and TMS. These small differences of MLTs would only be detectable by pairwise comparisons of TES and TMS used together in individual horses [9, 16, 26, 27].

Reproducibility of the technique.

Coil positioning in TMS has shown to significantly change MLT, which is not the case for TES as the electrodes stay in the same position. According to Nollet et al. [2] the effect of coil repositioning errors on MLTs is most critical in lateral directions. According to Table 1, both intra- and inter-individual coefficients of variation of MLTs were quite low: 0.059–0.081 and 0.033–0.051 respectively. Intra-individual coefficients of variation especially showed low values, underlining a good reproducibility of repeated measurements within the same horse, when using the TES technique.

Furthermore, TES predominantly bypasses the brain cortex by immediate activation of corticospinal tracts located in deeper regions. This minimizes motor cortical influence and possible influence of sedatives and anesthesia in the neural transmission across the UMN and thus may enhance reproducibility [5].

Comparison of MEP characteristics between sides.

Left/right differences were not found for any of the observed MEP characteristics, with the exception of the reported paired left/right difference for the recorded thoracic MEP amplitude (Table 1) with left being 3.61 ± 2.55 mV, and right: 3.10 ± 3.10 mV. Future studies including more horses may help to elucidate this issue.

Transcranial time window.

It is important to delineate a transcranial time window in which transcranial MEPs can be isolated to avoid interference with late MEPs that most likely result from reflexes that are elicited from extracranial current conduction [7]. As in previous studies [1, 2, 28, 29] late MEPs were also seen in all horses included in the current study. This occurrence of late MEPs is unique for horses. In human, similar effects are seen in a hyperactive spinal cord often resulting from cranially located lesions in the spinal cord or the brain. As previously proposed, these late MEPs in horses result most probably from reflex circuits, which are elicited by stimulation of extracranially located sensory axons [7]. The earlier manifestation of the transcranial MEPs of interest leaves a time window enabling a selective analysis of MEPs without contamination of MEPs from another origin. The window is about 16–20 ms in ECR and 15–18. 5 ms in TC muscles (95% confidence interval). It is important to realize that the duration of transcranial MEPs may exceed this defined time window so that interpretation of MEP characteristics in the last part of polyphasic patterns of the MEP wave outside the window may become inaccurate. These interfering effects outside the transcranial time window on phases pertain to TES and also TMS techniques. This will likely complicate its clinical interpretation in pathological conditions of the spinal cord.

Voltage dependency of MLTs

TES voltage dependent decreases of MLTs are visible in d-waves [30, 31]. Similar MLT decreases are also reported in muscle MEPs of dogs [32]. Table 2 shows comparable data in horses. Figure 2 shows the gradual decrease of MLTs in function of the applied TES voltage, for each extremity. These MLT reductions were observed in each horse individually without exceptions. The average decrease of MLTs over MT + 10 V to MT + 30 V in the thoracic limbs is about − 1 ms and − 1.7 ms in the pelvic limbs. A further decrease to nearly − 3 ms is achieved at MT + 50 V. The MLT reduction can partly be explained by deeper activation of motor tracts at higher stimulation intensities. This causes an earlier start of the epsp summation process at LMNs. The much larger mean muscular MLT reduction of − 7,45 ms at increasing TMS intensities of Nollet et al. [19], resembles the latency jumps in the transition region from extracranial to intracranial elicited MEPs in our study. In that study, no transcranial time window was considered. This entails that the reported MLT averages comprise a mix of transcranial and extracranial MEP components in all muscle groups. Therefore, this study is the first to report on stimulation voltage dependency of MLTs by taking the proposed transcranial time window into account.

One can anticipate on the intensity bias of MLTs of − 1 to − 2 ms by choosing the default intensity at fixed voltage above MT, e.g. MT + 20 V, or at fixed percentage above MT.

Influence of height at withers on TES induced MLTs

A trend of positive correlation was found between height at withers and MLTs in all 4 muscle groups (Table 3). However, only the correlation of the left TC MEPs with height at withers was significant. Nollet et al. reported that height at withers correlated well with the length of motor tracts in the spinal cord and peripheral nerves [3]. The correlation is ascribed to the linear relation between conduction times and axon length, which in turn is related to geometric dimensions of the horse when assuming equal action potential conduction velocities. Our observations are in reasonable agreement with those findings in TMS studies [3]. However, the number of horses in our study was probably too small to offer enough significant statistical power to demonstrate significant correlations in all 4 muscle groups, which is a limitation of our study.

Temperature effects

Axonal conduction velocities and related MLTs depend on temperature. The part of the motor conduction route that is involved in the TES procedure is mainly embedded in tissues well within central body temperature range. MLT changes under hypothermia in TES studies in pigs and rabbits are in a range of – 1 to – 5% at an increase of body temperature of 1 °C [22, 23]. In the normal range of body temperature in horses (37.4–38.0 °C), the expected inter-individual variation in MLT are for the ECR – 0.12 ms to – 0.5 ms and for the TC -0.22 ms to – 1 ms. This is well within the inaccuracy of transcranial MLTs.

Conclusions

TES is a novel and sensitive technique to assess motor function in horses. It is easily applied and highly reproducible. The current study provides normative data in healthy horses on TES induced MEPs in the extensor carpi radialis and tibialis cranialis muscles bilaterally. It is important to notice that extracranial elicited late MEPs appear to be a persistent side effect in horses undergoing electrical or magnetic transcranial stimulation, thus restricting reliable assessment of MEP characteristics to a transcranial time window of about 15–19 ms. For all MEP characterizing parameters no significant left to right differences were demonstrated. A significant effect of stimulation voltage on MLT's was found. No significant effect of height at withers could be found based upon the results of the current study. A study in which both TMS and TES are applied on the same group of horses is needed.

Abbreviations

$A_{n,i,m}$: Amplitude for the n-th MEP, case i and muscle group m; CV: Coefficients of variation; ECR: Musculus extensor carpi radialis; epsp: Excitatory postsynaptic potential; i: Case; LMN: Lower motor neuron; m: Muscle; MEP: Motor evoked potential; MLT: Motor latency time; MLT_m: Mean motor latency time; $MLT_{n,i,m}$: Motor latency times n denotes case number, i is one of 6 data points per case and m refers to the muscle group; $mSD_{intra,\ i,\ m}$: Mean intra-individual Standard Deviation; MT: Motor thresholds; n: n-th MEP; $SD_{intra,\ i,\ m}$: Intra-individual Standard Deviation; SD_m: Mean Standard deviation; TC: Musculus tibialis cranialis; TCW: Transcranial time window; TES: Transcranial electrical stimulation; TMS: Transcranial magnetic stimulation; UMN: Upper motor neuron

Acknowledgements

The authors like to thank Berit Boshuizen, DVM for her valuable contribution when finishing the manuscript.

Funding

This work has been financially supported by JS Center and Wolvega Equine Clinic.

Authors' contributions

SJ, HJ and MB designed and performed the study. Data collection was performed by SJ and HJ. Data analyses and interpretation was performed by SJ and HJ. SJ, HJ and CD were involved in creating the manuscript. CD and HL supervised the study. All authors critically revised the manuscript. All authors read and approved the final manuscript.

Consent for publication

Not applicable for this study.

Competing interests

The authors declare that they have no competing interests.

Author details

[1]Equine Diagnostics, Tergracht 2A, 9091 BG Wijns, The Netherlands. [2]Department of Neurosurgery, University Groningen, University Medical Center Groningen, Hanzeplein 1, 9713 GZ Groningen, The Netherlands. [3]Wolvega Equine Clinic, Stellingenweg 10, 8474 EA Oldeholtpade, The Netherlands. [4]Department of Comparative Physiology and Biometrics, Faculty of Veterinary Medicine, Ghent University, Salisburylaan 133, 9820 Merelbeke, Belgium.

References

1. Mayhew IG, Washbourne JR. Magnetic motor evoked potentials in ponies. J Vet Intern Med. 1996;10:326–9.
2. Nollet H, Van Ham L, Dewulf J, Vanderstraeten G, Deprez P. Standardization of transcranial magnetic stimulation in the horse. Vet J. 2003;166:244–50.
3. Nollet H, Deprez P, van Ham L, Dewulf J, Decleir A, Vanderstraeten G. Transcranial magnetic stimulation: normal values of magnetic motor evoked potentials in 84 normal horses and influence of height, weight, age and sex. Equine Vet J. 2004;36:51–7.
4. Nollet H, Deprez P, Van Ham L, Verschooten F, Vanderstraeten G. The use of magnetic motor evoked potentials in horses with cervical spinal cord disease. Equine Vet J. 2002;34:156–63.
5. Amassian VE, Quirk GJ, Stewart MA. Comparison of corticospinal activation by magnetic coil and electrical stimulation of monkey motor cortex. Electroencephalogr Clin Neurophysiol. 1990;77:390–401.
6. Houlden DA, Schwartz ML, Tator CH, Ashby P, MacKay WA. Spinal cord-evoked potentials and muscle responses evoked by transcranial magnetic stimulation in 10 awake human subjects. J Neurosci. 1999;19:1855–62.
7. Journée SL, Journée HL, de Bruijn CM, CJG D. Design and optimization of a novel method for assessment of the motor function of the spinal cord by multipulse Transcranial electrical stimulation in horses. J Equine Vet Sci. 2015;35:793–800.
8. Merton PA, Morton HB. Stimulation of the cerebral cortex in the intact human subject. Nature. 1980;285:227.
9. Ubags LH, Kalkman CJ, Been HD, Koelman JH, Ongerboer de Visser BW. A comparison of myogenic motor evoked responses to electrical and magnetic transcranial stimulation during nitrous oxide/opioid anesthesia. Anesth Analg. 1999;88:568–72.
10. Rothwell JC, Thompson PD, Day BL, Dick JP, Kachi T, Cowan JM, et al. Motor cortex stimulation in intact man. 1. General characteristics of EMG responses in different muscles. Brain. 1987;110:1173–90.
11. Amassian VE, Stewart M, Quirk GJ, Rosenthal JL. Physiological basis of motor effects of a transient stimulus to cerebral cortex. Neurosurgery. 1987;20:74–93.
12. Amassian VE, Cracco RQ. Human cerebral cortical responses to contralateral transcranial stimulation. Neurosurgery. 1987;20:148–55.
13. Deletis V. Intraoperative monitoring of the functional integrity of the motor pathways. Adv Neurol. 1993;63:201–14.
14. Li DL, Journee HL, van Hulzen A, Rath WT, Sclabassi RJ, Sun M. Computer simulation of corticospinal activity during Transcranial electrical stimulation in neurosurgery. Stud Health Technol Inform. 2007;125:292–7.
15. Merton PA, Hill DK, Morton HB, Marsden CD. Scope of a technique for electrical stimulation of human brain, spinal cord, and muscle. Lancet. 1982; 2:597–600.
16. Edgley SA, Eyre JA, Lemon RN, Miller S. Excitation of the corticospinal tract by electromagnetic and electrical stimulation of the scalp in the macaque monkey. J Physiol. 1990;425:301–20.

17. Edgley SA, Eyre JA, Lemon RN, Miller S. Comparison of activation of corticospinal neurons and spinal motor neurons by magnetic and electrical transcranial stimulation in the lumbosacral cord of the anaesthetized monkey. Brain. 1997;120:839–53.
18. Macdonald DB, Skinner S, Shils J, Yingling C. Intraoperative motor evoked potential monitoring - a position statement by the American society of Neurophysiological monitoring. Clin Neurophysiol. 2013;124:2291–316.
19. Nollet H, Van Ham L, Deprez P, Vanderstraeten G. Transcranial magnetic stimulation: review of the technique, basic principles and applications. Vet J. 2003;166:28–42.
20. Nollet H, Van Ham L, Gasthuys F, Dewulf J, Vanderstraeten G, Deprez P. Influence of detomidine and buprenorphine on motor-evoked potentials in horses. Vet Rec. 2003;152:534–7.
21. Hess CW, Ludin HP. [Transcranial cortex stimulation with magnetic field pulses: methodologic and physiologic principles]. EEG. EMG. Z. Elektroenzephalogr. Elektromyogr. Verwandte Geb. 1988;19:209–15.
22. Meylaerts SA, De Haan P, Kalkman CJ, Lips J, De Mol BAJM. The influence of regional spinal cord hypothermia on transcranial myogenic motor-evoked potential monitoring and the efficacy of spinal cord ischemia detection. J Thorac Cardiovasc Surg. 1999;118:1038–45.
23. Kakimoto M, Kawaguchi M, Sakamoto T, Inoue S, Takahashi M, Furuya H. Effect of nitrous oxide on myogenic motor evoked potentials during hypothermia in rabbits anaesthetized with ketamine/fentanyl/propofol. Br J Anaesth. 2002;88:836–40.
24. Luft AR, Kaelin-Lang A, Hauser TK, Cohen LG, Thakor NV, Hanley DF. Transcranial magnetic stimulation in the rat. Exp Brain Res. 2001;140:112–21.
25. Murakami H, Tsukube T, Kawanishi Y, Okita Y. Transcranial myogenic motor-evoked potentials after transient spinal cord ischemia predicts neurologic outcome in rabbits. J Vasc Surg. 2004;39:207–13.
26. Amassian VE, Cracco RQ, Maccabee PJ. Focal stimulation of human cerebral cortex with the magnetic coil: a comparison with electrical stimulation. Electroencephalogr Clin Neurophysiol. 1989;74:401–16.
27. Burke D, Hicks R, Gandevia SC, Stephen J, Woodforth I, Crawford M. Direct comparison of corticospinal volleys in human subjects to transcranial magnetic and electrical stimulation. J Physiol. 1993;470:383–93.
28. Bagley CJ. Cortical motor mechanism of the sheep brain. Arch Neurol Psychiatr. 1922;7:417–53.
29. Lemon RN, Griffiths J. Comparing the function of the corticospinal system in different species: organizational differences for motor specialization? Muscle Nerve. 2005;32:261–79.
30. Rothwell J, Burke D, Hicks R, Stephen J, Woodforth I, Crawford M. Transcranial electrical stimulation of the motor cortex in man: further evidence for the site of activation. J Physiol. 1994;481:243–50.
31. Burke D, Bartley K, Woodforth IJ, Yakoubi A, Stephen JP. The effects of a volatile anaesthetic on the excitability of human corticospinal axons. Brain. 2000;123:992–1000.
32. Sylvestre AM, Cockshutt JRPJ, Brooke JD, Holmberg DLPG. Magnetic motor evoked potentials for assessing spinal cord integrity in dogs with Intervertebral disc disease. Vet Surg. 1993;22:5–10.

18

Magnetic motor evoked potentials of cervical muscles in horses

Joke Rijckaert[1*], Bart Pardon[1], Luc Van Ham[2], Philip Joosten[3], Gunther van Loon[1] and Piet Deprez[1]

Abstract

Background: When surgical treatment of cervical vertebral malformation is considered, precise localization of compression sites is essential, but remains challenging. Magnetic motor evoked potentials (mMEP) from paravertebral muscles are useful in localizing spinal cord lesions, but no information about cervical muscle mMEP in horses is available yet. Therefore, the aim of this study was to determine the possibility, normal values, inter- and intra-observer agreement and factors that have an effect on cervical mMEP in healthy horses.

Methods: Transcranial magnetic stimulation was performed on 50 normal horses and 4 (2 left, 2 right) muscle responses were recorded at the middle of each cervical vertebra (C1-C7) and additionally just caudal to C7 to evaluate cervical nerves (Cn) Cn1 to Cn8. Latency time and amplitude of the recorded mMEP were defined by both an experienced and an unexperienced operator.

Results: Latency increased gradually from 14.2 ± 1.38 ms for Cn3 to 17.7 ± 1.36 ms for Cn8, was significantly influenced by cervical nerve ($P < 0.01$), gender ($P = 0.02$) and height ($P = 0.03$) and had a good intra-observer agreement. The smallest mean amplitude (4.35 ± 2.37 mV) was found at Cn2, the largest (5.99 ± 2.53 mV) at Cn3. Amplitude was only significantly influenced by cervical nerve ($P < 0.01$) and had a low intra-observer agreement. No significant effect of observer on latency ($P = 0.88$) or amplitude ($P = 0.99$) measurements was found.

Conclusion: mMEP of cervical muscles in normal horses are easy to collect and to evaluate with limited intra- and inter-observer variation concerning amplitude and should be investigated in future studies in ataxic horses to evaluate its clinical value.

Keywords: EMG, Neurologic test, Spinal ataxia, Surgery, Transcranial magnetic stimulation

Background

In human patients with compressive myelopathy, spinal cord vascular disorders, myelitis or spinal cord injury, medical diagnostic imaging provides detailed information, but often shows compression in asymptomatic lesions [1–4]. Also in horses, many studies highlight the controversy, difficulties and limitations of cervical radiography, myeolography, computed tomography (CT), magnetic resonance imaging (MRI) and myeloscopy to diagnose spinal cord disease. Sensitivities (47–50%) and specificities (70–78%) of cervical radiographs and sagittal ratio calculations are too low for adequate diagnosis of spinal cord compression [5, 6] and variation between observers is high [7]. Myelography also has a low sensitivity (43–85%) and additionally requires general anesthesia and intrathecal contrast injection [6, 8]. Most CT and MRI scanners can only image the cranial cervical spinal cord because of the limited diameter of the CT and MRI gantry. This is an important limitation since 37–54% of CVM lesions occur in the caudal (C5-C7) cervical vertebral column [6, 8]. Furthermore, no flexion or extension of the neck is possible in CT or MRI scanning [9–11]. Cervical vertebral canal endoscopy is not routinely performed as there is a high risk of complications associated with entering the spinal canal or due to neck movement during the procedure. In addition, the visual assessment of subarachnoid space narrowing may not be reliable in cases with mild to moderate stenosis [12].

On the other hand, non-infectious spinal ataxia and paresis is an important issue in horses. Major causes include trauma, neoplasia or equine degenerative

* Correspondence: Joke.Rijckaert@ugent.be
[1]Department of Large Animal Internal Medicine, Faculty of Veterinary Medicine, Ghent University, Salisburylaan 133, 9820 Merelbeke, Belgium
Full list of author information is available at the end of the article

myeloencephalopathy, but in European horses, spinal ataxia is most commonly caused by cervical vertebral malformation (CVM). CVM is a stenosis of the cervical vertebral canal with static or dynamic compression of the spinal cord [13] commonly seen in young, rapidly growing thoroughbreds and in warmblood horses [5, 6, 14]. Thoroughbreds (6 months–2 years) are prone to a dynamic compressive form (type 1), while the static form (type 2) typically affects older warmblood horses in the caudal cervical region and is caused by osteoarthritic enlargement of the cervical articular processes [5, 15].

Hoffman and Clark [16] described that some thoroughbreds (about 30%) were able to race at least once after CVM diagnosis and non-surgical management, but if bony malformations or soft tissue proliferations exist, neurological deficits remain present [13] and many horses are euthanized [6, 16]. Surgical treatment can improve prognosis: Moore, Reed [17] and Walmsley [18] described that 45–60% of the patients who underwent vertebral body fusion returned to use, but the clinical response to surgery depended strongly on the ability to identify all compressed sites [17, 18]. Although this precise localization is essential, it still remains challenging because of the limitations of medical imaging. Therefore, it is essential to correlate results of medical imaging with neurophysiological examinations [2, 19].

A highly accurate diagnostic test with a very high sensitivity in human patients is transcranial magnetic stimulation which evokes synchronized descending volleys in corticospinal pathways: magnetic motor evoked potentials (mMEP) [20]. MMEP with prolonged latencies indicate pathological slowing of the conduction through the corticospinal tract in a non-invasive way [21]. The test might be contra-indicated in epileptic patients and in patients with pacemakers or implanted metal structures in the brain but the incidence of side effects is low. By using specific muscles to record mMEP, such as paravertebral muscles, and by determination of central and peripheral motor conduction time, exact localization of lesions and distinction between central and peripheral neural pathology is possible in human patients [2, 22]. In ataxic or paralytic horses, lesions have already grossly been localized using mMEP conductions into thoracic and pelvic limbs [23–25]. Best results are obtained after sedation with detomidine (1 mg/100 kg) and buprenorphine (0.24 mg/100 kg) and stimulation with a round 70 mm diameter coil placed high on the frontal region of the horse, with a maximal output of the stimulator (maximal magnetic field of 4 Tesla) [26–28]. Coil current had no significant effect on latency values and no adverse effects have been reported [26]. Abnormal thoracic and pelvic limb muscle mMEP latency and amplitude values suggest cervical spinal cord disease [23] while pelvic muscle abnormalities alone, occur with thoracic or thoracolumbar pathology. However, no differentiation between etiology or central or peripheral lesions can be made [25]. Of course, it would be interesting to localize the lesion more precisely in horses, just like in human medicine, using cervical paravertebral muscles mMEP. These muscles are situated close to the vertebral column making the peripheral component of the nervous system small. This means that, if spinal root compression is absent, these cervical muscle mMEP will approximate the central motor conduction time, making distinction between central and peripheral pathology possible. However, this paravertebral muscles examination is currently unexplored in horses. Therefore, the aim of this study was to investigate whether paravertebral muscle mMEP recording is possible in horses and, if so, to determine normal values, inter- and intra-observer agreement and factors that might have an influence on mMEP recordings of paravertebral cervical muscles in healthy horses.

Methods

Animals

To determine reference values for mMEP in cervical muscles of horses, sample size was set at 50 as recommended [29]. Healthy horses (36 mares, 12 geldings and 2 stallions; 35 warmbloods, 11 trotters, 1 pony, 1 Friesian, 1 Arabian and 1 Andalusian) were conveniently selected. Thirty horses were owned by the faculty of veterinary medicine of Ghent University as laboratory animals, the other 20 horses were recipient mares for embryo transfers loaned by Keros plc. All horses returned to their owners 1 day after the test. The median age of the horses was 11.5 (range 3 to 22, 15 horses between 3 and 7, 14 between 8 and 12, 17 between 13 and 17 and 4 between 18 and 22) years, the median height160 (range 142 to 175) cm and median weight 553 (range 388 to 705) kg. All horses had a body condition score between 3/9 and 6/9. There were no significant age or height differences between males and females. The mean weight of male horses was significantly ($P < 0.01$) higher than the mean weight of the female horses (557 ± 79 versus 546 ± 76 kg). Rectal temperature was normal ranging from 37.1 to 37.9 °C. All horses were examined clinically and neurologically by a veterinarian with 3 years of experience in neurological examinations. The neurological evaluation form of Mayhew [30] was used as guideline. During the examination, special attention was paid to a normal mobility and the absence of any swelling of the neck. Only clinically and neurologically normal horses were included in this study.

Magnetic stimulation and mMEP recording

Each horse was sedated intravenously with a combination of detomidine (Domidine, Eurovet Animal Health, 12 μg/

kg bwt) and butorphanol (Dolorex, MSD Animal Health, 12 µg/kg bwt). After 5 min, the level of sedation of the horse was subjectively evaluated. Horses that were still alert and reactive to a hand clap, received an additional 6 µg/kg detomidine and 6 µg/kg butorphanol. For the magnetic stimulation and mMEP recording, the horses were all placed in the same examination room with an environmental temperature ranging from 18 to 24 °C. A magnetic stimulator (Magstim 200, The Magstim Company) and a round 70 mm coil were used to generate a maximal magnetic field of 4 Tesla at the coil surface. The coil was centered over the dorsal part of the frontal bone as described by Nollet, Van Ham [26] and maximal stimulus intensity (100%) was applied. The muscle responses were recorded by a standard electromyograph (EMG; Medelec Sapphire, Medelec) through needle electrodes at the level of the middle of each vertebra (C1-C7) and additionally just caudal to the 7th vertebra (C7) to evaluate cervical nerves (Cn) Cn1 to Cn8. The active needle electrode (disposable monopolar needle electrode, 37 mm, 26G, TECA Corporation) was placed as deep as possible (full length or until contact with the vertebral bone, when it was pulled back 2 mm) to reach the paravertebral *intertransversarii cervicii* muscles of C3-C7. The accessibility of these paravertebral muscles was confirmed with ultrasound based on the study of Berg, Nielsen [31]. At the level of the atlas and axis, the needle was placed as deep as possible in the *obliquus capitis cranialis* and *caudalis* muscle, as there are no paravertebral *intertransversarii* muscles at this level. The reference electrode (disposable monopolar needle electrode, 25 mm, 26G, TECA Corporation) was placed subcutaneously at the level of the active electrode. The ground electrode was always attached at the level of the tuber olecranon. Localization of the measurement points was done by palpating the transversal processes of the cervical vertebra and visually determining the middle between 2 sequential processes. At each vertebra, two responses were recorded at the left side and two at the right side of the horse.

Latency and amplitude were defined for each response. Latency (ms) was defined as the time between the stimulation and the onset of contraction, indicated by the first deflection from the baseline. Amplitude (mV) was defined as the difference between the two largest peaks of opposite polarity. All stimulations were carried out by observer 1. On all recorded mMEP, marker positioning for latency and amplitude were done independently by the same two operators. Observer 1 had 3 years of experience in neurological examinations and recording of mMEP, observer 2 had no experience.

Statistics

Data were entered on a spreadsheet (Excel, Microsoft Corporation) and transferred to SPSS 2.4 (IBM SPSS Statistics for Windows) for descriptive and statistical analysis. The continuous outcome variables latency and amplitude were checked for a normal distribution (Kolmogorov Smirnov test and inspection of Q-Q plots and histograms). To determine the 90% reference intervals (upper and lower bound) for latency and amplitude, an Excel add-in was used (Reference Value Advisor; Geffré et al., 2011) and the shortest latency time and the highest amplitude of the four stimulations per location per horse were used. The programme calculates untransformed, box transformed and non-parametric reference intervals and indicates which intervals comply best with the data set.

To determine factors which are significantly associated with latency and amplitude, linear mixed models were used with horse and cervical nerve as random effect to account for clustering of measurements within a horse. Predictors added to the model were cervical nerve [1–8], side (left or right), sedation dose, breed and the physiological parameters gender, age (years), body weight (kg) and withers height (cm). First, all parameters were tested univariably. Then, all parameters with $P < 0.20$ were retained for the final multivariable model, which was built stepwise backwards gradually, excluding non-significant factors. When predictor variables were highly correlated (Pearson correlation > 0.60), only the most significant variable was added to the model. Biologically relevant interactions of significant main effects were tested. For all significant categorical variables, pairwise comparisons were made using post-hoc tests with a Bonferroni correction to adjust for multiple comparisons.

Inter- and intra-observer agreements were determined for each location (four measurements per vertebra), using linear mixed model procedures and coefficients of variation (CV (%) = (SD/mean) × 100), respectively. CVs were calculated on horse level by taking the mean value of the CV per horse and on study population level by calculating the CV of the minimal latency and maximal amplitude values of 4 measurements per horse.

Results

A total of 1600 stimulations were performed and all delivered measurable mMEP. Latency and amplitude recordings for each cervical nerve are displayed in Figs. 1 and 2 and descriptive statistics and calculated 90% reference intervals are presented in Table 1. Factors univariably associated with latency were cervical nerve ($P < 0.001$), gender ($P = 0.07$), age ($P = 0.05$), height ($P < 0.001$), weight ($P < 0.001$) and sedation dose ($P < 0.001$). In the final multivariable model for latency, only the factors cervical nerve ($P < 0.01$), gender ($P = 0.02$) and height ($P = 0.03$) remained significantly associated. Interactions between the different significant main effects

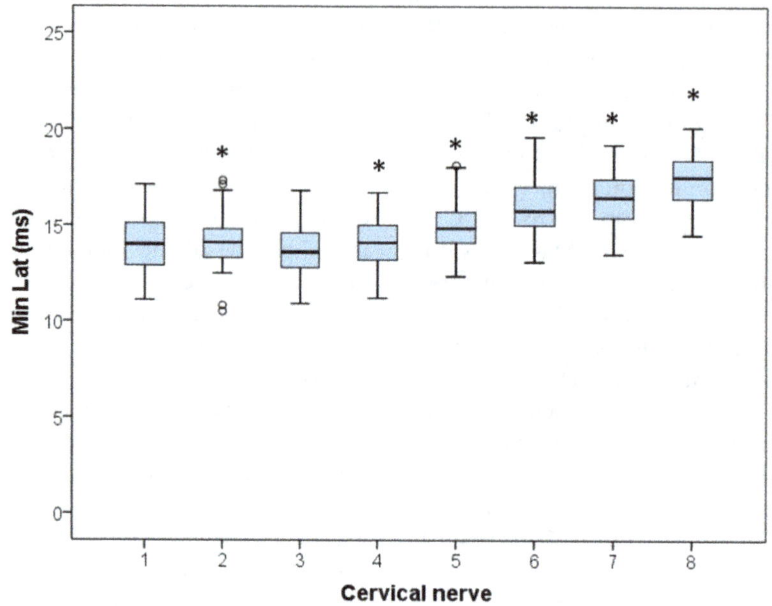

Fig. 1 Boxplots for all latency values per cervical nerve (8 times $n = 200$). Significant differences ($P < 0.01$) from group 3, the group with the lowest latency values, are indicated by *, outliers are indicated by a circle

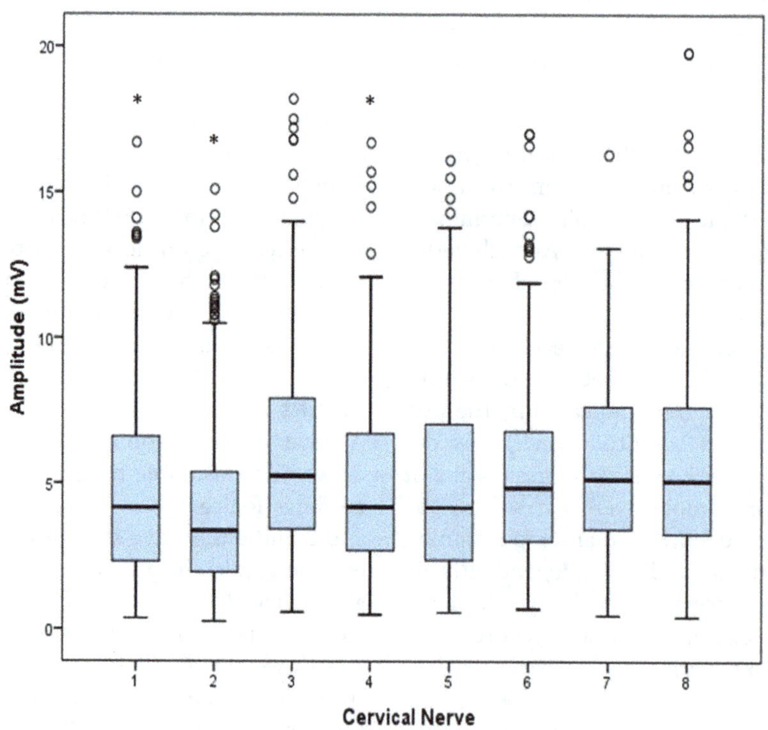

Fig. 2 Boxplots for all amplitude values per cervical nerve (8 times $n = 200$). Analogous to latency, significant differences ($P < 0.01$) from group 3 are indicated by *, outliers are indicated by a circle

Table 1 Mean observed values, standard deviations (SD), minimum (Min) and maximum (Max) values, and calculated reference intervals (RI) for latency (shortest latency of 4 observations per horse) and amplitude (maximum amplitude of 4 observations per horse) values for each cervical nerve in 50 healthy horses

	Cervical nerve	*n*	Mean	SD	Min	Max	90% RI
Latency (ms)	1	50	14.0	1.4	11.1	17.1	11.2–16.8
	2	50	14.1	1.4	10.5	17.3	10.6–17.2
	3	50	13.7	1.4	10.9	16.8	11.0–16.6
	4	50	14.1	1.2	11.2	16.7	11.4–16.6
	5	50	15.0	1.3	12.4	18.1	12.6–18.1
	6	50	15.9	1.5	13.1	19.6	13.2–19.4
	7	50	16.5	1.4	13.5	19.2	13.6–19.2
	8	50	17.4	1.3	14.5	20.1	14.6–20.1
Amplitude (mV)	1	50	8.2	3.7	0.9	16.7	1.2–16.2
	2	50	7.1	4.3	1.1	18.8	1.1–18.3
	3	50	9.3	4.0	2.0	18.2	2.2–18.0
	4	50	7.8	3.4	1.9	16.7	2.0–16.4
	5	50	8.4	3.9	1.5	16.1	1.6–15.9
	6	50	8.0	3.9	1.9	18.7	2.1–18.2
	7	50	8.3	2.9	1.8	16.3	2.1–15.4
	8	50	8.8	4.1	2.6	19.8	2.7–19.8

n, number of magnetic motor evoked potentials recorded

were tested, but only the interaction between cervical nerve and gender was significant ($P < 0.01$) (Fig. 3). This interaction signifies a different effect of the cervical nerve location on latency time for males and females. In male horses Cn2, Cn5, Cn6, Cn7 and Cn8 had significantly ($P < 0.01$) longer latency times with mean differences of respectively 0.7, 1.1, 1.0, 1.1 and 1.5 ms compared to females. Irrespective of gender, latency increases gradually from 14.2 ms in Cn3 to 17.7 ms in Cn8 with significant differences between the different locations. Cn1 and Cn2 were not significantly different, but Cn2 had significantly longer latency values than Cn3 (Fig. 1).

Data for amplitude needed to be log transformed to obtain a normal distribution. Factors univariably associated with amplitude were cervical nerve ($P < 0.01$) and sedation dose ($P = 0.15$). In the final multivariable model only cervical nerve was significant ($P < 0.01$). Amplitude was smallest (4.35 mV) in Cn2 and largest (5.99 mV) in Cn3. Cn2 had significantly different amplitude values compared to Cn3, Cn6, Cn7 and Cn8. Mean maximal amplitude for Cn3 was also significantly different from Cn1 and Cn4, and for Cn1 it was significantly different from Cn8.

Mixed models showed no significant effect of observer on latency ($P = 0.88$) or amplitude ($P = 0.99$). CV, on horse and on study population level, of latency and amplitude measurements for both observers are represented in Table 2.

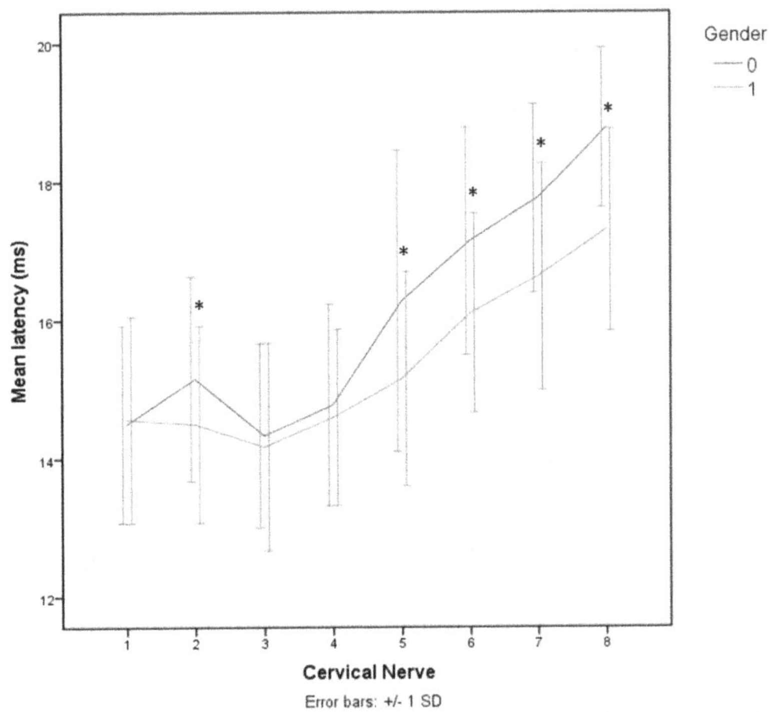

Fig. 3 Interaction between gender (0 = male and 1 = female) and cervical nerve on latency. Significant differences ($P < 0.05$) are demonstrated by *

Table 2 Coefficients of variation (CV (%) = SD/mean*100) per cervical nerve (Cn) of latency and amplitude on horse (mean of CVs calculated per horse) and study population (CV of minimal latency and maximum amplitude values per horse) level for observer 1 and 2

	Level	Observer	Cn1	Cn2	Cn3	Cn4	Cn5	Cn6	Cn7	Cn8	Mean
	Horse	1	3.10	3.00	2.70	3.19	3.76	2.48	3.16	2.24	2.79
		2	4.53	4.10	4.05	4.60	4.09	3.00	3.15	2.16	3.71
	Study population	1	9.71	9.87	10.14	8.81	8.76	9.31	8.36	7.67	9.08
		2	14.50	13.77	14.50	12.99	15.20	10.89	9.75	8.41	12.50
Amplitude	Horse	1	48.54	43.61	39.02	40.51	44.01	33.97	38.95	38.44	36.72
		2	49.61	44.57	39.95	40.39	43.18	36.96	39.31	38.44	41.55
	Study population	1	44.42	59.76	43.13	43.00	46.13	48.52	35.04	46.87	45.86
		2	57.26	60.32	43.23	44.22	46.83	46.02	36.78	61.21	49.48

Discussion

Transcranial magnetic stimulation with registration of mMEP in cervical muscles is possible and easy to perform in horses, as all stimulations resulted in muscle responses from which latency and amplitude could be measured. All measurements of latency and amplitude were carried out by an experienced and an unexperienced observer. For latency, the variation per cervical nerve within a horse was very small for each observer, indicating good intra-observer repeatability. General CVs in this population of horses were larger but still small enough to state that latency was sufficiently repeatable [32, 33]. These findings correspond to the small variations in repeated recordings found in previous equine mMEP studies [23, 28, 34, 35]. Also inter-observer reproducibility was very good as mixed models did not show a significant observer effect. So, in this study, no significant observer effects could be demonstrated suggesting that latency is a reproducible parameter for cervical mMEP, even for clinicians without experience.

Latency values were influenced by height, cervical nerve and gender with a significant interaction between cervical nerve and gender. The significant effect of height was already found in horses [28] and humans [36]. The increasing neural length along the spinal cord, results in a progressive increase in latency [37]. This was confirmed in our study although no measurements of exact neural or neck length were performed. In general, the increase in latency was relatively small (3.3 ms) and started only from Cn3. Mean values for Cn1 and Cn2 were significantly larger than for Cn3. Obviously the anatomy of the atlas and axis region is totally different compared to the more caudal parts of the neck. So, at the level of C1 and C2, a different muscle, which might also be different in composition and innervation, was tested than more caudally along the neck. The influence of gender was not found previously in horses [28] nor in calves [38], but has been described in human subjects [39, 40], though most studies showed no gender effect once corrected for height [41]. In the present study, no differences in height were found between males and females, but a significant weight difference was present. The most likely hypothesis is that male horses have a higher level of muscularity (hence the higher body weight) which might result in a longer distance from stimulation to recording site and hence to longer latencies. The longer latency times in male horses became even clearer in the caudal, stronger muscled, parts of the neck supporting this hypothesis.

The reference intervals for latency were calculated and can be used in clinical situations in future. The 5–6 ms variation in latency values in normal horses is relatively large and probably caused by the large range in horse height in this study population and a sample size at the lower half of the recommended number for reference interval determinations [29]. In addition, subjective localization of the measuring points, based on palpation of the transverse processes and subjectively determining the middle of each vertebra, differences in local temperature or subclinical lesions may have contributed to some variation. However, this variation is probably of limited clinically importance in horses with severe cervical spinal cord disease as in such horses latency times commonly double [when recorded from caudal to the lesion] compared to normal values [23]. Only in subtle or subclinical cases, the variation might result in false negative results. This needs to be determined by validation studies in future, by including acute and chronic and mild and severe clinical case material.

With regard to amplitude, intra-observer repeatability was poor for both horse and general level. The large CVs for amplitude are a logical consequence of the large standard deviations compared to the mean values. Large CVs for amplitude were also found in normal human patients [34, 36], dogs [38, 42, 43] and previous mMEP studies in large animals [23, 26–28, 35, 44]. This large variation is possibly due to physical changes in stimulation (inter-trial variations: output of the stimulator, position of the coil, position of the needle electrodes) or neurophysiological differences in the patient (inter- and intra-individual variations: level of relaxation or voluntary contraction, excitability variations) [28, 29, 36]. However, these factors are difficult or impossible to control in a clinical setting. As a consequence, the calculated reference intervals are wide. In contrast, inter-observer reproducibility of amplitude measurements was good as mixed models showed no significant influence of observer. Thus, results for amplitude measurements are similar for experienced and non-experienced clinicians, but the clinical value of this parameter remains limited because of its high variation.

Conclusion

Registration and measurement of latency and amplitude values from mMEP of cervical muscles in normal horses is easy, with limited intra- and inter-observer variation. The available reference values for healthy horses can be compared with values in horses with suspected cervical spinal cord disease to evaluate whether precise localization of lesions is possible.

Authors' contributions

JR and PD contributed to the study design. JR and PJ performed the measurements. JR and BP contributed to statistical data analysis and interpretation. JR, PJ, LVH and GVL contributed to the practical execution of the study. JR and BP wrote the manuscript. All authors read and critically revised and approved the final manuscript.

Consent for publication

Not Applicable.

Competing interests

The authors declare that they have no competing interests.

Author details

[1]Department of Large Animal Internal Medicine, Faculty of Veterinary Medicine, Ghent University, Salisburylaan 133, 9820 Merelbeke, Belgium. [2]Department of Obstetrics, Reproduction and Herd Health, Faculty of Veterinary Medicine, Ghent University, Salisburylaan 133, 9820 Merelbeke, Belgium. [3]Small Animal Department, Faculty of Veterinary Medicine, Ghent University, Salisburylaan 133, 9820 Merelbeke, Belgium.

References

1. Tani T, Yamamoto H, Kimura J. Cervical spondylotic myelopathy in elderly people: a high incidence of conduction block at C3-4 or C4-5. J Neurol Neurosur Ps. 1999;66(4):456–64.
2. Nardone R, Holler Y, Thomschewski A, Holler P, Bergmann J, Golaszewski S, et al. Central motor conduction studies in patients with spinal cord disorders: a review. Spinal Cord. 2014;52(6):420–7.
3. Barker AT, Jalinous R, Freeston IL. Non-invasive magnetic stimulation of human motor cortex. Lancet. 1985;1(8437):1106–7.
4. Boden SD, McCowin PR, Davis DO, Dina TS, Mark AS, Wiesel S. Abnormal magnetic-resonance scans of the cervical spine in asymptomatic subjects. A prospective investigation. J Bone Joint Surg Am. 1990;72(8):1178–84.
5. Levine JM, Adam E, MacKay RJ, Walker MA, Frederick JD, Cohen ND. Confirmed and presumptive cervical vertebral compressive myelopathy in older horses: a retrospective study (1992-2004). J Vet Intern Med. 2007;21(4): 812–9.
6. Levine JM, Scrivani PV, Divers TJ, Furr M, Mayhew IJ, Reed S, et al. Multicenter case-control study of signalment, diagnostic features, and outcome associated with cervical vertebral malformation-malarticulation in horses. J Am Vet Med A. 2010;237(7):812–22.
7. Hughes KJ, Laidlaw EH, Reed SM, Keen J, Abbott JB, Trevail T, et al. Repeatability and intra- and inter-observer agreement of cervical vertebral sagittal diameter ratios in horses with neurological disease. J Vet Intern Med. 2014;28(6):1860–70.
8. van Biervliet J, Scrivani PV, Divers TJ, Erb HN, de Lahunta A, Nixon A. Evaluation of decision criteria for detection of spinal cord compression based on cervical myelography in horses: 38 cases (1981–2001). Equine Vet J. 2004;36(1):14–20.
9. Yamada K, Sato F, Hada T, Horiuchi N, Ikeda H, Nishihara K, et al. Quantitative evaluation of cervical cord compression by computed tomographic myelography in thoroughbred foals. J Equine Sci. 2016; 27(4):143–8.
10. Mitchell CW, Nykamp SG, Foster R, Cruz R, Montieth G. The use of magnetic resonance imaging in evaluating horses with spinal ataxia. Vet Radiol Ultrasound. 2012;53(6):613–20.
11. Janes JG, Garrett KS, McQuerry KJ, Pease AP, Williams NM, Reed SM, et al. Comparison of magnetic resonance imaging with standing cervical radiographs for evaluation of vertebral canal stenosis in equine cervical stenotic myelopathy. Equine Vet J. 2014;46(6):681–6.
12. Prange T, Carr EA, Stick JA, Garcia-Pereira FL, Patterson JS, Derksen FJ. Cervical vertebral canal endoscopy in a horse with cervical vertebral stenotic myelopathy. Equine Vet J. 2012;44(1):116–9.
13. Nout YS, Reed SM. Cervical vertebral stenotic myelopathy. Equine Vet Educ. 2003;15(4):212–23.
14. Levine JM, Ngheim PP, Levine GJ, Cohen ND. Associations of sex, breed, and age with cervical vertebral compressive myelopathy in horses: 811 cases (1974-2007). J Am Vet Med A. 2008;233(9):1453–8.
15. Mayhew IG, Donawick WJ, Green SL, Galligan DT, Stanley EK, Osborne J. Diagnosis and prediction of cervical vertebral malformation in thoroughbred foals based on semi-quantitative radiographic indicators. Equine Vet J. 1993;25(5):435–40.
16. Hoffman CJ, Clark CK. Prognosis for racing with conservative management of cervical vertebral malformation in thoroughbreds: 103 cases (2002-2010). J Vet Intern Med. 2013;27(2):317–23.
17. Moore BR, Reed SM, Robertson JT. Surgical treatment of cervical stenotic myelopathy in horses: 73 cases (1983-1992). J Am Vet Med A. 1993;203(1): 108–12.
18. Walmsley JR. Surgical treatment of cervical spinal cord compression in horses: a European experience. Equine Vet Educ. 2005;17(1):39–43.
19. Chan KM, Nasathurai S, Chavin JM, Brown WF. The usefulness of central motor conduction studies in the localization of cord involvement in cervical spondylytic myelopathy. Muscle Nerve. 1998;21(9):1220–3.
20. Di Lazzaro V, Oliviero A, Profice P, Ferrara L, Saturno E, Pilato F, et al. The diagnostic value of motor evoked potentials. Clin Neurophysiol. 1999;110(7): 1297–307.
21. Dvorak J, Herdmann J, Theiler R. Magnetic transcranial brain stimulation: painless evaluation of central motor pathways. Normal values and clinical application in spinal cord diagnostics: upper extremities. Spine. 1990;15(3): 155–60.
22. Funaba M, Kanchiku T, Imajo Y, Suzuki H, Yoshida Y, Nishida N, et al. Transcranial magnetic stimulation in the diagnosis of cervical compressive myelopathy: comparison with spinal cord evoked potentials. Spine. 2015; 40(3):E161–7.
23. Nollet H, Deprez P, Van Ham L, Verschooten F, Vanderstraeten G. The use of magnetic motor evoked potentials in horses with cervical spinal cord disease. Equine Vet J 2002;34(2):156–163.
24. Nollet H, Vanschandevijl K, Van Ham L, Vanderstraeten G, Deprez P. Role of transcranial magnetic stimulation in differentiating motor nervous tract disorders from other causes of recumbency in four horses and one donkey. Vet Rec. 2005;157(21):656–8.
25. Nollet H, Van Ham L, Verschooten F, Vanderstraeten G, Deprez P. Use of magnetic motor-evoked potentials in horses with bilateral hind limb ataxia.

Am J Vet Res. 2003;64(11):1382–6.
26. Nollet H, Van Ham L, Dewulf J, Vanderstraeten G, Deprez P. Standardization of transcranial magnetic stimulation in the horse. Vet J. 2003;166(3):244–50.
27. Nollet H, Van Ham L, Gasthuys F, Dewulf J, Vanderstraeten G, Deprez P. Influence of detomidine and buprenorphine on motor-evoked potentials in horses. Vet Rec. 2003;152(17):534–7.
28. Nollet H, Deprez R, Van Ham L, Dewulf J, Decleir A, Vanderstraeten G. Transcranial magnetic stimulation: normal values of magnetic motor evoked potentials in 84 normal horses and influence of height, weight, age and sex. Equine Vet J 2004;36(1):51–57.
29. Wellek S, Lackner KJ, Jennen-Steinmetz C, Reinhard I, Hoffmann I, Blettner M. Determination of reference limits: statistical concepts and tools for sample size calculation. Clin Chem Lab Med. 2014;52(12):1685–94.
30. Mayhew IG. Large animal neurology - neurological evaluation form. 2nd ed. Chichester: Wiley-Blackwell; 2008. p. 453.
31. Berg LC, Nielsen JV, Thoefner MB, Thomsen PD. Ultrasonography of the equine cervical region: a descriptive study in eight horses. Equine Vet J. 2003;35(7):647–55.
32. Ashcroft T, Simpson JM, Timbrell V. Simple method of estimating severity of pulmonary fibrosis on a numerical scale. J Clin Pathol. 1988;41(4):467–70.
33. Mavrides E, Holden D, Bland JM, Tekay A, Thilaganathan B. Intraobserver and interobserver variability of transabdominal Doppler velocimetry measurements of the fetal ductus venosus between 10 and 14 weeks of gestation. Ultrasound Obstet Gynecol. 2001;17(4):306–10.
34. Hess CW, Mills KR, Murray NM. Magnetic stimulation of the human brain: facilitation of motor responses by voluntary contraction of ipsilateral and contralateral muscles with additional observations on an amputee. Neurosci Lett. 1986;71(2):235–40.
35. Rijckaert J, Pardon B, van Loon G, Deprez P. Agreement between needle and surface electrodes for magnetic motor evoked potential recording in horses. J Equine Veterinary Science. 2018; Under review.
36. Ellaway PH, Davey NJ, Maskill DW, Rawlinson SR, Lewis HS, Anissimova NP. Variability in the amplitude of skeletal muscle responses to magnetic stimulation of the motor cortex in man. Electroencephalogr Clin Neurophysiol. 1998;109(2):104–13.
37. Ertekin C, Uludag B, On A, Yetimalar Y, Ertas M, Colakoglu Z, et al. Motor-evoked potentials from various levels of paravertebral muscles in normal subjects and in patients with focal lesions of the spinal cord. Spine. 1998; 23(9):1016–22.
38. Sylvestre AM, Cockshutt JR, Parent JM, Brooke JD, Holmberg DL, Partlow GD. Magnetic motor evoked potentials for assessing spinal cord integrity in dogs with intervertebral disc disease. Vet Surg. 1993;22(1):5–10.
39. Tobimatsu S, Sun SJ, Fukui R, Kato M. Effects of sex, height and age on motor evoked potentials with magnetic stimulation. J Neurol. 1998;245(5): 256–61.
40. Chu NS. Motor evoked potentials with magnetic stimulation: correlations with height. Electroencephalogr Clin Neurophysiol. 1989;74(6):481–5.
41. Rossini PM, Burke D, Chen R, Cohen LG, Daskalakis Z, Di Iorio R, et al. Non-invasive electrical and magnetic stimulation of the brain, spinal cord, roots and peripheral nerves: basic principles and procedures for routine clinical and research application. An updated report from an I.F.C.N. committee. Clin Neurophysiol. 2015;126(6):1071–107.
42. Van Ham LM, Vanderstraeten GGW, Mattheeuws DRG, Nijs J. Transcranial magnetic motor evoked-potentials in sedated dogs. Prog Vet Neurol 1994; 5(4):147–154.
43. Van Ham LM, Nijs J, Mattheeuws DR, Vanderstraeten GG. Sufentanil and nitrous oxide anaesthesia for the recording of transcranial magnetic motor evoked potentials in dogs. Vet Rec. 1996;138(26):642–5.
44. Rijckaert J, Pardon B, Verryken K, Van Ham L, van Loon G, Deprez P. Motor evoked potentials in standing and recumbent calves induced by magnetic stimulation at the foramen magnum. Vet J. 2016;216:178–82.

19

Changes in biomarkers in equine synovial fluid two weeks after intra-articular hyaluronan treatment

Tytti M. Niemelä[*], Riitta-Mari Tulamo, Kaisa Aaltonen, Satu M. Sankari and Anna K. Hielm-Björkman

Abstract

Background: Inflammatory and degenerative activity inside the joint can be studied in vivo via analysis of synovial fluid (SF) biomarkers, which are molecular markers of inflammatory processes and tissue turnover. The aim of this study was to investigate the response of selected biomarkers in the SF after an intra-articular (IA) high-molecular-weight non-animal stabilized hyaluronic acid (NASHA) treatment. Our hypothesis was that prostaglandin E_2 (PGE_2), substance P, aggrecan chondroitin sulfate 846 epitope (CS846), and carboxypeptide of type II collagen (CPII) concentrations in SF would decrease more in the NASHA than in the placebo group. Twenty-eight clinically lame horses with positive responses to diagnostic IA anaesthesia of the metacarpophalangeal or metatarsophalangeal joints were randomized into treatment ($n = 15$) and control ($n = 13$) groups. After collection of baseline SF samples followed by IA diagnostic anaesthesia, horses in the treatment group received 3 ml of a NASHA product IA. Those in the placebo group received an equivalent volume of sterile 0.9% saline solution. The horses were re-evaluated and a second SF sample was obtained after a 2-week period.

Results: CS846 concentration decreased in the NASHA group only ($P = 0.010$). Both PGE_2 and CPII concentrations decreased within the groups (PGE_2, $P = 0.010$ for the NASHA group; $P = 0.027$ for the placebo group; CPII, $P < 0.001$ for NASHA group; $P = 0.009$ for placebo group). No significant treatment effect for any biomarker was found between groups. NASHA induced an increase in white blood cell count; this was significant compared with baseline ($P = 0.021$) and the placebo group ($P = 0.045$).

Conclusions: Although the SF concentration of the cartilage-derived biomarker CS846 decreased in the NASHA group, no statistically significant treatment effect of any of the biomarkers were observed between treatment groups. The significant increase in SF white blood cell count after IA NASHA may indicate a mild inflammatory response. However, as no clinical adverse effects were observed, we conclude that IA NASHA was well tolerated.

Keywords: Aggrecan chondroitin sulfate 846 epitope, Biomarkers, Carboxypeptide of type II collagen, Clinical study, Non-animal stabilized hyaluronic acid (NASHA), Placebo-controlled, Prostaglandin E_2, Substance P

* Correspondence: tytti.niemela@fimnet.fi
Department of Equine and Small Animal Medicine, Faculty of Veterinary Medicine, University of Helsinki, P.O. Box 57, 00014 Helsinki, Finland

Background

A majority of athletic horses suffer from lameness during their careers. Lameness resulting from joint disease is one of the major causes of poor performance [1, 2]. Intra-articular (IA) hyaluronan (HA) injection is a commonly used treatment for equine synovitis and osteoarthritis (OA), although only a few clinical studies have been conducted on IA HA treatment without any other medication in horses [3–7]. Hyaluronan is a glycosaminoglycan component of the synovial fluid (SF) and proteoglycan aggregates in the articular cartilage. The complete mechanism of HA action is not yet fully understood. HA reduces the sensitivity of articular nerve endings in the joint capsule by buffering transmission of mechanical forces to nociceptor nerve endings and thereby reduces pain [8]. HA also reduces impulse activity in the peripheral nociceptor endings by affecting receptor channels [9]. Furthermore, HA has an anti-inflammatory effect [8, 10–12]. However, repeated IA HA injections have also been found to induce a transitional IA inflammation reaction first [13–15], likely caused by low molecular weight breakdown products of HA [14].

Inflammatory and degenerative activity inside the joint can be studied in vivo via analysis of SF biomarkers, which are molecular markers of inflammatory processes and tissue turnover. Research into the biomarkers of equine SF has been focused on finding tools for early diagnosis and monitoring the progression of OA [16–21]. Furthermore, equine SF biomarkers have been used to measure responses to treatments [22, 23] and to evaluate any possible deleterious effects of IA medications [24, 25] and autologous platelet-rich plasma [26].

The aim of this study was to measure SF prostaglandin E_2 (PGE_2), substance P, aggrecan chondroitin sulfate 846 epitope (CS846), and carboxypeptide of type II collagen (CPII) concentrations before and 2 weeks after high-molecular-weight non-animal stabilized hyaluronic acid[1] (NASHA) or placebo (saline) injections in horses suffering clinically from pain in the metacarpophalangeal or metatarsophalangeal joints.

Prostaglandin E_2 (PGE_2) was chosen since it is the most important eicosanoid in joint diseases. Elevated SF PGE_2 levels and increased lameness in horses have been shown in several experimental studies after induction of synovitis or OA [23, 27–29]. Substance P is a pro-nociceptive neuropeptide [30] that has been shown to increase in osteoarthritic equine joints [21]. Furthermore, a relationship between elevated SF substance P concentration and pain and lameness in horses has been reported [31]. In the present study, substance P was chosen because in the first part of the study [32] joint pain and lameness and their response to NASHA[1] and placebo injections were examined.

The marker of collagen II synthesis has been shown to increase for a prolonged period in the SF of the LPS-induced synovitis model [28]. In contrast to that model and induced OA [17], joint pain was not related to SF CS846 or CPII and cartilage turnover in clinical patients [31]. However, CS846 and CPII were chosen as cartilage turnover markers for the present study.

In contrast with the short half-life of commonly used unmodified HA preparations [33, 34], NASHA has a long half-life (up to 32 days) [35] and remains in the synovial structures for a considerably longer period than other HA products [36–38]. This medication is thus intended for treating human arthritic conditions and potentially has a long-acting clinical effect on relieving pain and inflammation [39]. The pain-relieving effects of NASHA were also recently investigated clinically in lame horses [32]. Our hypothesis was that the decrease of selected SF biomarker concentrations would be greater in the NASHA group horses compared with the placebo group horses.

Methods

Horses were presented to the University of Helsinki Veterinary Teaching Hospital for the NASHA study. The study was approved by the Viikki Campus Research Ethics Committee of the University of Helsinki. All horse owners signed a study consent before the start of the study and owners were allowed withdraw from the study without giving any particular reason. Twenty-eight horses were included in the present trial.

The NASHA study was performed as a randomised double-blind and placebo-controlled trial with a parallel group design and equal allocation ratio [40]. Before starting the study, a non-blinded assisting technician created a computer-generated randomization list. Horses fulfilling the inclusion criteria were assigned to the treatment (NASHA) or control group according to the randomization list. The list and the NASHA[1] and placebo products were kept in a locked safe that only the non-blinded assisting veterinarian and the associated technician could access. The NASHA study was planned according to the CONSORT statement and the results of the clinical study have been reported earlier [32].

Horses with lameness due to synovitis of the metacarpophalangeal or metatarsophalangeal joint with or without mild OA and a positive response to diagnostic IA anaesthesia of the affected metacarpophalangeal or metatarsophalangeal joint but with no radiographic signs of OA (subchondral bone lucency or sclerosis, periarticular osteophyte formation, or narrowing of the joint space) of the affected joint were included in the study. Horses with severe or chronic OA were excluded. Mild remodelling of the joint and synovitis of all durations were acceptable. Adult, non-geriatric (age between 4 and 17 years), Finnhorse, Standardbred, Warmblood horses as well as large ponies (height 140–148 cm) of all disciplines were eligible. The ponies are referred to as horses in the text. In addition, horses with IA osteochondral or other fragments were excluded. Bilaterally lame horses and horses that had received IA medications (such as corticosteroids or HA within the previous 3 months or peroral NSAIDs within 15 days) were not eligible. Furthermore, horses with concurrent pathologies (such as clinically significant ligament, tendon, or other soft tissue injuries in the affected limb) were excluded. Treatment groups were equal at the first clinical (baseline) examination; no statistically significant difference between the two groups was found in signalment, use of the horse, radiograph findings, or clinical outcome measures. These measures included lameness, effusion of the affected joint, flexion test result, or pain in flexion. The pain score was created by the authors and recorded as follows: 0 = no pain on flexion, 1 = mild pain (i.e., the horse shows some reaction, such as moving the limb), 2 = moderate pain (i.e., the horse retracts the limb repeatedly during the 1-min flexion period), 3 = severe pain (i.e., the flexion test cannot be properly performed) [32].

The previously published clinical section [32] of the NASHA study provides more detailed data of the study population. Horses were subjected to a full lameness examination and radiographic examination of the affected joint with four standard views as described [32]. Prior to IA anaesthesia (mepivacaine hydrochloride[2]) of the metacarpophalangeal or metatarsophalangeal joint, which was performed to localize the source of lameness and to decide if the horse was eligible for the study (80–100% amelioration of lameness), 5 ml of SF was aspirated into a sterile 5-ml syringe for biomarker measurements. Arthrocentesis was performed through the lateral sesamoidean ligament and blood contamination was recorded if observed in the SF sample. The SF sample was immediately divided into a plain tube on ice (4 ml) and an EDTA (1 ml) tube. White blood cell (WBC) count and protein concentration measurements were performed from the fresh sample in the EDTA tube. Within 1 h of collection, the plain sample was centrifuged at 1700 g for 10 mins in 4 °C, after which it was aliquoted and stored at – 80 °C. If the horse fulfilled the inclusion criteria after examination, the horse received IA NASHA[1] (3 ml, 20 mg/ml into the affected joint) or an IA placebo injection (3 ml of a sterile 0.9% saline solution[3]) on the same day by the non-blinded assisting veterinarian. The horse was then sent home with the owner and asked to return in 2 weeks, when it was subjected to a second clinical examination [32]. Following the first clinical examination and treatment, the horse was allowed 30 min hand-walking per day and free access to a small paddock during the 2 weeks, after which the second clinical examination was performed and a second SF sample (5 ml) was collected and processed using the same techniques as described above.

SF samples were digested with 0.5 mg/ml hyaluronidase from bovine testes for 30 min at 37 °C prior to analyses of SF PGE_2, substance P, CS846, and CPII.

Prostaglandin E_2

Prostaglandin E_2 was measured using a commercial enzyme immunoassay kit.[4] Sample extraction was performed according to the manufacturer's instructions prior to the immunoassay. Briefly, SF samples were acidified by the addition of 1 M hydrochloric acid to pH 3.5 and then vortexed and centrifuged for 2 min at 12000 × g. The samples were applied to a C18 cartridge[5] previously conditioned with ethanol and water, and then flushed with water, 15% ethanol, and finally with hexane. PGE_2 was eluted from the cartridge with ethyl acetate and stored as an elution solution at – 80 °C until analysis. The extracted samples were analysed within 1 week. At the time of the assay, the samples were evaporated to dryness in a vacuum evaporator and reconstituted with assay buffer and analysed according to the manufacturer's instructions. The samples were extracted and analysed in duplicate. Parallelism was tested for dilutions between 1:2 and 1:50. An appropriate dilution was made for every sample. The detection range was 7.81 to 1000 pg/ml with a detection limit of 11 pg/ml. Recovery of the extraction was 81 to 114%. The intra-assay coefficient of variation (CV) was 14.6%.

Substance P

Substance P was measured using a commercial enzyme immunoassay kit[6] according to the manufacturer's instructions. Samples were analysed in duplicate. The detection range was 3.9 to 500 pg/ml with a detection limit of 10.5 pg/ml. The intra-assay CV was 12.5%.

Aggrecan chondroitin sulfate 846 epitope

CS846 epitope was measured using a commercial enzyme immunoassay kit[7] according to the manufacturer's instructions. The samples were then diluted 1:50 and added to plates in triplicate. The result was reported as the mean of triplicate values, unless the CV was over 20%; in this case the mean of the two closest values was calculated. The detection range was 20 to 1000 ng/ml with a detection limit of 20 ng/ml. The intra-assay CV was < 20%.

CPII

CPII was measured using a commercial enzyme immunoassay kit[8] according to the manufacturer's instructions. The samples were diluted 1:5 and added to plates in duplicate. The detection range was 50 to 2000 ng/ml with a detection limit of 50 ng/ml. The intra-assay CV was 8.1%.

Statistical methods

A sample size calculator [40] was used with 95% confidence level and 80% power. On the basis of 87% of cases showing clinical improvement in an earlier study on HA for the treatment of naturally occurring arthritic conditions in horses, the estimated sample size was 11 to 14 horses per group [5]. In the placebo group, the proportion that would improve was considered to be 20 to 30%, where 20% is 10% lower than the percentage that has been used in placebo groups in human studies [41, 42].

SF biomarker (substance P, CPII, PGE_2, CS846) concentrations, WBC count, and protein concentration measurements were analysed with analysis of covariance models. Changes between the baseline and follow-up measurements were used as the response, treatment was used as the fixed effect, and the corresponding baseline measurement as the covariate. For SF concentrations of substance P and CPII and SF WBC count, a logarithmic transformation was used to normalize the distributions. For PGE_2 concentration an inverse transformation was used to normalize the distributions. CS846 and TP were normally distributed.

The possible effects of background variables (age, gender, breed, use of the horse, lameness score, duration of clinical signs, previous incidences of the affected joint, radiograph findings) on the change in the different biomarker measurements from baseline were assessed with analysis of variance models. The models included the background variable of interest as the sole fixed effect and the change of the biomarker from the baseline as the response. If some of the background variables were statistically significant in these analyses, the effect was also included in the analysis of covariance model for treatment comparison.

We hypothesized that the decrease of these SF biomarker concentrations would be greater in the NASHA group than that of the placebo group. The difference in the change of each SF biomarker concentration after IA injection and a two-sided 95% confidence interval for the difference were estimated from the fitted analysis of covariance models using the contrast method. The estimates of the changes within groups were also calculated. Significance was set at $P < 0.05$ for all analyses. The same statistical analysis software[9] was used for all statistical analyses.

Results

Sixty-eight horse owners were interviewed; 36 horses were invited to the first clinical baseline examination. Altogether 30 horses fulfilled the inclusion criteria. Two horses were excluded due to an inadequate amount of high-quality SF for baseline and control samples; 28 horses were thus included in the study. The median age of the horses was 7 years in the NASHA ($n = 15$) and placebo ($n = 13$) groups (range 4–12 and 4–17 years, respectively). There were seven mares, five geldings, and three stallions in the NASHA group. There were six mares, five geldings, and two stallions in the placebo group. Of the horses in the NASHA group, 10 were harness racehorses and five were riding horses predominately used for general-purpose riding. In the placebo group there were seven harness racehorses and six riding horses. The breeds in the NASHA group were Finnhorse ($n = 8$), Standardbred ($n = 6$), and Warmblood ($n = 1$). The breeds in the placebo group were Finnhorse ($n = 5$), Standardbred ($n = 4$), Warmblood ($n = 2$), and pony ($n = 2$). At the first examination, the source of lameness was localized to the right metacarpophalangeal joint in 10 (NASHA group) and seven horses (placebo group), to the left metacarpophalangeal joint in four (NASHA group) and six horses (placebo group), and to the left metatarsophalangeal joint in one horse (NASHA group). No adverse effects of IA NASHA or placebo injections were observed at the second clinical examination or reported by the horse owners.

Background variables (age, gender, breed, use of the horse, lameness score, duration of clinical signs, previous incidences of the affected joint, radiograph findings) did not have any effect on the concentration changes of the different biomarkers.

NASHA induced a significant increase in SF WBC count when compared with baseline ($P = 0.021$) and the placebo group ($P = 0.045$) (Fig. 1). When the change in SF biomarker concentrations was compared between groups, no significant difference was detected (PGE_2, $P = 0.768$; substance P, $P = 0.662$; CS846, $P = 0.207$; CPII, $P = 0.155$) (Fig. 1). When examining SF biomarkers within groups, both PGE_2 and CPII concentrations decreased (PGE_2, $P = 0.010$ for the NASHA group; $P = 0.027$ for the placebo group; CPII, $P < 0.001$ for NASHA group; $P = 0.009$ for placebo group) (Fig. 1). However, for SF CS846 concentration, a statistically significant reduction from baseline was seen in the NASHA group ($P = 0.010$) but not in the placebo group ($P = 0.390$) (Fig. 1).

Discussion

In this study, the SF concentrations of selected biomarkers were measured before and 2 weeks after IA NASHA treatment in horses with lameness localized to the metacarpophalangeal or metatarsophalangeal joint.

IA NASHA caused an increase in SF WBC count. Blood contamination during sampling is an unlikely explanation since the arthrocentesis was performed through the lateral sesamoidean ligament, which has been shown to induce less synovial haemorrhage than arthrocentesis through the proximal palmar pouch [43]. In addition, no blood contamination in the analysed SF samples was observed. It seems more likely that IA

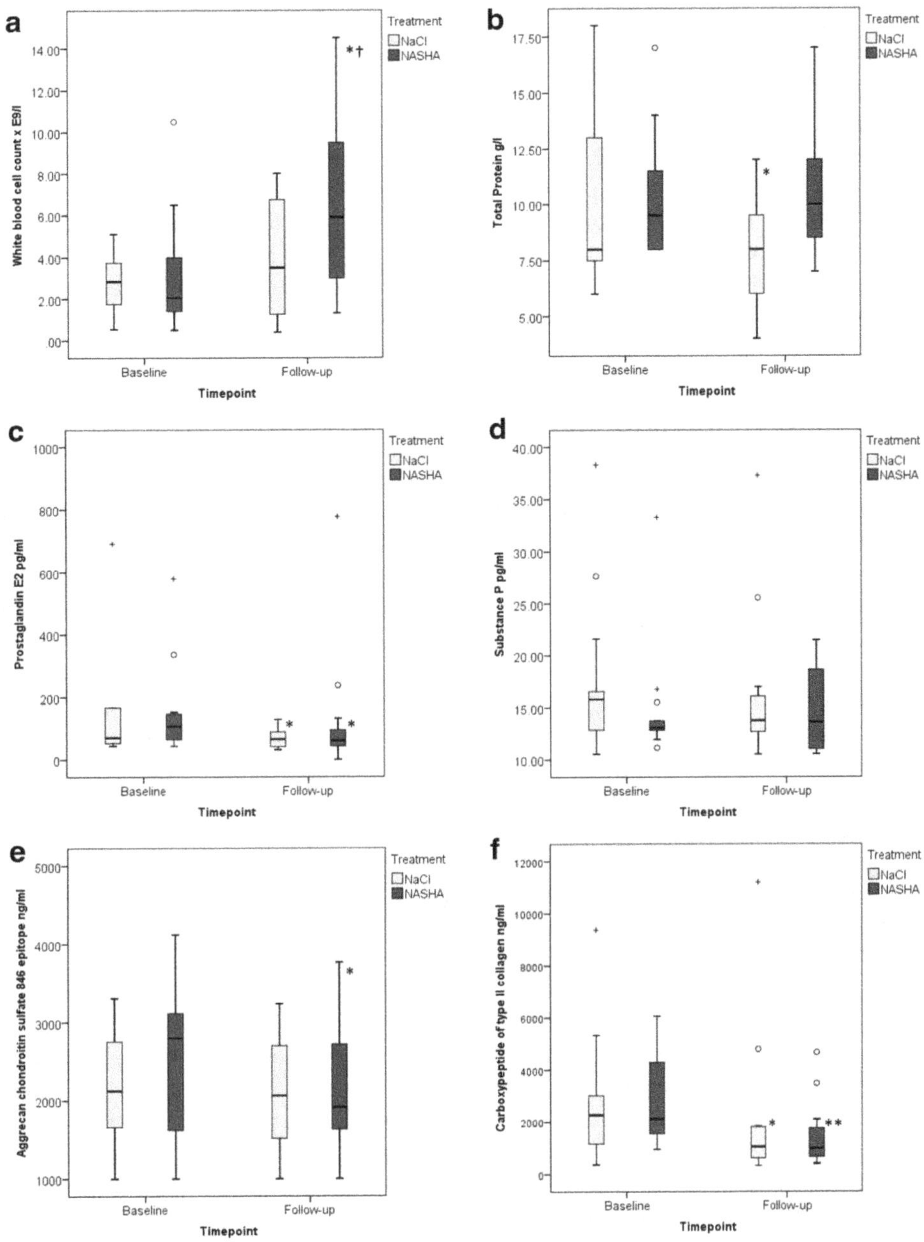

Fig. 1 Synovial fluid white blood cell count (**a**), concentrations of total protein (**b**), prostaglandin E_2 (outliers > 1000 pg/ml are removed to clarify figure) (**c**), substance P (**d**), aggrecan chondroitin sulfate 846 epitope (**e**) and carboxypeptide of type II collagen (**f**) before and after intra-articular NaCl (placebo) or non-animal stabilized hyaluronic acid (NASHA) injection. First and third quartiles are defined by the boxes and median by the band inside. The 2.5th and the 97.5th percentiles are shown as the lower and upper whiskers. $^*P < 0.05$, $^{**}P < 0.001$ between first and second sample in NaCl (placebo) and NASHA group respectively, † $P < 0.05$ NaCl (placebo) and NASHA groups

injection of NASHA induces a mild inflammatory response; this has also been reported after a combined injection of IA pentosane polysulfate and glucosamine injection [44], after repeated IA amikacin injection [45], and after IA gentamicin injection [46]. Moreover, arthrocentesis alone [46] and IA saline injection [44, 45] have been shown to cause significant increases in the SF WBC count. In humans, a transient IA inflammation has been reported after consecutive HA injections [13–15], likely caused by a cell-mediated hypersensitivity reaction [15] to the low-molecular-weight breakdown products of HA [14]. However, in the present study, no clinical signs (such as effusion or pain in the injected joint) were reported by the horse owners or trainers immediately after the injection. Moreover, in most of the samples the increased WBC count was within the normal reference range ($< 0.5 \times 10^9$/l) or very close ($< 1.0 \times 10^9$/l) [47]. One explanation for the difference in the

WBC count between groups could be decreased SF volume after NASHA injection, although no difference in the joint effusion score between groups was found [32].

When compared with the placebo group, the NASHA injection had no significant effect on SF PGE_2 concentration. The effect of various substances on PGE_2 concentration in equine SF has been evaluated previously mainly in experimental studies using induction models [22, 23, 27–29] or horses free of lameness or joint disease [24]. Only Carmona et al. [48] have studied SF markers and their response to treatment in clinical equine patients. As in the present study, they did not find a significant decrease between groups in the SF PGE_2 concentration when an oral HA formulation was evaluated in horses suffering from osteochondrosis.

PGE_2 concentration has been shown to increase in SF of equine osteoarthritic joints [19, 21]. Bertone et al. [18] reported SF PGE_2 concentration to be a good or excellent predictor of joint disease and thus a functional screening test tool in horses. However, high variability in concentrations limited discrimination among the types of joint disease. In contrast, Frisbie et al. [49] speculated that SF PGE_2 concentration may not be a true indicator of overall joint health, as no remarkable disease-modifying effects were detected after phenylbutazone treatment in their experimentally induced equine OA model despite decreased PGE_2 concentration. In the present study, we were unable to observe significantly decreased SF biomarker concentrations in the NASHA group compared with placebo. This may be a result of high variation in concentrations initially, and more specifically, high variations in responses to the treatment. In the case of synovitis, PGE_2 concentration may decrease more rapidly than in mild OA. Frisbie et al. [17] showed that there is a long-standing increase in PGE_2 concentration after arthroscopically induced OA while the increase was short-term in other studies using the LPS inflammation induction model [28, 29]. However, the lack of treatment effect by HA on SF PGE_2 concentration was also reported in experimental studies with more uniform osteoarthritic joints [12, 22]. Another study by de Grauw et al. [31] concluded that PGE_2 concentration might reflect joint pathology in general rather than specifically pain arising from the joint.

In the present study, no differences in SF substance P concentrations were observed within or between treatment groups. This is in contrast with the reported elevated concentrations in SF from osteoarthritic joints compared to normal equine joints [21]. Substance P concentration has been shown to be associated with joint pain [31]. In the equine LPS-induced synovitis model, substance P decreased following meloxicam treatment [28] but not after IA opioid analgesia [23]. Both medications resulted in decreased lameness. The differences in responses after the aforementioned medications can be explained by different mechanisms of action (i.e., opioid analgesia has presynaptic control while NSAIDs influence the release of substance P) [28, 31]. The complete mechanism of action of HA in the joint is not known but it has been shown that HA reduces the sensitivity of articular nerve endings by buffering transmission of mechanical forces to nociceptor nerve endings [8] and by affecting pain receptor channels [9]. The binding of neuropeptides could be one pain-reducing mechanism of HA. The results of the present study suggest, however, that intrasynovial NASHA injections do not have an effect on SF substance P concentration. The clinical section of this NASHA study showed reduction in pain sensation, as horses had a statistically milder response in the flexion test after they had received an IA NASHA injection [32]. This may be due to reducing sensitivity of nerve endings by the aforementioned mechanisms. However, the lameness score was not significantly different between the NASHA and placebo groups [32].

Frisbie et al. [17] showed a significant increase of SF CS846 and CPII concentrations in horses with induced OA compared to exercise-only horses. Although the change in SF CS846 concentration was not different between the treatment groups, the concentration decreased in the NASHA group after the IA injection in the present study. CS846 concentration has been shown to increase in SF following naturally occurring injury and OA in humans [50] and after surgically induced OA [51] and LPS-induced synovitis [52] in horses. Furthermore, exercise induces elevation of SF CS846 concentration in horses [17].

CS846 levels were reported to have a significant correlation with CPII [17]. However, such a correlation was not shown when the effects of meloxicam on cartilage turnover was studied in the equine LPS-induced synovitis model. While no treatment effect was seen on CS846 epitope levels, CPII concentration was significantly reduced compared to placebo [28]. In addition, phenylbutazone has been shown to reduce CPII levels in a comparable equine model [53]. Along with the increase of CPII, an increase in CS846 after IA lidocaine and bupivacaine injections in healthy equine joints was speculated to be the reparative response to the short chondrotoxic effect of these compounds [24]. As IA mepivacaine was injected on the same day (NASHA was also injected on the same day), it is possible that this IA anaesthetic was interfering with the biomarker concentrations to some extent. IA methylprednisolone was reported to elevate CS846 in horses free of joint disease, which suggests an increase in articular matrix turnover [25].

The cause for the decrease in CPII is unclear. SF CPII concentration decreased in both groups compared with pre-injection samples. Although the decrease could be interpreted as impaired synthesis of type II collagen, it may also reflect the fact that less damage to collagen has occurred in the joint after medication [28]. Unfortunately, the collagen degradation marker C2C was not measured in the present study to demonstrate this. It has been shown that CPII increases in equine joints after different types of insults, such as after LPS injection in the normal equine intercarpal joint [52] and after exercise or surgically induced OA [17]. The decreasing concentrations of SF CPII after IA injections in the present study could indicate compromised synthesis of type II collagen. This may also indicate less degradation of cartilage after the horses had discontinued training and rested due to participating in the study.

A 2-week period between SF sampling was chosen to optimize the clinical action of the NASHA injection [32]. The maximum effect of pain reduction of IA HA injection has been shown to be between 2 to 6 weeks post-treatment [7, 39]. On the other hand, some of the SF markers could have returned to baseline even earlier regardless of NASHA or saline injection. In the equine LPS induction model, PGE_2 and CS846 were reported to return to the baseline level before or at 168 h post-injection, while CPII stayed above the baseline level after that [52]. However, since our study population consisted of client-owned patients and many had to travel a long distance to the hospital, it was logistically difficult to organize additional SF sampling visits, either between the baseline and the final samplings or after 2 weeks. Frequent sampling of the SF also induces articular inflammation and therefore has an effect on the measured parameters, which would make assessment of these results challenging.

The absence of significant differences in the SF markers between groups could due to the wide variations in concentrations within groups. The intra-assay CV was also relatively high in some analyses (> 10% for PGE_2, substance P, and CS846). The disease stage and the intensity of inflammation influence concentrations of cartilage-derived markers [54]. Furthermore, time and type of primary insult, duration of lameness, disease, and the extent of joint effusion may have an effect on the SF concentrations of different markers. However, these variables were controlled as best as possible in the present study, as the demographic and clinical variables were similar between the treatment groups [32]. Also, demographic and clinical variables had no effect on the SF biomarker concentrations. Despite these precautions, inflammation may have been more acute and cartilage matrix degradation more advanced in some of the joints. The high variation in the initial SF baseline biomarker concentrations reflects this. Therefore, although we had calculated the group size according to previous studies, a much larger sample size is necessary to show possible differences between the groups.

Conclusions

Although cartilage-derived biomarker CS846 concentrations in SF decreased only in the NASHA group, no statistically significant change of any of the biomarkers was observed between the two treatment groups in this study. The IA NASHA injection induced significant increase in SF WBC count; this may indicate an inflammatory response akin to that also reported in human studies. However, IA NASHA injection was well tolerated, as no clinically adverse effects were observed.

Endnotes

[1]Durolane, Bioventus LLC, Durham, NC, USA
[2]Scandicain, Astra Zeneca, Cambridge, UK
[3]Sodium chloride 9 mg/ml, B Braun, Germany
[4]PGE_2 high sensitivity EIA kit, Enzo Life Sciences, Plymouth Meeting, PA, USA
[5]Sep-Pak, Waters, Milford, MA, USA
[6]Cayman Chemical, Ann Arbor, MI, USA
[7]IBEX Pharmaceuticals Inc., Montreal, Quebec, Canada
[8]IBEX Pharmaceuticals Inc., Montreal, Quebec, Canada
[9]SAS System for Windows, version 9.3, SAS Institute Inc., Cary, NC, USA

Abbreviations

CPII: Carboxypeptide of type II collagen; CS846: Aggrecan chondroitin sulfate 846 epitope; HA: Hyaluronan; IA: Intra-articular; NASHA: Non-animal stabilized hyaluronic acid; OA: Osteoarthritis; PGE_2: Prostaglandin E_2; SF: Synovial fluid; WBC: White blood cell

Acknowledgements

Financial support from Department of Equine and Small Animal Medicine and Veterinary Teaching Hospital, University of Helsinki is acknowledged. This study was supported in part by a grant from Finnish Foundation of Veterinary Research, the Finnish Veterinary Foundation, and the Erkki Rajakoski Foundation. The authors thank Jouni Junnila for statistical assistance and DVM Timo Paananen for his assistance in treatments.

Funding

The study was supported in part by a grant from the Finnish Foundation of Veterinary Research, the Finnish Veterinary Foundation, and the Erkki Rajakoski Foundation of the Finnish Trotting Association, which did not have any role in the design, collection, analysis, or interpretation of the data or in writing of the manuscript.

Authors' contributions

TMN performed the clinical study of all horses, evaluation of radiographs, and drafted the manuscript. KA performed biomarker analyses. R-MT, KA, SMS, and AKH-B participated in the design of the study and helped draft the manuscript. All authors read and approved the final manuscript.

Competing interests

The authors declare that they have no competing interests.

References

1. Jeffcott LB, Rossdale PD, Freestone JF. An assessment of wastage in thoroughbred racing from conception to 4 years of age. Equine Vet J. 1982; 14:185–98.
2. Morris EA, Seeherman HJ. Clinical evaluation of poor performance in the racehorse: the results of 275 evaluations. Equine Vet J. 1991;23:169–74.
3. Åsheim Å, Lindblad G. Intra-articular treatment of arthritis in racehorses with sodium hyaluronate. Acta Vet Scand. 1976;17:379–94.
4. Rose RJ. The intra-articular use of sodium hyaluronate for the treatment of osteoarthrosis in the horse. N Z Vet J. 1979;27:5–8.
5. Ruth DT, Swites BJ. Comparison of the effectiveness of intra-articular hyaluronic acid and conventional therapy for the treatment of naturally occurring arthritic conditions in horses. Equine Pract. 1985;7:25–9.
6. Aviad AD, Arthur RM, Brencick VA, et al. Synacid vs. Hylartin V in equine joint disease. J Equine Vet Sci. 1988;8:112–6.
7. Gaustad G, Larsen S. Comparison of polysulphated glycosaminoglycan and sodium hyaluronate with placebo in treatment of traumatic arthritis in horses. Equine Vet J. 1995;27:356–62.
8. Gomis A, Pawlak M, Balazs EA, et al. Effects of different molecular weight elastoviscous hyaluronan solutions on articular nociceptive afferents. Arthritis Rheum. 2004;50:314–26.
9. Caires R, Luis E, Taberner FJ, Fernandez-Ballester G, Ferrer-Montiel A, Balazs EA, Gomis A, Belmonte C, de la Penã E. Hyaluronan modulates TRPV1 channel opening, reducing peripheral nociceptor activity and pain. Nat Com. 2015;27:6.
10. Punzi L, Schiavon F, Cavasin F, et al. The influence of intra-articular hyaluronic acid on PGE_2 and cAMP of synovial fluid. Clin Exp Rheumatol. 1989;7:247–50.
11. Frean SP, Lees P. Effects of polysulfated glycosaminoglycan and hyaluronan on prostaglandin E_2 production by cultured equine synoviocytes. Am J Vet Res. 2000;61:499–505.
12. Frisbie DD, Kawcak CE, McIlwraith CW, et al. Evaluation of polysulfated glycosaminoglycan or sodium hyaluronan administered intra-articularly for treatment of horses with experimentally induced osteoarthritis. Am J Vet Res. 2009;70:203–9.
13. Leopold SS, Warme WJ, Colonel L, Pettis PD, Shott S. Increased frequency of acute local reaction, to intra-articular Hylan GF-20 (Synvisc) in patients receiving more than one course of treatment. J Bone Joint Surg. 2002;84: 1619–23.
14. Pullman-Mooar SI, Mooar P, Sieck M, Clayburne G, Schumacher HR. Are there distinctive inflammatory flares after Hylan GF-20 intra-articular injections? J Rheumatol. 2002;12:2611–4.
15. Marino AA, Waddell DD, Kolomytkin OV, Pruett S, Sadasivan S, Kalia K, Albright JA. Assessment of immunological mechanism for flare reactions to Synvisc®. Clin Ortop Relat Res. 2006;442:187–94.
16. Nicholson AM, Trumble TN, Merritt KA, et al. Association of horse age, joint type, and osteochondral injury with serum and synovial fluid concentrations of type II collagen biomarkers in thoroughbreds. Am J Vet Res. 2010;71:741–9.
17. Frisbie DD, Al-Sobayil F, Billinghurst RC, et al. Changes in synovial fluid serum biomarkers with exercise and early osteoarthritis in horses. Osteoarthr Cartil. 2008;16:1197–204.
18. Bertone A, Palmer JL, Jones J. Synovial fluid cytokines and eicosanoids as markers of joint disease in horses. Vet Surg. 2001;30:528–38.
19. Gibson KT, Hodge H, Whittem T. Inflammatory mediators in equine synovial fluid. Aust Vet J. 1996;73:148–51.
20. Todhunter PG, Kincaid SA, Todhunter RJ, et al. Immunohistochemical analysis of an equine model of synovitis-induced arthritis. Am J Vet Res. 1996;57:1080–93.
21. Kirker-Head CA, Chandna VK, Agarwal PK, et al. Concentrations of substance P and prostaglandin E_2 in synovial fluid of normal and abnormal joints of horses. Am J Vet Res. 2000;61:714–8.
22. Frisbie DD, McIlwraith CW, Kawcak CE, et al. Evaluation of intra-articular hyaluronan, sodium chondroitin sulfate and N-acetyl-D-glucosamine combination versus saline (0.9% NaCl) for osteoarthritis using an equine model. Vet J. 2013;197:824–9.
23. van Loon JPAM, de Grauw JC, van Dierendonck M, et al. Intra-articular opioid analgesia is effective in reducing pain and inflammation in an equine LPS induced synovitis model. Equine Vet J. 2010;42:412 9.
24. Piat P, Richard H, Beauchamp G, et al. In vivo effects of a single intra-articular injection of 2% lidocaine or 0.5% bupivacaine on articular cartilage of normal horses. Vet Surg. 2012;41:1002–10.
25. Robion FC, Doizè B, Bourè L, et al. Use of synovial fluid markers of cartilage synthesis and turnover to study effects of repeated intra-articular administration of methylprednisolone acetate on articular cartilage in vivo. J Orthop Res. 2001;19:250–8.
26. Moraes AP, Moreira JJ, Brossi PM, et al. Short- and long-term effects of platelet-rich plasma upon healthy equine joints: clinical and laboratory aspects. Can Vet J. 2015;56:831–7.
27. Schleining JA, McClure SR, Evans RB, et al. Liposome-based diclofenac for the treatment of inflammation in an acute synovitis model in horses. J Vet Pharmacol Ther. 2008;31:551–61.
28. de Grauw JC, van de Lest CHA, Brama PAJ, et al. In vivo effects of meloxicam on inflammatory mediators, MMP activity and cartilage biomarkers in equine joints with acute synovitis. Equine Vet J. 2009;41:693–9.
29. Owens JG, Kamerling SG, Stanton SR, et al. Effects of pre-treatment with ketoprofen and phenylbutazone on experimentally induced synovitis in horses. Am J Vet Res. 1996;57:866–7.
30. Marshall KW, Chiu B, Inman RD. Substance P and arthritis: analysis of plasma and synovial fluid levels. Arthritis Rheum. 1990;33:87–90.
31. de Grauw JC, van de Lest CHA, van Weeren R, et al. Arthrogenic lameness of the fetlock: synovial fluid markers of inflammation and cartilage turnover in relation to clinical joint pain. Equine Vet J. 2006;38:305–11.
32. Niemelä TM, Tulamo RM, Hielm-Björkman AK. A randomised, double-blinded, placebo-controlled clinical study on intra-articular hyaluronan treatment in equine lameness originating from the metacarpophalangeal joint. BMC Vet Res. 2016;12:60.
33. Brown TJ, Laurent UB, Fraser JR. Turnover of hyaluronan in the synovial joints: elimination of labelled hyaluronan from the knee joint of the rabbit. Exp Physiol. 1991;76:125–34.
34. Lindehayn HH, Heilmann HH, Niederhausen HUW, Pohlenz K. Elimination of tritium-labelled hyaluronic acid from normal and osteoarthritic rabbit knee joints. Eur J Chem Clin Biochem. 1997;35:355–63.
35. Edsman K, Hjelm R, Lärkner H, Nord LI, Karlsson A, Wiebensjö Å, Höglund AU, Kenne AH, Näsström J. Intra-articular duration of Durolane™ after single injection into the rabbit knee. Cartilage. 2011;2(4):384–8.
36. Dougados M, Nguyen M, Listrat V, Amor B. High molecular weight sodium hyaluronate (Hyalectin) in osteoarthritis of the knee; a 1 year placebo-controlled trial. Osteoarthr Cartil. 1993;1:97–103.
37. Åkermark C, Berg P, Björkman A, Malm P. Non-animal stabilised hyaluronic acid in the treatment of osteoarthritis of the knee: a tolerability study. Clin Drug Investig. 2002;22:157–66.
38. Lindqvist U, Tolmachev V, Kairemo K, Åström G, Jonsson E, Lundqvist H. Elimination of stabilised hyaluronan from the knee joint in healthy men. Clin Pharmacokinet. 2002;41(8):603–13.
39. Altman RD, Åkermark C, Beaulieu AD, et al. Efficacy and safety of a single intra-articular injection of non-animal stabilized hyaluronic acid (NASHA) in patients with osteoarthritis of the knee. Osteoarthr Cartil. 2004;12:642–9.
40. Working in Epidemiology. 2010. http://www.winepi.net/uk/index.htm. Accessed 1 Feb 2010.
41. Richette P, Ravaud P, Conrozier T, Euller_Ziegler L, Mazières B, Maugars Y, Mulleman D, Clerson P, Chevalier X. Effect of hyaluronic acid in symptomatic hip osteoarthritis: a multicenter, randomized, placebo-controlled trial. Arthritis Rheum. 2009;60:824–30.
42. Pham T, Le Henanff A, Ravaud P, Dieppe P, Paolozzi L, Dougados M. Evaluation of the symptomatic and structural efficacy of a new hyaluronic acid compound, NRD101, in comparison with diacerein and placebo in a 1 year randomised controlled study in symptomatic knee osteoarthritis. Ann Rheum Dis. 2004;63:1611–7.
43. Misheff MM, Stover SM. A comparison of two techniques for arthrocentesis of the equine metacarpophalangeal joint. Equine Vet J. 1991;23:273–6.
44. Kwan C, Koenig T, Bischofberger A, et al. Effects of intra-articular sodium pentosane polysulfate and glucosamine on the cytology, total protein concentration and viscosity of synovial fluid in horses. Aust Vet J. 2012;90: 15–20.

45. Sanchez Teran AF, Rubio-Martinez LM, Villarno NF, et al. Effects of repeated intra-articular administration of amikacin on serum amyloid a, total protein and nucleated cell count in synovial fluid from healthy horses. Equine Vet J. 2012;43:12–6.
46. Stover SM, Pool RR. Effect of intra-articular gentamicin sulfate on normal equine synovial membrane. Am J Vet Res. 1985;46:2485–91.
47. Caron JP. Osteoarthritis. In: Ross MW, Dyson SJ, editors. Lameness in the Horse. 2nd ed. St Louis: Saunders; 2011. p. 655–68.
48. Carmona JU, Argüelles D, Deulofeu R, et al. Effect of the administration of an oral hyaluronan formulation on clinical and biochemical parameters in young horses with osteochondrosis. Vet Comp Orthop Traumatol. 2009;22: 455–9.
49. Frisbie DD, McIlwraith CW, Kawcak CE, et al. Evaluation of topically administered diclofenac liposomal cream for treatment of horses with experimentally induced osteoarthritis. Am J Vet Res. 2009;70:210–5.
50. Lohmander LS, Ionescu M, Jugessur H, et al. Changes in joint cartilage aggrecan after knee injury and in osteoarthritis. Arthritis Rheum. 1999;42: 534–44.
51. Koenig TJ, Dart AJ, McIlwaith CW, et al. Treatment of experimentally induced osteoarthritis in horses using an intravenous combination of sodium pentosan polysulfate, N-acetyl glucosamine, and sodium hyaluronan. Vet Surg. 2014;43:612–22.
52. de Grauw JC, van Loon JPAM, van de Lest CHA, et al. In vivo effects of phenylbutazone on inflammation and cartilage-derived biomarkers in equine joints with acute synovitis. Vet J. 2014;201:51–6.
53. de Grauw JC, van de Lest CHA, van Weeren PR. Inflammatory mediators and cartilage biomarkers in synovial fluid after a single inflammatory insult: a longitudinal experimental study. Arthritis Res Ther. 2009;11:R35.
54. Johnson KA, Hay CW, Chu Q, et al. Cartilage-derived biomarkers of osteoarthritis in synovial fluid of dogs with naturally acquired rupture of the cranial cruciate ligament. Am J Vet Res. 2002;63:775–81.

20

Sero-epidemioloical survey on African horse sickness virus among horses in Khartoum State, Central Sudan

Siham T. Karamalla[1], Ahmed I. Gubran[1], Ibrahim A. Adam[1], Tamadur M. Abdalla[1], Reem O. Sinada[1], Eltahir M. Haroun[2] and Imadeldin E. Aradaib[1,2,3*]

Abstract

Background: African horse sickness virus (AHSV) is an infectious non contagious insect-transmitted double-stranded (ds) RNA orbivirus of the family *Reoviridae*. AHSV causes an often fatal hemorrhagic infection with high mortality among selected breeds of Arabian horses. This study was conducted to avail some information with regard to the prevalence and associated risk factors of AHSV among ecotype breeds of horses in central Sudan.

Methods: Sera were collected from 320 horses, which were selected randomly from four localities and employed in the study. A competitive enzyme-linked immunosorbent assay (cELISA) was used to screen sampled sera for AHSV-specific immunoglobulin G (Ig G) antibodies.

Results: Seropositivity to AHSV Ig G was detected in 275 out of the 320 horse sera, thus accounting for a prevalence rate of 85.9%. Potential risk factors to AHSV infection were reported to be associated with horse breed (OR = 5.0, CI = 0.07–2.104, *p*-value = 0.039) and activity of the horse (OR = 3.21, CI = 0.72–1.48, *p*- value = 0.008).

Conclusions: The high prevalence of AHSV in Khartoum State of Central Sudan necessitates the need for continuous surveillance for AHSV infection to prevent a possible disease outbreak in this region of the African continent.

Keywords: Epidemiology, Survey, equines, AHSV, ELISA, Sudan

Background

African horse sickness (AHS) is an acute disease of horses, which most often results in death of the infected animal. The disease is caused by the African horse sickness virus (AHSV), a member of the orbivirus genus in the *Reoviridae* family [1, 2]. In other equine species such as donkeys and mules, infection with AHSV is usually subclinical [3–5]. However, infected mules can amplify the virus and became seroconverted and thus play an important role in the epidemiology of the disease [6]. Nine serotypes of AHSV designated as AHSV-1 to AHSV-9 are recognized worldwide differentiated by serum neutralization test and molecular based assays [7].

* Correspondence: aradaib@yahoo.com; aradaib@uofk.edu
[1]Molecular Biology Laboratory (MBL), Department of Clinical Medicine, Faculty of Veterinary Medicine, University of Khartoum, P.O. Box 32, Khartoum North, Sudan
[2]Scientific Research Directorate, Al-Mughtaribeen University, Khartoum, Sudan
Full list of author information is available at the end of the article

An outbreak of AHS in a disease free region would have catastrophic effects on equine welfare and industry, particularly for international events such as the Olympic Games [8]. In areas of endemicity, AHSV is of concern to wildlife managers as an outbreak of the disease is likely to occur among the populations of zebra [9]. In addition, international trade of race horses is restricted to AHSV-free animals only [10]. AHSV is transmitted to horses by *Culicoides* midges, in particular by *Culicoides imicola* [11]. AHSV is related to bluetongue virus (BTV), epizootic hemorrhagic disease of deer virus (EHDV) and palyam serogroup of orbiviruses [11]. Whereas BTV, EHDV and Palyam viruses cause clinical diseases in ruminants, AHSV is mainly a disease of equines. AHSV induced a fatal infection in race horses in North Africa, the Middle East and different parts of the Arab world including the Sudan [12–14]. Serological evidence of AHSV infection in horses and donkeys is wide spread in the Sudan [6, 10, 12]. Multiple outbreaks and sporadic cases of AHSV were reported in Arabian horses in various states of the Sudan based on clinical presentation. However, the virus was isolated, for the first time, from whole blood and spleen of a mare in Khartoum State, Sudan [12]. Subsequently, AHSV was isolated from blood of infected horses in suckling mice (Aradaib, unpublished data). The two virus isolates were identified as AHSV serotype 9 (AHSV-9). Subsequently, sporadic cases and multiple outbreaks of AHSV were reported in different localities of Khartoum States. However, virus isolation attempts from blood and tissues of infected horses were largely unsuccessful.

Currently, the disease is diagnosed by conventional virus isolation, serology and molecular-based assays [15–19]. Virus isolation is tedious, time consuming, labor intensive and expensive [4, 19]. Serology is useful in epidemiologic studies to identify previous AHSV infection by detection of Ig G-specific antibodies or by detection of Ig M for detection of recent viral infections [20]. Several molecular-based assays were developed and evaluated for detection of AHSV serogroup and serotypes [21–26]. In previous studies, we have reported on a simple, rapid, sensitive and specific RT-PCR-assay for detection of AHSV serogroup in cell culture [6]. Subsequently, a more sensitive nested RT-PCR assay was also developed and evaluated for detection of AHSV RNA in a variety of clinical samples [10]. Currently, no information is available regarding the prevalence of AHSV or the potential risk factors associated with the disease among horses in Sudan. Therefore, the control of emerging viral pathogens, such as AHSV, is urgently needed in the country. The Sudan has a large numbers of horses, which play an important role in horse races and transport in remote areas. We believe further epidemiologic surveys including implementation of improved surveillance would be necessary to prevent further spread of the disease and to combat this important viral pathogen. The objectives of the present investigation were to determine the prevalence and identify risk factors associated with AHS among horses in Khartoum state, Central Sudan.

Methods

Study area

Khartoum State is one of the largest states in Sudan, which comprises three major cities. These cities are Khartoum, Khartoum North and Omdurman. Khartoum is the capital of Sudan and it is located in the middle of the country. The state covers an area of approximately 23,000 km^2 (km^2). The population of Khartoum state is composed of trips from different parts of the Sudan and estimated to be nearly 6 millions. The state is located at the junction of the White Nile and the Blue Nile. In Khartoum state, the 2 Niles unite to form the river Nile, which runs to the north throughout Sudan and Egypt. The state lies between longitudes 31.5 to 34 °E and latitudes 15 to 16 °N. The weather is very hot and dry in the summer season but cold dry in the winter season. Average rainfall reaches 150 mm in the north-eastern areas and 250 mm in the northwestern areas. The temperature in summer may reach up to 48 °C from April to June. In the winter, the temperature eventually declines to reach 15 °C between November and January. The horse population of Khartoum State is 6585 as estimated by the Sudan Ministry of Animal Resources, 2006 [9]. A map of Khartoum State representing the different localities is illustrated in (Fig. 1).

Study design

The present investigation was conducted as a cross sectional survey in Khartoum State of the Central Sudan. A multistage probability sampling method was applied in this study. Four localities in Khartoum state including Omdurman, East Nile, Bahri and Khartoum were selected randomly. Eight herds in each village of the four localities were selected. Finally, 10 blood samples were collected from horses in each herd using simple random sampling method, which accounts for a total of 320 blood sample size [27]. Horses over one year of age were considered for the purpose of this study to avoid detection of maternal AHSV antibodies in young animals.

Questionnaire

A structured questionnaire was employed for the survey and was applied to all animals participated in the study. The information required for the survey was obtained from the animal owners. Individual and management risk factor attributes were included in the questionnaire. The individual risk factors including age (younger animals < 2 years older animals 2 years and above), sex (male, female), breed (through breed, local breed), body condition (fair and thin); and the management risk factor attributes including insect vector (presence or absence), insect control measures (practiced or not), activity of the horse such as chaser (race horse), cart horse involved in transport of materials, and police horse involved in security of the state by the police at night. In addition, the four localities were also included in the study.

Ethics approval and consent to participate

The purpose of the study was made clear to the animal owners participated in the study. Those who agreed to participate in the study were requested to provide a written consent. All the information related to the AHSV risk factors was obtained from the animal owners. The ethical clearance for the study was obtained from the Research Board of the Faculty of Veterinary Medicine, University of Khartoum, Sudan.

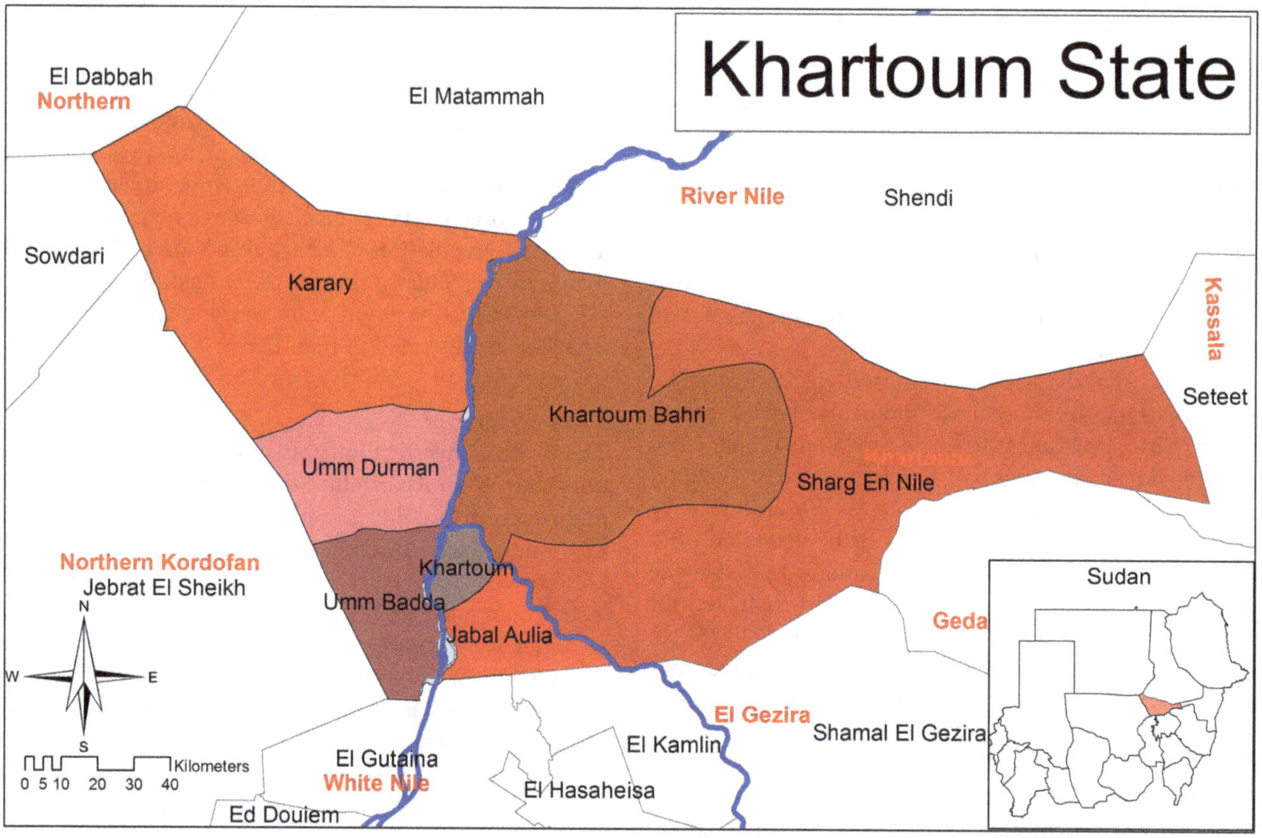

Fig. 1 A map of the localities included in the study area of Khartoum State, Sudan

Collection of blood samples

Blood samples were collected from horses by well trained veterinarians to ensure proper physical restraint of animals to avoid injury. Blood samples were collected from the jugular vein of the selected horses in the study area of Khartoum State, Central Sudan. A total number of 320 sera were collected randomly from the animals and employed in this study. Blood samples were allowed to clot and sera were separated and kept frozen at − 20 °C until used for screening of horses for seropositivity to AHSV-specific IgG antibodies using competitive indirect enzyme-linked immunosorbent assay (cELISA).

Enzyme-linked immunosorbent assay (ELISA)

Detection of AHSV-specific Ig G antibodies was made possible using a commercially available cELISA kit (Ingezim AHSV, Compact Plus, Spain). The cELISA was performed in antigen coated plates. A total of 100 μl (μl) test volumes were used in the cELISA assay. All incubations were performed for I h at 37 °C and washing of plates was performed three times with the provided washing buffer. The results of the cELISA were recorded using ELISA reader set at 630 nm. The test sample was considered positive when the optical density is less than 50% of the mean of the negative controls.

Statistical analyses

Statistical package for social sciences (SPSS) software package for window (version 21.0) was employed to enter the data in the computer. The univariable analysis using Chi-square (χ2) test was used to determine the associations between the outcome variable (status of AHSV seropositivity in horses) and its potential risk factors. Significant association between AHSV and risk factor was initially considered when P value < 0.25 (two tailed; $\alpha = 0.25$). The results of the univariable analysis were further subjected multivariable analysis using logistic regression. Results were expressed as odd ratios (OR) with 95% confidence intervals (C.I) for each risk factor. P value less than 0.05 ($p < 0.05$) represents significant association between the AHSV seropositivity and associated risk factors.

Results

AHSV seropositivity was recorded in 275 out of the 320 horses as detected by the cELISA, which accounts for prevalence rate of 85.9%. The highest rates of AHSV seropositivity was recorded in East Nile locality (94%) whereas the lowest rate of seropositivity was recorded in Bahry locality (81.5%). The univariate analysis using Chi-square test was conducted for the association between the potential risk factors and

AHSV seropositivity. The initial results using univariate analysis showed that the independent variables including, body condition, breed, activity of the horse, presence of insects and locality were statistically significant $p > 0.25$ (Table 1). The significant results in the univariable model were further re-entered into final multivariate model using logistic regression analysis to illuminate confounding factors. A *p*-value < 0.05 was considered statistically significant. Horse breed (OR = 5.0, CI = 0.07–2.104, *p*-value = 0.039) and activity of the horse (OR = 3.21, CI = 0.72–1.48, *p*- value = 0.008) were recorded as potential risk factors for contracting AHSV infection. The results are summarized in (Table 2). The rest of the risk factors did not show any significant association with AHSV seropositive horses.

Discussion

Infectious viral pathogens, such as AHSV, are reemerging as major veterinary problems in different parts of the African continent [13, 14]. Very little information is available about the epidemiology of AHSV in the Middle East and East Central Africa including the Sudan. To better predict and respond to AHSV outbreak, this cross sectional study has been initiated to estimate the prevalence of AHSV and to identify the potential risk factors associated with the disease among horses in Khartoum State of the Central Sudan. The study area of Khartoum state has been selected as it is considered the center for international trade of horses in the country. The routine surveillance for AHSV would be necessary to monitor incursion of the disease in other part of the country

Table 1 Univariate analysis for the association between potential risk factors and AHSV infection among horses in Khartoum state, Sudan, using chi-square test

Risk factors	Animals tested	Animals affected (%)	df	$\chi2$	*p*-value
Locality			3	6.7	0.079
East Nile	50	47(94%)			
Bahry	108	88(81.5%)			
Omdurman	35	33(94%)			
khartoum	127	107(84%)			
Age			1	0.29	0.58
young	89	78 (87.6%)			
Old	231	197(85.3%)			
Sex			1	0.70	0.48
Female	50	41(82%)			
Male	270	234(86.7%)			
Breed			2	7	0.031
Arabi	14	12(85.7%)			
Cross	30	21(70%)			
Local	276	242(87.7%)			
Body condition			1	4.6	0.03
Fair	294	249(84.7%)			
Thin	26	26(100%)			
Presence of insects			1	1.94	0.16
No	33	31(93.9%)			
Yes	287	244(85%)			
Control measures			1	0.49	0.48
No	193	168(87%)			
Yes	127	107(84.3%)			
Activity			2	6.01	0.049
Chaser	73	60(82.2%)			
Cart horse	108	88(81.5%)			
Police horse	139	127(91.4%)			

Table 2 Multivariate analysis using logistic regression model for significant association ($p > 0.05$) between risk factors and AHSV infection among Horses in Khartoum State, Sudan

Risk factors	OR	95%C I	*P*-Value
Breed			
Cross	Reference		
Arabi	5	0.07–2.104	0.039
Activity			
Cart horse	Reference		
Chaser	3.21	0.072–1.48	0.008

considered to be AHSV- free zones. The present study showed that the prevalence of AHSV seropositivity is gnificantly high (85.9%). The detection of AHSV antibodies indicated previous exposure of horses to AHSV. The high prevalence rate (85.9%), as indicted by detection of AHSV antibodies, showed an evidence of previous circulation of AHSV in the study area. There is no vaccination program for AHSV in the Sudan. Therefore, the detected antibodies were due to natural infections. It should also be noted that detection of maternal antibodies to AHSV was excluded as horses included in this study aged over one year.

The present study showed that there was a significant difference between the AHSV seropositivity rate and the breed of the horse. Exotic (Cross) breed of horses are at 5 times at risk compared to indigenous (local) breed of Sudanese horses. High seroprevalence was observed among cross breeds with high percentage of exotic blood. Exotic breeds are usually highly susceptible to bites of insect vectors and subsequent development of AHSV infection. In contrast, the indigenous breed of horses are relatively resistant to bites of insect vectors hence, they were at lower risk for the disease compared to cross breed. In addition, there was a significant difference between AHSV seropositivity and the activities of the horse, particularly those involve in horse racing. Race horses are at 3 times more likely to be at risk compared to other horses involved in transportation activities. Once again, this is attributed to the fact that almost all race horses are of the Arabian horse origin or imported from other countries. It is also possible that most race horses are not usually kept in insect-secured houses and are likely to be exposed to the insect vector as is the case in most horse houses in Khartoum State. The highest rates of AHSV seropositivity was recorded among horses in the East Nile locality (94%). This is most probably to construction of irrigation projects and agricultural schemes in this locality, which provide conducive environmental condition for the breeding of *Culicoides* midge, the insect vector. However, the lowest seropositivity rate was recorded among horses in Bahry locality (81.5), which is possibly attributed to dry climate condition and high variations in temperatures. The present study illustrated that AHSV is now becoming broadly distributed in Sudan with a very high prevalence rate of 85.9% in Khartoum state. It is recommended that the survey should be extended in the future to include virus isolation attempts and to identify the AHSV serotypes circulating in the country. Molecular epidemiological studies such as, viral sequence analysis and phylogeny, should be conducted to monitor the movement of the virus between these African countries. The rest of the individual or management risk factors did not show any significant association with HSV seropositivity. Male or female horses have no significant association with AHSV seropositivity. In addition, no significant difference was observed between AHSV seropositivity and the age of the animals. A Previous study on Seroprevalence of the disease in Ethiopia reported that age and sex were not significantly associated with seroprevalence of AHSV [14]. Early diagnosis during disease outbreak among non vaccinated equines would be necessary for prevention and control of the disease [28]. Complete viral genome sequencing and phylogeny would be necessary to determine the virus genetic lineages [29]. It should be noted that treatment of horses with insecticides be applied monthly to prevent insect bite. The animal owners should also be educated about the risks of the disease, and prevention of the infection through insect control program.

Conclusions

The prevalence of AHSV is significantly high (85.9%) among horses in Khartoum State, Sudan. Exotic Breed and activity of the horse particularly those involved in racing activity are considered to be at higher risk of contracting AHSV infection. This study would be expected to reduce the impact of the disease on horse breeders and subsequently avoid a possible AHSV outbreak among horses. Virus isolation attempts would be necessary for subsequent molecular characterization studies. It is recommended that complete viral genome sequencing and phylogenetic studies should be conducted to determine the genetic lineages of AHSV serotypes circulating in Sudan to follow the movement of the virus in the African continent.

Abbreviations

AHSV: African horse sickness virus; BTV: Blue tongue virus; CI: Confidence interval; EHDV: Epizootic hemorrhagic disese virus; ELISA: Enzyme-linked immunosorbent assay; HRP: Horse radish peroxidase; Ig G: Immunoglobulin G; OR: Odd ratio; RT-PCR: Reverse transcriptase polymerase chain reaction; Ml: Microliter

Acknowledgements

We thank the Police Department, Khartoum State for permission of blood collection from the police horses. The technical assistance of Mr. Abdalla M. Fadlelmoula is gratefully acknowledged.

Authors' contributions

STK, AIG, IAA helped with collection of blood samples from horses and the design of the study. TMA, STK and ROS performed the laboratory work including ELISA assay. IEA and EMH analyzed the data. All authors have read and approved the final version of this manuscript.

Consent for publication

Not applicable.

Competing interests

The authors declare that they have no competing interests.

Author details

[1]Molecular Biology Laboratory (MBL), Department of Clinical Medicine, Faculty of Veterinary Medicine, University of Khartoum, P.O. Box 32, Khartoum North, Sudan. [2]Scientific Research Directorate, Al-Mughtaribeen University, Khartoum, Sudan. [3]EBH Scientific Research Laboratory, Zamzam University College (ZUC), Khartoum, Sudan.

References

1. Borden EC, Shope RE, Murphy FA. Physicochemical and morphological relationships of some arthropod-borne viruses to bluetongue virus-anew taxonomic group. Physicochemical and serological studies. J Gen Virol. 1971;3:261–71.
2. Fenner F, Pereira HG, Porterfield JS. Family and generic names for virus approved by the International Committee on Taxonomy of Viruses. Intervirology. 1974;3:193–4.
3. Abuelzein EME, Mirghani ME, Ali BE. Observations on African horse sickness in donkeys in the Sudan. Rev Sci Tech Off Int Epiz. 1989;8:785–7.
4. El-Hasnaoui H, el Harrak M, Zientara S, Laviada M, Hamblin C. Serological and virological responses in mules and donkeys following inoculation with African horse sickness virus serotype 4. Arch Virol. 1998;14:29–36.
5. Fassi-Fihri O, el Harrak M, Fass-Fehri MM. Clinical, virological and immune responses of normal and immunosuppressed donkeys (*Equus asinus africanus*) after inoculation with African horse sickness virus. Arch Virol Suppl. 1998;14:49–56.
6. Aradaib IE, Mohammed EHM, Ali NOM, Majid AA, Idris SH, Karrar AE. A simple and rapid method for detection of African horse sickness virus serogroup using RT-PCR. Vet Res Comm. 2006;30:319–24.
7. Sailleau C, Hamblin C, Paweska JT, Zientara S. Identification and differentiation of nine African horse sickness virus serotypes by RT-PCR amplification of the serotype-specific genome segment 2. J Gen Virol. 2000;81:831–7.
8. Robin M, Page P, Archer D, Baylis M. African horse sickness: The potential for an outbreak in disease-free regions and current disease control and elimination techniques. Equine Vet J. 2016;48:659–69.
9. Becker E, Venter GJ, Greyling T, Molini U, van Hamburg H. Evidence of African horse sickness virus infection of *Equus zebra hartmannae* in the south-western Khomas Region, Namibia. Transbound Emerg Dis. 2018;65(1): 278–80. https://doi.org/10.1111/tbed.12651.
10. Aradaib IE. PCR detection of African horse sickness virus based on genome segment three sequence analysis. J Virol Method. 2009;159:1–5.
11. Mohammed EHM, Mellor PS. Further studies on bluetongue-related Orbiviruses in the Sudan. Epidemiol & infect. 1990;105:619–32.
12. Eisa M. The isolation and identification of type 9 African horse sickness virus in the Sudan. Br Vet J. 1974;130:606–10.
13. Ayelet G, Derso S, Jenberie S, Tigre W, Aklilu N, Gelaye E, Asmare K. Outbreak investigation and molecular characterization of African horse sickness virus circulating in selected areas of Ethiopia. Acta Trop. 2013;127:91–6.
14. Bitew M, Andargie A, Bekele M, Jenberie S, Ayelet G, Gelaye E. Serological survey of African horse sickness in selected districts of Jimma zone, Southwestern Ethiopia. Trop Anim Health Prod. 2011;43:1543–7.
15. Hamblin C, Mertens PPC, Mellor PS, Burroughs NJ, Crowther JR. A serogroup specific enzyme-linked immunosorbent assay for the detection and identification of African horse sickness viruses. J Virol Methods. 1991;31:285–92.
16. Maree S, Paweska JT. Preparation of recombinant African horse sickness virus VP7 antigen via a simple method and validation of a VP7-based indirect ELISA for the detection of group-specific IgG antibodies in horse sera. J Virol Methods. 2005;125:55–65.
17. Martinez-Torrecuadrada JL, Diaz-Laviada M, Roy P, Sanchez C, Vela C, Sanchez-Vizcaino JM, Casal JI. Serologic markers in early stages of African horse sickness virus infection. J Clin Microbiol. 1997;35:531–5.
18. Martinez-Torrecuadrada JL, Iwata H, Venteo A, Casal I, Roy P. Expression and characterization of the two outer capsid proteins of African horsesickness virus: the role of VP2 in virus neutralization. Virology. 1994;202:348–59.
19. Rodriguez M, Hooghuis H, Castano M. Current status of the diagnosis and control of African horse sickness. Vet Res. 1993;24:189–97.
20. Wade-Evans AM, Woolhouse T, O'Hara R, Hamblin C. The use of African horse sickness virus VP7 antigen, synthesised in bacteria, and anti-VP7 monoclonal antibodies in a competitive ELISA. J Virol Method. 1993;45:179–88.
21. Stone-Marschat M, Carville A, Skowronek A, Laegreid W. W: detection of African horse sickness virus by reverse transcription–PCR. J Clin Microbiol. 1994;32:697–700.
22. Williams CF, Inoue T, Lucus AM, Zanotto PM, Roy R. The complete sequence of four structural proteins of African horse sickness virus serotype 6: evolutionary relationships within and between the orbiviruses. Virus Res. 1998;53:53–73.
23. Zientara S, Sailleau C, Moulay S, Plateau E, Cruciere C. Diagnosis and molecular epidemiology of the African horse sickness virus by the polymerase chain reaction and restriction patterns. Vet Res. 1993;24:385–95.
24. Zientara S, Sailleau C, Moulay S, Cruciere C. Differentiation of African horse sickness viruses by polymerase chain reaction and segments 10 restriction patterns. Vet Microbiol. 1995;47:365–75.
25. Zientara S, Sailleau C, Moulay S, Wade-Evans A, Cruciere C. Application of the polymerase chain reaction to the detection of African horse sickness viruses. J Virol Methods. 1995;1995(53):47–54.
26. Zientara S, Sailleau C, Moulay S, Cruciere C, el- Harrak M, Laegreid WW, Hamblin C. Use of reverse transcriptase-polymerase chain reaction (RT-PCR) and dot-blot hybridization for the detection and identification of African horse sickness virus nucleic acids. Arch Virol. 1998;14:317–27.
27. Martin SW, Meek HA, Willeberg P. Veterinary Epidemiology: Principles and Methods. AMES: Iowa state University Press; 1987.
28. Koekemoer JJ. Serotype-specific detection of African horsesickness virus by real-time PCR and the influence of genetic variations. J Virol Methods. 2008; 154:104–10.
29. Martin LA, Meyer AJ, O'Hara RS, Fu H, Mellor PS, Knowles NJ, Mertens PP. Phylogenetic analysis of African horse sickness virus segment 10: sequence variation, virulence characteristics and cell exit. Arch Virol. 1998;14:281–93.

21

Expression of vascular endothelial growth factor (VEGF) in equine sarcoid

Manuela Martano*, Karen Power, Brunella Restucci, Ilaria Pagano, Gennaro Altamura, Giuseppe Borzacchiello and Paola Maiolino

Abstract

Background: Sarcoids are the mostcommon skin tumors in horses, characterized by rare regression, invasiveness and high recurrence following surgical intervention and Delta Papillomaviruses are widely recognized as the causative agents of the disease. In order to gain new insights into equine sarcoid development, we have evaluated, in 25 equine sarcoids, by immunohistochemistry and western blotting analysis, the expression levels of VEGF, Ki67 and bcl-2. Moreover, we have measured microvessel density and specific vessel parameters.

Results: All sarcoid samples showed a strong and finely granular cytoplasmatic staining for VEGF in the majority (90%) of keratinocytes, sarcoid fibroblasts and endothelial cells. Numerous small blood vessels, immunostained with Von Willebrand factor, often appeared irregular in shape and without a distinct lumen, with mean values of microvessel area and perimeter lower than normal. Moreover, in all sarcoid samples, Ki67 immunoreactivity was moderately positive in 5–10% of dermal sarcoid fibroblasts, while Bcl2 immunoreactivity was detected in 52% of the sarcoid samples, with a weak staining in 20–50% of dermal sarcoid fibroblasts. Biochemical analysis was consistent with immunohistochemical results.

Conclusions: This study has provided evidence that in equine sarcoid: VEGF was strongly expressed; the increased number of vessels was not associated with their complete maturation, probably leading to a hypoxic condition, which could increase VEGF synthesis; the levels of sarcoid fibroblasts proliferation were very low. Concluding, VEGF may have a role in equine sarcoid development, not only through the increase of angiogenesis, but also through the control of sarcoid fibroblast activity.

Keywords: Angiogenesis, BPV, Equine sarcoid, VEGF

Background

Sarcoids are the most common skin tumors in horses [1–3], with prevalence rates ranging from 12.9 to 67% of all equine tumors [4, 5]. They appear as benign fibroblastic skin tumors, and are characterized by rare regression, invasiveness and high recurrence following surgery [6–8]. Delta Papillomaviruses (Bovine Papillomavirus 1, Bovine Papillomavirus 2 and Bovine Papillomavirus 13) [9–11] are involved in the pathogenesis of this tumor, mainly through the biological activity of the E5 oncogene. It has also been reported that BPV alters DNA methylation status and oxidative stress parameters [12, 13].

Moreover, equine sarcoid may be considered one of the main long-term complications in the wound healing process of the horse [5, 14], consequent to abnormal fibroblast proliferation and changes in dynamics of the *extracellular matrix* (ECM) and its main components [15]. Altered turnover of the ECM deposition and degradation, as result of an altered expression of matrix metalloproteinases (MMPs) and tissue inhibitor of metalloproteinases (TIMPs), were reported as basic mechanism for these changes [15]. ECM remodeling is strictly correlated to angiogenesis [16], as MMPs production is stimulated by many of the same factors (VEGF; tumor necrosis factor alpha; *basic fibroblast growth factor*) implicated in endothelial migration and formation of new capillaries (angiogenesis) [17]. VEGF, also known as vascular permeability factor (VPF), is a member of the *platelet-derived growth factor* (*PDGF*) family of growth factors, having a potent angiogenic activity and an

* Correspondence: manuela.martano@unina.it
Department of Veterinary Medicine and Animal Productions, Naples University "Federico II", Via F. Delpino 1, 80137 Naples, Italy

important role in the modulation of ECM homeostasis and remodeling [18, 19]. It is involved in numerous physiological and pathological processes, such as embryonic development [20], bone formation [21] wound healing [22] and cancer [23–27], in which it is up-regulated by oncogene expression, growth factors and hypoxia [28–30]. Moreover, it has been reported that Human Papillomavirus type 16 E6 and E7 oncoproteins may contribute to tumor angiogenesis by direct activation of the VEGF gene promoter in human lung and cervical carcinoma [31–33].

Although the general role of VEGF in angiogenic processes has been intensively studied [23–27], its specific function in sarcoid development has not been investigated, so far. In this regard, the aim of this study was to evaluate in a subset of equine sarcoids, the levels of VEGF expression in association with angiogenesis (evaluation of microvessel density and specific vessel parameters), and with Ki67 and bcl-2 expression.

Results

Histological features

Haematoxylin and eosin staining of examined sarcoids ($n = 25$) showed the typical histological changes in their epidermal (when present) and dermal component, as reported by Martano et al. (2016) [15], such as: hyperkeratosis and epidermal hyperplasia often accompanied by rete pegs; dermal fibroblasts usually oriented perpendicular to the basal epidermal layer in a 'picket fence' pattern; abundant ECM; numerous small vessels irregular in shape.

Immunohistochemical and biochemical results

The expression patterns of VEGF, Ki67 and bcl-2 in 25 equine sarcoids and 5 normal skin samples are summarized in Table 1.

In all normal skin samples, weak granular cytoplasmatic VEGF immunopositivity was detected predominantly in the basal layer of normal epidermis (Fig. 1a), while normal fibroblasts were negative. Ki67 immunostaining was moderate and restricted to the basal layer of epidermis and hair follicle (Fig. 1b), while bcl-2 immunostaing was very weak and in 2/5 samples was negative (Fig. 1c). Moreover, in normal skin samples, blood vessels, immunostained with vWF, appeared regular in shape and size, with a distinct lumen (Fig. 1d).

In all sarcoid samples the majority (90%) of keratinocytes, neoplastic fibroblasts and endothelial cells showed a strong and finely granular cytoplasmatic staining for VEGF (Fig. 2a; secondary-only negative control Fig. 2b) and Ki67 immunoreactivity was strong in the majority (90%) of epidermal and hair follicle basal cells and endothelial cells, while only 5–10% of neoplastic dermal fibroblasts were moderately positive (Fig. 2c; secondary-only negative control Fig. 2d). In 18 out of 25 sarcoid samples (72%) bcl-2 immunoreactivity was moderate in basal and parabasal layer of epidermis and in 20–50% of fibroblasts located immediately under the epidermis (Fig. 2e; secondary-only negative control Fig. 2f)), while the percentage of bcl-2 positive dermal fibroblasts was very low (10%) (Fig. 2g; secondary-only negative control

Table 1 Immunoreactivity scoring of VEGF, Ki67 and Bcl2 in 25 equine sarcoid samples and 5 equine normal skins

Samples	Location	VEGF Staining Intensity	Ki67 Staining Intensity	bcl-2 Staining Intensity
S1	neck	++	+	+
S2	limb	++	+	+/−
S3	Pectoral region	++	+	+
S4	limb	++	+	+/−
S5	head	++	+	+/−
S6	abdomen	++	+	+/−
S7	head	++	++	−
S8	Pectoral region	++	+	+/−
S9	limb	++	+	+/−
S10	(para)-Genital	++	+	+/−
S11	Limb	++	+	+
S12	abdomen	++	+	n.a.
S13	Pectoral region	++	++	+/−
S14	head	++	+	+
S15	limb	++	++	−
S16	(para)-Genital	++	+	+
S17	Limb	++	+	+/−
S18	abdomen	++	+	+
S19	Pectoral region	++	+	−
S20	neck	++	+	+
S21	limb	++	+	+
S22	(para)-Genital	++	++	n.a.
S23	Limb	++	+	+/−
S24	abdomen	++	++	−
S25	Pectoral region	++	+/−	+/−
N1	head	+/−	+	+/−
N2	abdomen	+/−	+/−	−
N3	neck	+/−	+	−
N4	limb	+/−	+/−	+/−
N5	Pectoral region	+/−	+	+/−

N Normal skin sample, *S* sarcoid sample, *n.a.* not assessable; − negative staining; +/− weak immunolabelling; + moderate immunolabelling; ++ extensive and strong immunolabelling

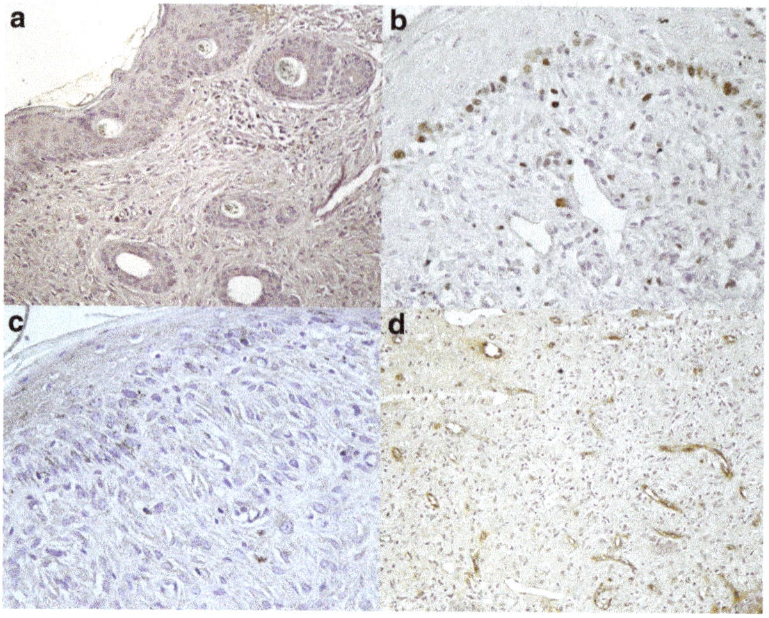

Fig. 1 Equine normal skin. Streptavidin-biotin-peroxidase stain. **a** weak granular cytoplasmatic VEGF immunostaining was detected in the basal layer of epidermis and hair follicle while normal fibroblasts were negative 20×; **b** Ki67 immunostaining was moderate and restricted to the basal layer of epidermis 40×; **c** bcl-2 immunostaining was very weak and restricted to the basal layer of epidermis 40×; **d** blood vessels, immunolabeled with vWF, appeared regular in shape, with a distinct lumen 20×

fig. h) and the intensity of staining was weak. Moreover, in all sarcoid samples, numerous small blood vessels often appeared irregular in shape (Fig. 2i; negative control Fig.l).

Microvessel density was lower in normal skin samples (39.5 ± 2.1) than in sarcoid samples (84.8 ± 65.06), with not statistically significant p value ($p > 0.05$), while vascular parameters mean values (area and perimeter) were higher in normal skins (418.02 ± 84.14; 78.01 ± 7.07) than in sarcoid samples (223.08 ± 55.92; 62.03 ± 6.08), with statistically significant p value ($p <$ 0,05) (Table 2).

Western blotting analysis was performed to check the specificity of the antibodies used throughout the study (Fig. 3a-h). A band of the expected molecular size for VEGF (25 Kda), vWF (250 Kda), bcl-2 (26 Kda) and Ki67 (110 Kda) was identified in the tested samples as well as in Hela or Saos-2 cell lines used as positive control (Fig. 3a, c, e, f). The densitometric analysis of the bands normalized for β-actin revealed variable levels of VEGF protein among the samples, with higher expression in two sarcoid samples (Fig. 3b). Moreover, Von Willebrand factor protein was over-expressed in each sarcoid sample compared to each of normal skin lysates, in which the specific band was almost undetectable (Fig. 3d). The biochemical expression of bcl-2 and Ki67 was variable among the samples and no different trends between normal skin and tumor samples could be pointed out as confirmed by densitometric analysis and normalization for β-actin levels (Fig. 3f, h).

Discussion

VEGF is a potent angiogenic factor, produced by a variety of cell types, including keratinocytes, endothelial cells, macrophages, mast cells, fibroblasts [29, 34, 35] and is involved in several types of tumors [23–27], where it has been shown to influence both tumor neovascularization and dissemination [36, 37]. Vascular endothelial growth factor can occur in at least six different isoforms, containing 121, 145, 165, 183, 189 and 206 amino acids. VEGF 121 is a freely diffusible isoform [38] and it has been proved to have a stronger angiogenic and tumorigenic activity when compared to the bigger isoforms [39–41].

In the present study, for the first time, we have demonstrated, by immunohistochemistry, the overexpression of VEGF (isoform 121) in equine sarcoid compared to normal skin, which was in part confirmed by biochemical analysis. It appeared as a strong and finely granular cytoplasmic staining pattern in the majority (> 90%) of keratinocytes, endothelial cells and sarcoid fibroblasts, suggesting a possible role in equine sarcoid development. Interestingly, in sarcoid samples we have also observed the presence of numerous small vessels, immunostained with vWF, which appeared often irregular in shape These findings were in agreement with other studies, which reported that tumor vasculature, formed under the influence of VEGF, is often structurally and functionally abnormal [42], probably as the results of the insufficient production or activation of other angiogenic factors, necessary for the formation of mature

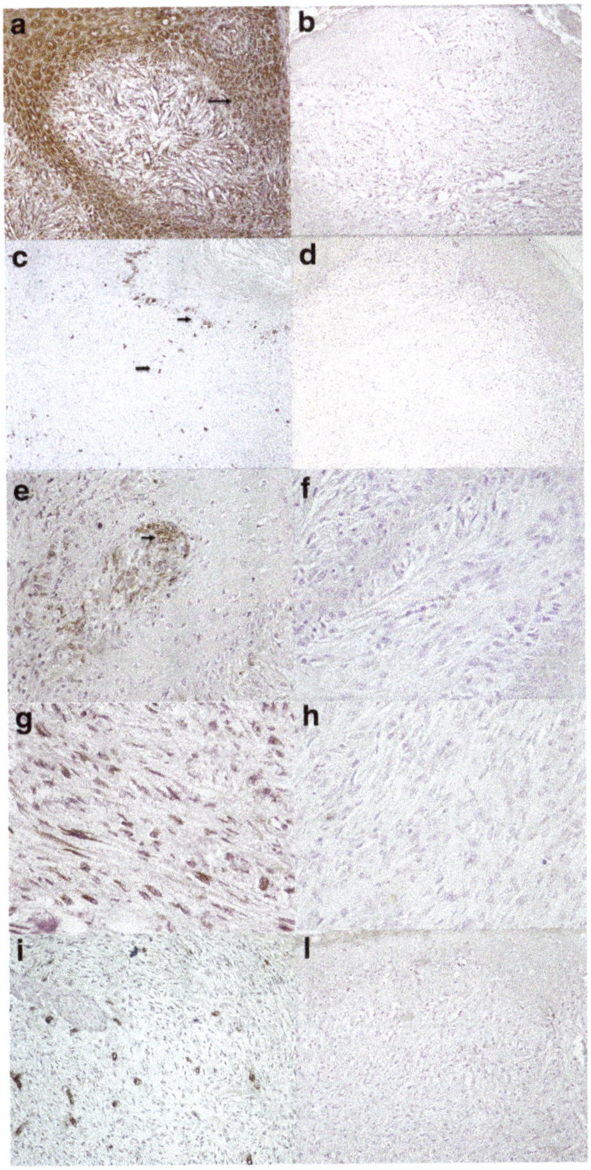

Fig. 2 Equine sarcoid. Streptavidin-biotin-peroxidase stain. **a** Keratinocytes and fibroblasts showed a strong and finely granular cytoplasmatic staining for VEGF (arrow). 20×; **b** Secondary-only negative control for VEGF. 20×; **c** Ki67 immunoreactivity was strong in the epidermal and hair follicle basal cells (little arrow), while only few dermal fibroblasts (big arrow) were moderately positive. 20×; **d** Secondary-only negative control for Ki67. 20×; **e** Fibroblasts located immediately under the epidermis were moderately positive for bcl2 (arrow). 40×; **f** Secondary-only negative control for bcl-2. 40×; **g** bcl-2 immunoreactivity was weak in few dermal fibroblasts (arrow). 40×; **h** Secondary-only negative control for bcl-2 40×; **i** Numerous small blood vessels, immunolabeled with vWF, often appered irregular in shape and without a distinct lumen (arrow). 20×; **l** Secondary-only negative control for bcl-2. 20×

and functioning new vessels [25, 26]. These data seem to strongly support the hypothesis that in sarcoid, a suboptimal blood flow could lead to a deficient oxygen gradient within the tissue that exacerbates angiogenesis [43]. It is well known that tissue mild hypoxia, an almost universal condition within wound healing, from which sarcoid could origin, is an effective inducer of VEGF synthesis [44]. Therefore, in sarcoid, a vicious circle may occur in which hypoxia upregulates VEGF synthesis, leading to an insufficient vascularization, which in turn probably exacerbates hypoxia. Despite numerous studies characterizing its angiogenic property, data on the role of VEGF in ECM homeostasis and remodeling are still scanty.

For this reason, we speculate that, in equine sarcoid, VEGF could be implicated not only in angiogenesis but also in ECM homeostasis and remodeling, through a deregulation of fibroblasts proliferation and apoptosis in a possible hypoxic condition. This mechanism was also reported during endochondral bone formation, in which VEGF couples hypertrophic cartilage remodeling, ossification and angiogenesis [21]. In this regard, a very low fibroblast growth rate has been reported in equine sarcoid, along with a low frequency of p53 mutations [45]. These last were generally associated with abnormalities in apoptotic pathways rather than abnormal cell cycle control mechanism [46].

In our sarcoids samples, the percentage of Ki67 positive fibroblasts ranged from 5 to 10% and, in agreement with previous studies [46–48], these results confirm that the rate of fibroblast proliferation in equine sarcoid was very low. Moreover, these observations correspond to the clinical evidence that equine sarcoids are slow growing tumors and can remain quiescent for years [47]. IHC and biochemical data did not prove an overall differential expression of Ki67 and bcl-2 in sarcoids compared to normal skin; however, the more frequent localization of BPV-positive cells, right near the dermo-epidermal junction [49, 50], could explain the higher expression of Ki67 and bcl-2 observed in epithelial portion and in dermo-epidermal junction.

Conclusion

Concluding, in this study we hypothesized that VEGF might have a role in sarcoid development, by altering ECM homeostasis, through a selection of a quiescent population of fibroblast, leading to an impaired degradation and excessive accumulation of ECM [14]. This also seems to be also supported by our previous study, which documented that the excessive and progressive deposition of connective tissue (collagen) in sarcoid is not only the result of elevated synthesis by fibroblasts, but it is also caused by a deficiency in matrix degradation due to an altered expression of MMPs and TIMPs [15].

Currently, despite the numerous *sarcoid treatment* choices available, *not* all *sarcoids* are responsive. Hence, the importance of a better knowledge of equine sarcoid development. Further studies in the near future are needed to investigate the association between equine sarcoid and tissue

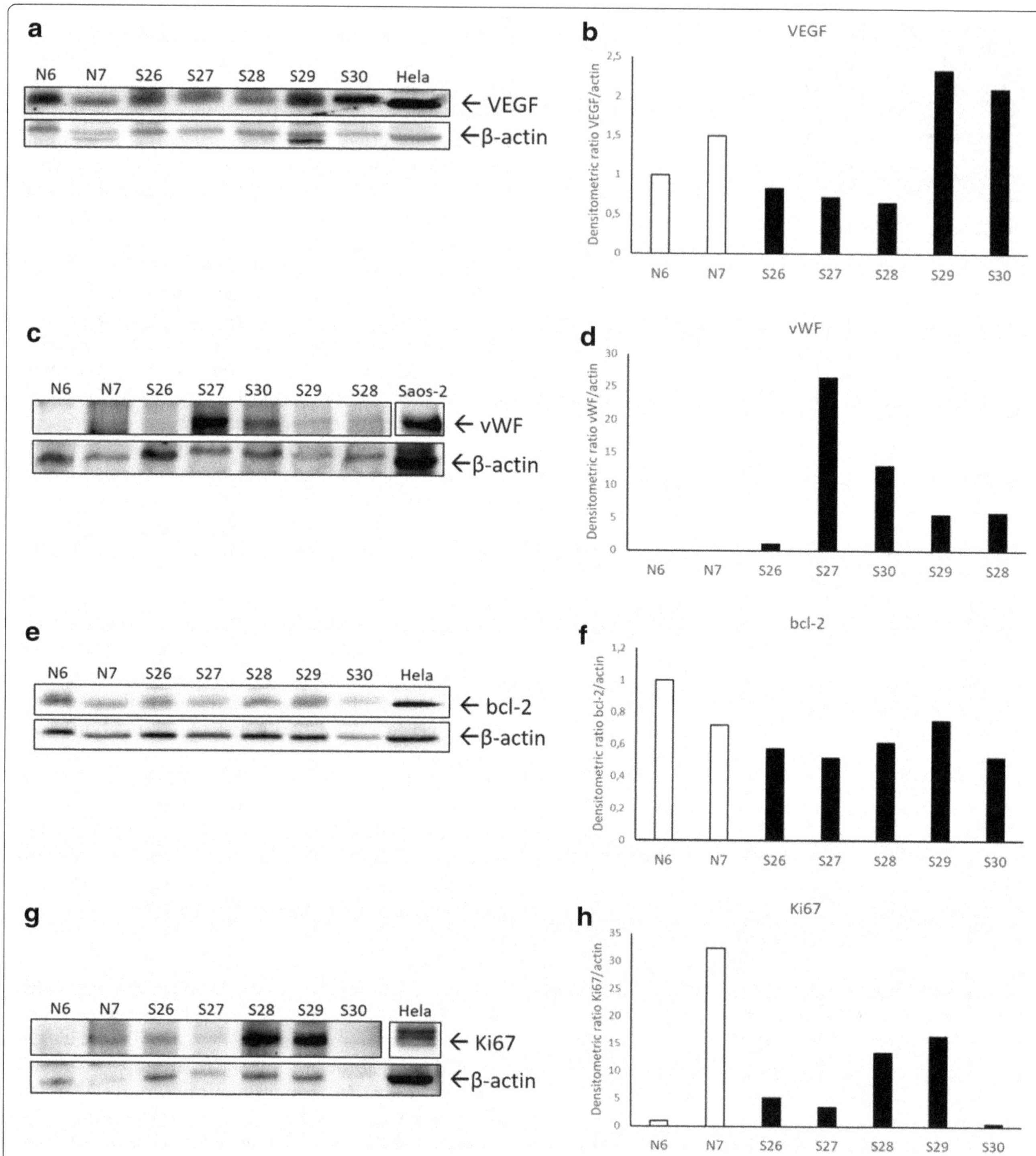

Fig. 3 (See legend on next page.)

(See figure on previous page.)
Fig. 3 Western blotting analysis of VEGF, vWF, bcl-2 and Ki67 protein expression in equine sarcoids (S) and normal skin samples (N). **a** VEGF was expressed in all the analysed samples, with higher protein levels in S29 and S30. Hela whole cell lysate was run along with equine samples as positive control. The membrane was re-probed for β-actin to allow normalization. **b** Densitometric values were measured and expressed as VEGF/actin ratio. **c** vWF was detectable in sarcoids but not in normal skin samples. Saos-2 whole cell lysate was run along with equine samples as positive control. The Saos-2 box is cut from the same membrane at a different exposure time and properly aligned according to the molecular standard loaded onto the gel. The membrane was re-probed for β-actin to allow normalization. **d** Densitometric values were measured and expressed as vWF/actin ratio. **e** bcl-2 was expressed at variable levels in the analysed samples. Hela whole cell lysate was run along with equine samples as positive control. The membrane was re-probed for β-actin to allow normalization. **f** Densitometric values were measured and expressed as bcl-2/actin ratio. **g** Variable expression of Ki67 protein in the analysed samples. Hela whole cell lysate was run along with equine samples as positive control. The Hela box is cut from the same membrane at a different exposure time and properly aligned according to the molecular standard loaded onto the gel. The membrane was re-probed for β-actin to allow normalization. **h** Densitometric values were measured and expressed as Ki67/actin ratio

hypoxia, which could have a crucial role for the development of new therapeutic strategies.

Methods

Tumor samples

A total of 25 (S1-S25) equine sarcoids (each from a different horse), clinically identified based on their gross morphology according to Pascoe and Knottenbelt [51], were obtained from affected horses, which underwent surgery routinely, adhering to a high standard (best practice) of veterinary care, after informed written consent of the owners, and according to Directives 2010/63/EU (art. 1 c. 4) and 2010/63/EU. Tumors were localized on the neck (2), limbs (8), pectoral region (5), head (3), abdomen (4), (para)-genital (3) (Table 1). Sarcoid tissues used in this study were known to be BPV positive [48].

As controls, tissues from 5 normal skin BPV positive samples (N1-N5), were taken during necropsy from five healthy horses. We did not seek committee approval as all samples analyzed were not collected as part of experimental clinical veterinary practices but as routine diagnosis and treatment, according to Directive 2010/63/EU (art. 1 c. 4) on protection of animals used for scientific purposes. All samples were 10% formalin fixed, paraffin-embedded for routine histological processing and stained with haematoxylin and eosin for light microscopy study.

Table 2 Microvessel density and vascular parameters (areas and perimeters), expressed as mean (X) and standard deviation (SD), in equine sarcoids and normal skins

	Normal skin (X ± SD)	Equine sarcoids (X ± SD)	*p* values (< 0,05)
Microvessel density	39.5 ± 2.1	84.8 ± 65.06	0,3
Areas (mm^2)	418.02 ± 84.14	223.08 ± 55.92	0,001
Perimeters (mm)	78.01 ± 7.07	62.03 ± 6.08	0,007

Additional five sarcoids (S26-S30) and 2 normal skin samples (N6-N7) were collected as above and immediately frozen at − 80 °C in order to allow Western blotting analysis.

Immunohistochemistry

Paraffin sections of equine sarcoids (S1-S25) and normal skin (N1-N5) from healthy horses were dewaxed in xylene, dehydrated in graded alcohols and washed in 0.01 M phosphate-buffered saline (PBS), pH 7.2–7.4. Endogenous peroxidase was blocked with hydrogen peroxide 0.3% in absolute methanol for 30 min. The immunohistochemical procedure (streptavidin biotin-peroxidase method) for the detection of VEGF, bcl-2, Ki67 and vWF was the same as that used by the authors in a previous study [15]. The immunolabelling procedure included negative control sections incubated with PBS instead of the primary antibodies (Fig. 2b, d, f, h, l). Primary antibodies, dilutions and antigen retrieval techniques used in this study are listed in Table 3. Primary antibodies were diluted in phosphate-buffered saline (PBS) and applied overnight at 4 °C. After 2 washes in PBS, MACH 1 mouse probe (Biocare Medical, LLC, Concord, CA, USA) was applied for 20 min at room temperature. After, MACH-1 Universal HPR-Polymer (Biocare Medical) was applied for 30 min at room temperature. To reveal immunolabelling, diaminobenzidine-tetrahydrochloride was used as a chromogen, and haematoxylin as counterstain.

Scoring of immunoreactivity

The intensity of immunolabelling in each specimen, for each antibody, was scored by two independent observers (MM and KP) under blinded conditions, as performed in a previous study [52]. Briefly, for each sample the immunoreactivity was scored from negative to strong, as follows: n.a., not assessable; − negative staining; +/− weak immunolabelling; + moderate immunolabelling; ++ extensive and strong immunolabelling. Moreover, the number of positively-labelled cells was established by counting 1.000 cells in 10 fields

Table 3 List of primary antibodies used for immunohistochemistry and western blotting analysis

Antibody	Manufacturer	Clone	Host species	Antigen retriever	IHC Dilution	WB Dilution
vWF	DAKO	Polyclonal	Rabbit	0.05% pepsin in 0.01 M HCl (pH 2) at 37 ° C for 15 min	1:400	1:1000
bcl-2	DAKO	124	mouse	Heated Citrate buffer, ph 6.0, 30 min	1:100	1:1000
VEGF	Thermoscientific	JH121	mouse	Heated Citrate buffer, ph 6.0, 30 min,	1:200	1:200
Ki67	Santa Cruz	D-6	mouse	Heated Citrate buffer, ph 6.0, 30 min,	1:100	1: 1000

at 400× magnification (40× objective 10× ocular) and results were expressed as percentage.

Microvessel density and vascular parameter measurements

Microvessel density (number of vessels per mm^2) and vascular parameter measurements (vessel area and perimeter) were performed on vWF immunostained sections, using a free image analysis software (Image J). For each tumor 10 fields, randomly selected, were captured at 400× magnification (40× objective 10× ocular) with a microscope (E-400; Nikon Eclipse, Tokyo, Japan) coupled to a videocamera (TKC1380E; JVC, Tokyo, Japan), stored in the digital memory, and shown on the monitor. The fields were examined and manual outlining of immunolabelled microvessels was performed; microvessel density, areas, perimeters were then calculated based on image analysis, and results were expressed as mean (X) and standard deviation values (±SD) (Table 2). Statistical assessment was performed using a Student t-test by analysis of variance (ANOVA) and p-value< 0.05 with 95% confidence interval (CI) was considered statistically significant.

Protein extraction and SDS PAGE/western blotting

Tissue samples N6-N7 and T26-T30 were homogenized in ice-cold RIPA buffer (50 mM Tris-HCl, pH 7.5, 150 mM NaCl, 1% Triton X100, 1 mM EDTA, deoxycholate 0.25%) added with phosphatase and protease inhibitor cocktails (Sigma-Aldrich, Milan, Italy) by using TissueLyser machinery (Qiagen, Milan, Italy) according to manufacturer's protocol. Tissue homogenates were incubated on a rocking wheel for 30′ at 4 °C. Protein extracts were clarified by high-speed centrifugation at 4 °C for 30'and total proteins were quantified by Bradford assay (Bio-Rad, Bio-Rad Laboratories, Segrate (MI), Italy). Equal amounts of lysates were resuspended in Laemmli sample buffer (Bio-Rad), boiled and analyzed by denaturing polyacrylamide gel electrophoresis (SDS PAGE). Proteins were blotted from gel onto nitrocellulose membranes using TransBlot Turbo apparatus (Bio-Rad, Bio-Rad Laboratories, Segrate (MI), Italy). The membranes were blocked with 5% non-fat dry milk in Tris buffered saline (10 mM Tris-HCl, pH 7.4, 165 mM NaCl) with 0.1% tween (TTBS), for 1 h (h) at room temperature (RT) and incubated over night at 4 °C with the primary antibodies at the indicated dilutions: anti- Bcl2 (1:1000), anti-VEGF (1:200), anti-Ki67 (1:1000), anti-vWF (1:1000). After four washing steps of 10 minutes, appropriate peroxidase-conjugated secondary antibodies were applied for 1 h at RT at 1:2000 dilution. Following further four washings in TTBS, bound antibodies were visualized by enhanced chemiluminescence (Cyanagen, Bologna, Italy). The blots were stripped and reprobed against mouse anti-β-actin antibody (CP01, Calbiochem, San Diego, CA, USA) (1:500) to allow normalization. Protein levels were quantitatively estimated by densitometric analysis using ChemiDoc gel scanner (Bio-Rad) equipped with a densitometric workstation (Image Lab software, (Bio-Rad Laboratories, Segrate (MI), Italy). Proteins concentrations were normalized to the β-actin levels.

Abbreviations

bcl-2: B-cell lymphoma 2; BPV: Bovine papillomavirus; BPV-2: Bovine papillomavirus type-2; ECM: Extracellular Matrix; MMP: matrix metalloproteinase; N: normal skin; PBS: phosphate-buffered saline; PDGF: platelet-derived growth factor; S: samples T: sarcoid samples; TIMP: Tissue inhibitor of metalloproteinase; VEGF: Vascular endothelial growth factor; vWF: Von Willebrandt factor

Acknowledgements

The authors thank Mr. Raffaele Ilsami (Department of Veterinary medicine and animal production) for his technical assistance, and Dr. Tommaso De Palma (veterinarian) for providing some sarcoid samples.

Funding

The authors received financial support from the research funding of the Department of Veterinary medicine and animal production, University of Naples, Italy.

Authors' contributions

PM has conceived the study, coordinated the group and drafted the manuscript; MM together with PM, has participated in the conception and design of the study, in analysis and interpretation of histological and immunohistochemical data and drafted the manuscript; BR and GB have been involved in revising the manuscript for important intellectual content; IP and KP carried out the histological and immunohistochemical studies, taking part in western blotting analysis; GA and IP carried out the molecular studies, taking part in western blotting analysis. All authors read and approved the final manuscript.

Author's information

MM is employed as a researcher at the Department of Veterinary medicine and animal production; **BR and GB** are employed as associate professors at the Department of Veterinary medicine and animal production; **PM** is employed as a full professor at the Department of Veterinary medicine and animal production; **IP** is a student trainee for the degree thesis; **GA** is a post-doc research fellow at Department of Veterinary medicine and animal production; **KP** is PhD fellow at Department of Veterinary medicine and animal production.

Consent for publication
Not applicable.

Competing interests
The authors declare that they have no competing interests.

References

1. Jackson C. The incidence and pathology of tumours of domesticated animals in South Africa. Onderstepoort J Vet Sci Anim Ind. 1936;6:375–85.
2. Pascoe RR, Summers PM. Clinical survey of tumours and tumor like lesions in horses in southeast. Equine Vet J. 1981;13:325–9.
3. Ragland WL, Keown GH, Spencer GR. Equine sarcoid. Equine Vet J. 1970;2:2–11.
4. Lavach JD, Sullins KE, Roberts SM, Severin GA, Wheeler C, Leuker DC. BCG treatment of periocular sarcoid. Equine Vet J. 1985;17:445–8.
5. Knottenbelt DC. A suggested clinical classification of the equine sarcoid. Clin Tech Equine Pract. 2005;4:278–95.
6. Borzacchiello G, Corteggio A. Equine sarcoid: state of the art. Ippologia. 2009;20:7–14.
7. Nasir L, Campo MS. Bovine papillomaviruses: their role in the aetiology of cutaneous tumours of bovids and equids. Vet Dermatol. 2008;19:243–54.
8. Nasir L, Brandt S. Papillomavirus associated diseases of the horse. Vet Microbiol. 2013;167(Suppl 1–2):159–67.
9. Borzacchiello G, Roperto F. Bovine papillomaviruses, papillomas and cancer in cattle. Vet Res. 2008;39:45.
10. Lunardi M, Alcântara B, Otonel R, Rodrigues W, Alfieri A, Alfieri A. Bovine papillomavirus type 13 DNA in equine sarcoids. J Clin Microbiol. 2013;51:2167–71.
11. Chambers G, Ellsmore VA, O'Brien PM, Reid SW, Love S, Campo MS, Nasir L. Association of bovine papillomavirus with the equine sarcoid. J Gen Virol. 2003;84:1055–62.
12. Potocki L, Lewinska A, Klukowska-Rötzler J, Bielak-Zmijewska A, Grabowska W, Rzeszutek I, Kaminska P, Roga E, Bugno-Poniewierska M, Slota E, Mählmann K, Koch C, Wnuk M. Sarcoid-derived fibroblasts: links between genomic instability, energy metabolism and senescence. Biochimie. 2014;97:163–72.
13. Potocki L, Lewinska A, Klukowska-Rötzler J, Bugno-Poniewierska M, Koch C, Mählmann K, Janda J, Wnuk M. DNA hypomethylation and oxidative stress-mediated increase in genomic instability in equine sarcoid-derived fibroblasts. Biochimie. 2012;94(9):2013–24.
14. Cochrane AC. Models in vivo of wound healing in the horse and the role of growth factors. Vet Dermatol. 1997;8:259–72.
15. Martano M, Corteggio A, Restucci B, De Biase ME, Borzacchiello G, Maiolino P. Extracellular matrix remodeling in equine sarcoid: an immunohistochemical and molecular study. BMC Vet Res. 2016;12:24.
16. Neve A, Cantatore FP, Maruotti N, Corrado A, Ribatti D. Extracellular matrix modulates angiogenesis in physiological and pathological conditions. Biomed Res Int. 2014;2014:756078.
17. Raza SL, Cornelius LA. Matrix metalloproteinases: pro- and anti-angiogenic activities. J Investig Dermatol Symp Proc. 2000;5(1):47–54.
18. Cornelius LA, Nehring LC, Roby JD, Parks WC, Welgus HG. Human dermal microvascular andothelial cells produce matrix metalloproteinases in response to agiogenic factors and migration. J Invest Dermatol. 1995;105(2):170–6.
19. Ucuzian AA, Gassman AA, East AT, Greisler HP. Molecular mediators of angiogenesis. J Burn Care Res. 2010;31(1):158.
20. Reichardt LF, Tomaselli KJ. Extracellular matrix molecules and their receptors: functions in neural development. Annu Rev Neurosci. 1991;14:531–70.
21. Gerber HP, Vu TH, Ryan AM, Kowalski J, Werb Z, Ferrara N. VEGF couples hypertrophic cartilage remodeling, ossification and angiogenesis during endochondral bone formation. Nat Med. 1999;5:623–8.
22. Chintalgattu V, Nair DM, Katwa LC. Cardiac myofibroblasts: a novel source of vascular endothelial growth factor (VEGF) and its receptors Flt-1 and KDR. J Mol Cell Cardiol. 2003;35:277–86.
23. Maiolino P, De Vico G, Restucci B. Expression of vascular endothelial growth factor in basal cell tumours and in squamous cell carcinomas of canine skin. J Comp Pathol. 2000;123(2–3):141–5.
24. Restucci B, Papparella S, Maiolino P, De Vico G. Expression of vascular endothelial growth factor in canine mammary tumors. Vet Pathol. 2002;39(4):488–93.
25. Restucci B, Maiolino P, Paciello O, Martano M, De Vico G, Papparella S. Evaluation of angiogenesis in canine seminomas by quantitative immunohistochemistry. J Comp Pathol. 2003;128(4):252–9.
26. Restucci B, Borzacchiello G, Maiolino P, Martano M, Paciello O, Papparella S. Expression of vascular endothelial growth factor receptor Flk-1 in canine mammary tumours. J Comp Pathol. 2004;130(2–3):99–104.
27. Martano M, Restucci B, Ceccarelli DM, Lo Muzio L, Maiolino P. Immunohistochemical expression of vascular endothelial growth factor in canine oral squamous cell carcinomas. Oncol Lett. 2016;11(1):399–404.
28. Lee SH, Jeong D, Han YS, Baek MJ. Pivotal role of vascular endothelial growth factor pathway in tumor angiogenesis. Ann Surg Treat Res. 2015;89(1):1–8.
29. Dvorak HF, Detmar M, Claffey KP, Nagy JA, van de Water L, Senger DR. Vascular permeability factor/vascular endothelial growth factor: an important mediator of angiogenesis in malignancy and inflammation. Int Arch Allergy Immunol. 1995;107:233–5.
30. Dvorak HF. Rous-Whipple Award Lecture. How tumors make bad blood vessels and stroma. Am J Pathol. 2003;162(6):1747–57.
31. López-Ocejo O, Viloria-Petit A, Bequet-Romero M, Mukhopadhyay D, Rak J, Kerbel RS. Oncogenes and tumor angiogenesis: the HPV-16 E6 oncoprotein activates the vascular endothelial growth factor (VEGF) gene promoter in a p53 independent manner. Oncogene. 2000;19(40):4611–20.
32. Li G, He L, Zhang E, Shi J, Zhang Q, Le AD, Zhou K, Tang X. Overexpression of human papillomavirus (HPV) type 16 oncoproteins promotes angiogenesis via enhancing HIF-1a and VEGF expression in non-small cell lung cancer cells. Cancer Lett. 2011;311(2):160–70.
33. Shao JS, Shiyu Wang JS, Chung K, Du JT, Wang J, Qiu X-S, Wang E-H, Guang-Ping W. HPV16 E6/E7 upregulates HIF-2α and VEGF by inhibiting LKB1 in lung cancer cells. Tumour Biol. 2017;39(7):1010428317717137.
34. Ferrara N, Davis-Smyth T. The biology of vascular endothelial growth factor. Endocr Rev. 1997;18:4–25.
35. Frank S, Hubner G, Breier G, Longaker MT, Greenhalgh DG, Werner S. Regulation of vascular endothelial growth factor expression in cultured keratinocytes. Implications for normal and impaired wound healing. J Biol Chem. 1995;270:12607–13.
36. Naumov GN, Akslen LA, Folkman J. Role of angiogenesis in human tumor dormancy: animal models of the angiogenic switch. Cell Cycle. 2006;5(16):1779–87.
37. Folkman J. Role of angiogenesis in tumor growth and metastasis. Semin Oncol 2002; (6 Suppl 16):15–18.
38. Park JE, Keller GA, Ferrara N. The vascular endothelial growth factor (VEGF) isoforms: differential deposition into the subepithelial extracellular matrix and bioactivity of extracellular matrix-bound VEGF. Mol Biol Cell. 1993;4(12):1317–26.
39. Zhang HT, Scott PA, Morbidelli L, Peak S, Moore J, Turley H, Harris AL, Ziche M, Bicknell R. Br J Cancer. 2000;83(1):63–8.
40. Jacobsen J, Grankvist K, Rasmuson T, Bergh A, Landberg G, Ljungberg B. Expression of vascular endothelial growth factor protein in human renal cell carcinoma. BJU Int. 2004;93:297–302.
41. van der Loos CM, Meijer-Jorna LB, Broekmans MEC, Ploegmakers HP, Teeling P, de Boer OJ, van der Wal AC. Anti-human vascular endothelial growth factor (VEGF) antibody selection for Immunohistochemical staining of proliferating blood vessels. J Histochem Cytochem. 2010;58(2):109–18.
42. Nagy JA, Chang SH, Dvorak AM, Dvorak HF. Why are tumour blood vessels abnormal and why is it important to know? Br J Cancer. 2009;100(6):865–9.
43. Deschene K, Céleste C, Boerboom D, Theoret CL. Hypoxia regulates the expression of extracellular matrix associated proteins in equine dermal fibroblasts via HIF1. J Dermatol Sci. 2012;65(1):12–8.
44. Bao P, Kodra A, Tomic-Canic M, Golinko MS, Ehrlich HP, Brem H. The role of vascular endothelial growth factor in wound healing. J Surg Res. 2009;153:347–58.
45. Bucher K, Szalai G, Marti E, Griot-Wenk ME, Lazary S, Pauli U. Tumour suppressor gene p53 in the horse: identification, cloning, sequencing and possible role in the pathogenesis of equine sarcoid. Res Vet Sci. 1996;61(2):114–9.
46. Nixon C, Chambers G, Ellsmore V, Campo MS, Burr P, Argyle DJ, Reid SW, Nasir L. Expression of cell cycle associated proteins cyclin a, CDK-2, p27kip1 and p53 in equine sarcoids. Cancer Lett. 2005;221(2):237–45.
47. Martens A, Moor ADE, Demeulemeester J, Ducatelle R. Histopathological characteristics of five clinical types of equine sarcoid. Res Vet Sci. 2000; 69(Suppl3):295–300.

48. Borzacchiello G, Russo V, Della Salda L, Roperto S, Roperto F. Expression of platelet-derived growth factor-β receptor and bovine papillomavirus E5 and E7 Oncoproteins in equine sarcoid. J Comp Pathol. 2008;139(4):231–7.
49. Lory S, von Tscharmer C, Marti E, Bestetti G, Grimm S, Waldvogel A. In situ hybridization of equine sarcoids with bovine papilloma virus. Vet Rec. 1993;132:132–3.
50. Teifke JP, Hardt M, Weiss E. Detection of bovine papillomavirus DNA in formalin-fixed and paraffin-embedded equine sarcoids by polymerase chain reaction and non-radioactive in situ hybridization. Eur J Vet Pathol. 1994;1:5–10.
51. Pascoe RR, Knottenbelt DC. Manual of Equine Dermatology pub. London: WB Saunders; 1999. p. 244–50.
52. Salem A, Assaf M, Helmy A, Nofal A, Ibrahim S, Eldeeb F, Youssef C. Role of vascular endothelial growth factor in keloids: a clinicopathologic study. Int J Dermatol. 2009;48(10):1071–7.

Salivary alpha-amylase activity and cortisol in horses with acute abdominal disease

María Dolores Contreras-Aguilar[1], Damián Escribano[1,2], María Martín-Cuervo[3], Fernando Tecles[1*] and Jose Joaquín Cerón[1]

Abstract

Background: The aim of this study was to evaluate salivary alpha-amylase (sAA), considered a non-invasive biomarker for sympathetic nervous system (SNS) activity, and salivary cortisol as possible pain-induced stress biomarker, in horses with acute abdominal disease. Therefore, a prospective observational study was performed in which both biomarkers were analyzed in a group of horses with acute abdomen syndrome, and compared with a group of healthy control horses by an unpaired Student's t-test. In addition, the possible relationship between both biomarkers, the score in Equine Acute Abdominal Pain scales version 1 (EAAPS-1 scale), Heart Rate (HR) and Respiratory Rate (RR), plasma lactate, the systemic inflammatory response syndrome (SIRS) score and serum amyloid A (SAA) concentration was assessed by a Spearman correlation test.

Results: A total of 30 horses were included in the study, 19 with acute abdominal disease diagnosed as large colon displacements, simple impactions of the pelvic flexure, spasmodic colics and enteritis and 11 healthy ones. sAA activity (24.5 median-fold, $P < 0.0001$) and salivary cortisol (1.7 median-fold, $P < 0.01$) were significantly higher in horses with acute abdomen than in healthy horses. sAA activity was significantly correlated with EAAPS-1 scale ($r = 0.78$, 95% confidence interval [CI] 0.38–0.89, $P < 0.001$) and SIRS score ($r = 0.49$, 95% CI 0.03–0.78, $P < 0.05$). Neither sAA nor salivary cortisol correlated with HR, RR, plasma lactate and SAA.

Conclusions: Although this study should be considered as preliminary one, alpha-amylase measurements in saliva could be a biomarker of pain-induced stress in horses with acute abdominal disease.

Keywords: Salivary alpha-amylase, Salivary cortisol, Horse, Pain, Colic

Background

Equine acute abdominal disease is one of the most important and relatively frequent diseases found in horses [1], being associated with different degrees of pain [2]. Currently, different scales have been developed for clinical use to evaluate the pain in the acute abdominal disease in horses such as the Equine Utrecht University Scale for Composite Pain Assessment (EQUUS-COMPASS) [1], the Equine Utrecht University Scale for Facial Assessment of Pain (EQUUS-FAP) [1], and the Equine Acute Abdominal Pain scales (EAAPS, version 1 and 2) [3]. In addition, physiological and endocrine measurements, such as heart (HR) and respiratory rate (RR), and blood catecholamines and cortisol levels have been used to assess pain in horses [4–6].

Saliva sampling is easy to obtain, non-invasive and less stressful than blood sampling [7]. Therefore, saliva would be an adequate sample for evaluating possible pain-induced stress level since reflects the activity of the sympathetic adrenal medullary system in individuals under stress. Plasma cortisol concentrations have a positive correlation with pain in horses [6] and a high correlation coefficient between blood and salivary cortisol

* Correspondence: ftecles@um.es
[1]Interdisciplinary Laboratory of Clinical Analysis (Interlab-UMU), Veterinary School, Campus of Excellence Mare Nostrum, University of Murcia, 30100, Espinardo, Murcia, Spain
Full list of author information is available at the end of the article

concentrations has been found in horses [8]. Salivary alpha amylase (sAA) is considered as non-invasive biomarker for sympathetic nervous system (SNS) activity [9] and increases in psychological and physical stress situations [9, 10]. Previous reports have indicated the potential of sAA as an indirect marker for pain in mice [7]. In addition, sAA has been used in horses as a stress biomarker in different situations of physical efforts such as walking, trotting and dressage exercises [11]. So it could be postulated that measuring biomarkers like sAA or salivary cortisol can give a more reproducible method and objective assessment of pain-induced stress level in horses to contribute to an integrated description of state of pain. However, to the authors` knowledge, sAA activity and salivary cortisol have not been evaluated in equine acute abdominal disease.

The main objective of this study was to evaluate sAA activity and salivary cortisol in horses with acute abdominal disease as pain-induced stress biomarkers. For this purpose, a prospective observational study was designed in which sAA and salivary cortisol were analyzed in a group of horses with acute abdomen syndrome, and the possible changes in both biomarkers depending of the pain degree evaluated by the EAAPS-1 scale were studied. In addition, possible relationships between these salivary biomarkers, physiological variables such as HR and RR, the severity of the process evaluated by plasma lactate and the systemic inflammatory response syndrome (SIRS) score [12] and also the inflammation evaluated by serum amyloid A (SAA) concentration were assessed.

Methods

Stability pilot study

To evaluate sAA and salivary cortisol stability at room temperature and in refrigeration, a pilot study was performed. Saliva from five horses with different levels of sAA (ranging from 15.5 U/L to 59.1 U/L) and saliva cortisol (ranging from 0.17 μg/dL to 0.71 μg/dL) were selected. From each sample two aliquots were made: one was kept at room temperature (25 °C) and the second one was refrigerated (4 °C). Measurements were made just after saliva collection, 24 h and 48 h later.

Clinical case and control population

The diseased population included private owned horses of two different provinces of Spain (Almería and Granada) showing abdominal pain that required the visit of a veterinarian and that were diagnosed as acute abdominal disease. Horses were evaluated by two veterinary specialists in equine clinic who visited the horses at their boxes. Information about age, gender, breed, treatment before presentation, heart rate, respiratory rate, pounding digital pulses and capillary refill time was collected. The clinical diagnosis was based on history, physical examination (abdominal auscultation, rectal examination and nasogastric intubation) and the results of additional diagnostics tests: (1) complete blood work by complete blood count (CBC) including hematocrit value (HCT), hemoglobin concentration, erythrocyte indices, platelet count, white blood cell (WBC) and differential WBC counts; (2) chemistry profile including plasma lactate and SAA; (3) abdominal ultrasound; (4) and abdominocentesis if it was necessary. Horses with pounding digital pulses or lameness that could indicate laminitis or synovitis [2] were not included in the study.

Eleven privately owned horses of the same provinces were selected as control group for being healthy based on history, physical examination, and a lack of abnormalities on CBC and serum biochemistry profile. Four females, two geldings and five stallions integrated this group, with a mean age of nine years (range of 2–15). The breeds included were six Spanish and five crossbred horses.

Sampling

The samples collection was taken at the time of the veterinarian examination of the horse. In addition, sample collection was obtained before any potentially painful procedures (jugular venipuncture, nasogastric intubation, etc.).

Saliva samples were collected by introducing a small sponge in the horses' mouth for at least 1 min, and they were placed in collection devices (Salivette, Sarstedt, Aktiengesellschaft & Co). Blood samples were collected after saliva sampling by jugular venipuncture. Saliva and blood were centrifuged at *4000 g* for 8 min at 4 °C and then transferred into 1.5 mL eppendorf tubes and stored at − 80 °C until analysis. Saliva and blood samples were referred in refrigeration to Interdisciplinary Laboratory of Clinical Analysis of UMU (*Interlab-UMU*) after 24–48 h. Horses that yielded serum samples with gross hemolysis and blood contaminated saliva samples were excluded from the study. No treatment was administered to the horses before the sample collection.

Pain behavior scale

EAAPS-1 [3, 13] was evaluated in the habitual box of the horses with a previously history of abdominal pain by the veterinarians immediately upon arrival and before sample collection. This is based on a 5 point-score, which grades the severity of pain the horse is showing by picking the most severe behavior manifested, and the score for that particular behavior is the pain score (Table 1). Pain scale was translated to Spanish language and it was described in detail to the veterinarians before the beginning of the experimental study.

Table 1 Equine acute abdominal pain scale-version 1 (EAAPS-1)

Behaviors	Score
Depression	1
Flank watching	1
Weight shifting	2
Restlessness	2
Kicking abdomen	3
Pawing	3
Stretching	3
Sternal recumbence	3
Attempting to lie down	3
Lateral recumbence	4
Rolling	4
Collapse	5

To grade the severity of pain the horse is showing, pick the most severe behavior manifested, and the score for that particular behavior is the pain score. Table according to Sutton et al., (12)

Assays for salivary biomarkers

sAA activity was measured using a colorimetric commercial kit (Alpha-Amylase, Beckman Coulter Inc.) following the International Medicine (IFCC) method [14], as previously reported and validated for horses [11], in an automatic analyser for biochemical assay (Olympus UA600, Olympus Diagnostica GmbH). It was expressed as U/L.

Salivary cortisol was analyzed with an immunoassay system (Immulite 1000, Siemens Healthcare Diagnostic), which uses a solid-phase competitive enzyme-amplified chemiluminescent immunoassay. The assay showed an intra-assay coefficient of variation lower than 15%, a parallel displacement to the standard linearly curve with serial sample dilutions and a analytical limit of detection of 0.016 μg/dL [15].

Statistical analysis

The statistical analyses were calculated using Graph Pad Prism 6 (Graph Pad Software). sAA activity and salivary cortisol concentration results, EAAPS-1 score, HR and RR, plasma lactate concentration and SAA concentration were checked using Shapiro-Wilk test to assess normality, showing all of them a non-normal distribution except plasma lactate. Then, sAA and salivary cortisol results were transformed logarithmically by applying the formula $\ln x = \ln (x + 1)$ [16] that restored normality before a unpaired Student's t test (2-tailed) to determine if sAA and salivary cortisol were statistically different between clinical cases and controls.

The minimum number of individuals necessary to be included in each group for reaching a significance level of $\alpha = 5\%$ ($P < 0.05$) and a power of 80% was calculated. For this purpose, means and standard deviations were initially calculated for the first 11 individuals received from the clinical cases and for the 11 control horses, and a stand-alone power programme for statistical testing commonly used in social and behavior research (G-Power) [17] was employed. This gave that a minimum number of seven individuals for each group get appropriate results for sAA and salivary cortisol. However, a post hoc analysis was performed with the final number of animals used in the study to guarantee that the significance level and power required were correctly obtained.

Additionally, a Spearman correlation between salivary biomarkers (sAA and salivary cortisol), pain scale, HR, RR, plasma lactate, the systemic inflammatory response syndrome (SIRS) score and SAA was performed. The SIRS is defined as having two or more abnormal results for any of the following: HR > 52 beats/min, RR > 20 breath /min, WBC above or below $5.0–12.5 \times 10^9$/L, and temperature below or above 37.0–38.5 °C [12]. SIRS score is obtained on the number of abnormal SIRS criteria (4 point-score).

To study the stability of the salivary analytes measured, a repeated measures ANOVA and the Friedman post hoc test were used to evaluate changes in mean sAA and salivary cortisol in five saliva samples after storage at room temperature (25 °C) and refrigeration (4 °C) for 48 h. The limit for considering an acceptable stability for a given storage conditions was set as differences in values between time points lower than two intra-assay coefficient of variation (CV) of the assays (7.2% × 2 = 14. 4% for sAA; and 12.5% × 2 = 25.1% for salivary cortisol) and no significant ($P < 0.05$) differences over time in relation to baselines levels (just after collection) [18].

Results

Clinical cases

Nineteen animals were included in the group of horses with acute abdominal pain, being seven females, four geldings and eight stallions. Average age was eight years (range of 1–19). The breeds included were nine Spanish horses, one Friesian horse, and nine were crossbred horses. Causes of the acute colic were diagnosed as large colon displacements ($n = 10$), simple impactions of the pelvic flexure ($n = 5$), spasmodic colics ($n = 3$) and enteritis ($n = 1$). All horses received medical treatment, since to the judgment of the clinicians it was considered more convenient. Of the 19 clinical cases, 17 survived while two horses with colon displacements died due to the disease. The two horses that did not survive showed the highest plasma lactate and SAA concentrations (one 18.08 mmol/L and 213.1 μg/mL, and the other 19.09 mmol/L and 308.5 μg/mL, respectively). Individual values about data required for the SIRS score calculation (HR, RR, temperature and WBC) in the disease horses are reported in the Additional file 1.

sAA and salivary cortisol in acute colic

The five saliva samples used in the pilot stability study did not show significant changes in their sAA and salivary cortisol values at 24 and 48 h of storage compared with baseline values. In addition, the values obtained between the different time points did not differ more than two times the intra-assay CV.

Median and quartiles values of sAA and cortisol appear in Fig. 1. Salivary cortisol was measured in 27 horses (16 of the acute abdomen group and 11 of the control group) due to insufficient saliva volume. sAA activity (U/L) in horses with acute abdomen was significantly higher than in healthy control horses (24.5 median-fold, $t_{25.44} = 7.27$, $P < 0.0001$). Salivary cortisol was also significantly higher in horses with acute colic than in healthy controls (1.7 median- fold, $t_{21.54} = 3.43$, $P < 0.01$). The highest values of sAA (706.7 U/L and 680.9 U/L) and salivary cortisol (2.9 μg/dL and 1.3 μg/dL) were presented in the two no-survivor horses. The post hoc analysis performed with the final number of individuals used in this study computed a power of 90% for the sAA results and 89% for salivary cortisol results.

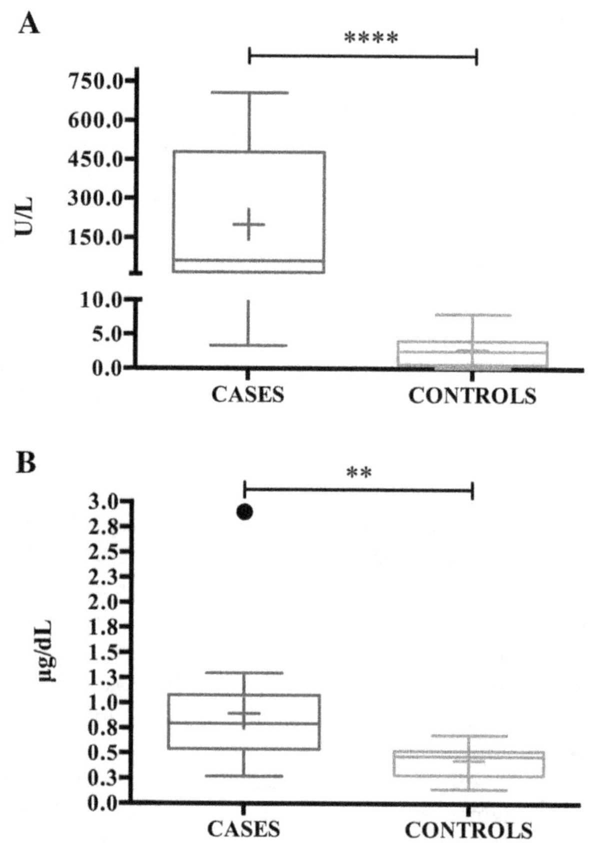

Fig. 1 Salivary alpha-amylase (sAA) activity (**a**) and salivary cortisol (**b**) from horses with acute abdominal pain (cases) and healthy horses (controls). The plot shows median (line within box), 25th and 75th percentiles (box), 5th and 95th percentiles (whiskers) and outliers (•). The cross inside the box shows the mean. Asterisk indicates statistically significant difference (**$P < 0.01$; **** $P < 0.0001$) between groups

Correlation between parameters

Coefficients of correlation between salivary biomarkers and pain scale, HR, RR, plasma lactate, SIRS score, SAA and salivary flow rate are shown in Table 2. A significant correlation between sAA activity and pain scale was observed ($n = 19$, $r = 0.78$, 95% confidence interval [CI] 0.38–0.89, $P < 0.001$), while salivary cortisol did not correlate with pain scale (Table 2). In addition, sAA activity was also correlated with SIRS score ($n = 19$, $r = 0.49$, 95% CI 0.03–0.78, $P < 0.05$). Both salivary biomarkers did not correlate between them, neither with plasma lactate or SAA.

Discussion

In veterinary practice, adequate diagnosis and treatment of painful conditions is dependent on accurate recognition of pain experienced by non-verbal animals [2], and represent an important way to improve the welfare and quality of care of the equine patient [19]. In horses, tools for objective assessment of pain such as cardiovascular measurements (HR and blood pressure) or biochemical determinations of plasma concentrations of β-endorphins, catecholamines and corticosteroids have been used for this purpose [1, 20]. In addition different scales based on external signs have been used to evaluate pain in horses; in this study EAAPS-1 scale was used because it is faster and easier to assess than EQUUS-COMPASS and EQUUS-FAP scales, being EAAPS-1 more reliable than EAAPS-2.

sAA activity was evaluated in our work as a potential indirect marker of pain showing a good correlation with EAAPS-1 and higher values in horses with acute abdominal disease compared to controls. Although comparisons should be made with caution due to the different species and nature of pain, the correlation found in our work was higher than those described in previous studies in humans such as heat pain perception [21], cancer with bone metastases [22] and chronic pain [23]. In addition, the magnitude of the increases of sAA found in colic cases compared to control group (24.5 median-fold) was higher than when pain was induced in mice (3.5 mean-fold) [7]. Overall, based in our results, it could be postulated that there is relation between pain and higher levels of sAA activity in horses with acute abdomen syndrome. Although further studies should be made to corroborate this, a possible cause of increasing of sAA would be the activation of SNS caused by pain [24]. No

Table 2 Salivary alpha-amylase (sAA, $n = 19$) and salivary cortisol ($n = 16$) coefficients of correlation between Equine acute abdominal pain scales-version 1 (EAAPS-1), heart rate (HR) and respiratory rate (RR), plasma lactate, systemic inflammatory response syndrome (SIRS) score and Serum Amyloid A (SAA)

	sAA (U/L)	*P* values	Salivary cortisol (μg/dL)	*P* values
EAAPS-1 score	0.78 (0.38, 0.89)	< 0.001	0.11 (−0.42, 0.58)	0.685
HR (beats/min)	0.22 (−0.27, 0.62)	0.362	0.24 (−0.31, 0.67)	0.370
RR (breaths/min)	0.32 (−0.17, 0.68)	0.184	0.26 (−0.28, 0.68)	0.320
SAA (μg/mL)	0.29 (−0.21, 0.67)	0.235	−0.08 (− 0.54, 0.42)	0.761
Plasma lactate (mmol/L)	0.44 (−0.05, 0.76)	0.069	0.17 (−0.38, 0.64)	0.532
SIRS score	0.49 (0.03, 0.78)	0.032	0.16 (−0.38, 0.62)	0.560

Results are expressed as Spearman r-value (95% confidence interval [CI]). SIRS score (4 point-score) is based on the number of abnormal SIRS criteria among the following: HR > 52 beats/min, RR > 20 breath/min, WBC above or below 5.0–12.5 × 10^9/L, and temperature below or above 37.0–38.5 °C

correlations were found between sAA and HR or RR. Although these parameters may be affected by pain and are often incorporated into composite pain scales as physiological parameters [2], several studies reported that, in general, physiological parameters are weakly associated with pain [4, 25, 26].

sAA was not correlated with plasma lactate and SAA, which are considered as markers of severity of disease [5] and acute inflammation in horses [27], as was moderately correlated with SIRS score. Overall this data would indicate that sAA is more linked with pain that with the inflammation that occurs in the cases of acute abdominal pain. Salivary cortisol did not correlate with pain scales in this preliminary study, although horses with colic showed higher values of cortisol than the healthy ones. However, previous reports showed a correlation between blood cortisol and a composite multifactorial pain scale (CPS) in acute orthopedic pain in horses [28]. Maybe the different nature of the pain stimulus could be the reason of this discrepancy. In addition, salivary cortisol did not correlate with sAA. The absence of correlation between sAA and salivary cortisol has been previously described [11, 29, 30]. One reason for this lack of correlation could be that sAA reflects the reaction of the SNS, while cortisol is related with the hypothalamic -pituitary-adrenal (HPA) axis [31, 32] having a different time of response, with the sAA release being faster than the cortisol. In all cases of our study, the colic were acute because they lasted lower than one day and the veterinarian attended the case as an emergency [33, 34], therefore it could be postulated that in some cases the cortisol could not reach its peak of concentration.

The pilot study made about sampling storage suggested that sAA activity and salivary cortisol were stable with the handling conditions of the saliva samples used in our study. Stability of the analyte is an important point when saliva is used as a sample since significant changes in concentrations can appear in some analytes under specific storage conditions, such as occurs with Norepinephrine in saliva after storage at 25 °C more than one hour [35].

This study has various limitations. One could be related with the accuracy of evaluation of the pain by the EAAPS-1 scale. Although EAAPS-1 was described in detail to the veterinarians before the study started and Sutton et al. [3] reported a good inter-rater reliability when scale was validated, it is important to point out that there are no standardized pain scale yet to assess the horses' pain. Other limitation is that, although horses with possible laminitis or synovitis were excluded from the study, other possible pain diseases that could influence sAA values were not controlled, such as oral wounds [36]. In addition, the results of this study could not be extrapolated to situations of pain produced by other diseases such as laminitis or synovitis, and specific studies to evaluate the dynamics of both salivary biomarkers in pain conditions should be performed.

In our study, the time of sample collection varied since depended of when the veterinarian attended the emergency case. Although ideally, in order to avoid circadian rhythms, sampling should have been always made at the same time, this was not possible from a practical point of view since the priority was to explore and attend the horses as soon as possible. In any case, although there is no data in horses about circadian rhythms of sAA, if we consider the data reported in humans [37] with a maximum of 1.76 fold of increase from basal time at 9:00 to the peak which was found 16:00, this would not have a major influence in the differences obtained in our study, since median values in the clinical cases were 24.5-fold higher in healthy horses. Regarding the salivary cortisol, it has demonstrated an acrophase at 10:00 in horses [38] with a difference only of 0.03 μg/dL between 10:00 at 22:00 which is much lower than the median difference found in our study between the two groups of horses (0.3 μg/dL).

Although the statistical analysis confirmed that the number of horses used in our study was enough to evaluate differences between clinical and control horses, further studies involving a larger number of horses with acute abdominal disease would be recommended in order to confirm the relationship between sAA and pain. It is important to point out that pain evaluation do not replaces clinical decision making (which is made based on physical examination, blood results, ultrasound, and other diagnostic tests), but its objective evaluation by biomarkers could help to better evaluate the patient at admission and also to improve the follow-up during the treatment. In addition, it could have importance as a prognostic factor for the severity of colic [1]. Overall, this study should be expanded using a larger population to assess possible differences in the biomarkers depending of the origin of the acute abdominal disease and to evaluate the possible use of sAA and cortisol as a prognostic factor since the two highest sAA values were presented in the two no-survivor horses. In addition, it would be of interest to analyze a population of horses admitted to a hospital for non-painful, elective procedures to investigate the effect of other variables that cause stress for horses, such as transport and arrival to an unfamiliar facility, in the salivary biomarkers assessing in this study. Eventually, these studies could even lead to include sAA in future pain scales as a pain-induced stress biomarker.

Conclusion

This study reports an increase of alpha-amylase activity in saliva of horses with acute abdominal disease, and it is correlated with EAPPS-1 pain scale. These preliminary results indicate that sAA could potentially be a biomarker of pain-induced stress in cases of horses with acute abdominal disease.

Additional file

Additional file 1: Individuals values of heart rate (HR), respiratory rate (RR), white blood cell (WBC), temperature and systemic inflammatory response syndrome (SIRS) score in the disease horses ($n = 19$). Individuals values about data required for the SIRS score calculation (HR, RR, temperature and WBC) in the disease horses. SIRS state is defined as having two or more abnormal results for any of the following: HR > 52 beats/min, RR > 20 breath /min, WBC above or below 5.0–12.5 × 10^9/L, and temperature below or above 37.0–38.5 °C. SIRS score is obtained on the number of abnormal SIRS criteria (4 point-score). non-SIRS: 0–1 abnormal criteria; SIRS2: 2 abnormal SIRS criteria; SIRS3/4: 3 or 4 abnormal SIRS criteria [12]. (XLSX 41 kb)

Abbreviations

CBC: Complete blood work by complete blood count; CI: Confidence interval; CPS: Composite multifactorial pain scale; CV: Coefficient of variation; EAAPS-1: Equine Acute Abdominal Pain scales version 1; EQUUS-COMPASS: Equine Utrecht University Scale for Composite Pain Assessment; EQUUS-FAP: Equine Utrecht University Scale for Facial Assessment of Pain; HCT: Hematocrit; HPA: Hypothalamic -pituitary-adrenal axis; HR: Heart Rate; RR: Respiratory Rate; sAA: Salivary Alfa-amylase; SAA: Serum amyloid A; SIRS: Systemic inflammatory response syndrome; SNS: Sympathetic nervous system; WBC: White blood cell

Acknowledgements

D. Escribano was granted by the postdoctoral program 'Juan de la Cierva' of the 'Ministerio de Economía y Competitividad', Spain. M.D. Contreras-Aguilar was granted by the predoctoral contract 'FPU' of University of Murcia (R- 605/2016), Spain. We wish to thank Carmina Martínez and Antonio Cruz for their help in the project. Preliminary results were presented as a Poster at the 7th International conference on the Assessment of Animal Welfare at Farm and Group Level, 5th-8th September 2017.

Funding

Seneca Foundation of Murcia Region (grant number: 19894/GERM/15).

Authors' contributions

JJC conceived and designed the study. MMC collected some samples. MDCA were involved in the chemical analysis. MDCA, DE, MMC, FT and JJC were involved in the data interpretation. MDCA drafted the manuscript and DE, MMC, FT and JJC critically read and edited the manuscript. All authors read and approved the final manuscript.

Competing interests

None of the authors has any financial or personal relationships that could inappropriately influence or bias the content of the paper.

Author details

[1]Interdisciplinary Laboratory of Clinical Analysis (Interlab-UMU), Veterinary School, Campus of Excellence Mare Nostrum, University of Murcia, 30100, Espinardo, Murcia, Spain. [2]Department of Food and Animal Science, School of Veterinary Medicine, Universitat Autònoma de Barcelona, 08193, Bellaterra, Barcelona, Spain. [3]Surgery Department, Faculty of Veterinary Medicine, University of Extremadura, 10005 Cáceres, Spain.

References

1. Van Loon JPAM, VanDierendonck MC. Monitoring acute equine visceral pain with the equine Utrecht University scale for composite pain assessment (EQUUS-COMPASS) and the equine Utrecht University scale for facial assessment of pain (EQUUS-FAP): a scale-construction study. Vet J. 2016;216:175–7.
2. de Grauw JC, van Loon JPAM. Systematic pain assessment in horses. Vet J. 2016;209:14–22.
3. Sutton GA, Paltiel O, Soffer M, Turner D. Validation of two behaviour-based pain scales for horses with acute colic. Vet J. 2013;197:646–50.
4. Gleerup KB, Lindegaard C. Recognition and quantification of pain in horses: a tutorial review. Equine Vet Educ. 2016;28:47–57.
5. Hinchcliff KW, Rush BR, Farris JW. Evaluation of plasma catecholamine and serum cortisol concentrations in horses with colic. JAVMA. 2005;227:276–80.
6. Pritchett LC, Ulibarri C, Roberts MC, Schneider RK, Sellon DC. Identification of potential physiological and behavioral indicators of postoperative pain in horses after exploratory celiotomy for colic. Appl Anim Behav Sci. 2003;80:31–43.
7. Tsuchiya K. Saidin MY bin, Inoue T, Kajiwara K, Kimura M. Qualitative measurement of pain by analysing the salivary alpha amylase. Precis Eng. 2014;38:257–60.
8. Kedzierski W, Strzelec K, Anna C, Kowalik S. Salivary cortisol concentration in exercised thoroughbred horses. J Equine Vet Sci. 2013;33:1106–9.
9. Nater UM, Rohleder N. Salivary alpha-amylase as a non-invasive biomarker for the sympathetic nervous system: current state of research. Psychoneuroendocrinology. 2009;34:486–96.
10. Granger DA, Kivlighan KT, El-Sheikh M, Gordis EB, Stroud LR. Salivary alpha-amylase in biobehavioral research - recent developments and applications. Ann N Y Acad Sci. 2007;1098:122–44.
11. Fuentes-Rubio M, Fuentes F, Otal J, Quiles A, Tecles F, Cerón JJ, et al. Measurements of salivary alpha-amylase in horse: comparison of 2 different assays. J Vet Behav. 2015;10:122–7.
12. Roy M, Kwong GPS, Lambert J, Massie S, Lockhart S. Prognostic value and development of a scoring system in horses with systemic inflammatory response syndrome. J Vet Intern Med. 2017;31:582–92.
13. Sutton GA, Dahan R, Turner D, Paltiel O. A behaviour-based pain scale for horses with acute colic: scale construction. Vet J. 2013;196:394–401.

14. van der Heiden C, Bais R, Gerhardt W, Lorentz K, Rosalki S. IFCC methods for measurement of catalytic concentration of enzymes - part 9. IFCC method for alpha-amylase {[]1,4-alpha-D-glucan 4-glucanohydrolase, EC 3.2.1.1]. Clin Chim Acta. 1999;281:S5–S39.
15. Escribano D, Fuentes-Rubio M, Ceron JJ. Validation of an automated chemiluminescent immunoassay for salivary cortisol measurements in pigs. J Vet Diagn Investig. 2012;24:918–23.
16. Rohleder N, Nater UM. Determinants of salivary α-amylase in humans and methodological considerations. Psychoneuroendocrinology. 2009;34:469–85.
17. Faul F, Erdfelder E, Lang A, Buchner A. G*power: a flexible statistical power analysis program for the social, behavioral, and biomedical sciences. Behav Res Methods. 2007;39:175–91.
18. Gröschl M, Wagner R, Rauh M, Dörr HG. Stability of salivary steroids: the influences of storage, food and dental care. Steroids. 2001;66:737–41.
19. VanDierendonck MC, van Loon JPAM. Monitoring acute equine visceral pain with the equine Utrecht University scale for composite pain assessment (EQUUS-COMPASS) and the equine Utrecht University scale for facial assessment of pain (EQUUS-FAP): a validation study. Vet J. 2016;216:175–7.
20. Valverde A, Gunkel CI. Pain management in horses and farm animals. J Vet Emerg Crit Car. 2005;15:295–307.
21. Wittwer A, Krummenacher P, La Marca R, Ehlert U. Salivary alpha-amylase correlates with subjective heat pain perception. Pain Med. 2016;17:1131–6.
22. Hong L, Wen-yan D, Jian-bo W, Tao W, Peng H, Shu-fang W, et al. Association between salivary alpha-amylase activity and pain relief scale scores in cancer patients with bone metastases treated with radiotherapy. Chinese Med J. 2013;126:4444–7.
23. Shirasaki S, Fujii H, Takahashi M, Sato T, Ebina M, Noto Y, et al. Correlation between salivary alpha-amylase activity and pain scale in patients with chronic pain. Region Anesth Pain M. 2007;32:120–3.
24. Mellor DJ, Stafford KJ, Todd SE, Lowe TE, Gregory NG, Bruce RA, et al. A comparison of catecholamine and cortisol responses of young lambs and calves to painful husbandry procedures. Aust Vet J. 2002;80:228–33.
25. Price J, Catriona S, Welsh EM, Waran NK. Preliminary evaluation of a behaviour-based system for assessment of post-operative pain in horses following arthroscopic surgery. Vet Anaesth Analg. 2003;30:124–37.
26. Raekallio M, Taylor PM, Bennett RC. Preliminary investigations of pain and analgesia assessment in horses administered phenylbutazone or placebo after arthroscopic surgery. Vet Surg. 1997;26:150–5.
27. Dondi F, Lukacs RM, Gentilini F, Rinnovati R, Spadari A, Romagnoli N. Serum amyloid a, haptoglobin, and ferritin in horses with colic: association with common clinicopathological variables and short-term outcome. Vet J. 2015;205:50–5.
28. Bussieres G, Jacques C, Lainay O, Beauchamp G, Leblond A, Cadore J, et al. Development of a composite orthopaedic pain scale in horses. Res Vet Sci. 2008;85:294–306.
29. Chatterton R, Vogelsong K, Lu Y, Ellman A, Hudgens G. Salivary alpha-amylase as a measure of endogenous adrenergic activity. Clin Physiol. 1996;16:433–48.
30. Nater UM, Rohleder N, Gaab J, Berger S, Jud A, Kirschbaum C, et al. Human salivary alpha-amylase reactivity in a psychosocial stress paradigm. Int J Psychophysiol. 2005;55:333–42.
31. Engert V, Efanov SI, Duchesne A, Vogel S, Corbo V, Pruessner JC. Differentiating anticipatory from reactive cortisol responses to psychosocial stress. Psychoneuroendocrinology. 2013;38:1328–37.
32. Sumter SR, Bokhorst CL, Miers AC, Van Pelt J, Westenberg PM. Age and puberty differences in stress responses during a public speaking task: do adolescents grow more sensitive to social evaluation? Psychoneuroendocrinology. 2010;35:1510–6.
33. Mair TS, Edwards GB. Chronic and recurrent colic: challenging clinical syndromes. Equine Vet Educ. 2007;19:130.
34. Mair TS, Hillyer MH. Chronic colic in the mature horse: a retrospective review of 106 cases. Equine Vet J. 1997;29:415–20.
35. Kennedy B, Dillon E, Mills PJ, Ziegler MG. Catecholamines in human saliva. Life Sci. 2001;69:87–99.
36. Ashley F, Waterman-Pearson A, Whay H. Behavioural assessment of pain in horses and donkeys: application to clinical practice and future studies. Equine Vet J. 2005;37:565–75.
37. Rohleder N, Wolf JM, Maldonado EF, Kirschbaum C. The psychosocial stress-induced increase in salivary alpha-amylase is independent of saliva flow rate. Psychophysiology. 2006;43:645–52.
38. Bohák Z, Szabó F, Beckers JF, Melo de Sousa N, Kutasi O, Nagy K, et al. Monitoring the circadian rhythm of serum and salivary cortisol concentrations in the horse. Domest Anim Endocrin. 2013;45:38–42.

23

Can heart rate variability parameters derived by a heart rate monitor differentiate between atrial fibrillation and sinus rhythm?

B. Broux*, D. De Clercq, L. Vera, S. Ven, P. Deprez, A. Decloedt and G. van Loon

Abstract

Background: Heart rate variability (HRV) parameters, and especially RMSSD (root mean squared successive differences in RR interval), could distinguish atrial fibrillation (AF) from sinus rhythm(SR) in horses, as was demonstrated in a previous study. If heart rate monitors (HRM) automatically calculating RMSSD could also distinguish AF from SR, they would be useful for the monitoring of AF recurrence. The objective of the study was to assess whether RMSSD values obtained from a HRM can differentiate AF from SR in horses. Furthermore, the impact of artifact correction algorithms, integrated in the analyses software for HRV analyses was evaluated. Fourteen horses presented for AF treatment were simultaneously equipped with a HRM and an electrocardiogram (ECG). A two-minute recording at rest, walk and trot, before and after cardioversion, was obtained. RR intervals used were those determined automatically by the HRM and by the equine ECG analysis software, and those obtained after manual correction of QRS detection within the ECG software. RMSSD was calculated by the HRM software and by dedicated HRV software, using six different artifact filters. Statistical analysis was performed using the Wilcoxon signed-rank test and receiver operating curves.

Results: The HRM, which applies a low level filter, produced high area under the curve (AUC) (> 0.9) and cut off values with high sensitivity and specificity. Similar results were obtained for the ECG, when low level artifact filtering was applied. When no artifact correction was used during trotting, an important decrease in AUC (0.75) occurred.

Conclusion: In horses treated for AF, HRMs with automatic RMSSD calculations distinguish between AF and SR. Such devices might be a useful aid to monitor for AF recurrence in horses.

Keywords: Arrhythmia, Artifact correction, Cardioversion, Equine

Introduction

With a prevalence of 0.3–2.5% of the population, atrial fibrillation (AF) is the most common clinically important arrhythmia in horses. Treatment, either by pharmacological or electrical cardioversion, is often successful, but recurrence rates are reported to be relatively high (16–43%) [1–5]. Most horses with AF have little or no detectable underlying cardiac diseases and clinical signs limited to different grades of poor performance. During strenuous exercise horses with AF can reach extremely high heart rates which may lead to R-on-T phenomenon and, in rare cases, even collapse or sudden death [6–8]. Timely diagnosis and treatment are important. After successful AF treatment, home monitoring by means of frequent auscultation or ECG is advised to check for AF recurrence. However, this cannot always be performed by lay people, requiring frequent veterinary visits or specialized equipment, which is time consuming and expensive.

Heart rate variability (HRV) describes and quantifies the beat-to-beat variability and the long-term variation in heart rate [9]. The heart rate is influenced by both the autonomic nervous system and the neuroendocrine

* Correspondence: Barbara.Broux@UGent.be
Equine Cardioteam, Department of Large Animal Internal Medicine, Faculty of Veterinary Medicine, Ghent University, Salisburylaan 133, 9820 Merelbeke, Belgium

system. Cyclical and beat-to-beat variations in heart rate are normal in the healthy individual. In horses, HRV has been used to study the autonomic regulation of the heart and animal welfare, quantifying stress and pain [10–12]. Aside from its use as indicator of autonomic tone, HRV is used in human medicine to diagnose arrhythmias [13, 14]. Since arrhythmia, especially AF, leads to an increased beat-to-beat interval variation, HRV parameters describing short-term variability are increased compared to sinus rhythm (SR) and algorithms using HRV parameters are implemented in devices detecting AF in humans [15–19]. In horses, HRV has already been evaluated for the detection of AF in horses before and after transvenous electrical cardioversion [20]. In that study, 6 different HRV variables were calculated from RR intervals after beat-to-beat QRS identification on the ECG trace, both during AF and during SR. RMSSD, the root mean squared successive differences in RR interval, yielded the best results with high sensitivity and specificity to distinguish AF from SR.

Different types of heart rate monitors (HRM) are increasingly being used in horses and some of them offer basic HRV calculations, including RMSSD [11, 21, 22]. They might be an accessible diagnostic tool for both veterinarians and horse owners to monitor horses for AF recurrence. Most HRMs, however, have not been validated for use in horses and significant differences between their RR registration and RR intervals from ECG recordings have been shown [23]. Therefore the purpose of this study was to assess whether AF and SR can be differentiated in horses based upon RMSSD generated from a HRM or automatically analyzed ECG trace, using that from manually identified RR intervals from an ECG as gold standard. Furthermore the impact of artifact correction prior to HRV analysis was evaluated.

Materials and methods

Study design and study population

Fourteen warmblood horses were presented to the Faculty of Veterinary Medicine, Ghent University for the treatment of AF. All horses were client-owned horses admitted to our clinic for cardiac examination and treatment of AF. AF was confirmed in all horses by an experienced cardiologist using an ambulatory ECG recording. All horses were warmblood horses with a mean ± SD age, bodyweight and height at the withers of 12 ± 6 years, 544 ± 62 kg and 167 ± 13 cm. The study population consisted of 5 mares, 8 geldings and 1 stallion. All horses were included in the study with written informed owner consent and cared for according to the principles outlined in the NIH Guide for the Care and Use of Laboratory Animals. Each horse was simultaneously equipped with a HRM and an ECG and subjected to a recording at rest and a standardized exercise test including 5 min of walk and 10 min of trot, both in AF (before cardioversion) and in SR (5 days after cardioversion). The recordings of both devices was started at the same time. After the examinations and AF treatment, all horses returned home with the owners.

Electrodes and heart rate detection

Three different systems of heart rate detection (electrodes + RR detection) were compared. A modified base apex ECG was recorded as described elsewhere [20], using adhesive electrodes (Skintact, Leonhard Lang GmbH, Innsbruck, Austria) and analyzed using a commercial ECG software program (Televet 100 software version 5.1.2, Engel Engineering Services GmbH, Heusenstamm, Germany) with a detection limit of 8%, meaning that all RR intervals differing more than 8% from the previous RR interval were detected as outliers, but included in the analysis. First, the RR intervals automatically detected by the ECG software, leaving errors in QRS detection in place, were exported (ECG_{Aut}). Subsequently, all RR intervals were checked by one experienced observer and manually corrected within the software in case of artifacts or wrong QRS detection to obtain manually corrected RR intervals (ECG_{Man}) which served as gold standard. Furthermore, a HRM using a commercial plastic electrode set (Polar equine heart rate electrode set, Polar Electro Benelux, Dendermonde, Belgium) and a heart rate sensor for RR detection (Polar heart rate sensor H7, Polar Electro Benelux, Dendermonde, Belgium) was attached according to the manufacturer's instructions. Also for this detection method, errors in RR detection by the HRM were left in the database.

Heart rate variability and artifact correction methods

From all 14 horses, RR intervals from both ECG_{Man} and ECG_{Aut} were imported in Kubios Software (Kubios Heart Rate Variability Analysis Software, Varsitie 22, 70,150 Kuopio, Finland) at default settings (smooth priors and Lambda 500) for HRV analysis, while RR data from the HRM were imported into its own commercial software program (Polar Flow Software, Polar Electro Benelux, Dendermonde, Belgium) (Table 1). Subsequently, a time-matched 2-min recording at rest, walk and trot, both in AF and SR, was selected for calculation of RMSSD using the following formula:

$$\mathrm{RMSSD} = \sqrt{\frac{1}{N-1}\sum_{j=1}^{N-1}\left(\mathrm{RR}_{j+1}-\mathrm{RR}_j\right)^2}.$$

Each recording was obtained 2 min after a change in gait, in order to exclude movement artifacts and stress reactions from the gait change.

Table 1 Median and range of the RMSSD values of 14 horses before (in atrial fibrillation (AF)) and after cardioversion (in sinus rhythm (SR))

Pace	Method	Artifact correction	RMSSD AF		RMSSD SR		*P*-value
			Median	Range	Median	Range	
Rest	ECG_{Man}	none	670	248–1409	85	26–378	0.024*
Rest	ECG_{Aut}	none	674	244–1409	118	26–580	0.024*
Rest	ECG_{Aut}	Kubios very low	216	194–293	87	26–181	.0.024*
Rest	ECG_{Aut}	Kubios low	195	160–233	82	16–175	0.024*
Rest	ECG_{Aut}	Kubios moderate	145	125–193	72	26–145	0.024*
Rest	ECG_{Aut}	Kubios high	78	61–112	61	25–94	0,79
Rest	ECG_{Aut}	Kubios very high	23	13–98	30	18–56	1
Rest	HRM	Polar Flow	233	72–329	78	32–169	0.024*
Walk	ECG_{Man}	None	229	84–495	43	11–185	0.024*
Walk	ECG_{Aut}	None	226	153–495	83	11–194	0.024*
Walk	ECG_{Aut}	Kubios very low	189	124–236	34	11–113	0.024*
Walk	ECG_{Aut}	Kubios low	163	117–219	34	11–104	0.024*
Walk	ECG_{Aut}	Kubios moderate	135	105–161	34	11–79	0.024*
Walk	ECG_{Aut}	Kubios high	82	62–102	28	11–63	0.024*
Walk	ECG_{Aut}	Kubios very high	33	11–52	22	10–45	1
Walk	HRM	Polar Flow	126	49–167	32	6–73	0.024*
Trot	ECG_{Man}	None	89	53–144	10	5–18	0.024*
Trot	ECG_{Aut}	None	125	34-377	86	7–221	1
Trot	ECG_{Aut}	Kubios very low	93	52–187	13	7–58	0.024*
Trot	ECG_{Aut}	Kubios low	84	48–124	13	7–53	0.024*
Trot	ECG_{Aut}	Kubios moderate	71	43–122	13	7–36	0.024*
Trot	ECG_{Aut}	Kubios high	52	34–85	13	7–32	0.024*
Trot	ECG_{Aut}	Kubios very high	22	14–49	11	5–32	0,22
Trot	HRM	Polar Flow	37	25–108	6	5–16	0.024*

Two-minute recordings at rest, walk and trot were analyzed using 4 different methods of RR detection and HRV analysis. The automatically analyzed ECG followed by beat-to-beat manual correction of QRS detection (ECG_{Man}) with HRV analysis using Kubios HRV Software without artifact filter was considered the gold standard method. *HRM* Polar heart rate monitor (Equine H7) with plastic electrodes and Polar Flow Software. *ECG_{Aut}* ECG with automatic RR interval detection (Televet 100) and Kubios HRV software with 5 different artifact correction levels. The artifact correction algorithm identifies every RR interval that differs from the average RR interval of the 2-min recording more than a specified threshold value as artifacts and replaces the corrupted RR interval by interpolated RR values. The threshold values used in this study were 0.45 s (very low artifact correction), 0.35 s (low), 0.25 s (moderate), 0.15 s (high) and 0.05 s (very high). * Indicates significant differences

Furthermore, for the ECG_{Aut} method, within the Kubios HRV software program, 5 different levels of artifact correction were applied. The artifact correction algorithm of this program compares every RR interval value against the average RR interval of the 2-min recording. The average is obtained by median filtering of the RR interval time series, and is therefore not affected by single outliers in RR interval time series. RR intervals that differ from the local average more than a specified threshold value, are identified as artifacts and corrected by replacing them by interpolated RR values using a cubic spline interpolation. The threshold values used in this study were 0.45 s (very low artifact correction; values that differ more than 0.45 s from the average), 0.35 s (low), 0.25 s (moderate), 0.15 s (high) and 0.05 s (very high). For example, the "Medium" correction level will identify all RR intervals that are 0.25 s longer/shorter compared to the local average. Detailed information about filtering methods is free available online in the Kubios user manual. For the ECG_{Man} method, no artifact correction was applied, while the commercial software program used for the RR intervals obtained with the HRM method, uses its own, unknown artifact correction algorithm.

Statistical analysis

Statistical analysis was performed using dedicated software (SPSS 24, IBM Analytics, Brussels, Belgium). Descriptive statistics, quantile-quantile plots and Shapiro-Wilk tests were used to check for normality of data.

Data were not normally distributed and therefore non-parametric related samples Wilcoxon signed-rank tests were used to detect significant differences in RMSSD between horses in AF and SR at different paces using the different detection methods and artifact correction levels. Bonferroni corrections were applied to account for multiple (× 24) comparisons. Receiver operating characteristic (ROC) curves were used to study the performance of each method and each artifact correction level as a discriminatory variable for the detection of AF. The coordinate points of the ROC curves were used to determine the most fitting cut off values for each parameter at each recording. Cut off values were chosen to maximize sensitivity whilst retaining good (≥80%) specificity, where possible.

Results

Mean values for RMSSD are displayed in Table 1. RMSSD values obtained from the ECG were significantly different ($P < 0.05$) between horses in SR and horses in AF, except when a high level of artifact correction was used and at trot if no artifact correction was applied. RMSSD values obtained with the HRM were significantly different between horses in SR and horses in AF, at all paces.

AUCs, cut off values and their sensitivity and specificity for the use of RMSSD as a discriminatory variable for the detection of atrial fibrillation are displayed in Table 2. Using the Polar Flow software in combination with a plastic electrode set (HRM), led to reliable cut off values, especially during exercise. ECG_{Aut}, without artifact correction, led to reliable results at rest and at walk (AUC 0.96), but there was an important decrease in AUCs during trotting exercise (AUC 0.75). Low level artifact correction during trotting exercise, led to a clear improvement in AUC (=1) and cut off values with very high sensitivity and specificity. High levels of artifact correction resulted in an important

Table 2 Area under the curve (AUC), cut off values and their sensitivity and specificity, and 95% confidence intervals (95% CI) for the use of RMSSD as discriminatory variable to distinguish atrial fibrillation from sinus rhythm in 14 warmblood horses

Pace	Method	Artifact correction	AUC	cut off	sens	95% CI	spec	95% CI
Rest	ECG_{Man}	none	0.99	215	1	0.77–1	1	0.77–1
Rest	ECG_{Aut}	none	0.96	383	0.93	0.66–1	0.93	0.66–1
Rest	ECG_{Aut}	1	1	188	1	0.77–1	1	0.77–1
Rest	ECG_{Aut}	2	0.99	131	1	0.66–1	0.93	0.66–1
Rest	ECG_{Aut}	3	0.94	111	1	0.77–1	0.93	0.66–1
Rest	ECG_{Aut}	4	0.77	65	0.93	0.66–1	0.69	0.42–0.92
Rest	ECG_{Aut}	5	0.37	24	0,5	0.23–0.77	0.38	0.13–0.65
Rest	HRM_{Elec}	Polar Flow	0.93	136	0.86	0.57–0.98	0.86	0.57–0.98
Walk	ECG_{Man}	none	0.97	121	0.93	0.66–1	0.93	0.66–1
Walk	ECG_{Aut}	none	0.96	164	0.93	0.66–1	0,86	0.57–0.98
Walk	ECG_{Aut}	1	1	119	1	0.77–1	1	0.77–1
Walk	ECG_{Aut}	2	1	111	1	0.77–1	1	0.77–1
Walk	ECG_{Aut}	3	1	92	1	0.77–1	1	0.77–1
Walk	ECG_{Aut}	4	0.99	57	1	0.77–1	0.93	0.66–1
Walk	ECG_{Aut}	5	0.74	22	0.78	0.49–0.95	0.57	0.29–0.82
Walk	HRM_{Elec}	Polar Flow	0.97	70	0.93	0.66–1	0.93	0.66–1
Trot	ECG_{Man}	none	1	36	1	0.77–1	1	0.77–1
Trot	ECG_{Aut}	none	0.77	90	0.86	0.57–0.98	0.72	0.42–0.91
Trot	ECG_{Aut}	1	1	51	1	0.77–1	0.93	0.66–1
Trot	ECG_{Aut}	2	1	42	1	0.77–1	0.93	0.66–1
Trot	ECG_{Aut}	3	1	40	1	0.77–1	1	0.77–1
Trot	ECG_{Aut}	4	1	33	1	0.77–1	1	0.77–1
Trot	ECG_{Aut}	5	0.93	15	0.93	0.66–1	0.93	0.66–1
Trot	HRM_{Elec}	Polar Flow	1	21	1	0.77–1	1	0.77–1

Two-minute recordings at rest, walk and trot were analyzed using 4 different methods of RR detection and HRV analysis. The automatically analyzed ECG followed by beat-to-beat manual correction of QRS detection (ECG_{Man}) with HRV analysis using Kubios HRV Software was considered the gold standard method. *HRM* Polar heart rate monitor (Equine H7) with plastic electrodes and Polar Flow Software. *ECG_{Aut}* ECG with automatic RR interval detection (Televet 100) and Kubios HRV software with 5 different artifact correction levels. The artifact correction algorithm identifies every RR interval that differs from the average RR interval of the 2-min recording more than a specified threshold value as artifacts and replaces the corrupted RR interval by interpolated RR values. The threshold values used in this study were 0.45 s (very low artifact correction), 0.35 s (low), 0.25 s (moderate), 0.15 s (high) and 0.05 s (very high)

drop in AUCs, especially at rest. Receiver operating curves (ROC) are available as Additional file 1.

Discussion

The goal of our study was to assess an easily applicable tool for home monitoring of AF recurrence after treatment. In the current study pre-treatment AF could be differentiated from post-treatment SR based upon RMSSD using a commercially available HRM. Investigation of different artifact filtering levels showed that, compared to no filtering, low levels of artifact correction improved sensitivity and specificity, especially during trotting exercise. However, sensitivity and specificity fell with higher levels of filtering.

In this study RMSSD was chosen as the HRV parameter to distinguish AF from SR. RMSSD is a time domain HRV parameter and especially useful in assessing short term HRV [9, 24]. In a previous study, using 6 different HRV parameters for the differentiation between AF and SR in horses, RMSSD yielded the best results with cut off values with high sensitivity and specificity, identifying all cases of AF with only a small chance of false positives [20]. Furthermore, RMSSD is a well-known and frequently used HRV parameter, available on a variety of HRMs, HRV software programs and mobile applications, which could make it a suitable tool for home monitoring of AF recurrence after treatment. However, if RMSSD calculations are not available, SDNN (the standard deviation of the RR intervals) and SD1 (nonlinear parameter, derived from Poincaré plot), other frequently used HRV parameters and inter-related with RMSSD, might also be useful to detect AF [20].

Correct QRS detection is important to obtain correct RR intervals but the algorithms used by devices is often unknown. Filtering of data is often used to eliminate erroneously detected artifacts from the dataset before RMSSD is calculated. Several methods to record RR intervals were used in this study. Automatic analysis followed by manual correction of identified QRS complexes of an ECG trace using adhesive electrodes and calculation of RMSSD by specialized software without filtering was used as gold standard. However, this requires specialized equipment, expertise for ECG interpretation and data handling (exporting, importing), which is time consuming and expensive. Automatic analysis of the ECG trace by dedicated software reduces analysis time, but also introduces error. HRMs are increasingly being used by both veterinarians and horse owners, because they are relatively cheap and easy to use. They automatically detect heart rate and some devices also generate HRV calculations, including RMSSD. Previous studies assessing precision and accuracy of HRMs both in horses and in other animals, however, reported variable results and many HRMs have not been thoroughly validated in horses [23, 25–28]. Furthermore, different HRMs with different electrode design and RR detection software are available. Although in our study the ECG and HRM recordings were started exactly at the same time, the HRM recording appeared to show a lag and therefore our data did not allow to evaluate the performance of HRMs in correctly detecting individual QRS complexes. Since large differences in RMSSD between horses in AF and in SR have been shown [20], we hypothesized that, even if the use of a HRM introduced some error in RR detection, differences were sufficiently large to allow for reliable differentiation.

For the data obtained by the HRM, we used Polar Flow commercial software for HRV analysis. There are, however, numerous other, often cheaper, software programs and mobile phone applications available automatically importing RR data from HRMs via Bluetooth, displaying them in real time and immediately generating some basic HRV calculations. These applications might be useful candidates for home monitoring of horses at risk for AF recurrence but need to be validated.

Different HRV software programs might apply a different artifact correction method. The second goal of this study was to assess the effect of artifact correction levels on RMSSD as a discriminatory parameter for the AF detection. Artifact filters eliminate outliers, i.e. RR intervals that strongly differ from other RR intervals, by deleting them or replacing them by interpolated values. Although this filtering helps to delete artifacts, it will also blunt beat-to-beat variation which is typical for AF. Low level artifact correction resulted in improved sensitivity and specificity approaching 100% at all paces. During SR, second degree atrioventricular block (AVB) is a common finding in horses at rest with a large impact on HRV [29]. In our study, low level artifact correction probably eliminated most AVB from the analysis, since AVB leads to a very large increase in RR interval, and may be important in distinguishing AF from SR with frequent AVB. The Polar Flow software also uses an algorithm for artifact correction, which cannot be adapted. Unfortunately the authors were not able to obtain the details of this algorithm, but mean Polar values were close to mean Kubios values after Low to Moderate filtering. We have chosen to use the Kubios software because it is often used in human and veterinary medicine, it is free online available, and it allows to apply different filter levels. Our data suggest that low level filtering is needed, but that higher filter levels decrease specificity and sensitivity. We tested a limited number of filters only and cannot conclude upon the optimal filter. A large number of HRV analysis software programs are commercially available but one should be aware that each of them uses its own, usually unknown, QRS detection algorithm and type of filtering, which may have a big effect on the obtained RMSSD value.

In human medicine, artifact correction algorithms are also used in AF detection devices [16, 17, 30]. Reported sensitivity and specificity of these human devices range from 86.6–100% and 84.3–99.9%, respectively [15, 18, 19, 30].

Cut off values determined in this study were chosen to optimize sensitivity whilst maintaining good specificity. Because early diagnosis positively affects outcome and AF may occasionally be associated with dangerous ventricular tachyarrhythmias, our focus was to identify all horses with AF, even if this potentially included some false positives. False positives, however, will most likely arise from either incorrect RR registration, electrical interference and movement artifacts, or from horses with frequent arrhythmias other than AF. If these horses remain positive at consecutive HRM sessions during walk and trot, further electrocardiographic examination is indicated as other arrhythmias might be present.

Despite the relatively small study population and the unknown level of error introduced by the heart rate detection method of the HRM, differences in HRV between SR and AF were large, leading to reliable cut off values. Also, power calculations based upon RMSSD differences between horses in AF and in SR from a previous study [20], indicated sufficient power to detect significant differences with 5–7 horses. An important limitation of the study was its self-control design. We used horses before and after cardioversion since our goal was to differentiate AF from SR after successful treatment. Atrial premature depolarizations were often found post-cardioversion in these horses which could potentially make differentiation more challenging than if a control group of normal horses had been used. In this study we did not specify the number of arrhythmias but our previous study already showed that a high number of AVB during SR has an important effect on RMSSD, while a high number of atrial premature depolarization has not. We did not include horses with other arrhythmias than AVB and atrial premature depolarizations in this study and it remains to be proven whether this technique can also be used to diagnose AF in a random population of horses.

Conclusions

We conclude that in horses before and after TVEC, AF can be differentiated from SR using RMSSD values obtained from automatically analyzed ECGs but also from an equine HRM. One should be aware that heart rate detection technique as well as level of artifact correction are important. Since we did not include horses with other arrhythmias in our study population, further studies are required before this technique can be used to differentiate AF from SR in a random population of horses.

Additional file

Additional file 1: Receiver Operating Curve (ROC) for the use of RMSSD to distinguish atrial fibrillation from sinus rhythm in 14 warmblood horses during a 2-min heart rate recording at rest, (A), walk (B) and trot (C). ECGman: RR intervals obtained from a surface ECG after manual correction of QRS detection, using a commercial ECG software program (Televet 100 software version 5.1.2, Engel Engineering Services GmbH, Heusenstamm, Germany) to calculate RMSSD within a commercial software program (Kubios Heart Rate Variability Analysis Software, Varsitie 22, 70,150 Kuopio, Finland). ECGaut: RR intervals after automatic analysis of the surface ECG by a commercial ECG software program (Televet 100) to calculate RMSSD within a commercial software program (Kubios Heart Rate Variability Analysis Software). Five different levels of artifact correction were applied for ECGaut, going from a very low to a very high level of filtering. HRM: RR intervals obtained from a heart rate monitor (Polar heart rate sensor H7, Polar Electro Benelux, Dendermonde, Belgium) using commercial plastic electrodes (Polar equine heart rate electrode set, Polar Electro Benelux, Dendermonde, Belgium) to calculate RMSSD within the manufacturer's software program (Polar Flow Software, Polar Electro Benelux, Dendermonde, Belgium). (TIF 636 kb)

Abbreviations

AF: Atrial fibrillation; AUC: Area under the curve; AVB: Atrioventricular block; HRM: Heart rate monitor; HRV: Heart rate variability; RMSSD: Root mean squared successive differences in RR interval; ROC: Receiver operating curves; SD: Standard deviation; SR: Sinus rhythm

Acknowledgements

No acknowledgements were declared by the authors.

Funding

Lisse Vera is funded by Fonds Wetenschappelijk Onderzoek, Award number 113491 N. The funding body had no role in design of the study and collection, analysis, and interpretation of data and in writing the manuscript.

Authors' contributions

BB contributed to the study design, acquisition of data, data analysis and the writing of the manuscript. DDC contributed to the study designs, the acquisition of data and the data analysis. LV and SV contributed to the acquisition of data, the data analysis and the writing of the manuscript. PD contributed to the study design and the writing of the manuscript. AD contributed to the study design, data analysis and the writing of the manuscript. GvL contributed to the study design, acquisition of data, data analysis and the writing of the manuscript. All authors have read and approved the manuscript.

Consent for publication

Not applicable.

Competing interests

The authors declare that they have no competing interests.

References

1. McGurrin MK, Physick-Sheard PW, Kenney DG. How to perform transvenous electrical cardioversion in horses with atrial fibrillation. J Vet Cardiol. 2005; 7(2):109–19.
2. McGurrin MK, Physick-Sheard PW, Kenney DG. Transvenous electrical cardioversion of equine atrial fibrillation: patient factors and clinical results in 72 treatment episodes. J Vet Intern Med. 2008;22(3):609–15.

3. Reef VB, Levitan CW, Spencer PA. Factors affecting prognosis and conversion in equine atrial fibrillation. J Vet Intern Med. 1988;2(1):1–6.
4. Decloedt A, Schwarzwald CC, De Clercq D, Van Der Vekens N, Pardon B, Reef VB, van Loon G. Risk factors for recurrence of atrial fibrillation in horses after cardioversion to sinus rhythm. J Vet Intern Med. 2015;29(3):946–53.
5. De Clercq D, Decloedt A, Sys SU, Verheyen T, Van Der Vekens N, van Loon G. Atrial fibrillation cycle length and atrial size in horses with and without recurrence of atrial fibrillation after electrical cardioversion. J Vet Intern Med. 2014;28(2):624–9.
6. Young L, van Loon G. Diseases of the heart and vessels. In: Hinchcliff KW, Kaneps AJ, Geor RJ, editors. Equine sports medicine and surgery : basic and clinical sciences of equine athlete. 2nd ed. USA: Saunders; 2013. p. 695–744.
7. Reef VB, Bonagura J, Buhl R, McGurrin MK, Schwarzwald CC, van Loon G, Young LE. Recommendations for management of equine athletes with cardiovascular abnormalities. J Vet Intern Med. 2014;28(3):749–61.
8. Verheyen T, Decloedt A, van der Vekens N, Sys S, De Clercq D, van Loon G. Ventricular response during lungeing exercise in horses with lone atrial fibrillation. Equine Vet J. 2013;45(3):309–14.
9. Bowen IM. Ambulatory electrocardiography and heart rate variability. In: Bowen MI, Marr CM, editors. Cardiology of the horse. Elsevier limited, Edinburgh; 2010. p. 127–37.
10. Kuwahara M, Hashimoto S, Ishii K, Yagi Y, Hada T, Hiraga A, Kai M, Kubo K, Oki H, Tsubone H, et al. Assessment of autonomic nervous function by power spectral analysis of heart rate variability in the horse. J Autonom Nerv Syst. 1996;60(1–2):43–8.
11. von Borell E, Langbein J, Despres G, Hansen S, Leterrier C, Marchant-Forde J, Marchant-Forde R, Minero M, Mohr E, Prunier A, et al. Heart rate variability as a measure of autonomic regulation of cardiac activity for assessing stress and welfare in farm animals - a review. Physiol Behav. 2007;92(3):293–316.
12. Smiet E, Van Dierendonck MC, Sleutjens J, Menheere PP, van Breda E, de Boer D, Back W, Wijnberg ID, van der Kolk JH. Effect of different head and neck positions on behaviour, heart rate variability and cortisol levels in lunged Royal Dutch Sport horses. Vet J. 2014;202(1):26–32.
13. Bruggemann T, Dahlke D, Chebbo A, Neumann I. Tachycardia detection in modern implantable cardioverter-defibrillators. Herzschrittmachertherapie Elektrophysiol. 2016;27(3):171–85.
14. Park J, Lee S, Jeon M. Atrial fibrillation detection by heart rate variability in Poincare plot. Biomed Eng Online. 2009;8:38.
15. Duverney D, Gaspoz JM, Pichot V, Roche F, Brion R, Antoniadis A, Barthelemy JC. High accuracy of automatic detection of atrial fibrillation using wavelet transform of heart rate intervals. Pacing Clin Electrophysiol. 2002;25(4 Pt 1):457–62.
16. Boon KH, Khalil-Hani M, Malarvili MB, Sia CW. Paroxysmal atrial fibrillation prediction method with shorter HRV sequences. Comput Methods Prog Biomed. 2016;134:187–96.
17. Yaghouby F, Ayatollahi A, Bahramali R, Yaghouby M, Alavi AH. Towards automatic detection of atrial fibrillation: a hybrid computational approach. Comput Biol Med. 2010;40(11–12):919–30.
18. Tateno K, Glass L. Automatic detection of atrial fibrillation using the coefficient of variation and density histograms of RR and Delta RR intervals. Med Biol Eng Comput. 2001;39(6):664–71.
19. Dash S, Chon KH, Lu S, Raeder EA. Automatic real time detection of atrial fibrillation. Ann Biomed Eng. 2009;37(9):1701–9.
20. Broux B, De Clercq D, Decloedt A, Ven S, Vera L, van Steenkiste G, Mitchell K, Schwarzwald C, van Loon G. Heart rate variability parameters in horses distinguish atrial fibrillation from sinus rhythm before and after successful electrical cardioversion. Equine Vet J. 2017;49(6):723–8.
21. Erber R, Wulf M, Becker-Birck M, Kaps S, Aurich JE, Mostl E, Aurich C. Physiological and behavioural responses of young horses to hot iron branding and microchip implantation. Vet J. 2012;191(2):171–5.
22. Munsters CC, de Gooijer JW, van den Broek J, van Oldruitenborgh-Oosterbaan MM. Heart rate, heart rate variability and behaviour of horses during air transport. Vet Rec. 2013;172(1):15.
23. Parker MG, Eager RA, Redhead ES, Marlin DJ. Comparison of polar heart rate interval data with simultaneously recorder ECG signals in horses. Comp Excer Physiol. 2009;6(04):137–42.
24. Camm AJ, Malik M. Heart rate variability. Standards of measurement, physiological interpretation, and clinical use. Task force of the European Society of Cardiology and the north American Society of Pacing and Electrophysiology. Eur Heart J. 1996;17(3):354–81.
25. Evans DL, Rose RJ. Method of investigation of the accuracy of four digitally-displaying heart rate meters suitable for use in the exercising horse. Equine Vet J. 1986;18(2):129–32.
26. Hopster H, Blokhuis HJ. Validation of a heart-rate monitor for measuring a stress-response in dairy-cows. Can J Anim Sci. 1994;74(3):465–74.
27. Marchant-Forde RM, Marlin DJ, Marchant-Forde JN. Validation of a cardiac monitor for measuring heart rate variability in adult female pigs: accuracy, artefacts and editing. Physiol Behav. 2004;80(4):449–58.
28. Jonckheer-Sheehy VSM, Vinke CM, Ortolani A. Validation of a polar (R) human heart rate monitor for measuring heart rate and heart rate variability in adult dogs under stationary conditions. J Vet Behav. 2012;7(4):205–12.
29. Eggensperger BH, Schwarzwald CC. Influence of 2nd-degree AV blocks, ECG recording length, and recording time on heart rate variability analyses in horses. J Vet Cardiol. 2017;19(2):160–74.
30. Vaes B, Stalpaert S, Tavernier K, Thaels B, Lapeire D, Mullens W, Degryse J. The diagnostic accuracy of the MyDiagnostick to detect atrial fibrillation in primary care. BMC Fam Pract. 2014;15:113.

Indicators of replicative damage in equine tendon fibroblast monolayers

Tina Rich[1*], Livia B Henderson[1], David L Becker[2], Hannah Cornell[1] and Janet C Patterson-Kane[1]

Abstract

Background: Superficial digital flexor tendon (SDFT) injuries of horses usually follow cumulative matrix microdamage; it is not known why the reparative abilities of tendon fibroblasts are overwhelmed or subverted. Relevant in vitro studies of this process require fibroblasts not already responding to stresses caused by the cell culture protocols. We investigated indicators of replicative damage in SDFT fibroblast monolayers, effects of this on their reparative ability, and measures that can be taken to reduce it.

Results: We found significant evidence of replicative stress, initially observing consistently large numbers of binucleate (BN) cells. A more variable but prominent feature was the presence of numerous gammaH2AX (γH2AX) puncta in nuclei, this being a histone protein that is phosphorylated in response to DNA double-stranded breaks (DSBs). Enrichment for injury detection and cell cycle arrest factors (p53 (ser15) and p21) occurred most frequently in BN cells; however, their numbers did not correlate with DNA damage levels and it is likely that the two processes have different causative mechanisms. Such remarkable levels of injury and binucleation are usually associated with irradiation, or treatment with cytoskeletal-disrupting agents.
Both DSBs and BN cells were greatest in subconfluent (replicating) monolayers. The DNA-damaged cells co-expressed the replication markers TPX2/repp86 and centromere protein F. Once damaged in the early stages of culture establishment, fibroblasts continued to express DNA breaks with each replicative cycle. However, significant levels of cell death were not measured, suggesting that DNA repair was occurring. Comet assays showed that DNA repair was delayed in proportion to levels of genotoxic stress.

Conclusions: Researchers using tendon fibroblast monolayers should assess their "health" using γH2AX labelling. Continued use of early passage cultures expressing initially high levels of γH2AX puncta should be avoided for mechanistic studies and ex-vivo therapeutic applications, as this will not be resolved with further replicative cycling. Low density cell culture should be avoided as it enriches for both DNA damage and mitotic defects (polyploidy). As monolayers differing only slightly in baseline DNA damage levels showed markedly variable responses to a further injury, studies of effects of various stressors on tendon cells must be very carefully controlled.

Keywords: Superficial digital flexor tendon, Tendon, Horses, Cell culture, Polyploidy, DNA damage, DNA repair, Replicative stress, GammaH2AX protein, Comet assay

Background

Superficial digital flexor tendon (SDFT) injury affects up to 30-33% of Thoroughbreds and event horses in racing or training (i.e. elite athletes) [1-3]. The consequent failure of regeneration with persistence of scar tissue leads to high rates of both re-injury (up to 50%) and retirement (up to 70%) [4-7]. It is generally agreed that injury usually follows a period of cumulative subclinical microdamage to the extracellular matrix that is both exercise- and age-associated; this damage includes reductions in collagen fibril diameter, increased amounts of weaker type III collagen (type I collagen predominates in normal adult tendon tissue), and reduced glycosaminoglycan levels [8-11].

Tenocytes are tendon fibroblasts with key responsibility for synthesis and degradation of the collagenous and noncollagenous matrix, and are thought to constantly

* Correspondence: Tina.Rich@glasgow.ac.uk
[1]Institute of Infection, Immunity and Inflammation, College of Medical, Veterinary and Life Sciences, University of Glasgow, 120 University Place, Glasgow G12 8TA, UK
Full list of author information is available at the end of the article

repair microdamage under normal circumstances [12]. In the adult SDFT the tenocytes are not highly active in collagen synthesis or turnover (relative to non-injury-prone digital tendons) [13-15]. This may explain why their reparative capacity is overwhelmed by factors occurring during high-speed exercise, including various potential combinations of high levels of mechanical strain, hypoxia, ischemia-reperfusion events, and hyperthermia (due to hysteresis in energy-storing tendons) [16-20]. Additionally, direct or indirect damage to tenocytes themselves and/or their detachment from collagen fibrils (resulting in mechanical understimulation) can instigate cell death or dysfunction; this dysfunctional activity may include upregulation of matrix metalloproteinase (MMP) activity, increased type III collagen synthesis, and cytokine production [18,21-23]. The result is a vicious cycle of cellular damage and production of mechanically weak matrix that is easily disrupted during normal activity [24].

Due to the limitations of *in vivo* work, appropriate cell culture models are required to more clearly define how tenocytes sense and respond to multiple environmental conditions occurring during galloping exercise, and how these processes might be modulated to reduce injury [25]. Tendon fibroblast monolayer (2-dimensional) culture systems are frequently used as tractable and easily analysed primary systems for experimentation / manipulation [13,21,26]. However, they are also necessary to obtain and expand these cells for use in (currently highly variable and poorly defined) 3-dimensional models, or for clinical purposes e.g. autologous tenocyte implantation into tendon injury sites [26-28]. There are many problems that might influence cellular stress and damage in these monolayers including the tissue extraction process: many researchers use enzymatic digestion rather than explant outgrowth due to the higher and more rapid yield of cells, without significant relative disadvantages in terms of phenotypic drift [13,26-29]. Importantly, levels of such damage can easily go unrecognized when using live/dead assays or simple phase contrast appearance for monitoring, as is common practice [25]. In our monolayers we noted high numbers of binucleate (BN) fibroblasts, a normally rare event in cell culture (excluding cardiomyocytes), that indicates cleavage failure during mitosis and has been associated with DNA damage and matrix surface type [30,31]. This prompted the present study, the objectives of which were to determine:

(i) a reliable read-out for DNA damage in equine cells;
(ii) the relationship between DNA damage and the replicative fraction;
(iii) whether the relationship between DNA damage and cellular replication altered when fibronectin was used as a surface rather than collagen;
(iv) if reparative activity could overcome any or all of the damage.

Our ultimate aim was to achieve "healthy" tendon fibroblast monolayers i.e. a baseline comprised of cells that were not already responding to stresses introduced by the culture system itself.

Results and discussion

Equine SDFT fibroblast monolayers contain abnormally high percentages of binucleate cells, indicating cleavage failure during mitosis

Specimens were obtained from an approved UK abattoir (abattoir group), and a veterinary post-mortem facility (post-mortem group; PM). Routine light microscopy examination of culture dishes and phase contrast microscopy of cells seeded onto collagen-coated coverslips revealed large numbers of BN (or occasionally multinucleate) fibroblasts in all monolayers (Figure 1A). In DAPI-labelled monolayers, these could only conclusively be identified where the nuclei were touching unless cytoplasmic or membrane elements were co-stained (Figures 1B,C). In confluent monolayers these comprised up to 7% of the total population and were not related to the age of the animal or the source group (abattoir versus PM) (Table 1). However, in subconfluent cultures the numbers were significantly higher i.e. up to 20%. In all equine tendon fibroblast monolayers, numbers of BN cells were higher than routinely seen in human fibroblast monolayers (~2%) or in equine palate fibroblasts (i.e. primary equine fibroblasts not of tendon-origin) [32], in which they did not exceed 3% (Table 1).

Binucleation indicates that there has been cleavage failure during mitosis; this is normally a rare event in cell culture for mammalian somatic cells with the exception of cardiomyocytes [30], but can be induced by application of anti-cytoskeletal drugs including cytochalasin B [31,33]. During division a cell rounds up, disassembles the cytoskeleton and redistributes cytoskeletal proteins and other molecules into the cleavage furrow that forms by assembly and contraction of an actomyosin ring to partition the cytoplasm [34,35]. The sister cells then re-spread and separate in the mid-body by removal of cytoskeletal structures from the intercellular bridge, constriction of the cell cortex (furrow ingression), and plasma membrane fission (the process of abscission) [34,35]. In cells where defects occur in cytokinesis (separation of the cytoplasm), furrow regression leads to BN cell formation.

In normal diploid fibroblast monolayers, approximately 70% of the mitotic fraction should be in the early mitotic phases (prophase (P) and metaphase (M)) with the remainder in anaphase (A) and telophase (T) when the daughter nuclei are formed and segregate [36].

Unusually, counts of mitotic indices in tendon-derived fibroblasts revealed a marked enrichment of the later mitotic phases; the A/T counts were 2–7 times those for P/M (Table 1; Figure 1D). This was particularly apparent in low-density cell cultures and was consistent with a delay in proceeding through the latter stages of mitosis. Late phase mitotic enrichment was not evident in human fibroblasts or in fibroblasts derived from equine palate. Previously it was shown that cells that could override a prolonged G2 arrest entered mitosis but

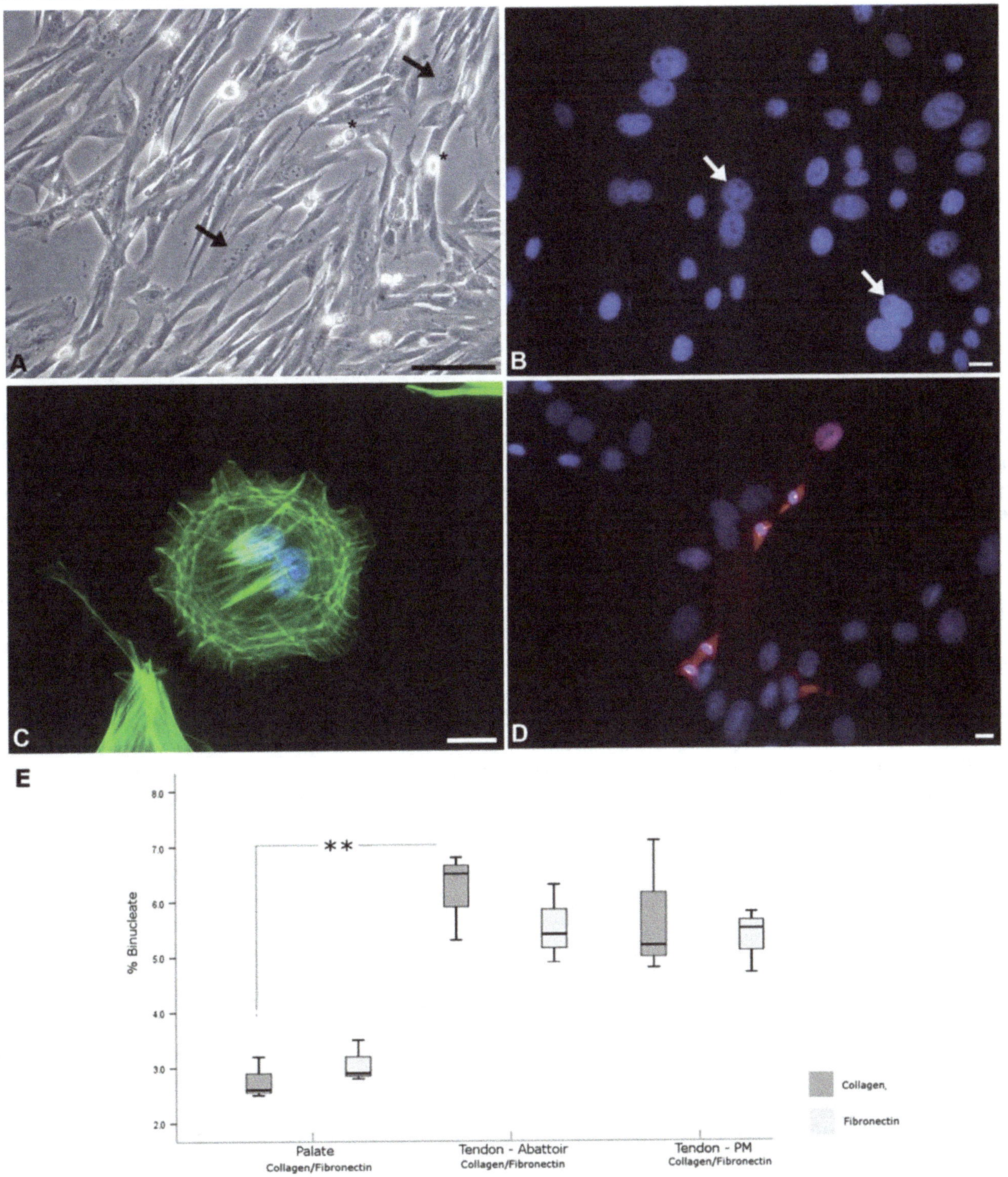

Figure 1 (See legend on next page.)

(See figure on previous page.)
Figure 1 Binucleate cells in equine tendon fibroblast monolayers. Phase contrast **(A)** and fluorescent **(B-D)** images of primary equine superficial digital flexor tendon (SDFT) fibroblasts, grown on collagen-coated surfaces. **(A)** Numerous binucleate cells in a typical monolayer. The arrows indicate two of the many bi- and multinucleate cells in the field. The asterisks indicate phase-bright mitotic figures just above the focal plane; these are not dead cells. Scale bar = 100 μm **(B)** Nuclei stained blue by DAPI; binucleate cells can most conclusively be identified when the nuclei are touching (arrows). Conservation in size of BN nuclei was commonly seen. Scale bar = 10 μm **(C)** Staining of actin using phalloidin reveals the cytoplasmic boundaries of this binucleate fibroblast. Scale bar = 10 μm **(D)** Two post metaphase dividing cells; this was a common observation and would be unlikely in normal circumstances given that the later phases of cell cycle are shorter than the proceeding prophase and metaphase. A slight dent between the daughter nuclei shows that the cleavage furrow is just beginning to compact the spindle in the lower of the two mitotic figures. The upper cells are further progressed through mitosis, with significant ingress of the central spindle which has compacted the midzone microtubules to form the typical midbody. Cells are labelled with the microtubule-binding protein TPX2 (red; a proliferation marker) and DAPI (blue; nuclear stain). Scale bar = 10 μm. **(E)** Percent binucleation in fibroblasts derived from equine palate or tendon (abattoir and PM group), cultured on either collagen or fibronectin. Cultures were 80% confluent.

remained tethered at the midbody at the end of cytokinesis [37]. Two thirds of those tethered cells became binucleate and the remainder either apoptosed (11%), or re-entered mitosis (22%) whilst still bridged to generate similarly bridged daughter nuclei and eventually, multinucleate cells [37]. Phase contrast images of our monolayer cultures revealed occasional multinucleated cells (Figure 1A), together with the binucleate fraction. The individual nuclei in each BN also showed a high correlation in terms of size (Figure 1B) and frequently the nuclei were enlarged, suggesting two tetraploid nuclei. A mechanism to describe the generation of tetraploid BN cells via successive rounds of failed cytokinesis has been described [38]; this together with the cell tethering described in [37] may be relevant to our monolayer cultures.

Normally, following furrow ingression there is a period when the (now) re-spreading and migrating daughter cells are still linked by the cytoplasmic bridge that narrows and then splits as they move apart [39], i.e. mechanical tension is involved [35]. In one study, 3T3 fibroblasts that were strongly adherent to high-concentration (versus low) fibronectin showed extensive stretching of the intercellular bridge and failure of the midbody to disassemble [33]. It was proposed that cells that cannot move apart from one another due to a too-adhesive substrate will be unlikely to undergo traction-mediated cytofission, i.e. this indicates a significant cell culture artefact [33]. In contrast, researchers using rat embryonic fibroblasts relieved cytochalasin D-induced arrest by growing them on fibronectin, possibly via an integrin-linked effect on the cytoskeleton following failed cytokinesis; it has subsequently been suggested that species-specific differences may contribute to susceptibility to BN formation [40,41]. These differences may be due to altered adhesion properties of fibroblasts on fibronectin versus collagen surfaces, and or their susceptibility to cytoskeletal disruption [42]. To investigate the relationship between failed cytokinesis and matrix substrate for our equine cells, we compared numbers of BN fibroblasts on collagen and fibronectin-coated coverslips but did not see significant differences for these or for palate-derived equine fibroblasts (Figure 1E). If matrix adherence properties are a factor contributing to a greater failure of abscission (separation) for equine tendon fibroblasts versus equine palatine or human foreskin fibroblasts, the difference might also be explained by the difference in tissue-origin; tendon cells in tissue are located within very small niches where they interact intimately with surrounding, densely packed collagen fibrils and other collagenous and noncollagenous matrix components [43].

Table 1 High binucleate cell numbers and prolongation of late stages of mitosis in tendon fibroblast monolayers

Source	Horse age (y)	Binucleate (%)	P/M (%)	A/T (%)
Abattoir	5	6.8	0.7	2.8
Abattoir	15	4.5	0.4	2.3
Post-mortem	Foal (stillborn)	4.2	0.4	2.7
Post-mortem	3	5.9	1.8	3.1
Equine palate	(stillborn)	2.9	2.6	2.5
Human Hs68	new-born	1.7	2.9	1.8

The percentage of binucleate cells and those in prophase or metaphase (P/M), or anaphase/telophase (A/T) was calculated from counts of 1000 fibroblasts in ~80% confluent fibroblast monolayers. Values for each parameter in tendon-derived monolayers could not be related to horse age or source. Data from fibroblasts derived from non equine (human Hs68) or equine non tendon (palate) tissue sources are included for comparison.

Binucleation occurs in tendon fibroblast monolayers regardless of the presence of DNA damage

Binucleation was originally proposed to be a "tetraploidy checkpoint" to protect against cell overgrowth and neoplastic transformation, and therefore invariably resulting in permanent p53-dependent G1 arrest [44]. However other researchers using human diploid fibroblasts showed that the p53 expression causing G1 arrest of BN cells was due to DNA damage (in those experiments caused by cell synchronisation treatments), rather than the tetraploidy itself [31]. It was suggested that cells that have failed to undergo cytokinesis are more likely to arrest because they simply have twice as much DNA in which the damage may be present [31]. The activity of a DNA damage checkpoint to prevent exit from mitosis has since been demonstrated [45]. The full DNA damage response (DDR) is suppressed in normal mammalian cells until the stages of telophase/cytokinesis (i.e. the late stages of mitosis, as enriched in our monolayers), by high activity of cyclin-dependent kinase 1 [46].

Because we documented abnormal accumulation of our equine tendon fibroblasts in the latter phases of mitosis, and due to this known link between DNA damage and binucleation, we immunolabelled the monolayers for the phosphorylated form of the H2AX histone protein variant (γH2AX) using the vertebrate specific monoclonal antibody, clone JBW301; this antibody has previously been used to stain the γH2AX fraction involved in chromatin remodelling in equine sex chromosomes [47]. H2AX is phosphorylated by ATM kinase in response to DNA double-strand breaks (DSBs; the most lethal lesion); this event results in the recruitment of downstream repair factors into a microscopically visible focus [48,49]. An additional kinase, ATR, has been shown to co-operate with ATM/γH2AX to protect collapsed replication forks [50]. The growing γH2AX focus is thought to open up the chromatin structure and forms a "platform" to stabilise accumulating damage response and repair factors; there is close correlation between numbers of foci (or puncta, each containing several hundred γH2AX molecules) and numbers of DSBs [49]. Phosphorylation of H2AX has also been shown in response to stress-induced chromatin reorganisation; this can occur without DNA breaks.

The S-phase transition in fibroblasts usually results in reparable DNA damage, visible as low numbers of large γH2AX puncta (Figure 2A); we only classified cells expressing 7 or more puncta as excessively damaged. In monolayers from the PM group we detected occasional puncta together with micropuncta of γH2AX (Figure 2A). Micropuncta have previously been shown to arise independently of DNA damage [51], possibly because of the reorganization of chromatin structure that accompanies replication and cell division; only the larger puncta have been associated with DNA damage [49]. In contrast, frequent large puncta were noted in fibroblast monolayers from the abattoir group (Figure 2B), in 8-25% of both BN and mononuclear cells; the highest percentages were seen in the more sparse monolayers i.e. the amount of DNA damage reduced as the fibroblasts became confluent. These levels of γH2AX puncta expression were remarkable, as they have previously only been demonstrated (to this extent) in cells injured using genotoxic agents or ionising radiation [49]. The difference between PM and abattoir groups may have related to the delay of at least 6–7 h prior to placement of specimens into medium (containing digestive enzymes) for the latter group, or subtle differences in digestion technique. We feel that a tissue digestion effect was unlikely, given that comparable

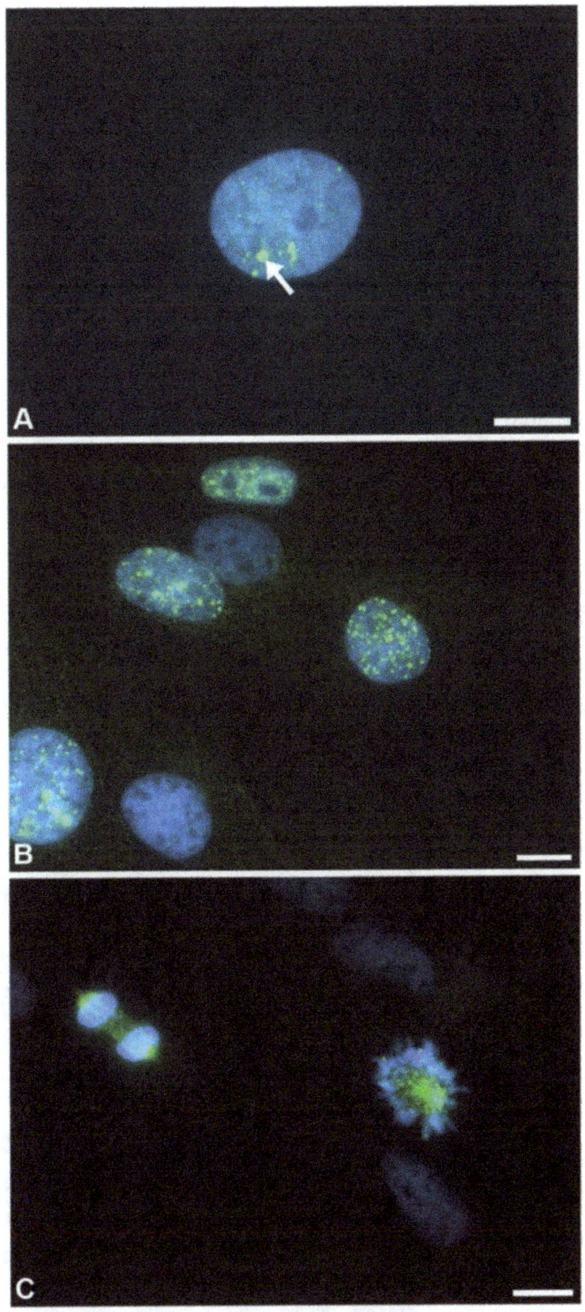

Figure 2 γH2AX staining patterns in equine tendon fibroblasts. **(A)** A fibroblast from the post-mortem (PM) group, in which little damage was noted. A few large γH2AX puncta (green; arrow) are considered an indicator of normal, reparable DNA damage that occurs during the S-phase transition. Numerous micropuncta (green) seen here in the remainder of the nucleus are not thought to be DNA damage-associated. DAPI nuclear counter-stain (blue). Scale bar = 10 μm **(B)** Fibroblasts from the abattoir group, containing remarkable numbers of γH2AX puncta (green) indicating severe DNA damage. Micropuncta can still be seen in the background. DAPI nuclear counter-stain (blue). Scale bar = 10 μm **(C)** Diffuse γH2AX labelling pattern (green) in mitotic fibroblasts, with labelling of the spindle poles and microtubules in the cell on the left. Scale bar = 10 μm.

levels of DNA damage and binucleation were evident in monolayer and explant cultures derived from the same tissue samples. Percentages of DNA-damaged cells were 15.7% ± 1.6 (mean ± standard error) and 12.8%±2.4 in ~70% confluent monolayer and explant cultures respectively, that were derived from an identical adult abattoir sample. Clearly the speed of cell processing post mortem requires further investigation, particularly as it has been considered acceptable to culture fibroblasts up to several days following death from both human and animal subjects [52,53].

Similar numbers of BN cells were detected in abattoir and PM group monolayers (and explant cultures). This suggested that BN cell formation was largely due to factors other than DNA damage (e.g. matrix substrate, as discussed above). In a previous study of human fibroblasts, not all arrested BN cells contained γH2AX puncta, again suggesting that DNA damage is not a necessary factor [31]. Interestingly, in both abattoir and PM tendon fibroblasts (i.e. those with and without large numbers of γH2AX puncta), diffuse or occasionally punctate γH2AX labelling was noted at mitosis at the spindle poles and microtubules (Figure 2C). In some interphase cells γH2AX labelling was also noted in small perinuclear foci consistent with localisation to the centrosome; this has been reported previously (in tandem with other DNA repair proteins) but is of unknown significance [54]. These distributions of γH2AX (puncta/micropuncta/centrosome-like and spindle) are identical to those previously described in other species [49].

In abattoir fibroblast monolayers labelled for p53 phosphorylated at serine 15 (a phosphorylation that occurs in response to DNA damage and replication stress), most of the positive nuclei were seen in BN cells i.e. although the numbers of BN formed were not influenced by DNA damage, they were more likely to contain an amount of damage visible in terms of stabilised p53 enrichment (Figure 3A,B). We did not see prominent p53 stabilisation in BN cells in monolayers from the PM group. Additional positive labelling for p21 (cyclin-dependent kinase inhibitor 1) confirmed cell cycle arrest in the p53-positive cells (Figure 3C,D); p21 mediates the cell cycle arrest (at G1), initiated and tightly controlled by stabilised p53. Some researchers have demonstrated the involvement of p21 in elevation of reactive oxygen species (ROS) levels in cultured (human) fibroblasts, feeding back to result in further γH2AX accumulation, continuation of cell cycle arrest and activation of cellular senescence [55]. Not all of the BN cells in the abattoir monolayers had p53-positive nuclei (in some cases only one of the 2 nuclei in one cell contained stabilised p53 (Figure 3B), and some of them were both p53- and p21-negative. Together with the fact

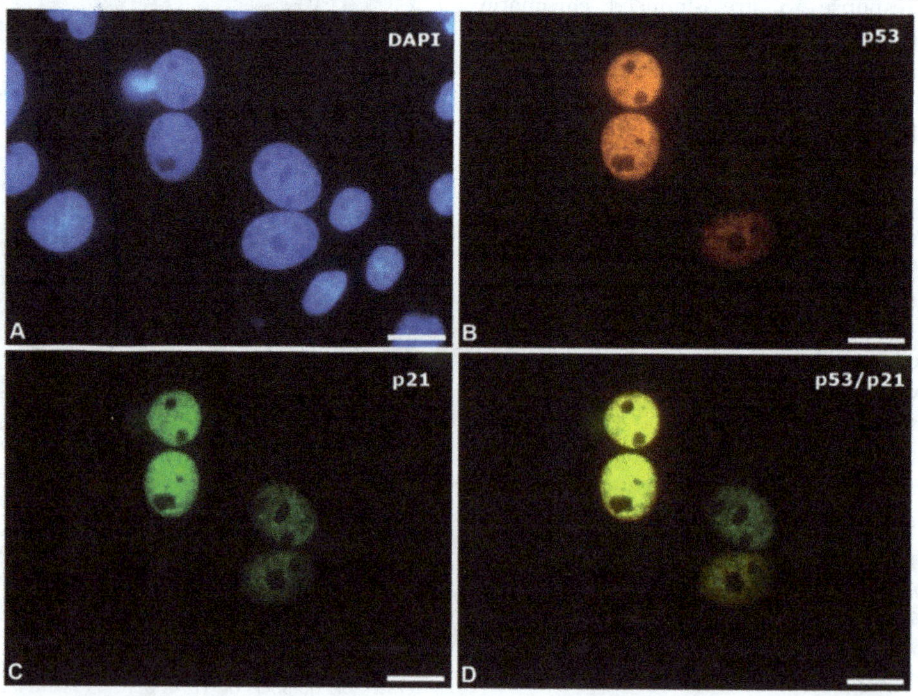

Figure 3 Cell cycle arrest in binucleate fibroblasts. These images are taken from the same field **(A)** Two of these fibroblasts are binucleate (BN), with larger nuclei that are almost touching. DAPI nuclear counter-stain (blue) **(B)** Nuclei in one of the BN cells show strong diffuse positive labelling for p53 (red), with faint staining of one of the nuclei in the closely adjacent cell; this indicates stabilisation of p53 to facilitate cell cycle arrest and is not seen in the mononuclear cells **(C)** Both nuclei in both BN cells also show labelling for p21 (green) i.e. the mediator of p53-induced cell cycle arrest **(D)** Colocalisation of p53 and p21. Scale bars = 10 μm.

that their numbers did not accumulate with time, this indicates survival and eventual re-entry into the cell cycle to complete mitosis. It has previously been demonstrated that if DNA damage does not reach a certain level, most BN cells will eventually finish mitosis and repair the DNA in the next G1 phase [45,46].

DNA double-strand breaks in tendon fibroblast cultures are replication-associated but do not result in significant cell death

Because in the abattoir group the numbers of large γH2AX puncta per nucleus were greatest in subconfluent monolayers, we proposed that DNA damage could be occurring in response to replication stress. During DNA replication the replication fork forms a Y-shaped structure at which DNA is unwound and copied. Erroneous replication can stall the replication fork complex, and the single-stranded DNA generated at that point activates cell cycle arrest [56]. If the stalling is prolonged, DNA damage will occur, and if the fork collapses, DSBs are generated that cannot be repaired by simply restarting the fork. However, the precise relationship between the formation of γH2AX puncta and DSBs at blocked replication forks is controversial. Some studies have shown that γH2AX puncta form some hours prior to fork breakage, after many hours of cell cycle arrest, i.e. the puncta may not necessarily represent breaks directly, but they do indicate replication stress and possibly the activities of different repair and chromatin modifying complexes [57,58]. Because we needed to determine if the high numbers of γH2AX puncta in abattoir fibroblasts were actually due to DSBs, we double immunolabelled the cells for γH2AX and two markers of replication-induced DNA damage, promyelocytic leukaemia protein (PML) and Rad51. We previously demonstrated that DSBs juxtapose (without co-localising) with nuclear puncta of PML; PML has since been shown to play a prominent role in the homologous recombination (HR) of DNA during DSB repair [59,60]. This repair process is favoured uniquely in the replicative fraction. The Rad51 protein searches for homologous sequence to act as a template for repair, having first bound to single stranded DNA generated by DNA resection at the breakage site [61]. Our co-staining experiments revealed the stereotypic juxtaposition of nuclear domains of PML protein with large γH2AX puncta in the abattoir fibroblast monolayers (Figure 4A) with co-localised foci of Rad51 (Figure 4B). The majority of the large γH2AX puncta in abattoir cells expressed co-localised puncta of γH2AX and Rad51 (evident in 84-90% of the cells expressing large γH2AX puncta). Rarer, large puncta of γH2AX in PM cells also co-localised with Rad51. However, not all γH2AX puncta contained Rad51 protein; these may have represented (as mentioned above) sites of γH2AX accumulation prior to breakage. Alternatively, some researchers have observed continued marking of resealed but poorly repaired DSB sites by γH2AX in order to recruit the more accurate HR repair machinery [62].

Having confirmed a strong association between γH2AX puncta and multiple DNA damage markers in these tendon fibroblasts, we then investigated the link with replication status. Double immunolabelling was performed for γH2AX and TPX2/repp86 or centromere protein F (CENPF) antigens respectively; both of these markers are expressed diffusely in the nucleus during the S and G2 phases of the cell cycle, with relocation to the spindle during mitosis (expression is absent in G1). There was almost exact matching of nuclei expressing increased numbers of γH2AX puncta with positive labelling for each of the replication markers (Figure 4C-F), with the exception of BN cells (arrested in G1). Other evidence of replication stress was noted morphologically, including the generation of nuclear blebs, microbodies, and aberrant multipolar mitoses (Figure 5A-C). There was one exception to this rule, found by comparing replicative and damaged fractions in coverslips from each of the abattoir horses (n = 5) at different levels of confluence on collagen or fibronectin surfaces (Figure 6). An effect of age of the donor (6 months, 3,5,14 and 15 years) was not shown, but for all horses, in the monolayers of the highest confluence level (in which fewer cells were replicating), the damage levels on fibronectin remained high i.e. there was damage-replication uncoupling on that matrix substrate. Confluence was not noted to be reached more rapidly on fibronectin versus collagen. Interestingly, recent data have indicated that fibronectin promotes DNA damage recognition (including H2AX phosphorylation) in an α5 integrin-dependent fashion [63]. This requires further investigation in three-dimensional cell culture systems and in tissue, as it has relevance for cellular therapies: fibronectin expression is markedly upregulated in damaged (and adjacent) tendon tissue, where it occurs pericellularly [64].

Another potential cause of DNA damage detectable by γH2AX staining is *Mycoplasma* sp. infection. Although this damage has never been linked to replicative status, it can be largely reversed by treatment with the free radical quenching agent N-acetyl cysteine (NAC) [65]. We routinely screen our cells for *Mycoplasma* infection and, additionally, we sent cells to a microbiology laboratory for testing (Veterinary Diagnostic Services, University of Glasgow). All isolates were negative. Despite this, we additionally 'treated' our cultures with a bacteriocidal agent (plasmocin) that targets mycoplasma protein synthesis and DNA replication, to see whether levels of DNA damage would be reduced. Following several weeks of treatment (i.e. the recommended time to achieve mycoplasma removal) we did not detect a reduction in the levels of γH2AX staining. Treatment with 1 mM NAC

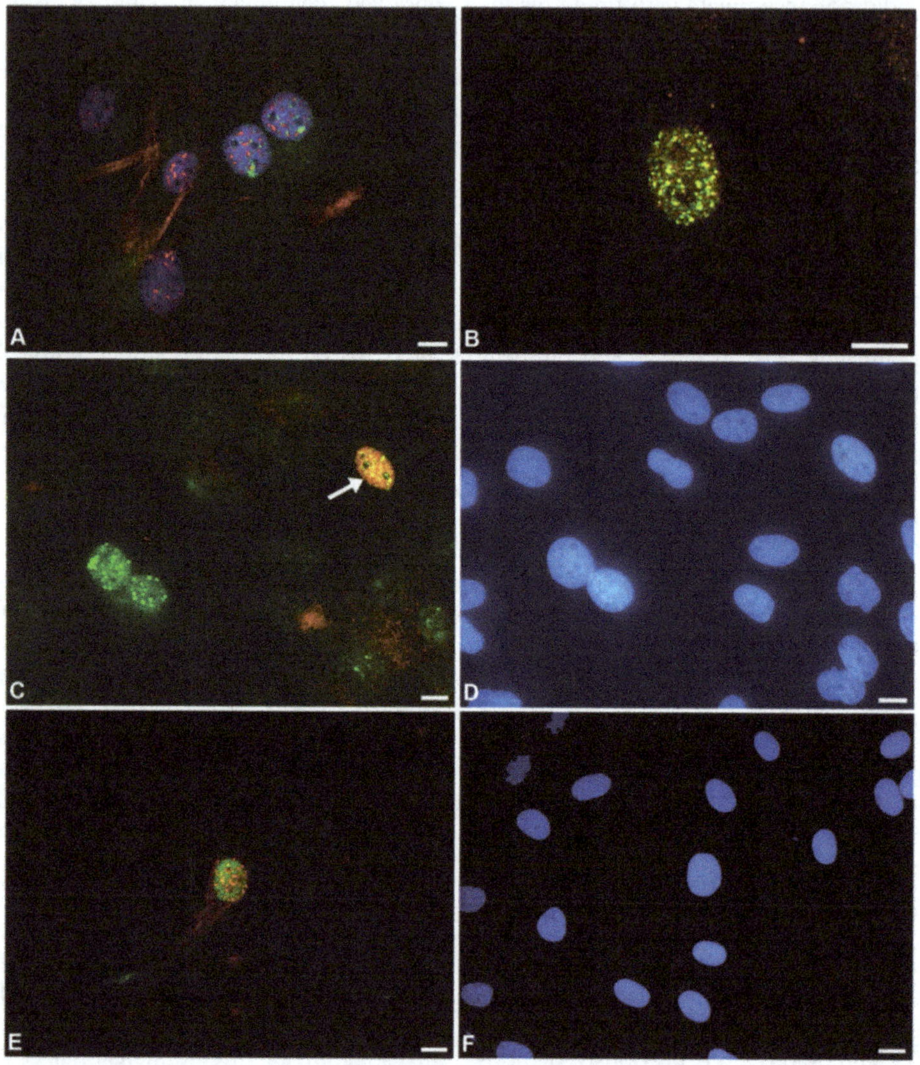

Figure 4 Association of DNA damage with the replicative fraction. (A) Promyelocytic leukaemia protein (PML) foci (red) juxtaposed with γH2AX puncta (green); as PML bodies are known to locate next to DNA double strand breaks (DSBs), this confirms that many of the γH2AX puncta in our culture system genuinely indicate the presence of DSBs **(B)** Co-localisation of Rad51 protein (red) and γH2AX (green) as yellow puncta, as further evidence of labelling of DNA breaks. **(C)** Co-localisation (yellow) of γH2AX puncta with positive labelling for the proliferation marker TPX2 in one mononuclear fibroblast (arrow), indicating a correlation between DNA damage and the replicative fraction. A binucleate cell in the same field contains typical, significant numbers of γH2AX puncta but is arrested **(D)** The associated DAPI counter-stain (blue) showing all fibroblast nuclei in the field; note the touching, enlarged nuclei in the BN cell **(E)** The nucleus of a cell that has entered the S/G_2 phase of the cell cycle, showing diffuse positive labelling for centromere protein F (green); the same nucleus is the only one in this field that contains γH2AX puncta (in this case, red) i.e. significant DNA damage **(F)** The associated DAPI counter-stain (blue) showing all of the fibroblast nuclei. Scale bars = 10 μm.

also failed to reduce levels of DNA damage. We therefore concluded that DNA damage in our cultures was not because of *Mycoplasma* contamination.

Despite the large amounts of replication-associated DNA damage in the abattoir fibroblast monolayers, there were not similarly significant levels of cell death. Morphologically, few apoptotic bodies were noted, and additionally there was no evidence of the diffuse, nuclear-wide γH2AX labelling that has been associated with apoptosis [57]. Importantly, because most researchers monitor the success of their monolayer cultures by observing and/or measuring cell death and viability, these differences in replication stress and DNA damage would not be identified routinely. We also rarely saw γH2AX puncta in mitotic figures as can occur when collapsed replication forks result in under-replicated loci [66]. These observations indicated that the tendon fibroblasts were largely repairing DNA lesions prior to mitosis.

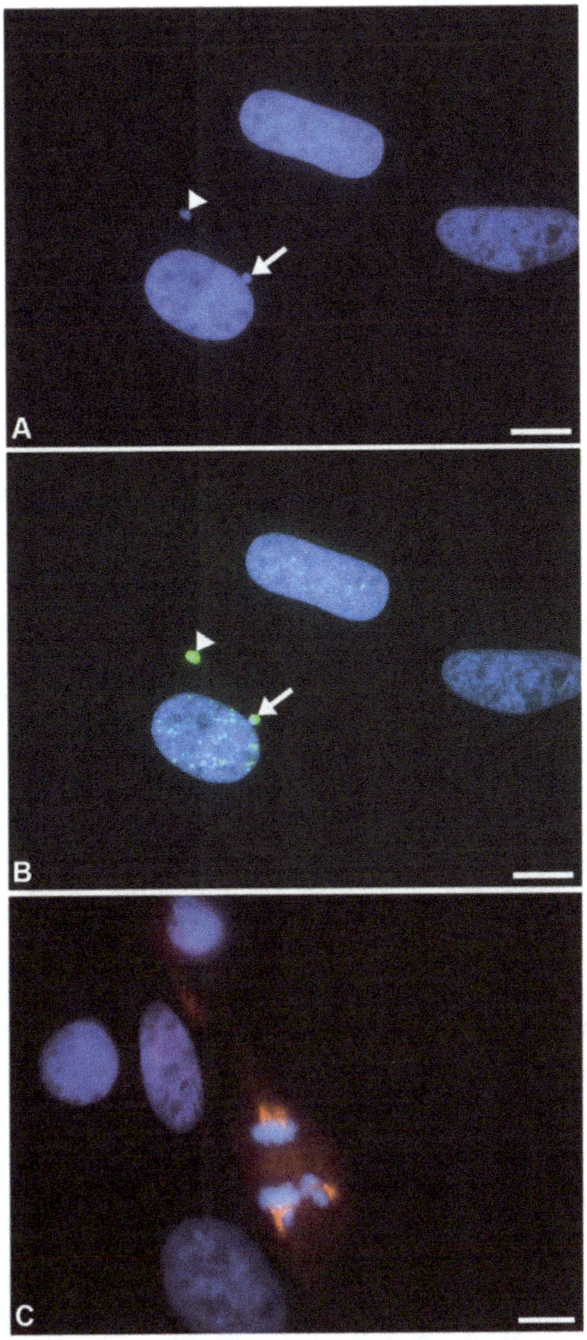

Figure 5 Morphological evidence of replication stress. (A) A nuclear bleb or bud (arrow; bleb/buds are nuclear material still attached but derived from the main nucleus) and a microbody (arrowhead; defined as separate or marginally overlapping with the nucleus, less than one third of its size and with a similar DAPI stain (criteria according to [67])); these structures are evidence of DNA damage, and mitotic stress that can give rise to unstable chromosomal material that is ejected from the cell at the subsequent interphase. DAPI counter-stain (blue). **(B)** The nuclear bleb and microbody show positive labelling for γH2AX (green) i.e. DNA damage **(C)** An abnormal, tripolar mitotic figure (TPX2 (red)) with DAPI counter-stain (blue). Scale bars = 10 μm.

Equine tendon fibroblasts have robust DNA repair activity, but the integrity of this repair is uncertain

There were now two reasons for investigating the reparative ability of these tendon fibroblasts: firstly the evidence that DNA damage even at remarkably high levels was not proceeding in most cases to cell death (or permanent arrest of BN cells in those monolayers) i.e. it was being repaired; and secondly due to the potential role of defective repair processes in the formation of DSBs in the first place. Given that SDFT fibroblasts have been shown to have low synthetic and degradative activity levels post-maturation and that they frequently allow accumulation of matrix microdamage [8-15], it was of interest to know if this extended to a poor ability to repair their own DNA.

Because γH2AX labelling only indicates DSB-type damage [49] and repair intermediates we used alkaline comet assays to assess damage and repair in these tendon cells. This assay involves lysing agarose-embedded cells and performing DNA unwinding and electrophoresis at an alkaline pH (12.1-12.4), to detect multiple types of DNA damage i.e. single and double strand breaks, incomplete excision repair sites and cross-links. These lesions often precede DSB formation. DNA migrates out of each cell in response to application of an electric field, and is visualised when fluorescently labelled, as a 'comet'; the comet tail size and shape correlate with the degree of DNA damage [67]. The equine genome is 2.7 Gb i.e. it is slightly smaller than the human genome at 3.2 Gb. As comet analysis is capable of measuring 0.06 to 3 breaks per 10^9 daltons, the lowest level of sensitivity would be approximately 100 breaks per equine genome; this is more than adequate to measure levels of background DNA damage in control cells [68]. We used hydrogen peroxide (H_2O_2) as a damaging agent because it is known to predominantly cause non-DSB lesions in DNA, particularly in replicating cells. Reactive oxygen species are also of practical relevance in tendon fibroblast research, as they are likely to be increased within the tissue of energy-storing tendons during high-speed exercise [18,19].

Significant damage was recorded for both abattoir and PM group cells following H_2O_2 treatment, but the majority of comet-tails (indicating broken DNAs) were lost after 1 h recovery i.e. these data showed robust repair activity for both groups (Figure 7A). We were particularly interested to see how subtle variation in initial DNA damage levels could alter damage and repair following the H_2O_2 treatment; to achieve this we reduced the biologic noise in our assay by comparing cells derived from the same animal. We used PM cells as they carried a lower amount of endogenous damage. Our assay involved two sets of cells; one early passage (P3) and the second, derived after several weeks in continuous culture (denoted

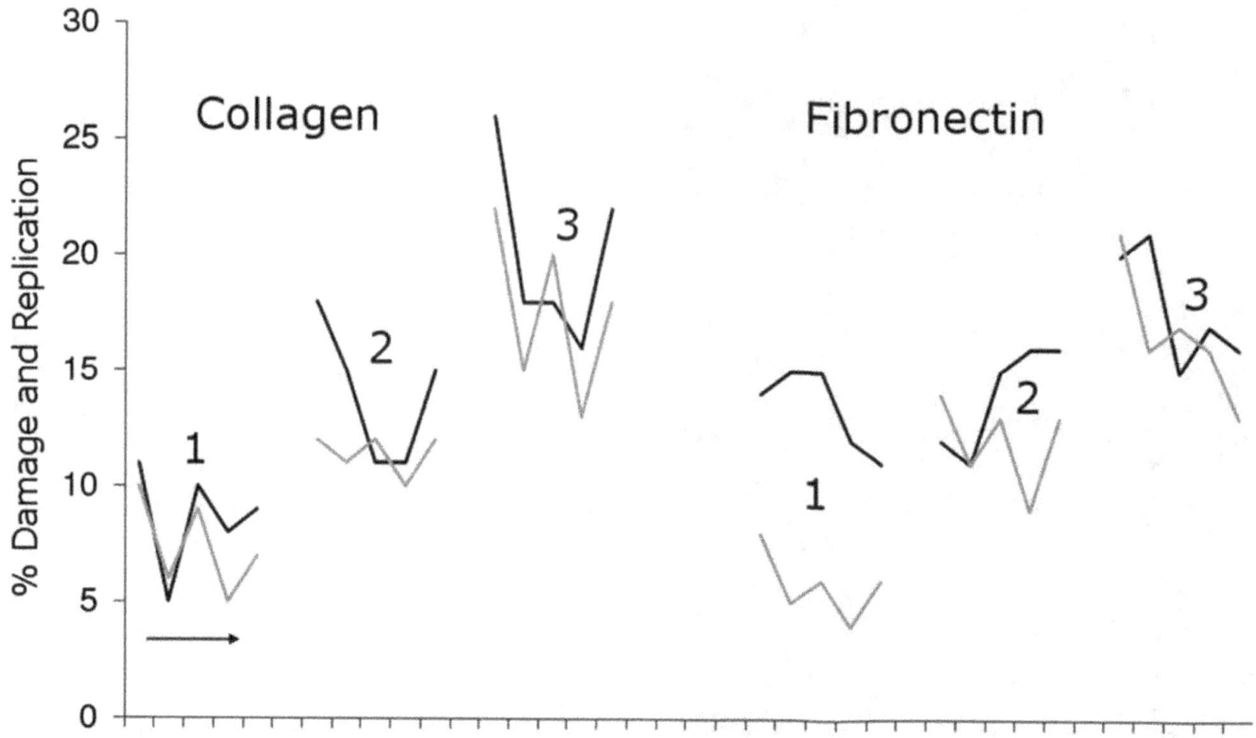

Figure 6 Close correlation between damaged and replicative fractions in tendon fibroblast monolayers is uncoupled on fibronectin. The percentages of damaged (black) and replicating (grey) cells are shown in monolayers with low (1), intermediate (2), or high replicative fractions (3) on both collagen and fibronectin surfaces. Each group comprises 5 data points collected from a different source animal. The ages of these animals were, from left to right: 6 months, 3, 5, 14 and 15 years. A close association of the two fractions can be seen on collagen, but on fibronectin the damage level remains relatively high regardless of confluence status i.e. there is an uncoupling of these two events.

EP/early passage and LP/late passage). To more accurately identify changes in repair capacity we used the CometScore software that allows analysis of individual comets with definition of their DNA distributions (i.e. percentage of DNA in the tail). The CometScore software generates histograms of fluorescence intensity across each comet which can then be quantified (Figure 7B). CometScore analyses from our two groups of cells (early and late passage) are shown in the box-whisker charts in Figure 7C. The upper chart shows EP cells; the lower, LP. The median values for control (initial) levels of DNA damage (% of DNA in the comet tail) in EP and LP cells were 1.2% and 3.0% respectively on collagen-coated surfaces and 0.4% and 2.5% on fibronectin. Following H_2O_2 treatment, the median values of these two groups diverged by more than 20% i.e. 60.7% for EP versus 82.6% for LP on collagen, with similar differentials when grown on fibronectin (Figure 7C). This difference was maintained following the 1 h recovery period. We could speculate that the increased injury generated by peroxide treatment of the LP cells delayed repair; the contribution of a minor increase in basal DNA injury prior to peroxide treatment remains to be established. However, if small differences in basal DNA damage can alter the injury thresholds for tendon fibroblasts, researchers will have to be wary of this possibility and carefully control for genotoxic stress in their experiments.

Interestingly, pairwise analyses to compare cells on either matrix surface within each of the EP and LP groups (i.e. comparing the EP controls on collagen and fibronectin) showed that DNA damage levels were not significantly different between cells on collagen versus fibronectin surfaces with one exception; for the LP cells there was a lower DNA damage level of 20.6% in the recovery group on fibronectin, versus 32.8% for collagen ($p < 0.001$). This finding is in keeping with previous work that indicates potentiation of DNA damage responses in cells growing on fibronectin [63], which might result in the altered repair kinetics that we observed. However, the integrity of this more rapid re-ligation is not certain given our previous measurements of high levels of γH2AX in cells growing on that surface, that occurred regardless of their replication status. High levels of γH2AX labelling have been shown to persist following DNA break re-ligation in situations where DNA repair has been inaccurate [62]. Our demonstration of a DNA damage-replication link would suggest that repair processes

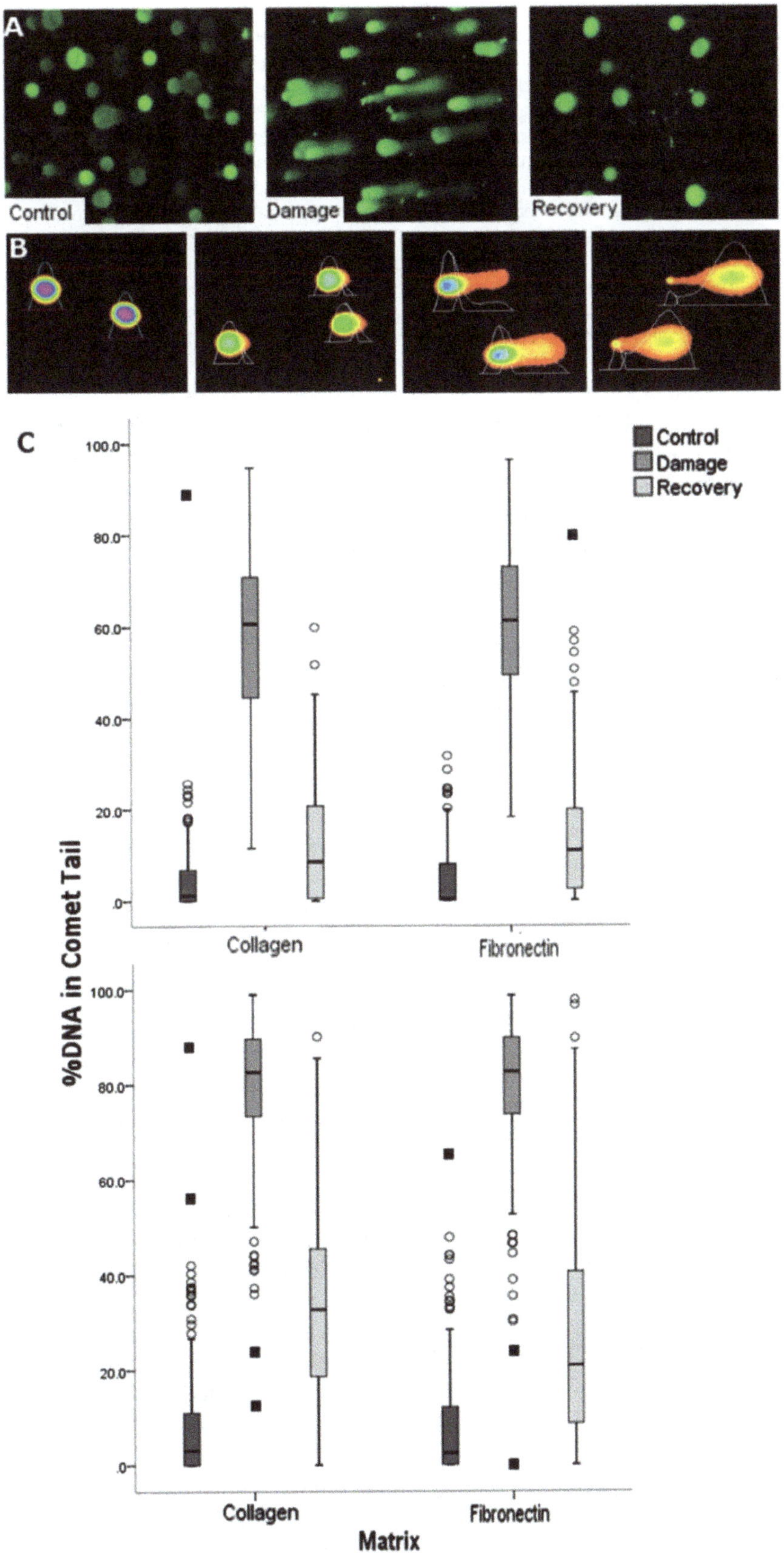

Figure 7 (See legend on next page.)

(See figure on previous page.)
Figure 7 Comet assays show that rate of DNA repair is linked to initial levels of DNA damage. (A) Comet assay showing efficient repair of peroxide-induced damage in an abattoir sample. The high level of DNA damage (indicated by long comet tails) in the middle panel is evident in cells collected immediately after peroxide treatment. Much of this damage is repaired after a 1 h recovery period with the result that the comet 'tails' are lost in the right hand panel. **(B)** CometScore analyses indicate cells which have been selected from bitmaps; these are converted into histograms by CometScore which quantifies %DNA in comet tails. The cells used in this panel are control cells. These are either undamaged (left hand panel) or have been treated with increasing concentrations of the DNA damaging agent etoposide (left to right). **(C)** CometScore analyses indicate levels of DNA damage following peroxide treatment of two populations from the same horse (PM group). The upper graph shows comet data for EP cells; the lower graph shows comet data for LP cells. The damage induced by peroxide treatment is markedly greater for the LP group; repair of DNA during the recovery period is also delayed for LP cells. Triplicate independent experiments were conducted with at least 50 comets analysed per condition. Outliers at 1.5 box-lengths or more from the edge of the box are indicated by spheres; extreme outliers at 3 or more box-lengths are indicated by black squares. The upper and lower boundaries of the box indicate the interquartile range; the line across the middle of the box represents the median value. Extreme outliers may indicate apoptotic cells or cells that have sustained irreparable damage; wide data distributions indicate these cell fate outcomes together with cells that are repairing, or have repaired, their DNAs.

that act in replicating cells, for example, HR, may be defective in the tendon fibroblasts. It is possible that this defect is enriched in monolayer cultures of tendon-derived cells due to the fact that they are generally post-replicative in their tissue niche [69]. This possibility will be investigated in future work.

Conclusions

Culturing equine tendon fibroblasts in monolayers resulted in two forms of cellular injury: numbers of binucleate cells at levels previously only documented in cells irradiated or treated with cytoskeletal poisons; and in cells from some sources, high initial levels of DNA damage including double strand breaks that did not resolve with further replicative cycling but did not result in significant cell death. We demonstrated that both forms of injury were replication-linked on collagen substrates, with uncoupling of the replication-DNA damage link on fibronectin. DNA repair mechanisms were robust, but increased DNA damage delayed repair; this effect was mitigated for cells carrying high levels of DNA damage but cultured on fibronectin. We would recommend that cells expressing these damage phenotypes at an early passage not be injected into injury sites or used for mechanistic injury studies due to problems with comparability. Additionally, ex-vivo cell expansion should be minimised in order to limit replication-induced cellular injury and mitotic disruption. The effects of fibronectin in uncoupling DNA damage from replication and accelerating DNA re-ligation (in monolayers with high DNA damage levels) require further investigation, given the high levels of this matrix glycoprotein in injury sites.

Methods

Sample collection

Mid-metacarpal segments (5 cm) of the SDFT were harvested under aseptic conditions from the forelimbs of Thoroughbred horses euthanized for reasons unrelated to tendon disease. Specimens from 5 adults (3, 5, 14, 15 years of age) and one foal (6 months of age) were obtained from an approved UK abattoir. Specimens from one adult (3-year-old) and one foal (full-term stillborn) were obtained from a veterinary post-mortem facility. All specimens were obtained and used in accordance with guidelines reviewed and approved by the Ethics and Welfare Committee, School of Veterinary Medicine, University of Glasgow. Equine palate fibroblasts were donated by Dr. L. Nasir (University of Glasgow) [32]. Human primary foreskin fibroblasts (Hs68) were purchased (CRL 1635; ATCC, Teddington, Middlesex, UK).

Cell preparation

The paratenon and peripheral tissue were removed from each tendon segment and the remaining tissue diced into 2 mm^3 pieces. These were incubated with constant agitation for 1 h at 37°C in sterile DMEM medium (10 mL per 1 g tissue) containing 1 mg/mL pronase and supplemented with 10% foetal calf serum (FCS) and 1% penicillin/streptomycin [13,21]. A second digestion for 1 h at 37°C with complete DMEM containing 0.25 mg/mL collagenase type VIII and 0.55 mg/mL dispase (40 mL per 1 g of tissue) was then performed [13,21]. Digested material was passed through a 70 μm cell strainer, and cells collected by centrifugation at 1000 rpm for 5 min; cell pellets were re-suspended in complete DMEM. The collagenase/dispase digestion was repeated to yield more cells. Routine expansion was carried out in flasks coated with 10 μg/cm^2 type I collagen. For experiments the cells were seeded onto glass coverslips coated with either 10 μg/cm^2 type I collagen or 1 μg/cm^2 fibronectin (as per manufacturers' instructions) and grown to 30-80% confluence in a standard humidified incubator (37°C, 21% O_2, 5% CO_2). Equine palate fibroblasts were processed as described previously [32]. Human fibroblasts were seeded onto collagen-coated coverslips in complete DMEM (10% serum; 1 g/L glucose) supplemented with penicillin/streptomycin, and maintained in the same incubator.

Culture of tendon explants

A 5 cm mid-metacarpal segment of the SDFT were aseptically retrieved and placed into pre-warmed DMEM (37°C). To retrieve tendon fibroblasts from the core of the mid-metacarpal region, a sharp single edged blade (HD Hardware) was used to excise peripheral tissue. The exposed core was diced into 2 mm^3 pieces that were placed onto collagen-coated 60 mm plastic culture dishes. The bottom of each dish was scored with a scalpel blade to create 5 or 6 parallel lines; this facilitated surface-adhesion of the tissue pieces. Pre-warmed (37°C) complete DMEM containing 10% bovine serum albumin and 1% penicillin / streptomycin was added to the dishes.

Imaging of binucleate fibroblasts and calculation of mitotic indices

Binucleate (BN) cells were quantified by phase contrast and fluorescent microscopy using an inverted Leica DM IRB microscope; CellMask (plasma membrane dye/Invitrogen) and AlexaFluor 488 Phalloidin were used to demarcate the cytoplasm. Mitotic indices were counted in multiple random fields by fluorescence microscopy using the DNA co-stain DAPI and the replicative marker TPX2. Numbers of prophase (P) and metaphase (M) cells were counted as one cohort and anaphase (A) and telophase (T) as the second.

Immunocytochemistry

Cells were fixed in 4% paraformaldehyde for 5 min, followed by permeabilization using 0.25% Triton-X 100 for 5 min. Non-specific binding was blocked using 10% milk powder/PBS for 30 min at room temperature (RT). Primary and secondary antibody incubations were carried out overnight at 4°C and 1 h at RT, respectively. Alexafluor conjugates (1:1000) were used to detect the primary antibodies. Slides were mounted using Prolong-Gold antifade containing DAPI (Invitrogen). Levels of DNA damage were assessed by labelling for phospho-H2AX (γH2AX) (clone JBW301 (1:250) Millipore, Watford, UK). p53 phosphorylated at serine 15 was immunolabelled using ab1431 (1:200; Abcam, Cambridge, UK). Cells were additionally labelled for p21 using EA10 (1:100; Calbiochem, Watford, UK). Double-stranded DNA breaks were more definitively identified by co-labelling for phospho-H2AX and proteins that respond to DNA damage, i.e. either promyelocytic leukaemia protein (PML; H-238 (1:100), Santa Cruz, Dallas, TX, USA) or Rad51 (H-92 (1:100), Santa Cruz, Dallas, TX, USA). Replication was assessed by labelling for the TPX/repp86 and centromere protein F (CENPF) antigens (ab71816 (1:100) and ab5 (1:100), Abcam, Cambridge UK), these being expressed diffusely in the nucleus during S and G2 phases of the cell cycle with relocation to the spindle during mitosis. Cells were examined and imaged using the 63x objective lens of an upright Axiophot2 (Zeiss) or inverted DM IRB microscope (Leica). Fluorescent micrographs were overlaid using GIMP digital software (version 2.6.1).

Mycoplasma testing

Cell culture samples were added to both solid and liquid mycoplasma media (Mycoplasma Experience, Reigate, UK), and incubated under microaerophilic conditions for up to 7 d. Cell cultures were also tested using the MycoProbe® Mycoplasma Detection Kit (R&D Systems Europe Inc., Abingdon, UK). Plasmocin (Invivogen, Toulouse, France) was used at a curative (rather than prophylactic) concentration of 25 µg/mL for two weeks.

Comet assay

The alkaline comet assay was performed as per the manufacturers' instructions using triplicate test samples (Trevigen Inc., Gaithersburg, MD, USA). DNA damage was induced by incubation with 200 µM H_2O_2 for 5 min on ice. To assess repair capacity, the H_2O_2 treatment was followed by a 1 h recovery period. The untreated controls were trypsinized immediately, counted and embedded in agarose. The "treatment" group was processed in this way directly following H_2O_2 incubation. The "recovery" group cells were rinsed with PBS, fresh DMEM was added, and they were then maintained for 1 h at 37°C in a 5% CO_2 incubator prior to processing. The processing was done as rapidly as possible to limit any further DNA repair that would result in under-estimation of the damage at that point. Cells at 1×10^5/mL were added to molten agarose (1:10 v/v). The CometSlides™ were evenly warmed to 37°C prior to application of cells in agarose (to improve adherence of cells); it was important to avoid spreading the cell mixture over the margins of each sample area (delineated in red). The lysis stage was performed at 4°C overnight to increase sensitivity; if the lysis solution crystallized over this period it was discarded. Electrophoresis (21 V, 30 min) at a high pH resulted in structures resembling comets as observed by fluorescence microscopy (using SybrGreen to stain DNA); comets form due to electrophoretic migration of broken DNA strands away from the nucleoid. Electrophoresis is one of the principal factors that can affect data reproducibility. If using a Trevigen CometAssay ES II tank it is crucial to add only 850 mL electrophoresis buffer such that the buffer height is held at 0.4 cm over the slide tray; changing this parameter will alter the efficiency of electrophoresis. Each run was standardized using control 'damaged' cells with expected comet tail grades. Images were viewed and captured using a Leica DM IRB microscope. Etoposide-damaged cells (Trevigen Inc., Gaithersburg, MD, USA) were used to establish damage reference groups and ensure that the control conditions were not themselves genotoxic. Treatment and recovery groups were electrophoresed at the same time as controls to reduce experimental variability; failure to visualize comet tails in etoposide-damaged cells was used to indicate failed electrophoresis, in which case the data was not used.

Analysis was performed using CometScore version 1.6.1.11 (TriTek Corp., Sumerduck, VA, USA). Individual "comets" were manually selected from monochrome bitmap images with all metrics saved. Overlapping comets in the images were not scored. Imaging and noise cut-off was as described in [70]. Values plotted were derived from 'percent DNA in the tail' as suggested by the COMET assay users group [71]. Each data point represented independent triplicate experiments with at least 50 comets scored per experiment.

Statistical analysis

All statistical analyses were performed using SPSS Statistics version 9 (IBM, New York, USA). Data normality was assessed using the Kolmogorov-Smirnov statistic. Probability values for significance between the treatment groups were assessed using the non-parametric Mann–Whitney U Test.

Abbreviations

SDFT: Superficial digital flexor tendon; BN: Binucleate; ATM: Ataxia telangiectasia mutated; ATR: Ataxia telangiectasia and Rad3-related protein; γH2AX: gammaH2AX; MMP: Matrix metalloproteinase; PM: Post mortem; DAPI: 4′,6-diamidino-2-phenylindole; P: Prophase; M: Metaphase; A: Anaphase; T: Telophase; DDR: DNA damage response; DSB: Double-strand break; ROS: Reactive oxygen species; PML: Promyelocytic leukaemia protein; HR: Homologous recombination; CENPF: Centromere protein F; NAC: N-acetyl cysteine; H_2O_2: Hydrogen peroxide; DMEM: Dulbecco's modified eagle medium; FCS: Foetal calf serum; RT: Room temperature; LDH: Lactate dehydrogenase.

Competing interests

The authors declare that they have no competing interests that could inappropriately influence or bias the content of this paper.

Authors' contributions

TR contributed to study design and creation and acquisition of funds, carried out the cell culture work, immunocytochemistry, microscopic imaging, comet assays, comet analysis, and assisted with statistical analysis. LBH and HC obtained the tendon specimens, derived the cells, and assisted with cell culture, immunocytochemistry, and comet assays. DLB participated in study design, acquisition of funds, data analysis, and drafting and revision of the manuscript. JPK contributed to study design and creation and acquisition of funds, assisted in overall supervision, contributed to statistical analysis, and drafted the manuscript. All authors read and approved the final manuscript.

Acknowledgements

We gratefully acknowledge the support of this study by The Equine Trust (Massey University, New Zealand), Petplan Charitable Trust, the Biotechnology and Biosciences Research Council (BBSRC; project grant BB/J000655/1) and the Horserace Betting Levy Board. None of the funding sources played any role in the study design, data collection, analysis, data interpretation, manuscript writing or the decision to submit the manuscript for publication. We also wish to thank the staff of the equine abattoir, and at The Animal Health Trust including Dr. Debbie Guest. We would also like to thank Elizabeth Gault for her assistance with primary culture; including handling of equine palate cells.

Author details

[1]Institute of Infection, Immunity and Inflammation, College of Medical, Veterinary and Life Sciences, University of Glasgow, 120 University Place, Glasgow G12 8TA, UK. [2]Department of Cell and Developmental Biology, University College London, Gower Street, London WC1E 6BT, UK.

References

1. Avella CS, Ely ER, Verheyen KL, Price JS, Wood JL, Smith RK: **Ultrasonographic assessment of the superficial digital flexor tendons of National Hunt racehorses in training over two racing seasons.** *Equine Vet J* 2009, **41**:449–454.
2. Goodship AE, Birch HL, Wilson AM: **The pathobiology and repair of tendon and ligament injury.** *Vet Clin North Am Equine Pract* 1994, **10**:323–349.
3. Singer ER, Barnes J, Saxby F, Murray JK: **Injuries in the event horse: training versus competition.** *Vet J* 2008, **175**:76–81.
4. Godwin EE, Young NJ, Dudhia J, Beamish IC, Smith RK: **Implantation of bone marrow-derived mesenchymal stem cells demonstrates improved outcome in horses with overstrain injury of the superficial digital flexor tendon.** *Equine Vet J* 2012, **44**:25–32.
5. O'Meara BO, Bladon B, Parkin TD, Fraser B, Lischer CJ: **An investigation of the relationship between race performance and superficial digital flexor tendonitis in the thoroughbred racehorse.** *Equine Vet J* 2010, **42**:322–326.
6. Lam KH, Parkin TD, Riggs CM, Morgan KL: **Descriptive analysis of retirement of thoroughbred racehorses due to tendon injuries.** *Equine Vet J* 2007, **39**:143–148.
7. Marr CM, Love S, Boyd JS, McKellar Q: **Factors affecting the clinical outcome of injuries to the superficial digital flexor tendon in National Hunt and point-to-point racehorses.** *Vet Rec* 1993, **132**:476–479.
8. Birch HL, Bailey JV, Bailey AJ, Goodship AE: **Age-related changes to the molecular and cellular components of equine flexor tendons.** *Equine Vet J* 1999, **31**:391–396.
9. Smith RK, Birch H, Patterson-Kane J, Firth EC, Williams L, Cherdchutham W, van Weeren WR, Goodship AE: **Should equine athletes commence training during skeletal development?: Changes in tendon matrix associated with development, ageing, function and exercise.** *Equine Vet J* 1999, **30**:201–209.
10. Patterson-Kane JC, Wilson AM, Firth EC, Parry DA, Goodship AE: **Comparison of collagen fibril populations in the superficial digital flexor tendons of exercised and nonexercised thoroughbreds.** *Equine Vet J* 1997, **29**:121–125.
11. Birch HL, Wilson AM, Goodship AE: **Physical activity: does long-term, high-intensity exercise in horses result in tendon degeneration?** *J Appl Physiol* 2008, **105**:1927–1933.
12. Ker RF: **The implications of adaptable fatigue quality of tendons for their construction, repair and function.** *Comp Biochem Physiol A Mol Integr Physiol* 2002, **133**:987–1000.
13. Young NJ, Becker DL, Fleck RA, Goodship AE, Patterson-Kane JC: **Maturational alterations in gap junction expression and associated collagen synthesis in response to tendon function.** *Matrix Biol* 2009, **28**:311–323.
14. Birch HL, Worboys S, Eissa S, Jackson B, Strassburg S, Clegg PD: **Matrix metabolism rate differs in functionally distinct tendons.** *Matrix Biol* 2008, **27**:182–189.
15. Smith RKW, Birch HL, Goodman S, Heingård D, Goodship AE: **The influence of ageing and exercise on tendon growth and degeneration – hypotheses for the initiation and prevention of strain-induced tendinopathies.** *Comp Biochem Physiol A Mol Integr Physiol* 2002, **133**:1039–1050.
16. Stephens PR, Nunamaker DM, Butterweck DM: **Application of a Hall-effect transducer for measurement of tendon strains in horses.** *Am J Vet Res* 1989, **50**:1089–1095.
17. Wang JH, Li Z, Yang G, Khan M: **Repetitively stretched tendon fibroblasts produce inflammatory mediators.** *Clin Orthop Relat Res* 2004, **422**:243–250.
18. Millar NL, Reilly JH, Kerr SC, Campbell AL, Little KJ, Leach WJ, Rooney BP, Murrell GA, McInnes B: **Hypoxia: a critical regulator of early human tendinopathy.** *Ann Rheum Dis* 2012, **71**:302–310.

19. Bestwick CS, Maffulli N: **Reactive oxygen species and tendinopathy: do they matter?** *Br J Sports Med* 2004, **38**:672–674.
20. Wilson AM, Goodship AE: **Exercise-induced hyperthermia as a possible mechanism for tendon degeneration.** *J Biomech* 1994, **27**:899–905.
21. Burrows S, Becker DL, Fleck RA, Patterson-Kane JC: **Gap junctional propagation of apoptosis in tendon fibroblast monolayers in response to physiological hyperthermia.** *Trans Orthop Res Soc* 2009, **34**:27.
22. Clegg PD, Strassburg S, Smith RK: **Cell phenotypic variation in normal and damaged tendons.** *Int J Exp Pathol* 2007, **88**:227–235.
23. Lavagnino M, Arnoczky SP, Egerbacher M, Gardner KL, Burns ME: **Isolated fibrillar damage in tendons stimulates local collagenase mRNA expression and protein synthesis.** *J Biomech* 2006, **39**:2355–2362.
24. Leadbetter WB: **Cell-matrix response in tendon injury.** *Clin Sports Med* 1992, **11**:533–578.
25. Patterson-Kane JC, Becker DL, Rich T: **The pathogenesis of tendon microdamage in athletes: the horse as a natural model for basic cellular research.** *J Comp Path* 2012, **147**:227–247.
26. Wagenhäuser MU, Pietschmann MF, Sievers B, Docheva D, Schieker M, Jansson V, Müller PE: **Collagen type I and decorin expression in tenocytes depend on the cell isolation method.** *BMC Musculoskelet Disord* 2012, **13**:140.
27. Taylor SE, Vaughan-Thomas A, Clements DN, Pinchbeck G, Macrory LC, Smith RKW, Clegg PD: **Gene expression markers of tendon fibroblasts in normal and diseased tissue compared to monolayer and three dimensional culture systems.** *BMC Musculoskelet Disord* 2009, **10**:27.
28. Chen J, Yu Q, Wu B, Lin Z, Pavlos NJ, Xu J, Ouyang H, Wang A, Zheng MH: **Autologous tenocyte therapy for experimental Achilles tendinopathy in a rabbit model.** *Tissue Eng Part A* 2011, **17**:2037–2048.
29. Durgam SS, Stewart AA, Pondenis HC, Yates AC, Evans RB, Stewart MC: **Responses of equine tendon- and bone marrow-derived cells to monolayer expansion with fibroblast growth factor-2 and sequential culture with pulverised tendon and insulin-like growth factor-I.** *Am J Vet Res* 2012, **73**:162–170.
30. Stephen MJ, Poindexter BJ, Moolman JA, Sheikh-Hamad D, Bick RJ: **Do binucleate cardiomyocytes have a role in myocardial repair? Insights using isolated rodent myocytes and cell culture.** *Open Cardiovasc Med J* 2009, **3**:1–7.
31. Wong C, Stearns T: **Mammalian cells lack checkpoints for tetraploidy, aberrant centrosome number, and cytokinesis failure.** *BMC Cell Biol* 2005, **6**:6.
32. Yuan ZQ, Gault EA, Gobeil P, Nixon C, Campo MS, Nasir L: **Establishment and characterisation of equine fibroblast cell lines transformed in vivo and in vitro by BPV-1: model systems for equine sarcoids.** *Virology* 2008, **373**:352–361.
33. Piel M, Nordberg J, Euteneuer U, Bornens M: **Centrosome-dependent exit of cytokinesis in animal cells.** *Science* 2001, **291**:1550–1553.
34. Fededa JP, Gerlich DW: **Molecular control of animal cell cytokinesis.** *Nature Cell Biol* 2012, **14**:440–447.
35. *Dividing normal adult rat fibroblasts in tissue cultures*, Warren H. Lewis. [http://www.youtube.com/watch?v=XhRX3vR474Y].
36. Sisken JE, Bonner SV, Grasch SD: **The prolongation of mitotic stages in SV40-transformed vs nontransformed human fibroblast cells.** *J Cell Physiol* 1982, **113**:219–223.
37. Huang H, Fletcher L, Beeharry N, Daniel R, Kao G, Yen TJ, Muschel RJ: **Abnormal cytokinesis after X-irradiation in tumor cells that override the G2 DNA damage checkpoint.** *Cancer Res* 2008, **68**:3724–3732.
38. Beams HW, King RL: **The origin of binucleate and large mono nucleate cells in the liver of the rat.** *Anat Rec* 1942, **83**:281–297.
39. Burton K, Taylor DL: **Traction forces of cytokinesis measured with optically modified elastic substrata.** *Nature* 1997, **385**:450–454.
40. Uetake Y, Sluder G: **Cell cycle progression after cleavage failure: mammalian somatic cells do not possess a "tetraploidy checkpoint".** *J Cell Biol* 2004, **165**:609–615.
41. Stukenberg PT: **Triggering p53 after cytokinesis failure.** *J Cell Biol* 2004, **165**:607–608.
42. Palaiologou AA, Yukna RA, Moses R, Lallier TE: **Gingival, dermal and periodontal fibroblasts express different extracellular matrix receptors.** *J Periodontol* 2001, **72**:798–807.
43. Ritty TM, Roth R, Heuser JE: **Tendon cell array isolation reveals a previously unknown fibrillin-2-containing macromolecular assembly.** *Structure* 2003, **11**:1179–1188.
44. Andreassen PR, Lohez OD, Lacroix FB, Margolis RL: **Tetraploid state induces p53-dependent arrest of nontransformed mammalian cells in G1.** *Mol Biol Cell* 2001, **12**:1315–1328.
45. Huang X, Tran T, Zhang L, Hatcher R, Zhang P: **DNA damage-induced mitotic catastrophe is mediated by the Chk1-dependent mitotic exit DNA damage checkpoint.** *Proc Natl Acad Sci USA* 2005, **102**:1065–1070.
46. Zhang W, Peng G, Lin S-Y, Zhang P: **DNA damage response is suppressed by the high cyclin-dependent kinase 1 activity in mitotic mammalian cells.** *J Biol Chem* 2011, **286**:35899–35905.
47. Baumann C, Daly CM, McDonnell SM, Viveiros MM, De La Fuente R: **Chromatin configuration and epigenetic landscape at the sex chromosome bivalent during equine spermatogenesis.** *Chromosoma* 2011, **120**:227–244.
48. Bekker-Jensen S, Mailand N: **Assembly and function of DNA double-strand break repair foci in mammalian cells.** *DNA Repair (Arnst)* 2010, **9**:1219–1228.
49. Bonner WH, Redon CE, Dickey JS, Nakamura AJ, Sedelnikova OA, Soller S, Pommier Y: **γH2AX and cancer.** *Nat Rev Cancer* 2008, **8**:957–967.
50. Chanoux RA, Yin B, Urtishak KA, Asare A, Bassing CH, Brown EJ: **ATR and H2AX cooperate in maintaining genome stability under replication stress.** *J Biol Chem* 2009, **284**:5994–6003.
51. Yosuke I, Ryo S, Naoyuki O, Kinji A, Shuki M, Hirobumi T: **Phosphorylation of histone H2AX at M phase in human cells without DNA damage response.** *Biochem Biophys Res Comm* 2005, **336**:807–812.
52. Silvestre MA, Saeed AM, Cervera RP, Escribá MJ, García-Ximénez F: **Rabbit and pig ear skin sampling cryobanking: effects of storage time and temperature of the whole ear extirpated immediately after death.** *Theriogenology* 2003, **59**:1469–1477.
53. Bliss LA, Sams MR, Deep-Soboslay A, Ren-Patterson R, Jaffe AE, Chenoweth JG, Jaishankar A, Kleinman JE, Hyde TM: **Use of post-mortem human dura mater and scalp for deriving human fibroblast cultures.** *PLoS One* 2012, **7**:e45282.
54. Rainey MD, Black EJ, Zachos G, Gillespie DAF: **Chk2 is required for optimal mitotic delay in response to irradiation-induced DNA damage incurred in G_2 phase.** *Oncogene* 2008, **27**:896–906.
55. Passos JF, Nelson G, Wang C, Richter T, Simillion C, Proctor CJ, Miwa S, Olijslagers S, Hallinan J, Wipat A, Saretzki G, Rudolph KL, Kirkwood TB, von Zglinicki T: **Feedback between p21 and reactive oxygen production is necessary for cell senescence.** *Mol Syst Biol* 2010, **6**:347.
56. Sabatinos SA: **Recovering a stalled replication fork.** *Nature Educ* 2010, **3**:31.
57. Cleaver JE: **γH2AX: biomarker of damage or functional participant in DNA repair "all that glitters is not gold".** *Photochem Photobiol* 2011, **87**:1230–1239.
58. Thompson LH: **Recognition, signaling, and repair of DNA double-strand breaks produced by ionizing radiation in mammalian cells: the molecular choreography.** *Mutat Res* 2012, **751**:158–246.
59. Varadaraj A, Dovey CL, Laredj L, Ferguson B, Alexander CE, Lubben N, Wyllie AH, Rich T: **Evidence for the receipt of DNA damage stimuli by PML nuclear domains.** *J Pathol* 2007, **211**:471–480.
60. Boichuk S, Hu L, Makielski K, Pandolfi PP, Gjoerup O: **Functional connection between Rad51 and PML in homology-directed repair.** *PLoS ONE* 2011, **6**:e25814.
61. Costanzo V: **Brca2, Rad51 and Mre11: performing balancing acts on replication forks.** *DNA Repair (Amst)* 2011, **10**:1060–1065.
62. Kinner A, Wu W, Staudt C, Iliakis G: **γ-H2AX in recognition and signaling of DNA double-strand breaks in the context of chromatin.** *Nucleic Acids Res* 2008, **36**:5678–5694.
63. De Wever O, Sobczak-Thépot J, Vercoutter-Edouart AS, Michalski JC, Ouelaa-Benslama R, Stupack DG, Bracke M, Wang JY, Gespach C, Emami S: **Priming and potentiation of DNA damage response by fibronectin human colon cancer cells and tumor-derived myofibroblasts.** *Int J Oncol* 2011, **39**:393–400.
64. Williams IF, McCullagh KG, Silver IA: **The distribution of types I and III collagen and fibronectin in the healing equine tendon.** *Connect Tissue Res* 1984, **12**:211–227.
65. Sun G, Xu X, Wang Y, Shen X, Chen Z, Yang J: ***Mycoplasma pneumoniae* infection induces reactive oxygen species and DNA damage in A549 human lung carcinoma cells.** *Infect Immun* 2008, **76**:4405–4413.
66. Lukas C, Savic V, Bekker-Jensen S, Doil C, Neumann B, Pedersen RS, Grøfte M, Chan KL, Hickson ID, Bartek J, Lukas J: **53BP1 nuclear bodies**

form around DNA lesions generated by mitotic transmission of chromosomes under replication stress. *Nat Cell Biol* 2011, **13**:243–253.
67. Fairbairn DW, Olive PL, O'Neill KL: **The comet assay: a comprehensive review.** *Mutat Res* 1995, **339**:37–59.
68. Collins AR, Oscoz AA, Brunborg G, Gaivão I, Giovannelli L, Kruszewski M, Smith CC, Stětina R: **The comet assay: topical issues.** *Mutagenesis* 2008, **23**:143–151.
69. Lundgreen K, Lian Ø, Scott A, Engelbretsen L: **Increased levels of apoptosis and p53 in partial-thickness supraspinatus tendon tears.** *Knee Surg Sports Traumatol Arthrosc* 2013, **21**:1636–1641.
70. *CometScore tutorial.* [http://www.autocomet.com/TutorialCometScore.pdf].
71. *Comet Assay Interest Group.* [http://www.cometassay.com/].

25

A spatiotemporal model to assess the introduction risk of African horse sickness by import of animals and vectors in France

C. Faverjon[1*], A. Leblond[2], P. Hendrikx[3], T. Balenghien[4], C. J. de Vos[5], E.A.J. Fischer[5] and A.A. de Koeijer[5]

Abstract

Background: African horse sickness (AHS) is a major, *Culicoides*-borne viral disease in equines whose introduction into Europe could have dramatic consequences. The disease is considered to be endemic in sub-Saharan Africa. Recent introductions of other *Culicoides*-borne viruses (bluetongue and Schmallenberg) into northern Europe have highlighted the risk that AHS may arrive in Europe as well. The aim of our study was to provide a spatiotemporal quantitative risk model of AHS introduction into France. The study focused on two pathways of introduction: the arrival of an infectious host (PW-host) and the arrival of an infectious *Culicoides* midge via the livestock trade (PW-vector). The risk of introduction was calculated by determining the probability of an infectious animal or vector entering the country and the probability of the virus then becoming established: i.e., the virus's arrival in France resulting in at least one local equine host being infected by one local vector. This risk was assessed using data from three consecutive years (2010 to 2012) for 22 regions in France.

Results: The results of the model indicate that the annual risk of AHS being introduced to France is very low but that major spatiotemporal differences exist. For both introduction pathways, risk is higher from July to October and peaks in July. In general, regions with warmer climates are more at risk, as are colder regions with larger equine populations; however, regional variation in animal importation patterns (number and species) also play a major role in determining risk. Despite the low probability that AHSV is present in the EU, intra-EU trade of equines contributes most to the risk of AHSV introduction to France because it involves a large number of horse movements.

Conclusion: It is important to address spatiotemporal differences when assessing the risk of ASH introduction and thus also when implementing efficient surveillance efforts. The methods and results of this study may help develop surveillance techniques and other risk reduction measures that will prevent the introduction of AHS or minimize AHS' potential impact once introduced, both in France and the rest of Europe.

Keywords: African horse sickness, Equine movements, Import risk assessment, Risk of introduction, *Culicoides*, Quantitative risk, Midge

Background

African Horse Sickness (AHS) is a highly fatal viral vector-borne disease that is transmitted among equine hosts by *Culicoides* midges (Diptera: Ceratoponidae) [1, 2]. It affects all extant Equidae, but morbidity and mortality vary among species: as many as 90 % of infected horses die within one week, while infection is largely subclinical in zebras [3, 4]. AHS virus (AHSV) is an orbivirus, and there are nine different ASHV serotypes that confer some degree of cross-protective immunity [4]. AHS is considered to be endemic in sub-Saharan Africa, where the zebra acts as a reservoir [5]. Rare outbreaks have occurred in North Africa, western Asia, and the Iberian Peninsula, where they have persisted for only a few years [6]. The last outbreak in Europe occurred in the Iberian Peninsula, between 1987 and 1990, and caused the death of more than 1,350 horses, either directly or as a result of control measures [7].

The recent introduction into northern Europe of bluetongue virus (specifically BTV-8, in 2006 [8]) and Schmallenberg virus (in 2011 [9]), both transmitted by

* Correspondence: celine.faverjon@vetagro-sup.fr
[1]INRA UR346 Animal Epidemiology, Vetagrosup, F-69280 Marcy l'Etoile, France
Full list of author information is available at the end of the article

Culicoides midges, highlights the relevance of assessing the risk that AHSV will be introduced to Europe [10]. It is particularly crucial to conduct a risk assessment analysis for France, as the country encompasses different ecosystems, including Mediterranean zones, where *Culicoides imicola*—considered to be the major vector of AHSV worldwide—is very abundant, and non-Mediterranean temperate zones, where *Culicoides obsoletus*—a potential AHSV vector—is dominant [11, 1, 12]. Moreover, France contains between 900,000 and 1 million equines, is the world's 4th largest exporter of horses, and has a horse industry that produces around 12 billion euros of revenue per year [13]. If AHS arrived in France, it could have devastating consequences, similar to those predicted for other EU members such as the United Kingdom (UK) [14], Ireland [15], and the Netherlands [16].

Introduction risks have recently been quantitatively assessed for similar vector-borne diseases, such as BTV [17–19], West Nile Virus [20, 21] and eastern and western equine encephalomyelitis [22], Venezuelan equine encephalitis [22], and Japanese encephalitis [22]. However, these studies mostly took into account only one pathway of introduction; different introduction pathways have rarely been examined in tandem. To explore AHSV in particular, a qualitative risk assessment analysis that accounted for multiple pathways of introduction was conducted in the UK [23]; the results suggested that the most likely pathway of introduction would be the arrival of an infectious host. This pathway of introduction was also examined by a quantitative risk assessment analysis of the likelihood that AHSV would be introduced to the Netherlands [24]. As AHSV is closely related to BTV and shares the same vectors, information on BTV introduction pathways could be helpful when assessing the risk that AHSV will be introduced to Europe. Several studies have indicated that long-distance, wind-mediated transport of *Culicoides* might have played a role in the introduction and spread of several BTV strains in Europe [25–27]. In particular, studies aimed at understanding the introduction of BTV-8 have indicated that the legal importation of an infectious host is unlikely to have caused the epidemic observed in 2006 [28, 29]. It is thought that the risk presented by other pathways of introduction, such as the introduction of a single *Culicoides* midge through intracontinental transport and trade networks [19], is low. Integrative studies are required to quantify and combine information on different pathways of introduction to better understand and confront the risks posed by vector-borne diseases [30].

In this study, we performed a quantitative risk assessment analysis of the introduction of AHSV to France. We focused on two pathways of introduction: the arrival of an infectious host and the arrival of an infectious *Culicoides* midge via the livestock trade. Introduction is defined here as the probability that an infectious host or vector will be released in such a way that at least one local host ends up infected by one local vector (establishment). The subsequent spread of the disease is not examined. As the initial infection of a local host will depend on spatial (e.g., the number of local hosts) and temporal factors (e.g., seasonal vector abundance), the probability of establishment will vary depending on location and time period. The objective of this study was to quantify the risk of introduction associated with a given time period and region for the two pathways of introduction under consideration, which could thus offer insight into temporal and regional variation in introduction risk. Furthermore, evaluating these two pathways of introduction could help optimize risk-mitigating control and surveillance measures.

Methods

Risk associated with introduction pathways and initial assumptions

To quantify the risk of AHSV introduction associated with the two introduction pathways, risk assessment analysis was conducted using the framework developed by de Vos et al. [31]. Although other potential pathways of introduction exist [23], we restricted ourselves to the two most probable: the arrival of an infectious equine and the arrival of an infectious *Culicoides* midge. Only the legal, registered horse trade was taken into account because no data exist on the illegal horse trade. In the analysis, only the introduction of an adult vector was considered since transovarial transmission of the virus has not been observed in *Culicoides* [1, 11, 15]. *Culicoides* midges are hematophagous and tend to stay close to their mammalian hosts (mainly large mammals [32, 33]). They are rarely found in vehicles of transport (such as aircraft or trucks) or merchandise when insect surveys are conducted [21, 34]. It is also uncommon to find *Culicoides* associated with plants or plant material [29, 35]. As a result, only *Culicoides* entering the country via the livestock trade were included in the analysis. Hence, the two main pathways of AHSV introduction examined in this study were: the legal importation of infectious equines (PW-host) and the arrival of infectious *Culicoides* as a consequence of livestock trade (PW-vector).

An introduction pathway was constructed to detail all the steps required for AHSV to be successfully released and become established in France (Fig. 1). This introduction pathway was evaluated using a stochastic risk simulation model. Monthly introduction probabilities were calculated using data from three consecutive years (2010 to 2012) for each area of arrival within France. A total of 22 such areas were defined.

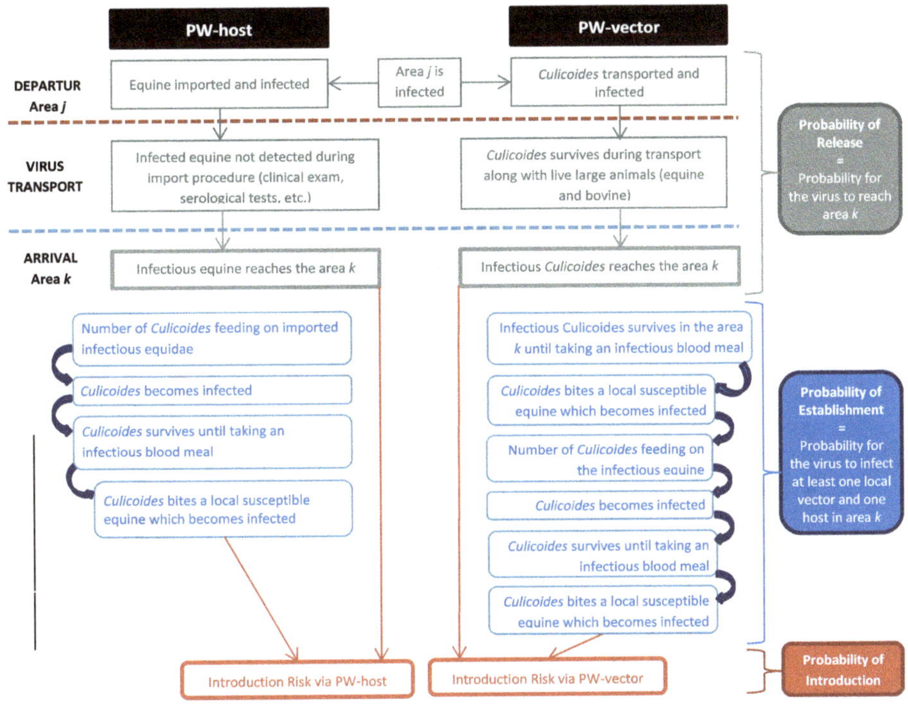

Fig. 1 Introduction pathways. Steps required for the successful release and establishment of AHSV resulting in at least one local host infected by one local vector

Sources of risk

First, the world's countries were grouped into three categories as per De Vos et al. [24]: (1) high-risk regions where the disease is considered to be endemic; (2) low-risk regions that have experienced AHS outbreaks in the past and/or where the main vector, *C. imicola*, is present; and (3) very-low-risk regions (all other countries). Since the main vector is not present in very-low-risk regions, we assumed that it is very unlikely that they would produce exports containing infectious vectors; consequently, very-low-risk regions were ignored for this pathway of introduction. In addition, because EU regulations differ for imports arriving from EU versus non-EU countries [36], we also distinguished between (a) EU members and (b) non-EU members. Five departure regions were thus defined (Fig. 2). Imports from non-EU countries were placed in one of two categories based on their point of arrival in Europe: whether they were shipped directly to France or whether they arrived via another EU country, because animals stopping in another country were considered to experience longer traveling times. Furthermore, equine imports were grouped according to species: (1) horses; (2) donkeys, mules, and hinnies; and (3) zebras.

The model

PW-host: introduction via an infectious host

The probability of AHSV being introduced by species i from region j to area k in month m via an infectious host (PW-host), ($introH_{ijkm}$), was defined as the probability of at least one infectious host of species i from region j arriving in area k in month m and of this arrival being followed by virus transmission to a local vector and host. This overall probability was defined as:

$$P(introH_{ijkm}) = 1 - \left[1 - P(relH_{ijkm}) \times P(estH_{ijkm})\right]^{eq_{ijkm}} \tag{1}$$

Where $P(relH_{ijkm})$ is the probability of an infectious equine of species i from region j being released in area k in month m; $P(estH_{ijkm})$ is the probability of an infection becoming established in month m given the release of one infectious equine of species i from region j in region k; and eq_{ijkm} is the number of equines of species i imported from region j arriving in area k in month m.

Release probabilities, $P(relH_{ijkm})$, were species specific since virus prevalence is different in different equines across the areas of origin, and different species show differences in their susceptibility to the disease. For instance, the release probability of horses is lower because horses have a shorter viremic period than do donkeys and zebras. $P(relH_{ijkm})$ also depended on the moment z of infection; the protective measures implemented before embarkation [36, 37]; and the duration of transport from region j to area k (t_{jk}). For imports coming from non-EU countries, t_{jk} was assumed to equal 1 day for

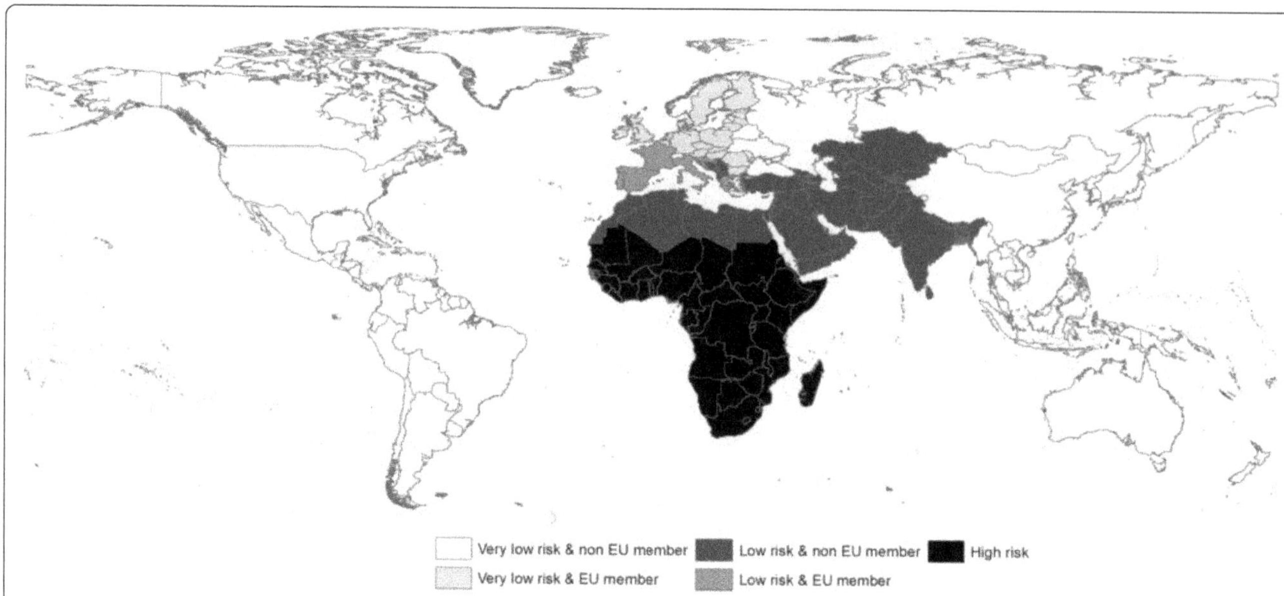

Fig. 2 Countries of the world classified regarding AHS occurrence and import regulations

animals coming directly to France (mainly air travel) and 2 days for animals arriving via another EU country (initial air travel followed by land transport or subsequent air travel). For intra-EU trade, t_{jk} was assumed to be between 1–2 days (uniform distribution) because air and land transport are supposed to be used with equal frequency and France is assumed to be a maximum of 2 days away from everywhere else in EU [38]. $P(relH_{ijkm})$ was defined as :

$$P(relH_{ijkm}) = \frac{\sum_{z=1}^{w}[(\text{length period z}) \times P(\text{relH}_{\text{ijkmz}})]}{\sum_{z=1}^{w}(\text{length period z})} \quad (2)$$

where $P(relH_{ijkmz})$ is the probability of release for an equine i infected during z. For a given region j, there were a total of w different time periods z during which an equine could become infected, depending on the importation procedures implemented for region j (e.g., before quarantine or during quarantine but before the first serological test, etc.). If j was a high-risk region, then $P(relH_{ijkmz})$ was defined as:

$$P(relH_{ijkmz}) = P(inf_{ijmz}) \times P(vir_{ijmz}) \times (1 - P(CF1_{iz})) \times (1 - P(CF2_{iz})) \times (1 - P(clin_{ijmz})) \times (1 - P(trans_{ijkz})) \quad (2.\text{bis})$$

Where $P(inf_{ijmz})$ is the probability of equine i being infected during time period z; $P(vir_{ijmz})$ is the probability of equine i infected during z becoming viremic after transport; $(1 - P(CF1_{iz}))$ and $(1 - P(CF2_{iz}))$ are the probabilities of equine i infected during z not being detected by the first and second serological tests, respectively; $(1 - P(clin_{ijmz}))$ is the probability of equine i infected during z not being detected by the clinical exam; and $(1 - P(trans_{ijkz}))$ is the probability of equine i infected during z not being detected during transport.

The probability of establishment via PW-host was defined as:

$$P(estH_{ijkm}) = 1 - [1 - \lambda_{HV} \times P(surv_{km}) \times b_{equi_k} \times \lambda_{VH}]^{culi_{km}} \quad (3)$$

where λ_{HV} and λ_{VH} are, respectively, the probabilities of a vector feeding on an infectious host becoming infected and of a host bitten by an infectious vector becoming infected; $P(surv_{km})$ is the probability of an infected *Culicoides* midge surviving until its first infectious blood meal; $culi_{km}$ is the number of vectors feeding on an infectious imported host; and b_{equi_k} is the probability of a *Culicoides* midge biting an equine in area k b_{equi_k} depends on the vector's preference for equines as hosts and on the cattle-to-equine ratio in area k.

The overall national and annual median probabilities were calculated based on the monthly regional values. The monthly national median probability of introduction was thus defined as:

$$P(introH_{ijm}) = 1 - \prod_{K=1}^{22}(1 - P(introH_{ijkm})) \quad (4)$$

and the annual national median probability of introduction was defined as:

$$P(introH_{ij}) = 1-\prod_{m=1}^{12}(1-P(introH_{ijm})) \quad (5)$$

The same formulas were used to define the probabilities of release and establishment at the national and annual levels. Using these formulas, the extreme values of these probabilities were determined by using the estimated the 5th and 95th percentiles for each region and month.

For a more detailed description of the probabilities and parameters used, see Additional files 1 and 2.

PW-vector: introduction via an infectious vector

Few data were found on the number of *Culicoides* midges transported with livestock (equines and cattle) over the distances of interest here; as a consequence, we assumed that the numbers could not be very high without having spurred notice and thus calculated the risk of release assuming that one *Culicoides* was transported with each animal. We defined the probability of establishment as the probability that this single vector was able to cause the infection of at least one local equine host by one local vector. $P(introV_{jkm})$ was thus define as:

$$P(introV_{jkm}) = 1-[1-P(relV_{jkm}) \times P(estV_{jkm})]^{n_{jkm}} \quad (6)$$

where $P(relV_{jkm})$ is the probability of a single infected *Culicoides* from region j being released in region k in month m; $P(estV_{jkm})$ is the probability of establishment; and n_{jkm} is the number of livestock (equines and bovines) transported from region j to area k during month m.

The probability of release was defined as:

$$P(relV_{jkm}) = P(inf\_culi_{jm}) \times P(trans_{culi_{jm}}) \times P\left(surv_{trans\,jkm}\right) \quad (7)$$

where $P(inf\_culi_{jm})$ is the probability of a vector in region j becoming infected in month m; $P(trans_{culi_{jm}})$ is the probability of a vector being transported post infection; and $P(surv_{trans_{jkm}})$ is the probability of a *Culicoides* surviving transport from region j to region k. $P(surv_{trans_{jkm}})$ was calculated assuming that transport conditions do not affect *Culicoides* viability (worst case scenario because the survival of insects is supposed to be optimal during transport). If pest control is implemented in region j, we reduced survival probabilities depending on the efficiency of the pest control product ($Prot_{vect}$) used. This was only the case for equines coming from high-risk regions [36]. Since bovines are not consistently and systematically disinfected before transport, we assumed that no pest control was implemented for them.

The probability of establishment via an infectied vector was defined as:

$$P(estV_{jkm}) = P(surv_{arrival_{jkm}}) \times b_{equi_k} \times \lambda_{VH} \times \left[1-[1-\lambda_{VH} \times P(surv_{km}) \times b_{equi_k} \times \lambda_{HV}]^{culi_{km}}\right] \quad (8)$$

where $P(surv_{arrival_{jkm}})$ is the probability of an infected vector surviving to its first infectious blood meal following its arrival in area k.

The overall national and annual median probabilities were calculated using the same procedures used to calculate the PW-host probabilities.

For a more detailed description of the probabilities and parameters used, see Additional files 2 and 3.

Input data

Because accurate registration data for horses were lacking, the ratio of bovines to equines per area k (ρ_k) was estimated by combining information from different databases. The 2010 census conducted by the French Ministry of Agriculture [39] was the source for cattle and equine abundances (horses kept in agricultural settings) for each area and the IFCE-SIRE database [40] provided additional estimates of equine abundance in each area. Because it became mandatory to identify all equines in France in 2012, this database is considered to include all of the country's equines; however, dead horses are still present in the database and, as a result, the number of equines is overestimated. Two ratios were calculated—one using each of the values of equine abundance—and ρ_k was estimated in our model as a uniform distribution that ranged from the smallest to the largest ratio calculated.

The number of bovines and equines transported to France were obtained from TRACES, the **TRA**de Control and **E**xpert **S**ystem, which monitors the transport of animals and products of animal origin both into and within the EU [41]. In our analysis, we only included animals whose final destination was France.

Vector abundance was estimated using data from the national surveillance system implemented in France from 2009 to 2012—approximately 160 locations were surveyed to follow the activity of *Culicoides* populations [42]. The number of competent vectors feeding on a given equine in area k during month m (C_{km}) was modeled using a truncated normal distribution; μ was the average monthly number of *Culicoides* collected per overnight trap (*Culicoides imicola* and members of the Obsoletus complex), σ was the standard deviation, and the minimum and maximum values observed were the lower and upper bounds of the distribution, respectively. Similar parameters were used in modeling efforts by de

Koeijer et al. [43]. The average monthly temperature during month m in area k (T_{km}) was modeled using a truncated normal distribution; μ was the average temperature of each month for each year (based on daily average temperatures obtained from MARS-Agri4cast), and σ was the standard deviation, and the 1st and 99th percentile values were the lower and upper bounds of the distribution, respectively.

Analyses were performed for the three consecutive years included in the study: 2010, 2011, and 2012.

Calculations

Model calculations were performed in Microsoft Office Excel 2010 and @Risk 6.1 [44]; 10,000 iterations were run. The sensitivity analysis tool in @Risk was used to evaluate the impact of stochasticity and uncertainty in the input parameters on model results. The correlation between the values of the input parameters and the pathway-specific probabilities of introduction were calculated (Spearman's rank correlation coefficients).

The sensitivity of the model to the values of the input parameters should have been very similar across all regions and months because we used the same model and input parameter estimates, except in the case of the bovine-to-equine ratio, the temperature data, and vector abundance. Indeed, the values of these three parameters varied across regions and months (i.e., in a given month, the vector abundance could vary greatly in one region and little in another). Larger amounts of variation could have a greater impact on the model than lesser amounts of variation. The reasoning is the same for the bovine-to-equine ratio, which also varied across regions. When determining the overall probability of introduction, we thus chose to focus our sensitivity analysis on the region-time period combinations associated with the highest levels of risk and/or uncertainty.

Results

Data on equine and bovine imports

TRACES data for 2010-2012 show that, on average, 1,300 equines arrived every year in France from non-EU countries, including about forty donkeys (and no zebras). Most of these animals (close to 80 %) passed through another EU country before arriving in France. Imports from high-risk regions represented an average of 1.6 % of the total imports; imports from low- and very-low-risk regions occurred at similar levels: 45.6 % and 52.4 %, respectively. By law, bovines cannot be imported from non-EU countries.

The trading of registered horses within the EU is not required to be reported to TRACES [36]. However, it is nonetheless regularly disclosed: in the TRACES database, more than 40 % of the equines traveling from other EU countries to France were registered horses. It is important to note that, in most of the data on the equine trade within the EU, no distinction is made between horses and donkeys. As a consequence, the TRACES database is somewhat limited in its ability to reveal equine movements within the EU. These concerns aside, according to the database, an average of 9,350 equines arrived in France every year from 2010 to 2012; 65 % came from very-low-risk regions, and 35 % came from low-risk regions. In the case of bovines, all movements are registered in the TRACES database. An average of 145,500 bovines arrived in France every year from 2010 to 2012; 61 % came from very-low-risk regions, and 39 % came from low-risk regions.

Probability of release

The probability of release is defined as the probability of an infectious equine or vector being released in a given area. The overall annual median probability of release in France was 3x10^{-3} for an infectious host (PW-host) and ranged from 1.4 x10^{-2} to 3.6x10^{-2} for an infectious vector (PW-vector). Seasonal variation mostly resulted from the fact that the risk of release is negligible during the first half of the year, when low- and very-low-risk regions are considered to be unlikely to experience AHS outbreaks and equine imports from high-risk regions are very rare. From July to December across all years, the probability of release remained relatively constant; the monthly median probability that an infectious host would be released (PW-host) varied from 2.6x10^{-4} to 9.5x10^{-4}, and the monthly median probability that an infectious vector (PW-vector) would be released ranged from 1.1x10^{-3} to 6.9x10^{-3}. An exceptionally high peak was observed in July 2011 due to arrival of several horses from a high-risk country.

Areas varied greatly in their median release probabilities due to differences in the type and number of imports, but the annual probability of release for a given area was similar over time. As a result, for a given pathway of AHSV introduction, the areas most at risk remained the same (see Fig. 3).

Probability of establishment

We determined the probability of establishment for each area of France, which was the probability that at least one local host would be infected by a local vector after the release of a single infectious host or vector. The probability of establishment varied as a function of temperature, vector abundance, the length of the equine host's viremic period, and the bovine-to-equine ratio in arrival area k. In the case of the infectious vector, $P(estV_{ijkm})$ also depended on the life span of the specific *Culicoides* being transported. The risk of establishment

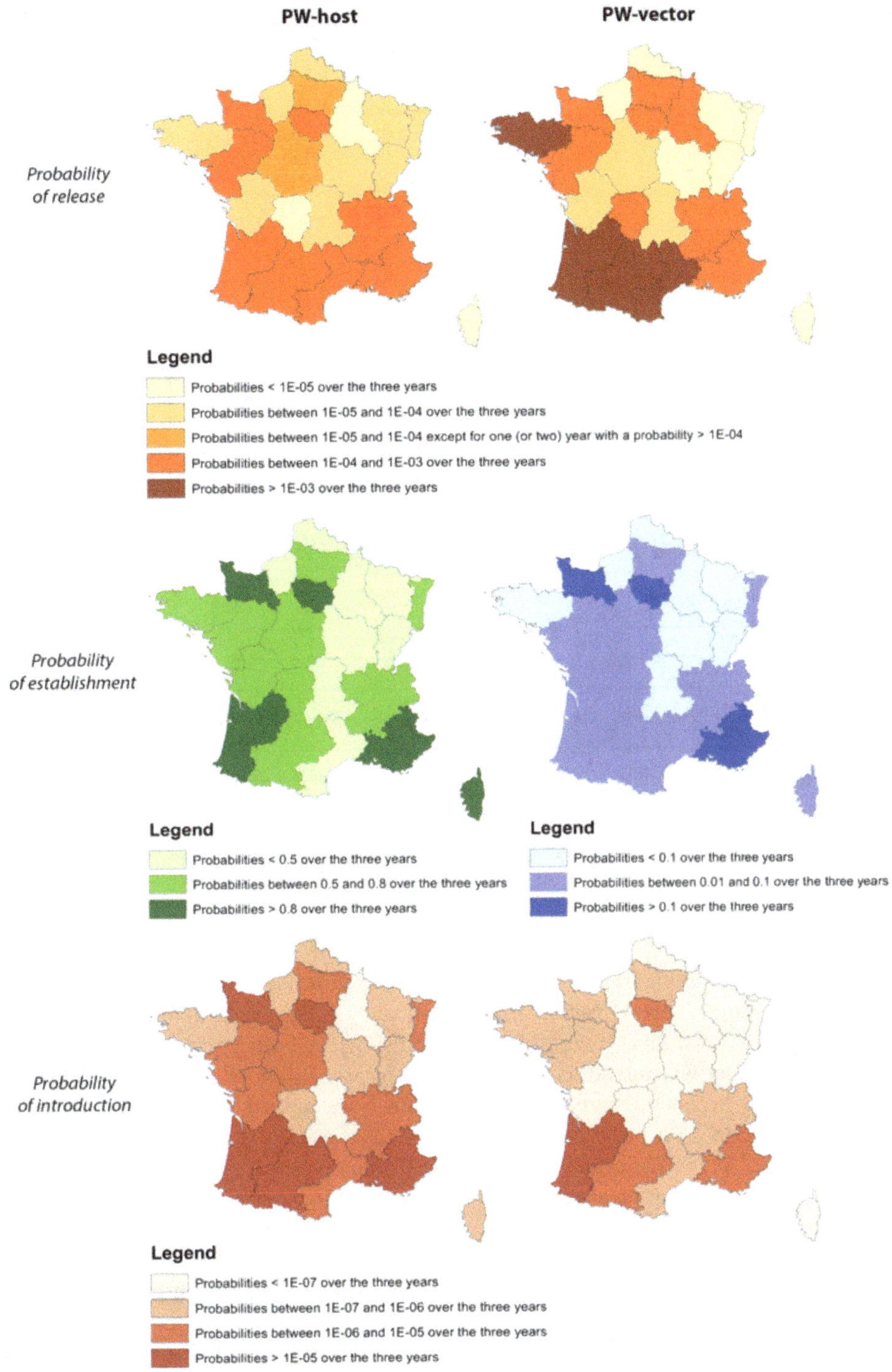

Fig. 3 Main at risk French areas for AHSV release, establishment and introduction per introduction pathways

was highest from May to October and peaked between June and August (Fig. 4). Temporal and regional differences were observed—owing to variation in temperature and relative host abundance—but some areas clearly faced greater risks than others (Fig. 3).

Overall risk assessment

The probability of introduction was obtained by combining the probability of release and the probability of establishment. The median annual risk of introduction due to an infectious host was almost constant across

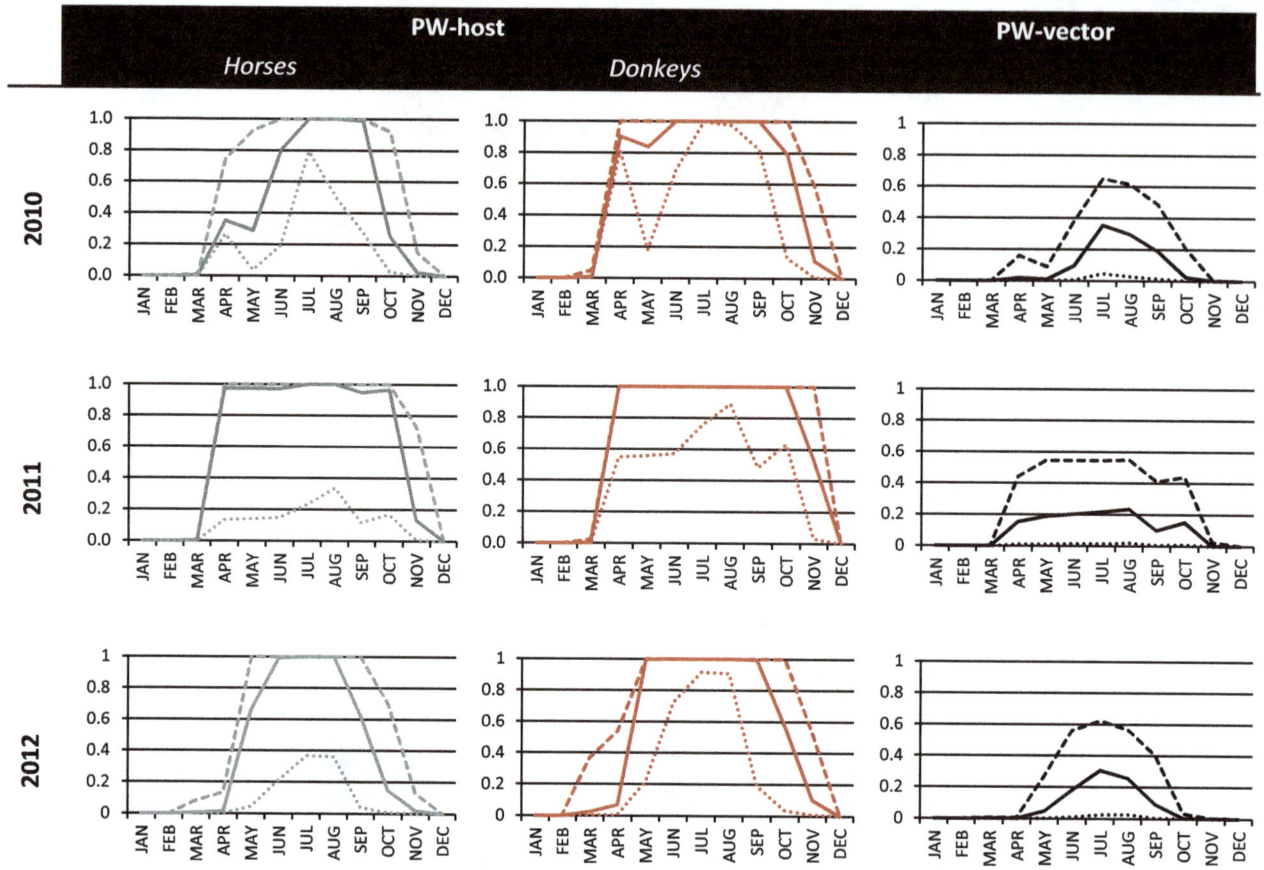

Fig. 4 National probabilities of AHS establishment per introduction pathway and per year for France. Solid lines are the median values, large dash lines the upper border and tiny dash lines the lowest border. NB: the results for zebras are similar to results for donkeys

time (approximately $5x10^{-4}$). The median annual risk of introduction due to an infectious vector varied from $4x10^{-5}$ to $6x10^{-5}$. These figures mean that, currently, the annual risk that an infectious host will introduce AHSV into France is approximately 1 in 2,000; there is a 1 in 16,666 to 25,000 chance that AHSV introduction will be caused by an infectious vector. At the national scale, the monthly probability of introduction was similar over time, but the level of uncertainty was large (Fig. 5). The probability of introduction was the highest in the summer; it peaked in July for both pathways of introduction and in all three years. From November to June, the probability of introduction was nil, except when animals were imported from high-risk regions to the warmest areas of France (e.g., Languedoc Roussillon in March 2012). When animals were imported to colder areas, the probability of establishment was zero, making the probability of introduction zero (e.g., Basse Normandie in March 2012). Introduction risk varied greatly across space and time (see, for example, year 2012 in Fig. 6 and Additional files 4 and 5) but, over the three years examined, some areas consistently had a higher probability of introduction (see Fig. 3). If it is assumed that an average of one midge accompanies each large animal being transported, both pathways can be combined to yield a single probability of introduction (Fig. 7), to which infectious hosts appear to be the main contributors.

The average contribution of each region of origin to introduction risk is shown in Table 1. Intra-EU trade contributes most to the risk of AHSV introduction via the infectious host pathway; low-risk EU countries are the largest contributors even though they are responsible for a lower volume of imports compared with very-low-risk EU countries. This pattern is explained by the high number of equines traded within the EU and by the fact that regulations governing intra-EU trade are less strict. No zebras were brought into France during the period we studied, and donkeys represented only 0.3 % of recorded equine imports. Their average relative contribution to AHSV introduction risk was 1.2 %. Animals imported from high-risk regions account for only 0.02 % of the large livestock arriving in France, and their average contribution to AHSV introduction risk via infectious vectors was 1.5 %. As a result, imports from

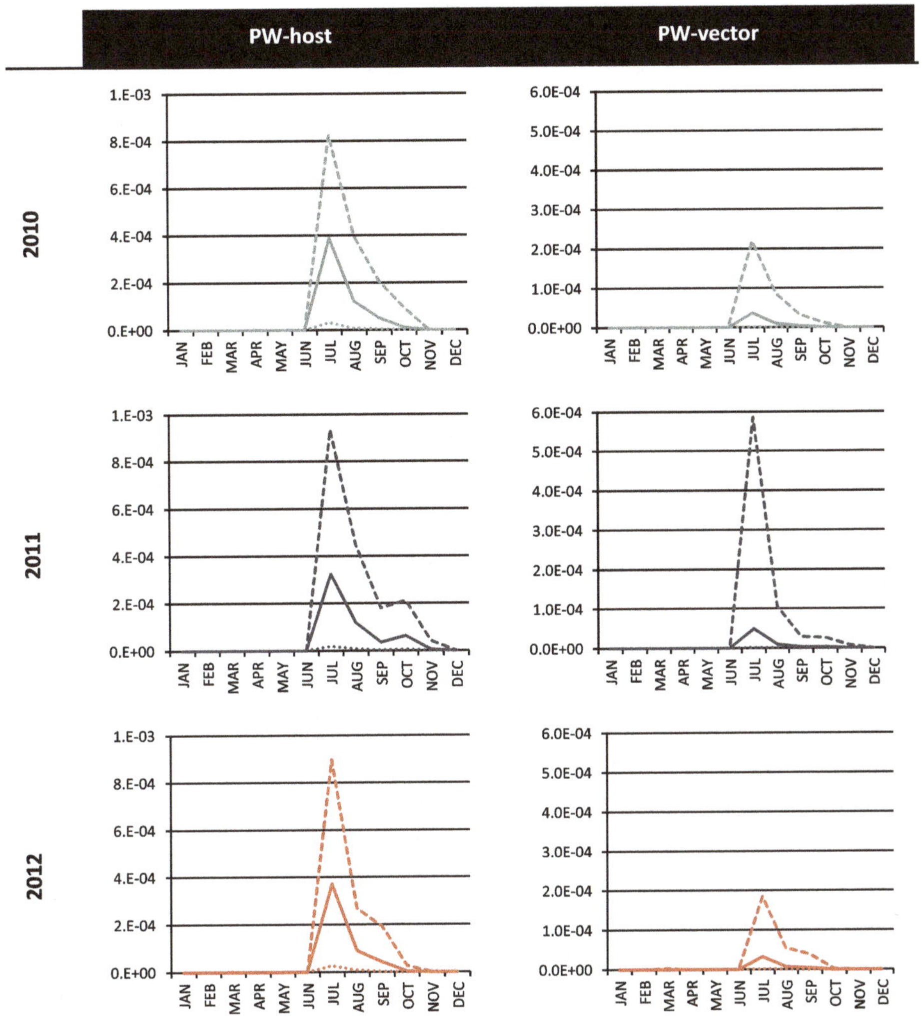

Fig. 5 National probabilities of AHS introduction per year and per introduction pathway for France. Solid lines are the median values, large dash lines the upper border and tiny dash lines the lowest border

low-risk regions made the largest contribution to AHSV introduction risk via infectious vectors. Furthermore, cattle cannot be imported from outside the EU and, consequently, most of the transport of large livestock takes place within the EU (99.3 %). Given this fact and the fact that regulations regarding vector control are identical in all low-risk regions (EU and non-EU countries alike), trade of large livestock within the EU is the main contributor when it comes to the risk of AHSV being introduced by an infectious vector.

Sensitivity analysis

A sensitivity analysis was performed for the two areas identified in Fig. 7 as being at risk for AHSV introduction via the two introduction pathways: Ile de France and Provence. The level of uncertainty surrounding the risk of introduction was rather constant for both areas, with one exception: the level of uncertainty was far higher than average in Provence in October 2012 as a result of major variation in local temperatures. The results of the analysis are summarized in Figs. 8 and 9, respectively, for the infectious host pathway and the infectious vector pathway for July (higher risk month) and October (late summer; characterized by lower risk and large uncertainty for one area) in 2012.

As expected, the values of the input parameters had a constant impact on the model's results over time and space, with only few exceptions. Furthermore, the most important input parameters mainly encompassed variability due to stochasticity (7 out of 10 parameters for PW-host and 6 out of 8 for PW-vector) and, to a lesser extent, uncertainty. Nevertheless, compared to its effects in other areas and months, average monthly temperature had a greater impact on the results for Provence in October for both pathways of introduction. This pattern was due to the fact that temperatures varied greatly in

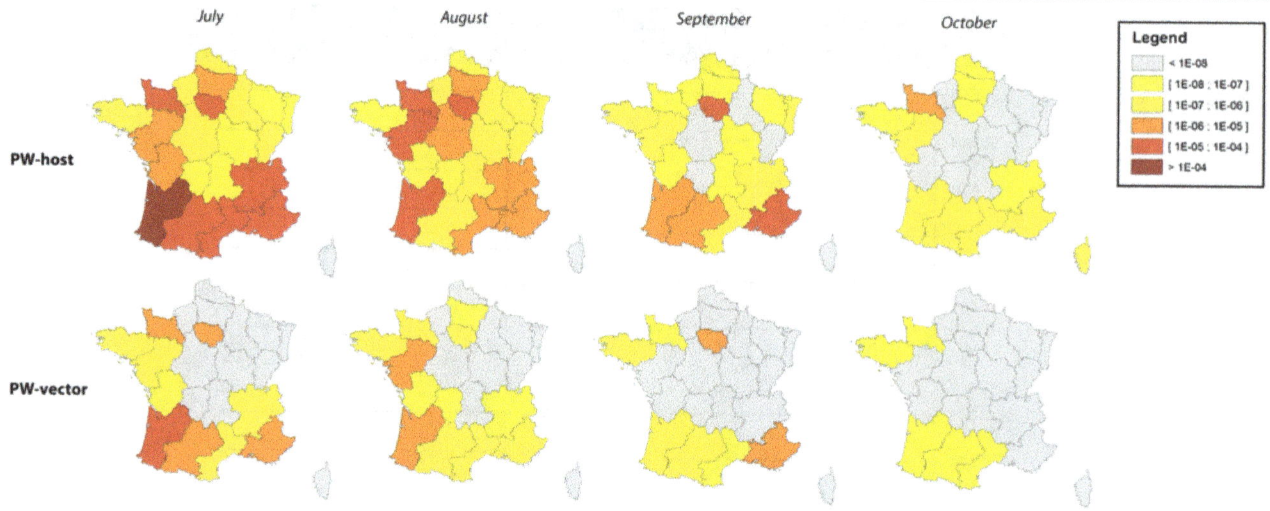

Fig. 6 Monthly regional probabilities of AHS introduction into France from July to October 2012. Results for PW-host are presented in the upper line and results for PW-vector in the lower line. Red: probability of introduction > 1E-05; Dark orange: probability of introduction >1E-06 and < 1E-05; Light orange: probability of introduction >1E-07 and < 1E-06; Yellow: probability of introduction >1E-08 and < 1E-07; White: probability of introduction <1E-08

this area during this month. This result explains the high level of uncertainty associated with the probability of introduction in this area in this month and highlights the large influence of temperature on the model's results.

Discussion

The model revealed that the annual risk of AHSV being introduced to France was very low and relatively constant for the pathways and years examined. The median value for the introduction risk via imported infectious equines (PW-host) was 0.0005; for infectious vectors (PW-vector), median introduction risk varied from $4x10^{-5}$ to $6x10^{-5}$ across years, assuming that one *Culicoides* midge arrived with each imported animal. The PW-host estimate was very similar to that obtained by de Vos and colleagues when they assessed the risk of AHSV being introduced to the Netherlands [24]. The latter study did not distinguish between EU countries and non-EU countries and only took into account competition horses; however, it did include horses traveling through the Netherlands to reach other countries. The PW-vector estimate was highly dependent on our assumption that only one *Culicoides* midge was associated with each imported animal. Indeed, the higher the number of associated *Culicoides*, the higher the probability of introduction. If it is the case that, on average, one *Culicoides* is associated with each imported animal, then the risk tied to this pathway of introduction is ten times lower than that tied to infectious hosts. As a result, AHS-free countries only face significant introduction risks if the number of *Culicoides* being transported is large as that required for BTV, as shown by Napp et al. for Spain [19]. On the one hand, our assumption of one *Culicoides* per animal could be overly pessimistic because midges could exit the transport vehicle after feeding and thus not reach the animal's final destination. On the other hand, it could be an overly optimistic assumption because large numbers of *Culicoides* may be found on large animals. Because data are lacking on the number of *Culicoides* being transported with mammalian hosts, it is difficult to determine how each pathway of introduction contributes to overall introduction risk.

Our study indicates AHSV establishment in France may be favored from May to October. This finding is consistent with the results obtained by Lo Iacono et al. for the UK [45], by Martinez-Lopez et al. for Spain [46] and by de Vos et al. for the Netherlands [24]. In France, the favorable period for AHSV establishment is longer than in the UK (June to September) and the Netherlands (June to August) but shorter than in Spain (April to December), which is a logical consequence of climatic differences. Such differences should be taken into account when AHSV introduction within Europe is addressed at a larger scale.

Major differences were found among French regions and between introduction pathways. As expected, the coldest regions with the smallest equine populations had the lowest risk of AHSV introduction (e.g., Centre and Auvergne). In contrast, the warmest regions were most at risk for AHSV introduction (e.g., Aquitaine and Midi-Pyrénées), as were colder regions with larger equine populations (e.g., Basse Normandie and Ile de France). Warmer regions faced higher levels of risk mostly

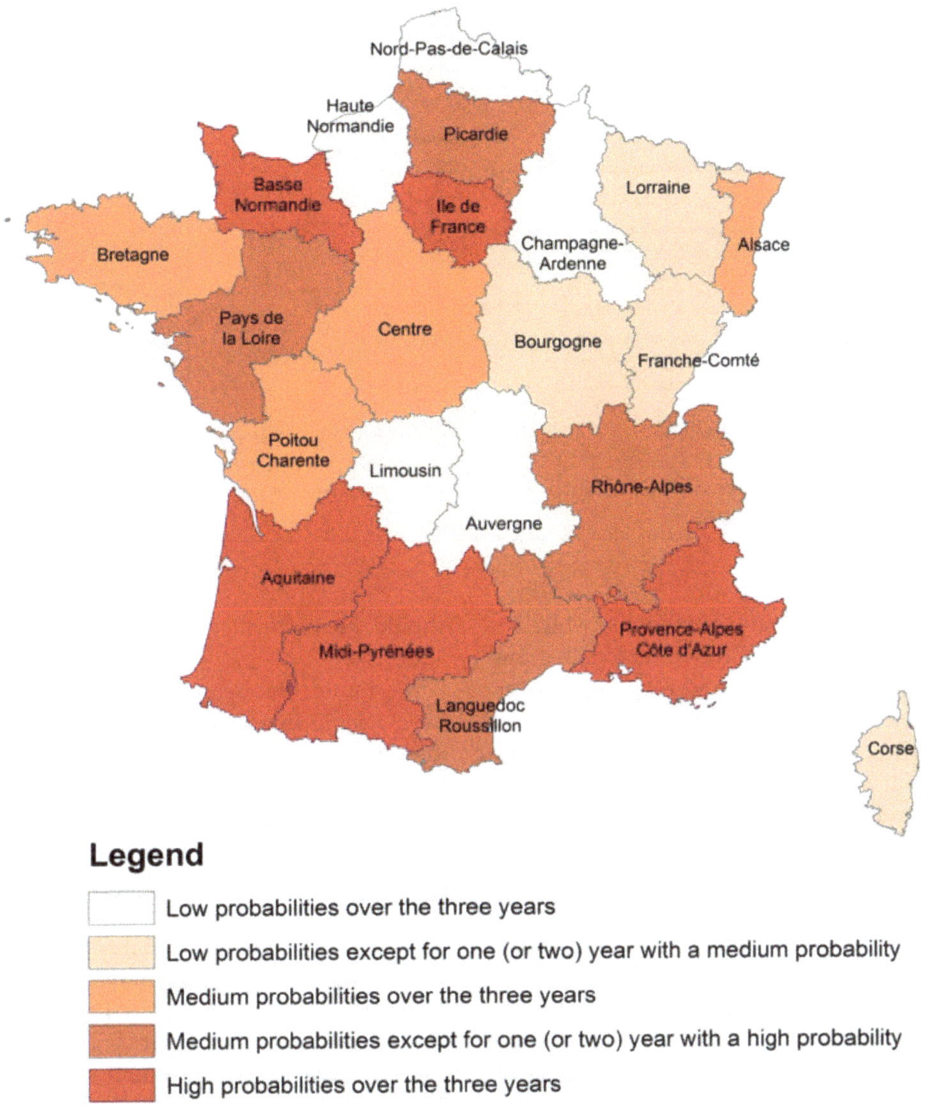

Fig. 7 Annual regional probabilities of AHSV introduction to France via PW-host and PW-vector. Low probabilities are defined as the probabilities < 1E-06, medium probabilities as the probabilities between 1E-06 and 1E-05, high probabilities as the probabilities > 1E-05

Table 1 Average contribution (%) of departure regions to the AHSV introduction risk for France. Results are presented for both pathways and compared to the total number of imports to France which are, for PW-host, the equine imports and, for PW-vector, the large animals imports (equine and bovine)

Exporting region		High risk	Low risk		Very low risk		TOTAL	
			non-EU member	*EU member*	*non-EU member*	*EU member*	*non-EU member*	*EU member*
PW-host	Risk	0.82	3.3	63.2	4.3	28	7.6	91.2
	Import	0.13	3.75	32.6	5.1	58.4	8.81	91
PW-vector	Risk	1.5	98.5		/		/	/
	Import	0.02	99.98		/		/	/

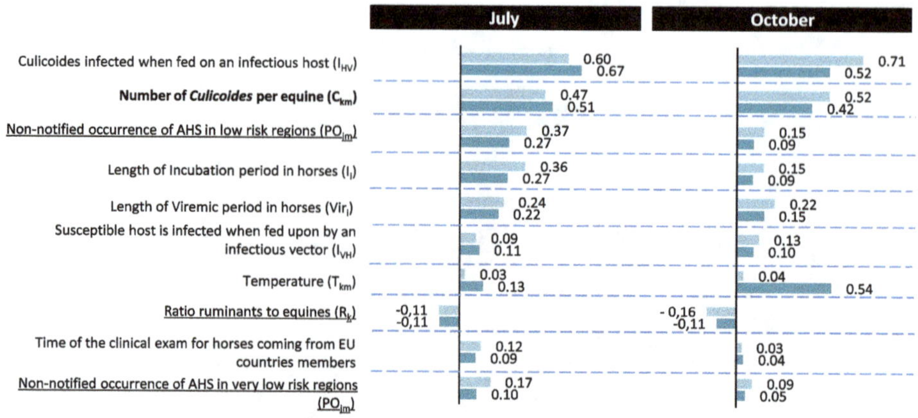

Fig. 8 Correlation of the model input parameters with the probability of introduction of AHSV via PW-host. Results are presented for Ile de France (light blue) and Provence (dark blue) in July and October 2012. Only input parameters with at least one correlation ≥ |0.1| have been included in the tornado charts. The underline parameters are the uncertain parameters; the bold parameters are both uncertain and variable due to stochasticity; the others are only variable due to stochasticity

because of their favorable climatic conditions, while larger equine populations increased risk in colder regions. Nevertheless, if spatial differences were mainly determined by the probability of establishment, import-related variation (number and species imported) also played an important role, as seen in the *Corse* region: even if climatic conditions are favorable, the probability of introduction will be low if there are very few imported animals. These results emphasize that it is important to analyze spatiotemporal variation in risk when developing efficient surveillance systems and optimizing control measures. For instance, if there is a high risk that a pathogen will be introduced by an infectious vector, insecticides should be applied before animals are imported. In contrast, if there is a high risk that a pathogen will be introduced by an infectious host, quarantine measures should be more stringent and/or extra tests should be performed on horses coming from low-risk regions.

We found that seasonal variation in temperature can have a large impact on the risk of introduction because it exerts a strong influence over vector abundance and biology, which, taken together, determine a vector's capacity to transmit AHSV [3, 47]. The risk of ASHV introduction was higher during periods characterized by higher than average temperatures. This finding concurs with results from work examining the introduction of BTV-8 to northwestern Europe: the extreme temperatures during July 2006 may have contributed to its widespread diffusion [48]. Therefore, rare, extreme climatic events and, more generally, global warming should have a large influence on the probability of AHSV establishment, as has been shown for BTV [49, 50]. Given the progression of global warming, risk assessments

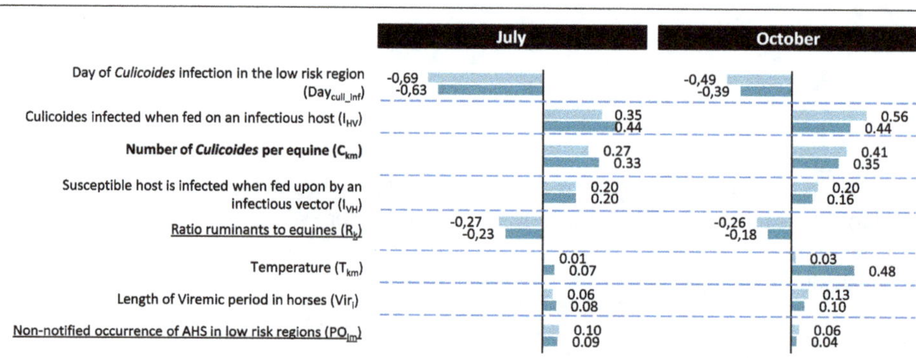

Fig. 9 Correlation of the model input parameters with the probability of introduction of AHSV via PW-vector. Results are presented for Ile de France (light blue) and Provence (dark blue) in July and October 2012. Only input parameters with at least one correlation ≥ |0.1| have been included in the tornado charts. The underline parameters are the uncertain parameters; the bold parameters are both uncertain and variable due to stochasticity; the others are only variable due to stochasticity

should be regularly updated to account for climatic changes.

Our study reveals that complete and accurate data on the movements and distribution of the EU's equine population are not available: it is hard to trace horses within the EU. The introduction of mandatory horse passports in 2008 improved the situation but, apart from rare exceptions [46], it is still difficult to follow the EU's equine population [51] and assessing the population's distribution and fluxes remains a challenge (see the UK [52]). for an example). This is a major concern given that the distribution of the equine population had an important impact on our results (see the ratio of bovines to equines in Figs. 8 and 9); moreover, the number of equines being imported is obviously highly correlated with introduction probabilities. Furthermore, several equine viruses are zoonotic (e.g., eastern and western equine encephalomyelitis viruses, Venezuelan equine encephalitis virus, and West Nile virus), and the risk that they will be introduced to and spread within the EU is definitely not negligible [22]. It is, in fact, currently increasing; indeed, West Nile virus has already become endemic in some regions [53]. Improving the traceability of horses within the EU would thus be advantageous when it comes to better assessing the risk posed by AHSV and other zoonotic diseases.

The risk assessment model described in this paper addresses the risk of AHSV being introduced to France by two pathways of introduction considered to be of importance [23]. However, other pathways may also substantially contribute to introduction risk. Several studies have highlighted that the wind may efficiently transport *Culicoides* over long distances, both across sea [25, 54] and land [55]; it might have been involved in the spread of BTV in Europe [25–27]. Wind-mediated dispersal of infected vectors might also have resulted in AHSV being introduced to Cape Verde Island in 1944, Cyprus in 1960, the Middle East in 1960 and Spain in 1966 [56]. An extensive assessment of the role played by the wind in spreading *Culicoides* midges and *Culicoides*-borne infections across the Mediterranean Basin would elucidate the importance of this pathway for AHS introduction. However, the wind-mediated dispersal of AHSV is most likely to occur in the south of France close to low-risk regions, which is also where AHSV introduction is most likely to occur via the pathways examined in this study. Therefore, we think that this study accurately identifies the regions of France that face the greatest risk of AHSV introduction. Furthermore, the risk that AHSV will be introduced via wind-borne infectious *Culicoides* cannot be mitigated by direct preventive measures, such as importation restrictions. Instead, to be effective, control measures would have to influence the probability of establishment; for instance, insecticides could be used to protect local hosts against wind-borne vectors.

Our model provides a basis for creating a risk-based surveillance system in France that focuses on the regions and time periods associated with higher levels of AHSV introduction risk. The model could also be used for assessing risk and establishing surveillance procedures in other European countries. This application is especially important because our study has revealed that European countries make the largest contribution to France's AHSV introduction risk (e.g., PW-host: 91.2 %). Indeed, if an infection occurs in one European country but is not detected, then it can easily spread to other European countries because there is little verification and tracking of equine movements within the EU. By implementing a risk-based surveillance strategy in each country in the EU, infections would have a higher probability of being detected early on; as a consequence, the contribution of fellow EU countries to introduction risk would decline (see the probabilities of non-notified AHS occurrence in low- and very-low-risk regions in Figs. 8 and 9). By reinforcing the tracking of equine movements within the EU, infection would also have less chance to disseminate and the policy implications of an AHS introduction will be more limited. Such strategies could be a means of minimizing the risk and impact of an AHSV outbreak for the entire European equine industry.

Conclusion

We have developed a quantitative risk assessment model to estimate the risk of AHSV being introduced to France via the importation of infectious equines and infectious *Culicoides* midges associated with large livestock. The risk that AHS will be introduced to France is very low; however, risk varies tremendously among the different regions of the country due to variation in temperature and equine population size. The regions most at risk are those with the warmest climates as well as those that are colder but that harbor larger equine populations. Introduction risk is greatest from July to October and peaks in July. Despite the low probability that AHSV is present in the EU, intra-EU trade of equines contributes most to the risk of AHSV introduction to France because it is responsible for a large number of horse movements. Spatiotemporal differences need to be addressed when assessing the risk that AHSV will be introduced to a given location and when developing and implementing risk-based surveillance procedures. The methods and results of this study may help guide surveillance programs and other risk-reduction measures aimed at preventing the introduction of AHSV or minimizing its potential impact once it has been introduced, both in France and in other European countries.

Competing interests
The authors declare that they have no competing interests.

Authors' contributions
CF participated in the design of the study, performed the statistical analysis and drafted the manuscript; AL participated in data acquisition and interpretation and contributed to the writing of the manuscript; PH participated in acquisition of the data and contributed to the improvement of the manuscript; TB participated in acquisition of the data and contributed to the improvement of the manuscript; CDV participated in in the interpretation of data and contributed to the writing of the manuscript; EF participated in the interpretation of data and contributed to the writing of the manuscript; ADK participated in the design and coordination of the study and contributed to the writing of the manuscript. All authors read and approved the final manuscript.

Acknowledgements
Entomological data were collected by the National entomological surveillance system that is funded by the French Ministry in charge of agriculture and implemented by CIRAD, the *Entente interdépartementale pour la démoustication du littoral méditerranéen* (EID-Med), and the *Institut de parasitologie et de pathologie tropicale de Strasbourg* (IPPTS) with the support of the *Directions départementales de la protection des population*. Authors want to thank all persons involved in this network and especially those in charge of insect identification: Claire Garros, Xavier Allène, Ignace Rakotarivony, Jonathan Lhoir (Cirad), Jean-Claude Delécolle, Delphine Delécolle, Bruno Mathieu (IPPTS), Marie-Laure Setier-Rio, Bethsabée Scheid and Roger Venail (EID-Med). Temperature data were kindly provided by MARS-Agri4cast at the Institute for Environment and Sustainability, European Commission. Data on trade in live animals were provided by the *Bureau de l'identification et du contrôle des mouvements des animaux* (BICMA) and the *service d'inspection vétérinaire et phytosanitaire aux frontières* (SIVEP) at the General Direction for Food (DGAl) of the French Ministry of Agriculture. The authors want to thank all these institutes for providing these data.
This research was carried within the VICE project funded under the FP7 EMIDA ERA-NET initiative. National funding within ERA-Net was provided by the Dutch Ministry of Economic Affairs (Project nr. BO-20-009-009). This work was also partially financially supported by IFCE (Institut Français du Cheval et de l'Equitation) and Vetagro Sup (National Veterinary School of Lyon).

Author details
[1]INRA UR346 Animal Epidemiology, Vetagrosup, F-69280 Marcy l'Etoile, France. [2]INRA UR346 Animal Epidemiology et Département Hippique, VetAgroSup, F-69280 Marcy L'Etoile, France. [3]ANSES, Direction scientifique des laboratoires – unité Survepi, 94700 Maisons-Alfort, France. [4]CIRAD, UMR CMAEE, F-34398 Montpellier, France ; INRA, UMR1309 CMAEE, F-34398 Montpellier, France. [5]Central Veterinary Institute, part of Wageningen UR, PO Box 658200 AB Lelystad, The Netherlands.

References
1. Mellor PS. African horse sickness: transmission and epidemiology. Vet Res. 1993;2:199–212.
2. Du Toit RM. The transmission of bluetongue and horse sickness by Culicoides. Onderstepoort J Vet Sci Anim Ind. 1944;19:7–16.
3. Wilson A, Mellor PS, Szmaragd C, Mertens PPC. Adaptive strategies of African horse sickness virus to facilitate vector transmission. Vet Res 2009;40(2):16
4. Mellor PS, Hamblin C. African horse sickness. Vet Res. 2004;35:445–66.
5. Barnard BJ. Circulation of African horsesickness virus in zebra (Equus burchelli) in the Kruger National Park, South Africa, as measured by the prevalence of type specific antibodies. Onderstepoort J Vet Res. 1993;60:111–7.
6. MacLachlan NJ, Guthrie AJ. Re-emergence of bluetongue, African horse sickness, and other Orbivirus diseases. Vet Res. 2010;41(6):35
7. Rodriguez M, Hooghuis H, Castaño M. African horse sickness in Spain. Vet Microbiol. 1992;33:129–42.
8. Zientara S, Sánchez-Vizcaíno JM. Control of bluetongue in Europe. Vet Microbiol. 2013;166:33–7.
9. Doceul V, Lara E, Sailleau C, Belbis G, Richardson J, Breard E, et al. Epidemiology, molecular virology and diagnostics of Schmallenberg virus, an emerging orthobunyavirus in Europe. Vet Res. 2013;44:31.
10. Carpenter S. Editorial: Bluetongue, Schmallenberg virus... African horse sickness? Vet Rec. 2014;174:299–300.
11. Lefèvre P-C, Blancou J, Chermette R, Uilenberg G: *Infectious and Parasitic Diseases of Livestock. Volume 1*. Paris: Lavoisier; 2010;2010.
12. Venail R, Balenghien T, Guis H, Tran A, Setier-Rio M-L, Delécolle J-C, Mathieu B, Cêtre-Sossah C, Martinez D, Languille J, Baldet T, Garros C: Assessing Diversity and Abundance of Vector Populations at a National Scale: Example of Culicoides Surveillance in France After Bluetongue Virus Emergence. In *Arthropods Vectors Emerg Dis. Volume 3*, Chapter 4. Springer-Verlag, Berlin Heidelberg; 2012:77–102. [*Parasitology Research Monographs*]
13. Lebrun J: *Les enjeux et les perspectives de la filière équine en France. Rapport public*. Conseil économique, social et environnemental. Section de l'agriculture et de le l'alimentation; 2010. Available at: http://www.ladocumentationfrancaise.fr/var/storage/rapports-publics/104000387.pdf
14. Allison K, Taylor N, Upton M, Wilsmore T: *African Horse Sickness, Impact on the UK Horse Industry*. Veterinary Epidemiology and Economics Research Unit, University of Reading; 2009. Available at: http://www.veeru.reading.ac.uk/documents/AHS%20-%20HT%20-%20Report%20final%20301109.pdf (accessed 31.05.13)
15. Thompson GM, Jess S, Murchie AK. A review of African horse sickness and its implications for Ireland. Ir Vet J. 2012;65:9.
16. Mourits MCM, Saatkamp HW: *Kostenberekening van een uitbraak met Afrikaanse paardenpest in Nederland*. Bedrijfseconomie Wageningen Universiteit; 2010. Available at: http://edepot.wur.nl/168958 (accessed 10.06.14 in Dutch)
17. Sutmoller P, Wrathall AE. A quantitative assessment of the risk of transmission of foot-and-mouth disease, bluetongue and vesicular stomatitis by embryo transfer in cattle. Prev Vet Med. 1997;32:111–32.
18. Hoar B, Carpenter T, Singer R, Gardner I. Probability of introduction of exotic strains of bluetongue virus into the US and into California through importation of infected cattle. Prev Vet Med. 2004;66:79–91.
19. Napp S, García-Bocanegra I, Pagès N, Allepuz A, Alba A, Casal J. Assessment of the risk of a bluetongue outbreak in Europe caused by Culicoides midges introduced through intracontinental transport and trade networks. Med Vet Entomol. 2012;27:19–28.
20. Kilpatrick AM, Gluzberg Y, Burgett J, Daszak P. Quantitative risk assessment of the pathways by which west Nile virus could reach Hawaii. EcoHealth. 2004;1:205–9.
21. Brown EBE, Adkin A, Fooks AR, Stephenson B, Medlock JM, Snary EL. Assessing the risks of west Nile virus-infected mosquitoes from transatlantic aircraft: implications for disease emergence in the united kingdom. Vector-Borne Zoonotic Dis. 2012;12:310–20.
22. Durand B, Lecollinet S, Beck C, Martínez-López B, Balenghien T, Chevalier V. Identification of hotspots in the european union for the introduction of four zoonotic arboviroses by live animal trade. PLoS One. 2013;8:e70000.
23. Sabirovic M, Lopez M, Patel K, Kingston A, Hall S: *African Horse Sickness: Potential Risk Factors and the Likelihood for the Introduction of the Disease to the United Kingdom*. Food and Farming Group, Department of Environment Food and Rural Affairs; 2008. Available at: http://webarchive.nationalarchives.gov.uk/20130402151656/http://archive.defra.gov.uk/foodfarm/farmanimal/diseases/monitoring/documents/ahs_uk081106.pdf (accessed 12.11.12)
24. De Vos CJ, Hoek CA, Nodelijk G. Risk of introducing African horse sickness virus into the Netherlands by international equine movements. Prev Vet Med. 2012;106:108–22.
25. Burgin LE, Gloster J, Sanders C, Mellor PS, Gubbins S, Carpenter S. Investigating incursions of bluetongue virus using a model of long-distance culicoides biting midge dispersal. Transbound Emerg Dis. 2012;60:263–72.
26. Ågren ECC, Burgin L, Lewerin SS, Gloster J, Elvander M. Possible means of introduction of bluetongue virus serotype 8 (BTV-8) to Sweden in August 2008: comparison of results from two models for atmospheric transport of the Culicoides vector. Vet Rec. 2010;167:484–8.
27. Ducheyne E, De Deken R, Bécu S, Codina B, Nomikou K, Mangana-Vougiaki O, et al. Quantifying the wind dispersal of Culicoides species in Greece and Bulgaria. Geospatial Health. 2007;1:177–89.

28. Carpenter S, Wilson A, Mellor PS. Culicoides and the emergence of bluetongue virus in northern Europe. Trends Microbiol. 2009;17:172–8.
29. Mintiens K, Méroc E, Mellor PS, Staubach C, Gerbier G, Elbers ARW, et al. Possible routes of introduction of bluetongue virus serotype 8 into the epicentre of the 2006 epidemic in north-western Europe. Prev Vet Med. 2008;87:131–44.
30. De La Rocque S, Balenghien T, Halos L, Dietze K, Claes F, Ferrari G, et al. A review of trends in the distribution of vector-borne diseases: is international trade contributing to their spread? Rev Sci Tech Int Off Epizoot. 2011;30:119–30.
31. De Vos CJ, Hoek M, Fischer E, De Koeijer A, Bremmer J: *Risk Assessment Framework for Emerging Vector-Borne Livestock Diseases*. Netherlands: Central Veterinary Institute of Wageningen UR; 2011. Available at: https://www.wageningenur.nl/en/Publication-details.htm?publicationId=publication-way-343232303431 (accessed 05.01.13)
32. Ninio C, Augot D, Delecolle J-C, Dufour B, Depaquit J. Contribution to the knowledge of culicoides (diptera: ceratopogonidae) host preferences in France. Parasitol Res. 2011;108:657–63.
33. Viennet E, Garros C, Gardès L, Rakotoarivony I, Allène X, Lancelot R, et al. Host preferences of Palaearctic Culicoides biting midges: implications for transmission of orbiviruses. Med Vet Entomol. 2013;27:255–66.
34. Gratz NG, Steffen R, Cocksedge W. Why aircraft disinsection? Bull World Health Organ. 2000;78:995–1004.
35. Mellor PS, Boorman J, Baylis M. Culicoides biting midges: their role as arbovirus vectors. Annu Rev Entomol. 2000;45:307–40.
36. CEC (Commission of the European Communities). Council Directive 2009/156/EC of 30 November 2009 on Animal Health Conditions Governing the Movement and Importation from Third Countries of Equidae. Off J Eur Union. 2010 L192/1
37. Commission Decision (EC) 2004/211 of 6 January 2004 *establishing the List of Third Countries and Parts of Territory Thereof from Which Member States Authorise Imports of Live Equidae and Semen, Ova and Embryos of the Equine Species, and Amending Decisions 93/195/EEC and 94/63/EC* [2004] OJ L73/1
38. Stevenson P, Formosinho J: *Long Distance Animal Transport in Europe: A Cruel and Unnecessary Trade*. Compassion in World Farming; 2008. Available at: https://www.ciwf.org.uk/media/3818249/transport-in-europe-report.pdf (accessed 06.06.14)
39. Agrest, 2010. Recensement Agricole 2010. Available at: http://agreste.agriculture.gouv.fr/recensement-agricole-2010/resultats-donnees-chiffrees/ (accessed 11.12.12 in French)
40. REFErences, 2011. Les effectifs d'équidés présents en France. Available at: http://www.haras-nationaux.fr/information/accueil-equipaedia/filiere-economie/chiffres-cles-sur-les-entreprises-ressources-et-territoire/les-effectifs-dequides-en-france.html?type=98 (accessed 11.12.12 in French)
41. Commission Decision (EC) 2003/623 of 19 August 2003 *concerning the Development of an Integrated Computerised Veterinary System Known as Traces* [2003] OJ L216/58
42. Balenghien T, Delécolle J-C, Setier-Rio M-L, Rakotoarivony I, Allène X, Venail R, et al. Vecteurs du virus de la fièvre catarrhale ovine: suivi des populations de culicoides en 2011 en France. Bull Epidémiologique Santé Anim Aliment. 2012;54:35–40.
43. De Koeijer A, Hartemink N, Boender GJ, Elbers A, Heesterbeek H: *Epidemiological Analysis of the 2006 Bluetongue Virus Serotype 8 Epidemic in North-Western Europe : A Risk Map for Epidemic Potential in the Netherlands*. Animal Science group. Wageningen UR; 2007. Available at: http://www.efsa.europa.eu/fr/efsajournal/doc/34r.pdf (accessed 06.06.14)
44. Palisade Corporation. Guide to using @Risk. Risk Analysis and Simulation Add-In for Microsoft Excel, Version 6.1. Newfield, NY, USA; Palisade Corporation; 2013
45. Lo Iacono G, Robin CA, Newton JR, Gubbins S, Wood JLN. Where are the horses? With the sheep or cows? Uncertain host location, vector-feeding preferences and the risk of African horse sickness transmission in Great Britain. J R Soc Interface. 2013;10:20130194–4.
46. Martínez-López B, Perez AM, Sánchez-Vizcaíno JM. Identifying equine premises at high risk of introduction of vector-borne diseases using geo-statistical and space-time analyses. Prev Vet Med. 2011;100:100–8.
47. Carpenter S, Wilson A, Barber J, Veronesi E, Mellor P, Venter G, et al. Temperature dependence of the extrinsic incubation period of orbiviruses in Culicoides biting midges. PLoS One. 2011;6:e27987.
48. Wilson AJ, Mellor PS. Bluetongue in Europe: past, present and future. Philos Trans R Soc B Biol Sci. 2009;364:2669–81.
49. Purse BV, Mellor PS, Rogers DJ, Samuel AR, Mertens PPC, Baylis M. Climate change and the recent emergence of bluetongue in Europe. Nat Rev Microbiol. 2005;3:171–81.
50. Guis H, Caminade C, Calvete C, Morse AP, Tran A, Baylis M. Modelling the effects of past and future climate on the risk of bluetongue emergence in Europe. J R Soc Interface. 2012;9:339–50.
51. Liljenstolpe C: *Horses in Europe*. Conference EU Equus 2009: Swedish University of Agricultural Sciences; 2009. Available at: http://www.wbfsh.org/files/EU%20Equus%202009.pdf (accessed 10.12.12)
52. Boden LA, Parkin TD, Yates J, Mellor D, Kao RR. An online survey of horse-owners in Great Britain. BMC Vet Res. 2013;9:188.
53. Calistri P, Giovannini A, Hubalek Z, Ionescu A, Monaco F, Savini G, et al. Epidemiology of West Nile in Europe and in the Mediterranean Basin. Open Virol J. 2010;4:29–37.
54. Eagles D, Walker PJ, Zalucki MP, Durr PA. Modelling spatio-temporal patterns of long-distance Culicoides dispersal into northern Australia. Prev Vet Med. 2013;110:312–22.
55. Garcia-Lastra R, Leginagoikoa I, Plazaola JM, Ocabo B, Aduriz G, Nunes T, et al. Bluetongue Virus Serotype 1 Outbreak in the Basque Country (Northern Spain) 2007–2008. Data Support a Primary Vector Windborne Transport. Plos One 2012;7(3):e3442
56. Sellers RF, Pedgley DE, Tucker MR. Possible spread of African horse sickness on the wind. J Hyg (Lond). 1977;79:279–98.

Permissions

All chapters in this book were first published in VR, by BioMed Central; hereby published with permission under the Creative Commons Attribution License or equivalent. Every chapter published in this book has been scrutinized by our experts. Their significance has been extensively debated. The topics covered herein carry significant findings which will fuel the growth of the discipline. They may even be implemented as practical applications or may be referred to as a beginning point for another development.

The contributors of this book come from diverse backgrounds, making this book a truly international effort. This book will bring forth new frontiers with its revolutionizing research information and detailed analysis of the nascent developments around the world.

We would like to thank all the contributing authors for lending their expertise to make the book truly unique. They have played a crucial role in the development of this book. Without their invaluable contributions this book wouldn't have been possible. They have made vital efforts to compile up to date information on the varied aspects of this subject to make this book a valuable addition to the collection of many professionals and students.

This book was conceptualized with the vision of imparting up-to-date information and advanced data in this field. To ensure the same, a matchless editorial board was set up. Every individual on the board went through rigorous rounds of assessment to prove their worth. After which they invested a large part of their time researching and compiling the most relevant data for our readers.

The editorial board has been involved in producing this book since its inception. They have spent rigorous hours researching and exploring the diverse topics which have resulted in the successful publishing of this book. They have passed on their knowledge of decades through this book. To expedite this challenging task, the publisher supported the team at every step. A small team of assistant editors was also appointed to further simplify the editing procedure and attain best results for the readers.

Apart from the editorial board, the designing team has also invested a significant amount of their time in understanding the subject and creating the most relevant covers. They scrutinized every image to scout for the most suitable representation of the subject and create an appropriate cover for the book.

The publishing team has been an ardent support to the editorial, designing and production team. Their endless efforts to recruit the best for this project, has resulted in the accomplishment of this book. They are a veteran in the field of academics and their pool of knowledge is as vast as their experience in printing. Their expertise and guidance has proved useful at every step. Their uncompromising quality standards have made this book an exceptional effort. Their encouragement from time to time has been an inspiration for everyone.

The publisher and the editorial board hope that this book will prove to be a valuable piece of knowledge for researchers, students, practitioners and scholars across the globe.

List of Contributors

Jorge U. Carmona, Diana L. Ríos and Catalina López
Grupo de Investigación Terapia Regenerativa, Departamento de Salud Animal, Universidad de Caldas, Manizales, Colombia

María E. Álvarez
Grupo de Investigación Terapia Regenerativa, Departamento de Salud Animal, Universidad de Caldas, Manizales, Colombia
Grupo de investigación Biosalud, Departamento de Ciencias Básicas para la Salud, Universidad de Caldas, Manizales, Colombia

Jorge E. Pérez
Grupo de investigación Biosalud, Departamento de Ciencias Básicas para la Salud, Universidad de Caldas, Manizales, Colombia

Mabel E. Bohórquez
Grupo de Investigación en Citogenética, Filogenia y Evolución de Poblaciones, Universidad del Tolima, Ibagué, Colombia

Liza Wittenberg-Voges, Florian Geburek, Charlotte Hopster-Iversen and Sabine B. R. Kästner
Equine Clinic, University of Veterinary Medicine Hanover, Foundation, Bünteweg 9, D-30559 Hanover, Germany

Klaus Hopster
Equine Clinic, University of Veterinary Medicine Hanover, Foundation, Bünteweg 9, D-30559 Hanover, Germany
Department of Clinical Studies-NBC, School of Veterinary Medicine, University of Pennsylvania, 382 West Street Road, Kennett Square, PA 19348, USA

Roberto Nardini, Gian Luca Autorino, Ida Ricci, Raffaele Frontoso, Francesca Rosone and Maria Teresa Scicluna
Istituto Zooprofilattico Sperimentale del Lazio e della Toscana "M. Aleandri", Via Appia Nuova 1411, 00178 Rome, Italy

Charles J. Issel and R. Frank Cook
Department of Veterinary Science, Gluck Equine Research Center, University of Kentucky, Lexington, KY, USA

Jeong-Min Hwang
Veterinary Research Center, Green Cross Veterinary Products Co., Ltd., Kugal-dong 227-5, Giheung-gu, Yongin-si, Gyeonggi-do 17066, Republic of Korea

Myung-Ji Seo
Division of Bioengineering, Incheon National University, Academy-ro 119, Incheon 22012, Republic of Korea
Department of Bioengineering and Nano-Bioengineering, Graduate School of Incheon National University, Academy-ro 119, Incheon 22012, Republic of Korea

Jung-Yong Yeh
Department of Life Sciences, College of Life Sciences and Bioengineering, Incheon National University, Academy-ro 119, Yeonsu-gu, Incheon 22012, Republic of Korea
Emerging & Exotic Diseases Research Laboratory, Foreign Animal Diseases Division, Animal, Plant and Fisheries Quarantine and Inspection Agency, Anyang-ro 175, Manan-gu, Anyang-si, Gyeonggi-do 14089, Republic of Korea

Christin Schoppe, Maren Hellige, Bernhard Ohnesorge and Astrid Bienert-Zeit
Clinic for Horses, University of Veterinary Medicine Hannover, Foundation, Buenteweg 9, 30559 Hannover, Germany

Karl Rohn
Institute for Veterinary Biometry and Epidemiology, University of Veterinary Medicine Hannover, Foundation, Buenteweg 2, 30559 Hannover, Germany

Mette Flethøj, Maria M. Haugaard, Helena Carstensen and Rikke Buhl
Department of Large Animal Sciences, Faculty of Health and Medical Sciences, University of Copenhagen, Hoejbakkegaard Allé 5, 2630 Taastrup, Denmark

Jørgen K. Kanters
Laboratory of Experimental Cardiology, Department of Biomedical Sciences, Faculty of Health and Medical Sciences, University of Copenhagen, Blegdamsvej 3B, 2200 Copenhagen N, Denmark
Department of Cardiology, Herlev & Gentofte University Hospitals, Copenhagen, Denmark

Philip J. Pedersen
Department of Veterinary Clinical and Animal Sciences, Faculty of Health and Medical Sciences, University of Copenhagen, Dyrlaegevej 100, 1870 Frederiksberg C, Denmark

Lisbeth H. Olsen
Department of Veterinary Disease Biology, Faculty of Health and Medical Sciences, University of Copenhagen, Groennegaardsvej 15, 1870 Frederiksberg C, Denmark

B. A. McGivney, K. F. Gough, C. L. McGivney, J. A. Browne and E. W. Hill
UCD School of Agriculture and Food Science, Section of Animal & Crop Sciences, University College Dublin, Belfield, Dublin 4, Ireland

M. E. Griffin and L. M. Katz
UCD School of Veterinary Medicine, Section of Veterinary Biomedical Sciences, University College Dublin, Belfield, Dublin 4, Ireland

Patrick Page and Johan Schoeman
Department of Companion Animal Clinical Studies, Faculty of Veterinary Science, University of Pretoria, Onderstepoort 0110, South Africa

Andre Ganswindt
Endocrine Research Laboratory, Department of Anatomy and Physiology, Faculty of Veterinary Science, University of Pretoria, Onderstepoort 0110, South Africa

Gert Venter
PVVD, ARC-Onderstepoort Veterinary Institute, Onderstepoort 0110, South Africa

Alan Guthrie
Equine Research Centre, Faculty of Veterinary Science, University of Pretoria, Onderstepoort 0110, South Africa

Catherine T. Gunther-Harrington, Alexandra Sinnott, Eric Ontiveros and Joshua A. Stern
Department of Medicine & Epidemiology, School of Veterinary Medicine, University of California Davis, Davis, CA 95616, USA

Rick Arthur
School of Veterinary Medicine, University of California Davis, Davis, CA 95616, USA

Anita Varga
William R. Pritchard Veterinary Medical Teaching Hospital (VMTH), University of California Davis, Davis, CA 95616, USA
Gold Coast Veterinary Service & Consulting, Esparto, CA 95627, USA

Krista Estell
William R. Pritchard Veterinary Medical Teaching Hospital (VMTH), University of California Davis, Davis, CA 95616, USA
Marion duPont Scott Equine Medical Center, Virginia-Maryland College of Veterinary Medicine, Leesburg, VA 20176, USA

Beatriz Martinez Lopez
Center for Animal Disease Modeling And Surveillance (CADMS), Department of Medicine & Epidemiology, School of Veterinary Medicine, University of California Davis, Davis, CA 95616, USA

Claudio Henríquez and Gabriel Morán
Pharmacology and Morphophysiology Department, Faculty of Veterinary Sciences, Universidad Austral de Chile, Valdivia, Chile

Miguel Barría and Hugo Folch
Immunology Department, Faculty of Medicine, Universidad Austral de Chile, Valdivia, Chile

Cristian Carrasco
Pathology Department, Regional Hospital of Valdivia, Valdivia, Chile

José Sarmiento
Physiology Department, Faculty of Medicine, Universidad Austral de Chile, Valdivia, Chile

Benjamin Uberti
Veterinary Clinical Sciences Department, Faculty of Veterinary Sciences, Universidad Austral de Chile, Valdivia, Chile

K. Burnheim, K. J. Hughes, D. L. Evans and S. L. Raidal
School of Animal and Veterinary Sciences, Charles Sturt University, Wagga Wagga 2650, NSW, Australia

Mariana Castro Martins and Luis M. Rubio-Martinez
Department of Equine Clinical Studies, Institute of Veterinary Science, University of Liverpool, Leahurst Campus, Chester High Road, Neston CH64 7TE, UK

Mandy J. Peffers and Katie Lee
Department of Musculoskeletal Biology, Institute of Ageing and Chronic Disease, University of Liverpool, Liverpool, UK

Maria K. Johansson, Kim Jäderkvist Fegraeus and Gabriella Lindgren
Department of Animal Breeding and Genetics, Swedish University of Agricultural Sciences, -750 07 Uppsala, SE, Sweden

Björn Ekesten
Department of Clinical Sciences, Swedish University of Agricultural Sciences, -750 07 Uppsala, SE, Sweden

Lucjan Witkowski and Magdalena and Jerzy Kita
Laboratory of Veterinary Epidemiology and Economics, Faculty of Veterinary Medicine, Warsaw University of Life Sciences, Nowoursynowska 159c, 02-776 Warsaw, Poland

Kizerwetter-Świda, Małgorzata Feret, Marta Gawryś, Magdalena Rzewuska and Dorota Chrobak-Chmiel
Department of Preclinical Sciences, Faculty of Veterinary Medicine, Warsaw University of Life Sciences, Ciszewskiego 8, 02-786 Warsaw, Poland

Shinji Takai
Department of Animal Hygiene, School of Veterinary Medicine, Kitasato University, Higashi 23-35-1, Towada, Aomori 034-8628, Japan

Maciej Witkowski
University Center of Veterinary Medicine UJ-UR, Mickiewicza 24/28, 30-059 Cracow, Poland

L. M. Rubio-Martínez, E. Rioja, M. Castro Martins and P. Clegg
Institute of Veterinary Science, University of Liverpool, Leahurst Campus, Chester High Road, CH647TE Neston, UK

S. Wipawee
Faculty of Veterinary Science, Rajamangala University of Technology Srivijaya (Thailand) and Institute of Aging and Chronic Disease, University of Liverpool, Liverpool, UK

M. J. Peffers
Institute of Aging and Chronic Disease, University of Liverpool, Liverpool, UK

Una Pongratz
Equine Clinic, University of Veterinary Medicine Vienna (Vetmeduni Vienna), Veterinaerplatz 1, 1210 Vienna, Austria

Theresia Licka
Department of Veterinary Clinical Science, Royal (Dick) School of Veterinary Studies, University of Edinburgh, Easter Bush, Edinburgh EH25 9RG, UK

Sanne Lotte Journée
Equine Diagnostics, Tergracht 2A, 9091 BG Wijns, The Netherlands

Henricus Louis Journée
Department of Neurosurgery, University Groningen, University Medical Center Groningen, Hanzeplein 1, 9713 GZ Groningen, The Netherlands

Cornelis Marinus de Bruijn
Wolvega Equine Clinic, Stellingenweg 10, 8474 EA Oldeholtpade, The Netherlands

Cathérine John Ghislaine Delesalle
Department of Comparative Physiology and Biometrics, Faculty of Veterinary Medicine, Ghent University, Salisburylaan 133, 9820 Merelbeke, Belgium

Joke Rijckaert, Bart Pardon, Gunther van Loon and Piet Deprez
Department of Large Animal Internal Medicine, Faculty of Veterinary Medicine, Ghent University, Salisburylaan 133, 9820 Merelbeke, Belgium

Luc Van Ham
Department of Obstetrics, Reproduction and Herd Health, Faculty of Veterinary Medicine, Ghent University, Salisburylaan 133, 9820 Merelbeke, Belgium

Philip Joosten
Small Animal Department, Faculty of Veterinary Medicine, Ghent University, Salisburylaan 133, 9820 Merelbeke, Belgium

Tytti M. Niemelä, Riitta-Mari Tulamo, Kaisa Aaltonen, Satu M. Sankari and Anna K. Hielm-Björkman
Department of Equine and Small Animal Medicine, Faculty of Veterinary Medicine, University of Helsinki, Helsinki, Finland

Siham T. Karamalla, Ahmed I. Gubran, Ibrahim A. Adam, Tamadur M. Abdalla and Reem O. Sinada
Molecular Biology Laboratory (MBL), Department of Clinical Medicine, Faculty of Veterinary Medicine, University of Khartoum, Khartoum North, Sudan

Imadeldin E. Aradaib
Molecular Biology Laboratory (MBL), Department of Clinical Medicine, Faculty of Veterinary Medicine, University of Khartoum, Khartoum North, Sudan
Scientific Research Directorate, Al-Mughtaribeen University, Khartoum, Sudan
EBH Scientific Research Laboratory, Zamzam University College (ZUC), Khartoum, Sudan

Eltahir M. Haroun
Scientific Research Directorate, Al-Mughtaribeen University, Khartoum, Sudan

Manuela Martano, Karen Power, Brunella Restucci, Ilaria Pagano, Gennaro Altamura, Giuseppe Borzacchiello and Paola Maiolino
Department of Veterinary Medicine and Animal Productions, Naples University "Federico II", Via F. Delpino 1, 80137 Naples, Italy

María Dolores Contreras-Aguilar, Fernando Tecles and Jose Joaquín Cerón
Interdisciplinary Laboratory of Clinical Analysis (Interlab-UMU), Veterinary School, Campus of Excellence Mare Nostrum, University of Murcia, 30100, Espinardo, Murcia, Spain

Damián Escribano
Interdisciplinary Laboratory of Clinical Analysis (Interlab-UMU), Veterinary School, Campus of Excellence Mare Nostrum, University of Murcia, 30100, Espinardo, Murcia, Spain
Department of Food and Animal Science, School of Veterinary Medicine, Universitat Autònoma de Barcelona, 08193, Bellaterra, Barcelona, Spain

María Martín-Cuervo
Surgery Department, Faculty of Veterinary Medicine, University of Extremadura, 10005 Cáceres, Spain

B. Broux, D. De Clercq, L. Vera, S. Ven, P. Deprez, A. Decloedt and G. van Loon
Equine Cardioteam, Department of Large Animal Internal Medicine, Faculty of Veterinary Medicine, Ghent University, Salisburylaan 133, 9820 Merelbeke, Belgium

Index

www.ingramcontent.com/pod-product-compliance
Lightning Source LLC
LaVergne TN
LVHW080914210926
848485LV00004B/649